T0202001

OXFORD MEDICAL PUBLICATIONS

Emergencies in Critical Care

Published and forthcoming titles in the Emergencies in... series:

Emergencies in Adult Nursing
Edited by Philip Downing

Emergencies in Anaesthesia
Edited by Keith Allman, Andrew McIndoe, and Iain H. Wilson

Emergencies in Cardiology
Edited by Saul G. Myerson, Robin P. Choudhury, and Andrew Mitchell

Emergencies in Children's and Young People's Nursing
Edited by E.A. Glasper, Gill McEwing, and Jim Richardson

Emergencies in Clinical Surgery
Edited by Chris Callaghan, Chris Watson and Andrew Bradley

Emergencies in Critical Care, 2e
Edited by Martin Beed, Richard Sherman, and Ravi Mahajan

Emergencies in Gastroenterology and Hepatology
Marcus Harbord and Daniel Marks

Emergencies in Mental Health Nursing
Edited by Patrick Callaghan

Emergencies in Obstetrics and Gynaecology
Edited by S. Arulkumaran

Emergencies in Oncology
Edited by Martin Scott-Brown, Roy A.J. Spence, and Patrick G. Johnston

Emergencies in Paediatrics and Neonatology, 2e
Edited by Stuart Crisp and Jo Rainbow

Emergencies in Palliative and Supportive Care
Edited by David Currow and Katherine Clark

Emergencies in Primary Care
Chantal Simon, Karen O'Reilly, John Buckmaster, and Robin Proctor

Emergencies in Psychiatry, 2e
Basant Puri and Ian Treasaden

Emergencies in Radiology
Edited by Richard Graham and Ferdia Gallagher

Emergencies in Respiratory Medicine
Edited by Robert Parker, Catherine Thomas, and Lesley Bennett

Emergencies in Sports Medicine
Edited by Julian Redhead and Jonathan Gordon

Head, Neck and Dental Emergencies
Edited by Mike Perry

Medical Emergencies in Dentistry
Nigel Robb and Jason Leitch

Emergencies in Critical Care

Second edition

Edited by

Martin Beed

Consultant in Critical Care and Anaesthesia
Nottingham University Hospitals, UK

Richard Sherman

Consultant in Critical Care and Anaesthesia
Nottingham University Hospitals, UK

Ravi Mahajan

Professor and Honorary Consultant in Anaesthesia
and Intensive Care Medicine
University of Nottingham
Nottingham University Hospitals, UK

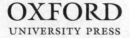

OXFORD
UNIVERSITY PRESS

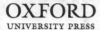

OXFORD
UNIVERSITY PRESS

Great Clarendon Street, Oxford, OX2 6DP,
United Kingdom

Oxford University Press is a department of the University of Oxford.
It furthers the University's objective of excellence in research, scholarship,
and education by publishing worldwide. Oxford is a registered trade mark of
Oxford University Press in the UK and in certain other countries

© Oxford University Press 2013

The moral rights of the authors have been asserted

First Edition published in 2007
Second Edition published in 2013

British Library Cataloguing in Publication Data
Data available

ISBN 978–0–19–969627–7

Printed in Great Britain by
Ashford Colour Press Ltd.

Preface to the second edition

This book is intended to be useful to doctors and nurses based on the intensive care unit (ICU) and on the wards, containing the key elements of how to manage critically ill patients in those first few crucial hours. Where possible the book follows an 'ABC' format, the commonest approach to dealing with emergencies; and this new edition has been updated to try and make that 'ABC' management as simple as possible. Key history and examination findings are listed as often as possible, as are drug doses and investigation results. There is even some deliberate duplication, so that the reader doesn't have to jump to different parts of the book to get that crucial piece of information.

For those based on the ICU or high dependency unit, this book also contains details of how to deal with common conditions that are managed in subtly different ways within a critical care environment; as well as conditions which are peculiar to ICU (e.g. complications associated with mechanical ventilation). Emergencies in critical care are often surprisingly predictable, and the knowledge of who is likely to be at risk, and how they may be best managed, will provide those involved with a rational approach for these stressful situations.

Guidelines are reviewed and updated regularly, and wherever possible the latest versions have been included in this new edition. We have also included references to key documents, high-quality review articles, or seminal ICU articles.

We have continued to include a broad spectrum of diseases and emergencies, expanding in some areas and simplifying in others, in order to try and present the clearest and most concise summary of all the essential information.

The first half of the book describes the management of emergencies affecting various systems, whilst the second half concentrates on various groups of patients or conditions. Most chapters begin with a generic description of how to manage emergencies affecting that system or patient group. This is followed by details of specific diagnoses and how they should be managed.

In short we hope that this new edition will prove invaluable to you, no matter what your position, grade, or experience, whenever you are faced with a critically ill patient, either as a guide to management or an aide-memoire for those hard-to-remember facts.

M.B.
R.S.
R.M.
March 2013

Contents

Contents

Contributors

Steve Beed
Teacher and artist

Victoria Banks
SpR in Critical Care and
Anaesthesia
Nottingham University Hospitals
Nottingham, UK

Thearina De Beer
Consultant in Critical Care and
Anaesthesia
Nottingham University Hospitals
Nottingham, UK

Myles Dowling
Consultant in Anaesthesia
Nottingham University Hospitals
Nottingham, UK

Lewis Gray
SpR in Critical Care and
Anaesthesia
Nottingham University Hospitals
Nottingham, UK

Dan Harvey
Consultant in Critical Care and
Anaesthesia
Nottingham University Hospitals
Nottingham, UK

Mandy Haughton[1]
Senior Staff Nurse
Nottingham University
Hospitals
Nottingham, UK

Lina Hijazi
Consultant in Genito-urinary
and HIV Medicine
Whipps Cross Hospital
Barts NHS Trust
London, UK

Martin Levitt
Consultant in Critical Care and
Anaesthesia
Nottingham University Hospitals
Nottingham, UK

Gareth Moncaster[1]
Consultant in Critical Care and
Anaesthesia
Sherwood Forest Hospitals
Nottinghamshire, UK

Matt O'Meara
SpR in Critical Care and Anaesthesia
Nottingham University Hospitals
Nottingham, UK

Rajkumar Rajendrum[1]
SpR in Anaesthesia and
Intensive Care
John Radcliffe Hospital
Oxford, UK

Andrew Sharman
Consultant in Critical Care and
Anaesthesia
Nottingham University Hospitals
Nottingham, UK

Suzanne Wallace
Consultant Obstetrician
Nottingham University Hospitals
Nottingham, UK

Sandy Whitehead[1]
Senior Staff Nurse
Nottingham University Hospitals
Nottingham, UK

Jonny Wilkinson
Consultant in Critical Care and
Anaesthesia
Northampton General Hospital
Northampton, UK

[1] Contributors to the first edition only

Symbols and abbreviations

📖	cross reference
↑	increased
↓	decreased
1°	primary
2°	secondary
⬥	website
~	approximately
2,3 DPG	2,3-diphosphoglycerate
5HIAA	hydroxy-indole acetic acid
βHCG	human chorionic gonadotropin beta-subunit
A&E	accident and emergency (see also ED)
A-a	alveolar/arterial [oxygen gradient]
AAA	abdominal aortic aneurysm
ABC	airway, breathing, circulation
ABGs	arterial blood gases
AC	alternating current
ACA	anterior cerebral artery
ACE	angiotensin-converting enzyme
ACh	acetylcholine
AChR	acetylcholine receptor
ACS	abdominal compartment syndrome or acute coronary syndrome
ACT	activated clotting time
ACTH	adrenocorticotropic hormone
ADH	anti-diuretic hormone
AF	atrial fibrillation
AFB	acid-fast bacilli
AFE	amniotic fluid embolism
AIDS	acquired immune deficiency syndrome
AKI	acute kidney injury
ALI	acute lung injury
ALL	acute lymphocytic leukaemia
ALP	alkaline phosphatase
ALS	advanced life support
ALT	alanine aminotransferase
AMPLE history	Allergies, Medication, Past medical history, Last meal, Environment

ANA	antinuclear antibodies
ANCA	antinuclear cytoplasmic antibodies
AP	antero-posterior [X-rays]
APACHE (II)	acute physiology and chronic health evaluation [score, version II]
APH	antepartum haemorrhage
APP	abdominal perfusion pressure
APTT	activated partial thromboplastin time
ARB(A)s	angiotensin receptor blockers (or antagonists)
ARDS	acute respiratory distress syndrome
ARF	acute renal failure
ASB	assisted spontaneous breathing
ASD	atrial septal defect
AST	aspartate aminotransferase
ATLS	advanced trauma life support
ATN	acute tubular necrosis
AVM	arteriovenous malformation
AVPU	Alert, responds to Voice, responds to Pain, Unresponsive [consciousness assessment]
AXR	abdominal X-ray
BAL	broncho-alveolar lavage
BBB	blood–brain barrier
BE	base excess
BIPAP	biphasic positive airways pressure
BIS	bispectral index
BLS	basic life support
BM	bone marrow or blood monitoring [glucose]
BMI	body mass index
BNF	*British National Formulary*
BOS	base of skull [fracture]
BP	blood pressure
BPF	bronchopleural fistula
BSA	body surface area
Ca^{2+}	calcium
CALS	cardiac surgery advanced life support
CAM-ICU	confusion assessment method for the ICU
cAMP	cyclic adenosine monophosphate
CAP	community-acquired pneumonia
CAPD	continuous ambulatory peritoneal dialysis
CAVH	continuous arterio-venous haemofiltration

CCF	congestive cardiac failure
CCHF	Crimean-Congo haemorrhagic fever
CCU	coronary care unit
CDT	*Clostridium difficile* toxin
CFI	cardiac function index
CF (A) M	cerebral function (analysing) monitor
CHF	congestive heart failure
CI	cardiac index
CIN	contrast induced nephropathy
CIWA-Ar	Clinical Institute withdrawal assessment of alcohol (revised) scale
CJD	Creutzfeld–Jakob disease
CK	creatine kinase
CKMB	CK myocardial bound [portion]
CLL	chronic lymphocytic leukaemia
CMV	cytomegalovirus *or* continuous mandatory ventilation
CNS	central nervous system
CO	cardiac output *or* carbon monoxide
CO_2	carbon dioxide
COHb	carboxyhaemoglobin
COPD	chronic obstructive pulmonary disease
CPAP	continuous positive airways pressure
CPIS	clinical pulmonary infection score
CPP	cerebral perfusion pressure
CPR	cardiopulmonary resuscitation
CPT	cryoprecipitate
CRBSI	catheter-related blood stream infection
CRP	C-reactive protein
CRT	capillary refill time
CSL	compound sodium lactate [fluid]
C-spine	cervical spine
CSF	cerebrospinal fluid
CSU	catheter specimen urine
C_T	lung compliance (thoracic compliance)
CT	computed tomography
CTG	cardiotocograph
CTPA	CT pulmonary angiogram
CURB-65	[a pneumonia scoring system]
CVA	cerebrovascular accident
CVC	central venous catheter

CVP	central venous pressure
CVS	cardiovascular system
CVVH	continuous veno-venous haemofiltration
CXR	chest X-ray
DAP	diastolic aortic pressure
DC	direct current
DCI	delayed cerebral ischaemia
DDT	dichloro diphenyl tricholoethane
DHI	dynamic hyperinflation
DI	diabetes insipidus
DIC	disseminated intravascular coagulopathy
DKA	diabetic ketoacidosis
DLT	double lumen [ET] tube
DM	diabetes mellitus
DMPS	sodium 2,3-dimercapto-1-propane sulphonate
DMSA	dimercaptosuccinic acid
DNAR	do not attempt resuscitation
DO_2	oxygen delivery
DOB	date of birth
DOH	department of health
DNA	deoxyribonucleic acid
DPL	diagnostic peritoneal lavage
DRESS	drug rash with eosinophilia and systemic symptoms
ds-DNA	double stranded DNA
DTs	delirium tremens
DVT	deep vein thrombosis
EBV	Epstein–Barr virus
$ECCO_2R$	extracorporeal carbon dioxide removal
ECG	electrocardiogram
ECHO	echocardiogram (TOE or TTE)
ECMO	extracorporeal membrane oxygenation
ED	emergency department (see also A&E)
EDTA	ethylene diamine tetraacetic acid
EEG	electroencephalogram
EF	ejection fraction
eGFR	estimated glomerular filtration rate
EMG	electromyograph
ENT	ear, nose, and throat
ERCP	endoscopic retrograde cholangiopancreatography
ESR	erythrocyte sedimentation rate

ETCO$_2$	end-tidal carbon dioxide
ETT	endotracheal tube
EVLWI	extravascular lung water index
EWS	early warning score
FAST	focused assessment with sonography for trauma
FBC	full blood count
FDPs	fibrinogen degradation products
Fe	iron
FES	fat embolism syndrome
FEV$_1$	forced expiratory volume in 1 second
FiO$_2$	fraction of inspired O$_2$
FFP	fresh frozen plasma
FOB	faecal occult blood
FOI	fibreoptic intubation
Fr	French gauge
FRC	functional residual capacity
FTc	corrected flow time
FVC	forced vital capacity
G	gauge
G&S	group and save
GBM	glomerular basement membrane
GBS	Guillain–Barré syndrome
GCS	Glasgow coma score
GEDVI	global end diastolic volume index
GFR	glomerular filtration rate
GGT	gamma-glutamyl transpeptidase
GHB	gammahydroxybutyric acid
GI(T)	gastrointestinal (tract)
GnRH	gonadotrophin releasing hormone
GP	general practitioner
GP2b3a	glycoprotein 2b3a [receptor inhibitor]
GSW	gunshot wounds
GTN	glyceryl trinitrate
GU	genitourinary
HAART	highly active antiretroviral therapy
HAI	hospital-acquired infection
HAP	hospital-acquired pneumonia
HAS	human albumin solution
HAV	hepatitis A virus
HAV-IgM	hepatitis A antibody

Hb	haemoglobin
HbA$_{1c}$	glycosylated haemoglobin
HBcore-IgM	hepatitis B core antibody
HbsAg	hepatitis B surface antigen
HBV	hepatitis B virus
hCG	human chorionic gonadotrophin
HCAP	healthcare-associated pneumonia
Hct	haematocrit
HCV	hepatitis C virus
HD	haemodialysis
HELLP	haemolysis, elevated liver enzymes, low platelets
HEPA [mask]	high-efficiency particulate air
HFOV	high-frequency oscillatory ventilation
HHS	hyperosmolar hyperglycaemic state
HiB	*Haemophilus influenzae* type b
HIT (S)	heparin-induced thrombocytopaenia (syndrome)
HIV	human immunodeficiency virus
HMMA	hydroxymethylmandelic acid
HOCM	hypertrophic obstructive cardiomyopathy
HONK	hyperosmolar non-ketotic [coma]
HPA (CFI)	Health Protection Agency (centre for infections)
HR	heart rate
HRS	hepatorenal syndrome
HSP	Henoch–Schönlein purpura
HSV	herpes simplex virus
HUS	haemolytic uraemic syndrome
IABP	intra-aortic balloon pump
IAH	intra-abdominal hypertension
IAP	intra-abdominal pressure
IBC	iron binding capacity
IBW	ideal body weight
ICP	intracranial pressure
ICU	intensive care unit
ID card	identification card
IDDM	insulin dependent diabetes mellitus
I:E ratio	inspired:expired [air] ratio
IgE	immunoglobulin E
IHD	ischaemic heart disease
IJ	internal jugular
IM	intramuscular

INR	international normalized ratio
IO	intraosseous
IOP	intraocular pressure
IPPV	intermittent positive pressure ventilation
IRIS (or IRS)	immune reconstitution inflammatory syndrome
ITBVI	intrathoracic blood volume index
ITP	idiopathic thrombocytopaenic purpura
ITU	intensive therapy unit
IUFD	intrauterine fetal death
IV	intravenous
IVC	inferior vena cava
IVIG	intravenous immunoglobulin
IVU	intravenous urogram
IVF	*in vitro* fertilization
JVP	jugular venous pressure
K^+	potassium
K_{co}	transfer coefficient
LACS	lacunar syndrome
LAP	left atrial pressure
LBBB	left bundle branch block
LDH	lactate dehydrogenase
LFTs	liver function tests
LH	luteinizing hormone
LiDCO™	lithium dilution cardiac output [monitor]
LMA	laryngeal mask airway
LMWH	low-molecular-weight heparin
LP	lumbar puncture
LRTI	lower respiratory tract infection
LSD	lysergic acid diethylamide
LV	left ventricle/ventricular
LVAD	left ventricular assist device
LVEDP	left ventricular end-diastolic pressure
LVF	left ventricular failure
LVSWI	left ventricular stroke work index
MAHA	microangiopathic haemolytic anaemia
MAOI	monoamine oxidase inhibitor
MAP	mean arterial pressure
MARS	molecular adsorbent recirculating system
MBA	motorbike accident
MCA	middle cerebral artery

MCH	mean cell haematocrit
MCV	mean cell volume
MDMA	methylenedioxymethamphetamine (ecstasy)
MDR	multiple drug resistance
MEN	multiple endocrine neoplasia
MERiT	medical emergency response team
MET	medical emergency team
MH	malignant hyperpyrexia
MI	myocardial infarction
MIBG	metaiodobenzylguanidine [scan]
MODS	multiple organ dysfunction syndrome
MOF	multiple organ failure
MPAP	mean pulmonary artery pressure
MR	mitral regurgitation
MRDT	malaria rapid detection test
MRI	magnetic resonance imaging
MRSA	meticillin-resistant *Staphylococcus aureus*
MSSA	meticillin-sensitive *Staphylococcus aureus*
MSU	mid-stream urine
MuSK	muscle specific kinase
MUST	malnutrition universal screening tool
Na^+	sodium
$NaHCO_3$	sodium bicarbonate
NBM	nil by mouth
NG/NGT	nasogastric (tube)
NIBP	non-invasive blood pressure
NIHSS	National Institute of Health stroke score
NIV	non-invasive ventilation
NJ	naso-jejunal
nNRTI	non-nucleotide reverse transcriptase inhibitors
NPAs	nasopharyngeal airways
NPIS	national poisons information service
NRTI	nucleotide reverse transcriptase inhibitors
NSAIDs	non-steroidal anti-inflammatory drugs
NSTEMI	non-ST elevation myocardial infarction
O_2	oxygen
OCP	oral contraceptive pill
OD	overdose
ODC	oxygen dissociation curve
OGT	oro-gastric tube

OHSS	ovarian hyperstimulation syndrome
OPAs	oropharyngeal airways
$P_{0.1}$	airway occlusion pressure at 0.1 seconds
P_{INSP}	inspiratory pressure (mechanical ventilation)
PA	pulmonary artery
$PaCO_2$	partial pressure of arterial cardon dioxide
PACS	partial anterior circulation syndrome
PAFC	pulmonary artery flotation catheter
PAN	polyarteritis nodosa
PaO_2	partial pressure of arterial oxygen
PAOP/PAWP	pulmonary artery occlusion [or wedge] pressure
PAP	pulmonary artery pressure
PBO_2	brain tissue oxygen tension
PC	platelet concentrate
PCA	posterior cerebral artery
PCA(S)	patient controlled analgesia (system)
PCI	percutaneous coronary intervention (e.g. angioplasty)
PCP	*Pneumocystis jiroveci (carinii)* pneumonia
PCR	polymerase chain reaction or [urinary] protein:creatinine ratio
PCT	procalcitonin
PCWP	pulmonary capillary wedge pressure
PE	pulmonary embolus or phenytoin equivalents
PEA	pulseless electrical activity
PEEP	positive end-expiratory pressure
PEEPi	intrinsic positive end-expiratory pressure
PEFR	peak expiratory flow rate
PEG	percutaneous endoscopic gastrostomy
PET	pre-eclamptic toxaemia
PFTs	pulmonary function tests
PI	protease inhibitor
PICC	peripherally inserted central catheter
PICH	primary intracerebral haemorrhage
PIH	pregnancy-induced hypertension
PMH	past medical history
PMR	polymyalgia rheumatica
PN	parenteral nutrition
PO	per os (orally)
POCS	posterior circulation syndrome
PPE	personal protective equipment

PPH	postpartum haemorrhage
PR	per rectum (rectally)
PRN	pro re nata (as required)
PSV	pressure support ventilation
PT	prothrombin time
PTH	parathyroid hormone
PUO	pyrexia of unknown origin
PV	per vagina
PVL	Panton–Valentine leucocidin
PVR	pulmonary vascular resistance
PVRI	pulmonary vascular resistance index
QTc	corrected QT interval
RA	rheumatoid arthritis *or* right atrium
RAP	right atrial pressure
RASS	Richmond agitation sedation assessment
RBBB	right bundle branch block
RBC	red blood cell
REJ	right external jugular
RIJ	right internal jugular
ROSC	return of spontaneous circulation
RPP	rate pressure product
RR	respiratory rate
RRT	renal replacement therapy
RS	respiratory system
RSI	rapid sequence intubation
RSV	respiratory syncytial virus
RSVP	Reason Story Vital signs Plan
RTA	road traffic accident *or* renal tubular acidosis
R-tPA	recombinant tissue plasminogen activator
RUQ	right upper quadrant
RV	right ventricle/ventricular
RVEDP	right ventricular end-diastolic pressure
SAFE	Shout for help, Approach with caution, Free from danger, Evaluate ABC
SAH	subarachnoid haemorrhage
SaO_2	arterial oxygen saturation
SARS (-CoV)	severe acute respiratory syndrome (corona virus)
SBAR	Situation Background Assessment Recommendation
SBP	spontaneous bacterial peritonitis
SBT	Sengstaken–Blakemore tube

SC	subcutaneous
$ScvO_2$	central venous O_2 saturation
SGC	Swan–Ganz catheter
SIADH	syndrome of inappropriate ADH [secretion]
SICH	spontaneous intracerebral haemorrhage
SIRS	systemic inflammatory response syndrome
SjO_2	Jugular venous bulb O_2 saturation
SJS	Stevens–Johnson syndrome
SK	streptokinase
SL	sublingual
SLE	systemic lupus erythematosus
SNP	sodium nitroprusside
SOB	shortness of breath
SpO_2	plethysmographic [skin] O_2 saturation
SSRI	selective serotonin reuptake inhibitor
STD	sexually transmitted disease
STEMI	ST elevation myocardial infarction
SV	stroke volume
SVC	superior vena cava
SVI	stroke volume index
SvO_2	venous O_2 saturation
$S\bar{v}O_2$	mixed venous O_2 saturation
SVR	systemic vascular resistance
SVRI	systemic vascular resistance index
SVT	supraventricular tachycardia
SVV	stroke volume variation
T3	tri-iodothyronine
T4	thyroxine
T_{INSP}	inspiratory time (mechanical ventilation)
TACO	transfusion associated circulatory overload
TACS	total anterior circulation syndrome
TAD	transfusion associated dyspnoea
TB	tuberculosis
TBI	traumatic brain injury
TBV	total blood volume
TCA	tricyclic antidepressants
TCD	transcranial Doppler
TCRE	transcervical resection of the endometrium
TEN	toxic epidermal necrolysis
TFTs	thyroid function tests

TGI	tracheal gas insufflation
TIA	transient ischaemic attack
TICA	terminal internal carotid artery
TICTAC	a tablet identification database
TIPSS	transjugular intrahepatic porto-systemic shunting
TLC	total lung capacity
TLS	tumour lysis syndrome
TOD	transoesophageal Doppler
TOE	transoesophageal echocardiogram
Toxbase	a toxicology database
t-PA	tissue plasminogen activator
TPN	total parenteral nutrition (see PN)
TR	tricuspid regurgitation
TRALI	transfusion related acute lung injury
TSH	thyroid-stimulating hormone
T-spine	thoracic spine
TT	thrombin time
TTE	transthoracic echocardiogram
TTP	thrombotic thrombocytopaenic purpura
TUR(P)(T)	transurethral resection (of prostate or tumour)
T_V	tidal volume
U&Es	urea and electrolytes
UOP	urine output
URTI	upper respiratory tract infection
US	ultrasound
UTI	urinary tract infection
VAP	ventilator-associated pneumonia
VC	vital capacity
V_E	minute volume
VE	ventricular ectopic
VF	ventricular fibrillation
VHF	viral haemorrhagic fever
VMA	vanillylmandelic acid
VO_2	systemic oxygen consumption
V-P shunt	ventriculo-peritoneal shunt
VQ mismatch	ventilation perfusion mismatch
VISA	vancomycin insensitive *Staphylococcus aureus*
VRE	vancomycin resistant enterococcus
VRSA	vancomycin resistant *Staphylococcus aureus*
VRSS	vasopressor resistant septic shock

VSD	ventricular septal defect
VT	ventricular tachycardia
vWF	von Willebrand factor
WBC	white blood cell
WCC	white cell count
WFNS	World Federation of Neurological Surgeons
WHO	World Health Organization
WPW	Wolff–Parkinson–White [syndrome]

Assessment and stabilization

Assessment and immediate management of an emergency 2
Early further management 10

☠ / ☢ / ⚠ Assessment and immediate management of an emergency

The assessment and immediate management of critically ill patients follows the established ABC approach (**A**pproach/**A**irway, **B**reathing, **C**irculation). What follows is a brief summary of the ABC approach adapted for patients within a critical care environment, further details on each system are considered in individual chapters. Any deterioration during assessment and resuscitation should prompt a return to 'A'.

Some interventions may need to be performed *whilst continuing assessment and emergency treatment,* particularly when emergencies are acute and life threatening (e.g. BLS/ALS, see 📖 p.98; needle thoracocentesis of a tension pneumothorax, 📖 p.80).

Approach

- In all cases it is essential to ensure that those treating the patient are safe to carry out their work.
- C-spine immobilization is often required where trauma is involved.
- Give 100% oxygen in acute emergencies, in less acute scenarios titrate the oxygen required to keep SpO_2 94–98%.
- Connect any monitoring available—aim to have SpO_2, continuous ECG, and non-invasive BP monitoring as a minimum:
  - Review any information from the monitoring devices (e.g. SpO_2, ventilatory parameters, heart rate and rhythm, BP) alongside physical findings when examining the patient
  - Be alert for equipment malfunction (e.g. airway occlusion, ventilator failure, or infusion pump failure); and/or alarms from the monitoring systems which may indicate the cause or extent of problem
- Obtain a history and detailed information about the patient:
  - From the patient where possible—the minimum history should include the 'AMPLE' template advocated in trauma resuscitation
  - From attending staff or from any associated documentation
  - Review notes, observation charts, imaging and blood results—fluid balance, blood gases, electrolytes
  - Physiological scoring systems (e.g. early warning scores, EWS, or 'track and trigger' systems) may be used to 'flag' up patients at high risk of deterioration (see 📖 p.9)
  - Assess the existing level of support required by the patient (e.g. requirement for inotropes or haemofiltration)

The 'AMPLE' history
- A Allergies
- M Medication
- P Past medical history
- L Last meal
- E Event (and environment)

Airway

The commonest cause of airway emergencies is *airway obstruction*. It may be partial or complete.

In the unintubated patient

- Assess the ability of the patient to breathe, or in conscious patients the ability to speak, listening for:
  - Silence (caused by apnoea or complete obstruction), or abnormally quiet breath sounds
  - Stridor, wheeze, or gurgling
  - A hoarse voice (associated with laryngeal oedema)
- In unconscious or uncooperative patients feel for breath with your hand or cheek, check for misting on an oxygen mask.
- Look for evidence of airway obstruction:
  - Bleeding, vomit, secretions, tissue swelling, or foreign bodies
  - Obstruction of the pharynx by the tongue
  - Look for neck swelling or bruising, surgical/subcutaneous emphysema, or crepitus
- Look/listen for chest and other signs of airway obstruction, including:
  - Paradoxical chest and abdominal movements, tracheal tug
  - Reduced air entry in chest
  - Use of accessory muscles of respiration
  - Hypoxia is a late sign and indicates extreme emergency
- Exclude obstruction of pharynx by the tongue:
  - Chin lift: useful for infants, edentulous or unconscious patients
  - Jaw thrust: generally more effective than chin lift, and can be done one-handed (skilled) or two-handed (unskilled)
- Consider airway adjuncts:
  - Oropharyngeal ('Guedel') airways are normally only tolerated by unconscious patients
  - Nasopharyngeal airways are tolerated by conscious patients but may cause nasal bleeding on insertion worsening airway problems
  - Laryngeal mask airways (LMAs) require basic training to use, are only tolerated by unconscious patients, and offer limited protection from aspiration
  - Orotracheal intubation is the gold-standard for protecting and maintaining the airway but is only tolerated by anaesthetized or unconscious patients and requires a skilled operator to insert (the nasotracheal route is rarely required outside operating theatres)
- Using a self-inflating bag and mask to assist ventilation, if possible, may allow time to look for or treat causes of obstruction.
- Consider endotracheal intubation or an emergency needle cricothyroidotomy/tracheostomy (see 📖 pp.522 and 528):
  - Specialist anaesthetic and/or ENT airway skills will also be required at this point
- In patients who are unconscious, but maintaining an airway, endotracheal intubation should be considered, or the recovery position should be adopted (or alternatively 'head-down, left lateral' if they are lying on a trolley/bed).

In the intubated, mechanically ventilated patient

Work methodically from the ventilator to the patient:

- Check the ventilator is working (with adequate pressures, tidal volumes, and minute volumes) and that O_2 is connected, check that ventilator tubing is still connected and not obstructed.
- High airway pressure ventilator alarms may indicate obstruction.
- Low pressure, or low expired volume alarms may indicate a leak.
- Listen for any air leaks from ventilator tubing or endotracheal cuff.
- Check the endotracheal tube (ETT):
  - ETT position is normally 20–22cm at lips (compare with any previously noted length), ↑ insertion depth may indicate endobronchial placement. If immediately available, review CXR films to confirm correct placement of tube
  - Check tube patency (by passing a suction catheter through the endotracheal tube to exclude obstruction)
  - Laryngoscopy may be required to confirm correct placement
  - Check end-tidal CO_2 to confirm ETT position (provided there is also adequate cardiac output)
- Disconnect from ventilator and try ventilating with a self-inflating bag (successful ventilation indicates obstruction at the level of ventilator tubing):
  - If unsuccessful then there is an obstruction within or beyond the ETT, consider re-intubating with a fresh ETT and/or passing a fibreoptic scope; also consider causes for failure to expand the lungs (e.g. tension pneumothorax or bronchospasm)
  - Unilateral chest movement may be associated with pneumothorax or endobronchial intubation.

Breathing

Common causes of breathing difficulties include pleural diseases (pneumothorax, haemothorax, or pleural effusion), airway diseases (asthma, secretions, acute exacerbation of COPD), parenchymal disease (collapse, consolidation, ARDS) and cardiogenic disease (cardiogenic pulmonary oedema). Evidence of inadequate breathing should be looked for and corrected, including:

- Hypoxia—reduced PaO_2 or SaO_2.
- Dyspnoea and/or tachypnoea (bradypnoea or Cheyne–Stokes breathing are late/severe signs).
- Obvious problem, e.g. regurgitation with aspiration, massive bleeding.
- Absent or abnormal chest movement:
  - Unilateral movements may indicate pneumothorax, pleural effusion, collapse
  - Paradoxical chest-abdominal movement may indicate airway obstruction or flail chest
  - Use of accessory muscles of respiration
- Raised JVP may be visible.
- Apex beat or tracheal shift may be seen towards areas of collapse or away from pneumothoraces or pleural effusions.

- Percussion may reveal effusions or pneumothoraces.
- Abnormal breath sounds may be heard on auscultation:
  - Silent chest or wheeze may be due to acute severe asthma/ bronchospasm (pulmonary oedema may also cause wheeze)
  - Rattling noises suggests secretions
  - Absent unilateral sounds may be due to pleural effusion
  - Bronchial breathing suggests underlying consolidation
- Patients should be asked to cough to assess their ability to clear secretions which may be limited by neuromuscular problems or pain.
- Secretions themselves should be examined where possible, and patients encouraged to 'cough up' samples
- Check any intercostal drains—check if drains are still swinging or bubbling, and check the volume of blood or serous discharge
- Emergency management should be aimed at:
  - Excluding/treating life-threatening conditions (e.g. acute severe asthma, tension pneumothorax, pulmonary oedema, massive haemothorax)
  - Keeping SaO_2 94–98%,[1] PaO_2 >9 kPa, and $PaCO_2$ within the normal limits for the patient with respiratory rate <35 breaths/ minute
- Treatments which can be rapidly commenced include:
  - A trial of bronchodilators if bronchospasm is suspected
  - Chest physiotherapy to clear secretions
  - Non-invasive ventilation in conscious and cooperative patients who do not respond to previous treatment (see 📖 p.53)
  - Endotracheal intubation and mechanical ventilation

In the mechanically ventilated patient
- Check the degree of any respiratory support:
  - Oxygen, peak pressures, PEEP and minute volume measurements
  - ↑airway pressures or ↓tidal volumes may be due to ↑airway resistance or reduced lung compliance
  - If bronchospasm is present, check the length of the expiratory wheeze (in order to set I:E ratios), and check intrinsic PEEP
- Tracheal suction may reveal the amount and quality of secretions, and clear mucous plugs (critical care charts also often record the amount and character of secretions).
- Alveolar recruitment manoeuvres may be helpful in ARDS, atelectasis, or pulmonary oedema.
- Consider ventilating with a self-inflating bag in order to manually assess compliance.
- Urgent bronchoscopy may help clear obstructions/secretions.

Investigations such as ABGs and CXR will be needed to guide initial management. Where rapidly available, chest US may help diagnose effusions or occult pneumothoraces.

---

[1] Or SaO_2 88–92% where there is a risk of hypercapnic respiratory failure (see 📖 p.74).

Circulation

Cardiovascular emergencies often present as severe hypotension and shock, heart failure with pulmonary oedema, or cardiac arrest.

Inadequate circulation may be caused by low-output states such as severe hypovolaemia or cardiogenic shock, and high-output states due to peripheral vasodilatation (e.g. sepsis). Non-cardiovascular causes (e.g. endocrine disorders, electrolytes, pneumothorax) should also be considered. In addition, certain interventions such as positive pressure ventilation or epidural analgesia can lead to relative hypovolaemia.

In critical care ECG, arterial BP, and cardiac output monitoring may already be connected to the patient, giving clues to the nature of emergency. Signs of cardiovascular compromise include:

- Cardiovascular signs:
  - Thready pulse, tachycardia, and hypotension
  - Cold peripheries, prolonged capillary refill (>2 seconds)
  - Alternatively a bounding pulse may occur with hypotension in individuals capable of compensating
  - Bradycardia is a pre-terminal sign, or a sign of vagal stimulation, (e.g. from intraperitoneal blood)
  - JVP may be raised
- Other signs:
  - Tachypnoea, altered mental state
  - ↓urine output (<0.5 ml/kg/hour)
  - Peripheral oedema
- Look for obvious or concealed blood/fluid loss.
- Check any abdominal or wound drains—check they are still *in situ* and measure the volume of any blood loss.
- Check the status of any inotropic infusions.
- Other signs of circulatory insufficiency may include lactataemia or metabolic acidosis.
- Non-specific signs may be present in ventilated patients, including chest pulsation (indicating a hyperdynamic state), the presence of $ETCO_2$ (indicating both patent endotracheal access and that cardiac output is present), a swinging arterial line trace (a non-specific indicator of hypovolaemia in ventilated patients).
- Measured variables may also include:
  - CVP, pulmonary artery occlusion pressure (using PAFC)
  - Stroke volume and cardiac output estimation (via echocardiography, PAFC, TOD, pulse contour analysis); these will also allow an estimation of systemic vascular resistance
  - Echocardiography will also allow rapid diagnosis of tamponade (and other signs such as regional wall motion abnormality)
  - TOD may give an estimation of cardiac filling and/or afterload changes by measuring the corrected flowtime (FTc)
  - Stroke volume variation may give an indication of cardiac filling in ventilated patients
  - Hb and haematocrit (often available as part of ABG analysis)
  - Venous blood saturations (either from the pulmonary artery, $S\bar{v}O_2$, or from a central line, $ScvO_2$) low values indicate a low

arterial oxygen supply or tissues which are extracting more
oxygen than usual; a high value may be indicative of a shunt
- Emergency management should consist of:
  - Exclude/treat life-threatening conditions such as cardiac
    tamponade (raised CVP/JVP, pulsus paradoxus, diminished
    heart sounds, low voltage ECG, globular heart on CXR,
    echocardiographic diagnosis), haemorrhage, or arrhythmia that
    compromises circulation
  - Adequate fluid/blood replacement for hypovolaemic shock; give
    500 ml of colloid/crystalloid within 5–10 minutes and reassess
  - For severe hypotension with a low-output state, consider starting
    an infusion of adrenaline until the cause is established
  - For severe hypotension with a high-output state, start with IV
    fluids and vasoconstrictive agents such as noradrenaline
  - Cardiogenic shock should be treated with appropriate inotropes
    (e.g. dobutamine or adrenaline), and the management of
    any associated condition such as acute coronary syndrome,
    arrhythmias, or pulmonary oedema
  - Exclude and treat acid–base and electrolyte abnormalities—in
    particular severe metabolic acidosis, hypo-/hyperkalaemia,
    hypomagnesaemia, and hypocalcaemia
- In patients with sepsis and hypotension or elevated serum lactate
  suggested resuscitation goals include:
  - Central venous pressure of 8–12 mmHg
  - Mean arterial pressure ≥65 mmHg
  - Urine output ≥0.5 ml/kg/hour
  - $S\bar{V}O_2$ or $ScvO_2$ ≥70%

Disability/neurology

Changes in neurological state may be related to neurological disease
(head injury, space-occupying lesion, subarachnoid haemorrhage), or
worsening respiratory, circulatory, or metabolic disorders. Exclude and
treat hypoglycaemia, hypoxia, hypotension, or hypercapnia.

The immediate management aims for patients with altered neurology should be to protect airway, ensure adequate breathing and gas
exchange, and prevent hypo-/hypertension. Tracheal intubation may be
necessary in unconscious patients (GCS <8, or P/U in AVPU).
- A rapid assessment of the patient's neurological status should
  be made by assessing GCS (see 🕮 p.153) or AVPU scale (Alert,
  responds to Voice, responds to Pain or is Unresponsive).
- Signs of altered neurological state may include:
  - Drowsiness, agitation, incoherence, or incontinence
  - Lack of response to verbal command and/or pain
- Other neurological signs may include seizures, focal neurological
  signs, pupil signs, or lack of gag/cough reflex.
- Check ICP if being monitored (see 🕮 p.186).

- Jugular bulb saturation and/or transcranial Doppler measurements may be available.

Unless the neurological signs resolve rapidly, an urgent CT scan may be required for diagnosis and management (see 🕮 p.155). Where there is evidence of acutely raised ICP (e.g. head injury with a fixed dilated pupil) treatment with hypertonic saline or mannitol may be required as a temporizing measure until more definitive measures are employed

Exposure/general

Other signs and symptoms include:
- Temperature.
- Rashes and stigmata.
- Evidence of DVT.
- Abdominal examination.
- Trauma survey (including burns assessment).

Further emergency investigations should be guided by the general condition of the patient. If sepsis is suspected, 2 or more blood cultures should be obtained. Other cultures may be indicated (including cerebrospinal fluid, respiratory secretions, urine, wounds, and other body fluids). IV antibiotics should then be started as soon as possible.

Pitfalls/difficult situations

- Certain groups of patients will be sicker than others with the same acute problem, including those patients who:
  - Are at the extremes of age
  - Have multi system disease (e.g. diabetes or rheumatoid arthritis)
  - Have chronic organ failures (e.g. heart, lung, kidney or liver)
  - Are immunosuppressed or malnourished (e.g. those on steroids or chemotherapy, or those with liver disease or cancer)
- Others may compensate for longer despite being more sick:
  - Children, young adults, athletes, and pregnant women

Early warning scores

These score basic physiological variables (heart rate, BP, respiratory rate, temperature, urine output, neurological status) as a means of identifying developing critical illness (Table 1.1). Patients with high EWS scores often need only basic management such as fluids, analgesia, or physiotherapy. An obstetric EWS is also available (see 🕮 p.428).

Further reading

Dellinger RP, et al. Surviving sepsis campaign: international guidelines for management of severe sepsis and septic shock: 2008. *Crit Care Med* 2008; **36**(1): 296–327.

Morgan R, et al. An early warning scoring system for detecting developing critical illness. *Clin Intensive Care* 1997; **8**: 100.

Prytherch DR et al. ViEWS—Towards a national early warning score for detecting adult inpatient deterioration. *Resuscitation* 2010; **81**: 932–7.

Riley B, et al. Critical care outreach: rationale and development. *BJA CEPD Rev* 2001; **1**(5): 146–9.

Smith G, et al. ABC of intensive care: criteria for admission. *Br Med J* 1999; **318**: 1544–7.

Table 1.1 Early warning score details

	Score					
	3	2	1	0	1	2	3
Respiration rate (resps/minute)	≤8		9–11	12–20		21–24	≥25
SpO₂ (%)	≤91	92–93	94–95	≥96			–
Inspired O₂				Air			Any O₂
Heart rate (BPM)		≤40	41–50	51–90	91–110	111–130	≥131
Systolic blood pressure (mmHg)	≤90	91–100	101–110	111–249	≥250		
Temperature (°C)	≤35.0		35.1–36	36.1–38	38.1–39.0	≥39.1	
Neurological status			–	Alert & orientated			Responds only to Voice or Pain or Unresponsive

A graded system of responses is recommended with a score of 6 or more triggering a medical response and a score of 9 or more triggering an immediate medical response.
ViEWS early warning score: Reprinted from *Resuscitation*, 81, 8, Prytherch DR et al., 'ViEWS—Towards a national early warning score for detecting adult inpatient deterioration', pp. 932–937, copyright 2010, with permission from Elsevier.

⑦ Early further management

After the initial assessment and management of any emergency there may be further aspects of patient care to consider or plan for. Details on the further management of specific emergencies are considered in individual chapters; more generic areas of further management are discussed in this section.

General

Following resuscitation, patients should be nursed in an appropriate environment according to the level of care required: level 2 patients require a minimum of HDU care whilst level 3 patients require ICU care; some diseases may require specialist care (e.g. coronary care, cardiothoracic intensive care, neurosurgical, burns, spinal injury, or liver units).

Levels of care

Level 0   Normal ward-care patients

Level 1   Patients who remain on a normal ward but who require a minimum of 4-hourly observations to avoid deterioration[1]

Level 2   Patients with, or at immediate risk of, single-organ[2] failure (e.g. requiring FiO_2 >50% or non-invasive ventilation, or requiring advanced cardiovascular support with vasoactive drugs). This may include patients requiring preoperative optimization, extended postoperative care, or patients 'stepping down' from level 3 care. There should be a 2:1 nurse/patient ratio in the UK

Level 3   Patients requiring the support of 2 or more failing organs, or those who require advanced respiratory support alone. 1:1 nurse patient ratios are the norm within the UK

Patient location does not determine their level of care.

↑care (including level 3) may still be appropriate even where resuscitation after cardiac arrest is not considered appropriate.

[1] Other factors can also determine the need for level 1 care, (e.g. the presence of an epidural or tracheostomy, the need for continuous O_2 therapy, or for regular PEFR measurement).

[2] Patients requiring basic respiratory and basic cardiovascular support simultaneously may be regarded as level 2. Any patient requiring advanced respiratory support is at level 3.

Reproduced from the Intensive Care Society. Levels of critical care for adult patients: Standards and guidelines. London: Intensive Care Society, 2009, with permission. For further, more detailed explanation please refer to these guidelines: ℛ http://www.ics.ac.uk/professional/standards_and_guidelines/levels_of_critical_care_for_adult_patients.

Where referral is required, it should follow the SBAR format (or similar) to ensure that all critical information is conveyed (see Box 1.1).

Box 1.1 SBAR method of referring patients
- Situation:
  - Confirm that you are talking to the correct person
  - Introduce yourself by name and position
  - Briefly explain the reason for the referral
  - Background
  - Identify the patient by name and age
- Summarize details of their past medical history of note
- Summarize details of their admission and relevant treatment
- Assessment:
  - Summarize the patient's current clinical condition using an ABCDE approach
  - Include relevant clinical findings and investigations
- Recommendation:
  - State your opinion of the current situation, including any treatment you think is required
  - Check whether or not your plan is appropriate, including any changes/suggestions made to you
  - Agree a timescale for observing whether treatment is effective, combined with plans for further treatment or re-referral
  - Document the discussion

A similar structure for referring patients is RSVP (Reasons, Story, Vital signs, Plan).

Ongoing management

Continuous respiratory and cardiovascular monitoring, combined with regular observations of physiological variables, such as temperature and urine output, should be carried out after resuscitation, along with the following management:

Airway

Airway patency should be continually monitored. Where patients have undergone endotracheal intubation:
- Review CXR (confirm correct positioning of ETT).
- The tube position at the teeth should be regularly checked/recorded.
- In patients who are expected to require prolonged endotracheal intubation, the insertion of a tracheostomy should be considered.

Breathing

Continuous saturation monitoring should be maintained. Where patients have undergone endotracheal intubation and mechanical ventilation:
- There is no definitive evidence as to which mode of ventilation (pressure controlled or volume controlled) is best, but modes which allow patients to breathe alongside the ventilator (e.g. SIMV or BIPAP) may be better tolerated.
- Modes such as ASB or PSV (with or without a mandatory element, e.g. SIMV or BIPAP) may allow respiratory support to be titrated to a patient's needs.

- Moderate hypercapnia should be tolerated, except in those at risk of raised intracranial pressure.
- Initial ventilator settings should be adjusted to ensure a lung-protective ventilation strategy is maintained (ARDSnet guidelines, 🕮 p.53):
  - Suggested initial ventilator settings can be found in the box of this title, 🕮 p.12.
- The head of bed should be raised to 30–45° (semi-recumbent) if possible in mechanically ventilated patients to help prevent ventilator-associated pneumonia.
- Regular chest physiotherapy should be attempted unless it is likely to worsen cardiovascular instability.
- A weaning protocol should be initiated as soon as practicable.
- End-tidal CO_2 monitoring has been recommended for all ventilated patients.

Indications for endotracheal intubation

To protect the airway
- From risk of aspiration (e.g. blood/vomit).
- From risk of obstruction.
- Loss of protective airway reflexes.
- Because sedation/anaesthesia is required to allow assessment or treatment, particularly in agitated or combative patients.

To permit mechanical ventilation
- Apnoea.
- Hypoxia or inadequate respiratory effort.
- Hypercapnia or requirement for hyperventilation.
- Cardiovascular instability, to maximize oxygenation.

Suggested initial ventilator settings

- Start with a high FiO_2 (0.9–1) and titrate according to SaO_2/PaO_2
- PEEP should be titrated to thoraco-pulmonary compliance and oxygen requirements, 5–10 cmH_2O is appropriate initially (bronchospastic patients may require less/none at all; see 🕮 p.79).
- Ventilator settings should be adjusted to achieve a minute volume which allows adequate oxygenation with moderate hypercapnia (if possible), a reasonable initial minute volume would be ~80 ml/kg (a tidal volume of 4–6 ml/kg [ideal body-weight] × respiratory rate, i.e. in an 80kg patient settings of 400 ml TV with a rate of 16 breaths/minute); where pressure-controlled ventilation is used an initial inspiratory pressure of 20 cmH_2O may be used, and then adjusted to achieve acceptable tidal volume.
- Initial I:E ratios should be of the order of 1:2–1:1.5 (except in bronchospasm, 🕮 p.79).
- Volume, pressure, apnoea, low minute volume, and oxygen failure alarms should all be activated; a maximum upper pressure limit of 40 cmH_2O should be set initially for all modes of ventilation.

Circulation

- Consider inserting an arterial line and central line for invasive cardiovascular monitoring.
- Review CXR to confirm correct positioning of any thoracic CVCs.
- Cardiac output monitoring may allow targeted fluid therapy or inotrope usage (although evidence to support this is limited).
- Severe haemodynamic compromise may respond to bicarbonate therapy, but this should not be used if pH ≥7.15.

Neurology

- Neurological status (GCS and pupil size/response) should be regularly assessed and recorded.
- Sedation protocols should be used and the level of sedation and delirium measured against a recognized scoring system (e.g. RASS, CAM-ICU).
- Where continuous infusions of sedation are used, daily interruptions of sedation should be undertaken whenever possible.
- Patients at risk of spinal trauma should be nursed supine with a whole-bed tilt and assessed and stabilized as soon as possible; hard collars should be removed according to protocol (🕮 p.408).
- Patients at risk of raised ICP should be positioned 30–45° head up to improve venous drainage.
- Avoid continuous muscle relaxants/neuromuscular blockade if possible (especially if there is seizure activity), unless refractory hypoxia is present—continuous infusions require train-of-four monitoring.

Richmond agitation sedation scoring

+4	Combative (overtly combative or violent; immediate danger to staff)
+3	Very agitated (pulls on or removes tube/tubes or catheter/catheters or has aggressive behaviour toward staff)
+2	Agitated (frequent non-purposeful movement or patient-ventilator dyssynchrony)
+1	Restless (anxious or apprehensive but movements not aggressive or vigorous)
0	Alert and calm
−1	Drowsy, not fully alert, but has sustained (>10 seconds) awakening, with eye contact, to voice
−2	Light sedation (briefly, <10 seconds, awakens with eye contact to voice)
−3	Moderate sedation (any movement, but no eye contact, to voice)
−4	Deep sedation (no response to voice, but any movement on physical stimulation)
−5	Unrousable (no response to voice or physical stimulation).

Reprinted with permission of the American Thoracic Society. Copyright © 2013 American Thoracic Society. Sessler et al., 2002, 'The Richmond Agitation–Sedation Scale', *American Journal of Respiratory and Critical Care Medicine*, 166, 10, pp. 1338–1344. Official Journal of the American Thoracic Society.

Endocrine/metabolism

- Managing blood glucose:
  - Regularly check blood glucose, at least every 4 hours
  - Targets for glycaemic control have been controversial, but hyperglycaemia should be avoided, particularly in patients with neurological or cardiac injury, and hypoglycaemia should be rapidly corrected. A target of <10mmol/L has previously been advocated
- Adrenal support:
  - Continue steroid support in patients who take long-term steroids
  - Commence steroids in patients with Addison's disease (see 📖 p.236)
  - Steroid support for inotrope-dependent patients at risk of adrenal suppression (e.g. those with sepsis, or following induction with etomidate; see 📖 p.525) is not well supported by evidence (some centres continue this practice, either indefinitely whilst on inotropes, or limited to 3 days; whilst other centres do not).

Insulin sliding scale
See Table 1.2. Hourly monitoring is recommended in unstable patients. This may be reduced to every 2–4 hours when patients are under stable control.

Table 1.2 Sample insulin sliding scale

Blood glucose (mmol/L)	Insulin infusion (units/hour)[1]
<3.9	0 (treat hypoglycaemia)
<10	0
10.1–12	1
12.1–15	2
15.1–18	3
>18	4 (and review)

[1] Add 50 units soluble insulin to 50 ml saline 0.9%

From Joslin EP (1934) A Diabetic Manual for the Mutual Use of Doctor and Patient. Philadelphia, PA: Lea & Febiger.

Renal

- Catheterization of critically ill or immobile patients will allow accurate monitoring of hourly urine output.
- Strict measurement of fluid balance should be maintained.
- Where renal replacement therapy is required (📖 p.266) intermittent haemodialysis or continuous veno-venous haemofiltration (CVVH) are considered equally effective; haemodynamic stability *may* be better using CVVH.

Gastrointestinal and hepatic

- Inserting a NGT will facilitate enteral feeding; base-of-skull fractures or nasal trauma may necessitate an orogastric tube.
- Review CXR to confirm correct positioning of NGT.

- Institute enteral feeding where possible (it may not be possible in cases of small bowel injury, or upper GI perforation or obstruction).
- Provide stress ulcer prophylaxis in high-risk patients (e.g. previous GI bleeding, coagulopathy, lack of enteral feeding, mechanical ventilation for >48 hours, renal failure, and burns), choices include:
  - H_2 receptor antagonists (e.g. ranitidine 50 mg IV 8-hourly, reduced to 12-hourly in renal failure); NG/oral dose 150 mg 12-hourly
  - IV proton pump inhibitors (e.g. omeprazole 40 mg IV/PO daily)—alternative to H_2 antagonists with no proven superiority in prophylaxis, dose reduction not required in renal failure
  - Alternatively sucralfate 2g NG 8-hourly, but provides less protection against clinically significant GI haemorrhage, may block NGTs or result in bezoars, and care is required in renal failure.

Haematology
- Consider DVT prophylaxis in all patients who are immobile or otherwise at high risk of developing DVT:
  - Subcutaneous low-molecular-weight heparin (e.g. enoxaparin 40 mg SC daily, or dalteparin 5000 units SC daily)
  - Alternatively subcutaneous heparin 5000–10,000 units SC 12-hourly, may be easier to reverse should the patient develop active bleeding
  - Prophylaxis may be withheld in coagulopathic, anticoagulated or actively bleeding patients; or in patients at high risk of catastrophic bleeding (e.g. following neurosurgery)
  - Use antithromboembolic stockings or an intermittent pneumatic compression device alongside pharmacologic prophylaxis, or where heparin is contraindicated
- Treatment of anaemia and clotting abnormalities:
  - In the absence of coronary artery disease, significant tissue hypoperfusion, or ongoing haemorrhage, haemoglobin may safely be allowed to fall to 7.0 g/dl
  - If transfusing red blood cells aim for a haemoglobin of 7.0–9.0 g/dl
  - Where coronary artery disease or active bleeding are present a suggested alternative transfusion 'trigger' is ~10 g/dl
  - Avoid correcting clotting if possible unless there is bleeding or invasive procedures are planned
  - Platelets should be transfused if: counts are $<50 \times 10^9$/L and surgery or invasive procedures are planned; or counts are $<30 \times 10^9$/L and there is a significant bleeding risk; or whenever counts are $<5 \times 10^9$/L

Microbiology
- Antimicrobial therapy should be commenced rapidly based on the broad-spectrum coverage for the most likely local pathogens.
- After 48 hours therapy should be adjusted, guided by culture results, to a narrow-spectrum regimen—some antimicrobials require regular serum concentration measurement.
- Universal precautions should be adopted for all patients.
- Where necessary patients should be isolated; routine surveillance swabs may be needed (see 📖 p.382).

Analgesia

- Analgesia should be used when required—as a bare-minimum patients should be able to cough and deep breathe with no or minor pain only.
- Epidurals should be examined daily for any complications (📖 p.401).

General care

- Pressure area care, oral toilet, and eye care should be attended to.
- Contact lenses should be removed and corneas should be kept moist.

Surgical patients

- Wound drain/stoma output, and stoma perfusion, should be monitored.
- In cases where abdominal compartment syndrome is possible (📖 p.284) intra-abdominal pressures should be measured.
- In vascular patients regular monitoring of the appropriate peripheral pulses may be required.

Trauma patients

- Trauma and burns patients admitted to ICU/HDU should undergo tertiary surveys to identify injuries missed during initial resuscitation.

Obstetric patients

- Obstetric patients require intermittent or continuous fetal monitoring.

Discussion of care

- The mental capacity of the patient should be assessed.
- Discussions with the patient and/or their family covering the likely progression of the illness should take place as soon as is practicable.
- Where appropriate, the resuscitation status of the patient should be discussed with the patient and/or their relatives.

Further reading

Chu YF, et al. Stress-related mucosal disease in the critically ill patient: Risk factors and strategies to prevent stress-related bleeding in the intensive care unit. *W J Emerg Med* 2010; **1**(1): 32–6.

Dellinger RP, et al. Surviving sepsis campaign: international guidelines for management of severe sepsis and septic shock: 2008. *Crit Care Med* 2008; **36**(1): 296–327.

Haig KM, et al. National Patient Safety Goals. SBAR: a shared mental model for improving communication between clinicians. *Jt Comm J Qual Patient Saf* 2006; **32**(3): 167–75.

Hebert PC, et al. A multicenter, randomized, controlled clinical trial of transfusion requirements in critical care (TRICC). *N Engl J Med* 1999; **340**: 409–17.

Intensive Care Society. *Levels of critical care for adult patients. Standards and guidelines.* London: Intensive Care Society, 2009.

Kress JP, et al. Daily interruption of sedative infusions in critically ill patients undergoing mechanical ventilation. *N Engl J Med* 2000; **342**: 1471–7.

Kumar A, et al. Duration of hypotension before initiation of effective antimicrobial therapy is the critical determinant of survival in human septic shock. *Crit Care Med* 2006; **34**(6): 1589–96.

National Institute for Health and Clinical Excellence. *Venous thromboembolism: reducing the risk.* London: NICE, 2010.

Sprung CL, et al. Hydrocortisone therapy for patients with septic shock (CORTICUS). *N Engl J Med* 2008; **358**: 111–24.

The Acute Respiratory Distress Syndrome Network. Ventilation with lower tidal volumes as compared with traditional tidal volumes for acute lung injury and the acute respiratory distress syndrome. *N Engl J Med* 2000; **342**: 1301–8.

The NICE-SUGAR Study Investigators. Intensive versus conventional glucose control in critically ill patients. *N Engl J Med* 2009; **360**: 1283–97.

Chapter 2

Airway

:☒: Airway obstruction

An obstructed airway is a medical emergency requiring immediate treatment. Where possible, patients at risk should be identified early so that airway obstruction can be prevented. Although upper airway obstruction may be gradual in onset it more commonly progresses very rapidly. Continuous assessment is required to identify signs of impending airway obstruction.

Whilst the ultimate aim when managing airway disorders is to obtain a definitive airway, patients die because of failed oxygenation and ventilation—not failed intubation. Basic airway management skills (e.g. bag and mask ventilation using simple airway adjuncts) are crucial.

Causes

Internal obstruction
- Foreign body or tumour.
- Airway bleeding/trauma.
- Aspirated vomit.
- Upper airway infection (e.g. epiglottitis, retropharyngeal abscess).
- Swelling/oedema:
  - Angio-oedema (ACE inhibitors, aspirin, hereditary C1-esterase deficiency)
  - Anaphylaxis
  - Following upper airway interventions or surgery (including post-extubation laryngeal oedema)
  - Airways burns or inhalation of smoke/toxic fumes

External obstruction
- Swelling/oedema: neck trauma, external mass, or tumour.
- Haematoma (especially in coagulopathic or anticoagulated patients).
  - Neck trauma
  - Following thyroid or carotid surgery
  - Following internal jugular line insertion

Neurological causes
- Diminished level of consciousness (e.g. intoxication, head injury/CVA, cardiac arrest).
- Laryngospasm (especially in semi-conscious patients).
- Paralysis of vocal cords.
  - Neurological disease (e.g. myasthenia gravis, Guillain–Barré, polyneuritis, or recurrent laryngeal nerve damage)
  - Inadequate reversal of muscle relaxants

Presentation and assessment

Partial obstruction
- Anxiety.
- Patient prefers sitting, standing, or leaning forward.
- Inability to speak or voice change (muffled or hoarse voice).
- Stridor (inspiratory noise accompanying breathing) or noisy breathing.
- Obvious neck swelling.
- Lump in throat, difficulty in swallowing.

- Choking.
- Coughing.
- Drooling.
- Respiratory distress:
  - Tachypnoea and dyspnoea
  - Use of accessory muscles of respiration
  - Paradoxical breathing: indrawn chest and suprasternal recession
  - Tracheal tug
  - 'Hunched' posture

Total or near-total obstruction
- Hypoxia, cyanosis, hypercapnia.
- Bradycardia, hypotension.
- Diminished or absent air entry.
- ↓consciousness.
- Cardiac/respiratory arrest, where bag and mask ventilation impossible.

Investigations

Diagnosis is mainly clinical and some investigations may have to wait until the patient is stabilized with a secure airway.
- ABGs (hypoxia, hypercapnia).
- FBC (↑WCC in infection).
- Clotting screen (coagulopathy).
- Blood cultures and oropharyngeal swabs[1] where appropriate.
- Imaging: neck X-ray (AP & lateral), CXR, or CT scan may be required (may reveal neck or mediastinal masses or foreign bodies).
- Fibreoptic endoscopy or direct laryngoscopy.[1]
  - Although nasendoscopy will potentially allow a view of the airway and aid diagnosis, it requires skill to be done safely
  - Direct laryngoscopy should not be attempted unless the airway is already secured, or all preparations are in place to immediately secure the airway (see 📖 pp.20–21).

Differential diagnoses

- Equipment failure (e.g. incorrectly assembled self-inflating ambu-bag).
- ETT or tracheostomy obstruction (see 📖 pp.40 and 45).
- Conditions which result in noisy breathing:
  - Bronchospasm
  - Hysterical stridor
- Conditions which result in difficulty breathing spontaneously or high airway pressures when ventilating patient:
  - Bronchospasm
  - Tension pneumothorax
- Conditions which result in patients adopting a sitting or leaning forward position:
  - SVC obstruction
  - Cardiac tamponade

---

1 Airway interventions in a patient with a partially obstructed airway can provoke complete airway obstruction.

Immediate management

- 100% O_2, pulse oximetry.
- Assess condition of patient and likely cause of airway obstruction .
- Support ventilation with bag and mask if required.

If patient has suffered cardiac/respiratory arrest:
- Follow BLS guidelines (📖 p.98).
- Support/open airway; use adjuncts (oropharyngeal or nasopharyngeal airways) and suction.
- Remove obvious obstruction and commence CPR.

If patient is peri-arrest:
- Call for skilled help: anaesthetist, ENT surgeon.
- Obstruction requires immediate laryngoscopy/tracheal intubation.
- Surgical airway, i.e. cricothyroidotomy or tracheostomy for total obstruction if the previous points fail.

If airway obstruction is due to diminished consciousness:
- Call for skilled anaesthetic assistance.
- If traumatic: assume C-spine injury and asses for other injuries.
- Consider replacing hard-collar with manual in-line stabilization (often helpful when supporting airway, required prior to intubation).
- *Ensuring an adequate airway always overrides concerns about potential C-spine injuries.*
- Support/open airway; use adjuncts (oropharyngeal or nasopharyngeal airways) and suction.
- Support ventilation with bag and mask if required.
- Proceed to definitive airway, most commonly using a rapid sequence intubation (📖 p.522).
- Cricothyroidotomy or tracheostomy is indicated in the event of failed intubation.

If airway obstruction is due to airway swelling, infection, or physical obstruction:
- Call for senior help (anaesthetic and ENT).
- Formulate an airway management plan and arrange for equipment to be available (e.g. plan A: endotracheal intubation; plan B: laryngeal mask airway; plan C: temporary cricothyroidotomy); see 📖 pp.26 and 27 for difficult airway equipment and failed intubation drill.
- Arrange equipment for inhalational induction (anaesthetic machine with an anaesthetic gas: sevoflurane or halothane):
  - Consider transferring patient to an operating theatre where this equipment is present if the patient is stable
- Temporary measures which may be used whilst arranging the equipment/transfer include: nebulized adrenaline (5 mg/5 ml 1:1000 in a nebulizer) and/or humidified oxygen or Heliox.
- *Early intubation should be considered to reduce the risk of sudden deterioration and airway obstruction:*
  - Cricothyroidotomy or tracheostomy is indicated in the event of failed intubation and ventilation, or as initial management plan under local anaesthesia.

Other considerations requiring simultaneous treatment:
• Anaphylaxis (p.110): IV or IM adrenaline, steroids, antihistamines.
• Haematoma after neck surgery: remove dressings, cut open sutures.
• Airway bleeding (p.36): correct coagulopathy.
• Facial trauma (p.28): simultaneous assessment of C-spine and other associated trauma.
• Laryngospasm: support ventilation with bag and mask ventilation, apply PEEP (easier using a Water's or C-circuit); although low-dose propofol, 10–20 mg IV, and low-dose suxamethonium, 10–15mg IV have been successfully used, intubation must be immediately available.
• Inadequate reversal of muscle relaxants: treat for laryngospasm, consider reversal with IV neostigmine 2.5 mg mixed with glycopyrronium bromide 0.5 mg (only works if reversing a non-depolarizing muscle relaxant that is already beginning to wear off); alternatively sugammadex 2–4 mg/kg IV may reverse muscle relaxation with vecuronium or rocuronium.
• Postextubation oedema: nebulized adrenaline, IV steroids.
• Angio-oedema which is non-allergic: this should be treated as allergic in the first instance (see earlier in list), where there is a clear history of hereditary angio-oedema consider C1 esterase inhibitor concentrate, icatibant, tranexamic acid, or danazol (seek specialist advice first).

In stable patients where diagnosis/degree of obstruction is in doubt, nasal endoscopy performed by an experienced ENT surgeon may help. Be prepared to intubate or perform cricothyroidotomy/tracheostomy if total airway obstruction is provoked.

Once **A**irway and **B**reathing are stabilized, continue **ABC** approach:
• Transfer to critical care environment for close observation.

Further management
Only if condition is stable and the airway obstruction has been relieved:
• Nurse patient 30–45° head up to promote venous drainage.
• Consider IV dexamethasone to reduce any further airway swelling.
• Ventilation and sedation for a number of days on ICU may be required for intubated patients until the cause of obstruction resolves.
• Adopt a lung-protective ventilation strategy (p.53).
• Surgical or microbiology opinions may be required.
• Supportive measures for sepsis may be required (see p.322).
• Assess airway swelling (laryngoscopy and/or cuff-leak test) prior to extubation.
• Where intubation is likely to be prolonged, or airway obstruction may recur after extubation, consider elective tracheostomy.

Pitfalls/difficult situations

- Delaying intubation may make a difficult intubation impossible.
- Deterioration to complete obstruction may progress rapidly over a few hours.
- Cardiovascular collapse may mask airway signs.
- Airway interventions in a patient with a partially obstructed airway can provoke complete airway obstruction.
- Insertion of oropharyngeal or nasopharyngeal airway in patients with retropharyngeal abscess may burst the abscess and soil the airway.
- Other, non-airway, indications for intubation also exist (see 📖 p.12).
- It is important to recognize patients in whom endotracheal intubation is likely to be difficult (see 📖 p.24).
- Obtaining a definitive airway via endotracheal intubation or surgical tracheostomy can be challenging in the face of airway obstruction; the priority is always to maintain oxygenation.
- Cricothyroidotomy (see 📖 p.528) should only be attempted by inexperienced operators in circumstances where the patient is otherwise likely to die.
- The commonest technique of intubation, the rapid sequence intubation, is described on 📖 p.522 so that non-anaesthetic trained critical care practitioners are familiar with a technique they may be required to assist with.
- Anyone who may be required to manage an airway or intubate patients in elective or emergency settings must be able to recognize a misplaced ETT (see 📖 p.26) and be aware of what to do in the event of a failure to intubate (see 📖 p.27).

Complications at intubation

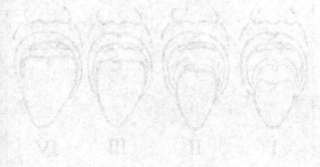

I   II   III   IV

☠: **Complications at intubation**

- Failed intubations occur in approximately 1 in 2000 routine intubations and up to 1 in 250 rapid sequence intubations.
- Difficult intubation may lead to failure to maintain oxygenation, airway protection, or trauma from repeated intubation attempts.
- 'Can't intubate/can't ventilate' situations account for 25% of all anaesthetic deaths.
- Studies have highlighted the importance of proper airway assessment, combined with the creation of an airway management plan based on a plan A, plan B, plan C approach.

Features predictive of difficult endotracheal intubation:
- Current airway obstruction, inflammation, or haemorrhage.
- Previous difficult intubation.
- Previous neck/jaw surgery/radiotherapy or previous tracheostomy.
- Receding jaw, or cannot protrude bottom incisors over top incisors.
- Limited mouth opening (≤3 cm or 2 finger breadths).
- Prominent front teeth.
- Unable to extend neck: C-spine injury/collar, rheumatoid arthritis, ankylosing spondylosis.
- Obesity, bull neck, large breasts.
- Mallampati class 3 or 4: with mouth full open and tongue protruding the back of the mouth, uvula and faucal pillars cannot be seen (Fig. 2.1).

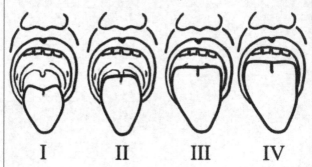

I   II   III   IV

Fig. 2.1 Mallampati classes. Data from Samsoon GL, Young JR. Difficult tracheal intubation: a retrospective study. *Anaesthesia* 1987; **42**(5): 487–90.

Ways to reduce intubation difficulties

(See Fig. 2.2.)
- Thorough assessment of airway and previous anaesthetic history.
- Formulate and communicate airway management strategy: plan A, plan B, plan C as per DAS guidelines (see 🕮 p.27).

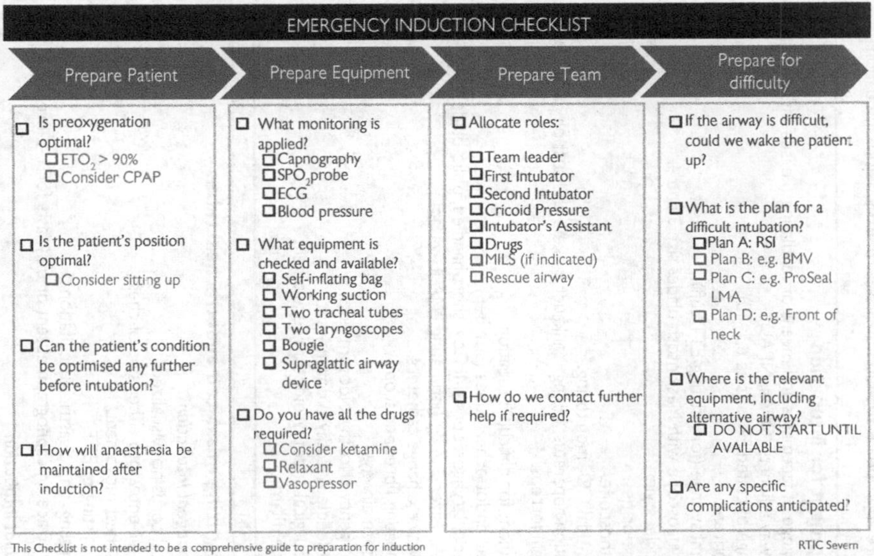

EMERGENCY INDUCTION CHECKLIST

Prepare Patient

- Is preoxygenation optimal?
  - ETO₂ > 90%
  - Consider CPAP

- Is the patient's position optimal?
  - Consider sitting up

- Can the patient's condition be optimised any further before intubation?

- How will anaesthesia be maintained after induction?

Prepare Equipment

- What monitoring is applied?
  - Capnography
  - SPO₂ probe
  - ECG
  - Blood pressure

- What equipment is checked and available?
  - Self-inflating bag
  - Working suction
  - Two tracheal tubes
  - Two laryngoscopes
  - Bougie
  - Supraglottic airway device

- Do you have all the drugs required?
  - Consider ketamine
  - Relaxant
  - Vasopressor

Prepare Team

- Allocate roles:
  - Team leader
  - First Intubator
  - Second Intubator
  - Cricoid Pressure
  - Intubator's Assistant
  - Drugs
  - MILS (if indicated)
  - Rescue airway

- How do we contact further help if required?

Prepare for difficulty

- If the airway is difficult, could we wake the patient up?

- What is the plan for a difficult intubation?
  - Plan A: RSI
  - Plan B: e.g. BMV
  - Plan C: e.g. ProSeal LMA
  - Plan D: e.g. Front of neck

- Where is the relevant equipment, including alternative airway? DO NOT START UNTIL AVAILABLE

- Are any specific complications anticipated?

RTIC Severn

This Checklist is not intended to be a comprehensive guide to preparation for induction

Fig. 2.2 Checklist for induction of anaesthesia/intubation. Adapted from the reports and findings of the 4th National Audit Project of The Royal College of Anaesthetists 2011. Reproduced with the permission of The Royal College of Anaesthetists.

- Consider awake fibreoptic intubation (if appropriate) if potential exists for difficult laryngoscopy with difficult bag–mask ventilation.
- Prepare equipment.
- Ensure senior help available.
- Position patient appropriately and pre-oxygenate.
- Ensure appropriate abolition of airway reflexes before intubation.

Equipment for intubation

- A range of facemasks and means of ventilating (i.e. self-inflating bag).
- Airway adjuncts (OPAs, NPAs).
- Range of cuffed ETTs (size 6.5–10).
- Lubricant.
- 10-ml syringe (for inflating ETT cuff).
- Laryngoscope with Mackintosh blades size 3 and 4.
- Bougie, stylet.
- Tape or ties.
- Stethoscope.
- End-tidal CO_2 monitoring.
- Suction apparatus, tubing; Yankauer suckers and suction catheters.
- Magill forceps.

Equipment for difficult intubation
- Small endotracheal tubes (size 5–6).
- Special laryngoscopes (McCoy, short-handled, polio blade).
- LMAs (sizes 3, 4, 5) (intubating LMA if available).
- Airway exchange catheters.
- Intubating fibreoptic scope.
- Berman airways.
- Emergency cricothyroidotomy kits:
  - Needle cricothyroidotomy set
  - Surgical cricothyroidotomy equipment
- Jet ventilator.

Recognizing misplaced endotracheal tube

Oesophageal intubation
- Vocal cords not visualized.
- No air-entry into either side of chest.
- No chest movement.
- No misting of ETT.
- 'Gurgling' on epigastric auscultation.
- CO_2 trace on capnograph absent or only lasts for 1–2 breaths.

Bronchial intubation
- Unilateral air entry (listen with stethoscope in both axillae).
- Hypoxia (may be gradual onset).
- High airway pressures.
- Position of ETT at lips too far (*average* position at the lips for females = 20–22 cm, for males = 22–24 cm).

Auscultation may be unreliable, particularly in the obese.

Further reading

Cook TM, et al. Fourth National Audit Project. Major complications of airway management in the UK: results of the Fourth National Audit Project of the Royal College of Anaesthetists and the Difficult Airway Society. Part 2: intensive care and emergency departments. Br J Anaesth 2011; **106**: 632–42.

⊙: Failed intubation, increasing hypoxia, and difficult ventilation in the paralysed anaesthetized patient: rescue techniques for the 'can't intubate, can't ventilate' situation

See Fig. 2.3.

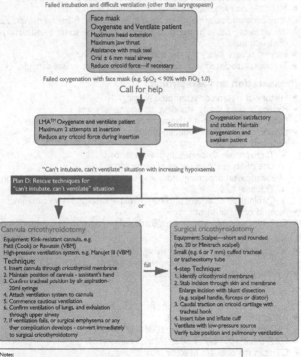

Failed intubation, increasing hypoxaemia and difficult ventilation in the paralysed anaesthetised patient: Rescue techniques for the "can't intubate, can't ventilate" situation

Failed intubation and difficult ventilation (other than laryngospasm)

Face mask
Oxygenate and Ventilate patient
Maximum head extension
Maximum jaw thrust
Assistance with mask seal
Oral ± 6 mm nasal airway
Reduce cricoid force—if necessary

Failed oxygenation with face mask (e.g. SpO₂ < 90% with FiO₂ 1.0)

Call for help

LMA™ Oxygenate and ventilate patient
Maximum 2 attempts at insertion
Reduce any cricoid force during insertion

Succeed → Oxygenation satisfactory and stable: Maintain oxygenation and awaken patient

"Can't intubate, can't ventilate" situation with increasing hypoxaemia

Plan D: Rescue techniques for "can't intubate, can't ventilate" situation

or

Cannula cricothyroidotomy
Equipment: Kink-resistant cannula, e.g. Patil (Cook) or Ravussin (VBM)
High-pressure ventilation system, e.g. Manujet III (VBM)
Technique:
1. Insert cannula through cricothyroid membrane
2. Maintain position of cannula - assistant's hand
3. Confirm tracheal position by air aspiration—20ml syringe
4. Attach ventilation system to cannula
5. Commence cautious ventilation
6. Confirm ventilation of lungs, and exhalation through upper airway
7. If ventilation fails, or surgical emphysema or any other complication develops - convert immediately to surgical cricothyroidotomy

fail →

Surgical cricothyroidotomy
Equipment: Scalpel—short and rounded (no. 20 or Minitrach scalpel)
Small (e.g. 6 or 7 mm) cuffed tracheal or tracheostomy tube
4-step Technique:
1. Identify cricothyroid membrane
2. Stab incision through skin and membrane Enlarge incision with blunt dissection (e.g. scalpel handle, forceps or dilator)
3. Caudal traction on cricoid cartilage with tracheal hook
4. Insert tube and inflate cuff
Ventilate with low-pressure source
Verify tube position and pulmonary ventilation

Notes:
1. These techniques can have serious complications—use only in life-threatening situations
2. Convert to definitive airway as soon as possible
3. Postoperative management—see other difficult airway guidelines and flow-charts
4. 4mm cannula with low-pressure ventilation may be successful in patient breathing spontaneously

Difficult Airway Society guidelines Flow-chart 2004 (use with DAS guidelines paper)

Fig. 2.3 Difficult Airway Society guidelines flowchart, 2004. Reproduced from the Difficult Airway Society guidelines 2004, with permission.

⚙ Airway/facial trauma

Trauma to the face and neck can directly damage airway structures or compress the airway as a result of swelling/haematoma formation; or it may cause airway obstruction because of blood, bone, or tooth debris.

Causes
• Blunt force trauma: commonly car crash or assault or hanging.
• Penetrating trauma: commonly stabbing or shooting.

Airway and facial trauma are associated with severe head and C-spine injury and/or intoxication. Injuries include:
• Midface: LeFort fractures, associated with base-of-skull fractures (these can collapse soft palate against pharynx and obstruct the airway).
• Mandible or zygoma: both may occasionally disrupt the temporomandibular joint limiting mouth opening. Bilateral mandibular fractures can cause posterior displacement of the tongue and airway obstruction.
• Larynx: severe injury rapidly leads to asphyxiation.
• Trachea: associated with severe thoracic or great vessel damage.

Presentation and assessment
• History of trauma or attempted hanging.
• Patient prefers sitting, standing, or leaning forward.
• Facial disruption, airway haemorrhage, spitting blood, epistaxis.
• Dental malocclusion, reduced mouth opening.
• Respiratory distress:
  • Tachypnoea, dyspnoea, hypoxia, cyanosis
  • Use of accessory muscles of respiration
  • Paradoxical breathing: indrawing chest and suprasternal recession
  • Tracheal tug
  • Diminished or absent air entry, minimal respiratory excursions
• Altered consciousness.
• CSF rhinorrhoea, racoon eyes, Battle's sign, haemotympanum.

Laryngeal/tracheal trauma:
• Surgical emphysema, neck swelling, bruising, or palpable fracture.
• Inability to speak or vocal changes (muffled or hoarse voice).
• Stridor (inspiratory noise accompanying breathing) or noisy breathing.

Investigations
Diagnosis is clinical; investigations may have to wait until airway is secure
• ABGs (hypoxia, hypercapnia).
• FBC, crossmatch, coagulation, U&Es, LFTs.
• CXR/trauma X-rays (if other injuries suspected).
• CT scan (to evaluate head or facial injuries).
• Fibreoptic laryngoscopy (vocal cord paralysis, mucosal/cartilage disruption, haematoma, laceration).

Differential diagnoses
• Epistaxis.
• Tension pneumothorax.

Immediate management

- 100% O_2, pulse oximetry.
- Assess degree of airway disruption, obstruction, bleeding.
- Assume C-spine injury and apply collar.
- If patient is in extremis or injury is severe:
  - Call for senior help (anaesthetic and maxillofacial/ENT)
  - Assist ventilation via bag and mask if required (oropharyngeal airways may be needed but could provoke bleeding)
  - Avoid nasal airways/intubation if possible in facial injuries because of the possible risk of disrupting the dura in base-of-skull fractures
  - Anterior traction on mobile segment (midface fracture, mandible or tongue) may relieve obstruction
  - Total obstruction requires immediate laryngoscopy/intubation (use uncut ETTs in case of later facial swelling)
  - Two suction devices may be needed if bleeding is rapid
  - Surgical airway (i.e. cricothyroidotomy or tracheostomy) is indicated for total obstruction if these listed points fail
- If difficult intubation is likely, prepare equipment for inhalational induction (anaesthetic machine with anaesthetic gas: sevoflurane or halothane); and prepare difficult airway equipment (see 📖 p.26):
  - Emergency surgical tracheostomy by a skilled surgeon is indicated in the event of a 'failed intubation', or as the first-line technique
- To stem bleeding in the case of torrential haemorrhage:
  - Anterior nasopharyngeal packs or Foley catheters into the posterior nasopharynx may help
  - Consider external carotid ligation, or angiographic embolization
- If laryngeal/tracheal disruption is likely:
  - Fibreoptic laryngoscopy may help in determining degree of injury
  - Avoid blind intubation as it may create a false passage
  - Avoid cricoid pressure as it may cause laryngo-tracheal separation
  - Allow spontaneous ventilation until tube tip is distal to the injury
  - Tracheostomy under local anaesthesia with C-spine control is the definitive airway of choice.

Once **A**irway and **B**reathing are stabilized, continue **ABC** approach.

Further management

- Complete 2° surveys and trauma screen: X-rays.
- Assess and treat other traumatic injuries.
- Consider ventilation/sedation on ICU until inflammation has resolved.
- Consider antibiotics and check tetanus status.
- Delay extubation until after any surgical repairs, and assess airway swelling (laryngoscopy and/or cuff-leak test) prior to extubation.

Pitfalls/difficult situations

- Associated head, chest, and C-spine injuries are common; perform a tertiary survey.

Further reading

Curran JE. Anaesthesia for facial trauma. *Anaesth Intens Care Med* 2005; **6**: 258–62.

☼ Airway/facial burns

(See also 📖 pp.68 and 416.)

Airway burns can rapidly cause airway obstruction within hours. Corrosive/toxic gases may also cause impaired gas exchange and oxygenation.

Causes

- Direct contact thermal burns to the face or airway:
  - Airway fires (rare outside operating theatres)
  - Self-immolation
  - Trapped/unconscious near a heat source
- Inhalation of hot or corrosive gas:
  - Entrapment near a burning substance (house fire, car fire)
  - 'Flashbacks' of hot gases (foundry accidents, aerosol can fires)
- Inhalation of steam or drinking hot fluids:
  - Drinking corrosive fluids (e.g. bleach)

Airway and facial burns are associated with alcoholism, chronic ill health, psychiatric illness, trauma, and extremes of age.

Presentation and assessment

The following features indicate a high risk of airway oedema leading to obstruction:

- On examining the face:
  - Facial oedema is already present
  - Marked facial burns are present (blistering, peeling skin)
- On examining the inside of the mouth and nose:
  - Airway oedema or blistering/peeling of mucosal membranes is present, or soot is present in the oropharynx
- On examining the neck:
  - Circumferential or marked anterior neck burns are present
  - Laryngeal structures are no longer palpable
- Difficulty swallowing, drooling.
- Carbonaceous sputum.
- Inability to speak or vocal changes (muffled or hoarse voice).
- Inspiratory stridor or noisy breathing.
- Respiratory distress:
  - Tachypnoea, dyspnoea, wheeze, cough
  - Use of accessory muscles of respiration, tracheal tug
  - Paradoxical breathing
  - Patient prefers sitting, standing, or leaning forward

Investigations

Diagnosis is clinical; investigations may have to wait until airway is secure:

- ABGs (hypoxia, metabolic acidosis).
- Lactate (may be ↑).
- Carboxyhaemoglobin using co-oximetry (COHb may be ↑).
- FBC, crossmatch, U&Es.
- CXR (if aspiration or ALI is suspected).
- C-spine and trauma-series X-rays (if appropriate).

Immediate management

- 100% O_2, pulse oximetry.
- Assess degree of burn and airway obstruction.
- If associated trauma simultaneously assess C-spine and other injuries.
- If patient already has evidence of airway obstruction:
    - Call for senior help (anaesthetic and ENT)
    - Consider nebulized adrenaline (5 mg/5 ml 1:1000 in a nebulizer)
    - Consider nasal endoscopy to assess degree of airway oedema
    - Prepare equipment for rapid sequence intubation or inhalational induction (anaesthetic machine with anaesthetic gas: sevoflurane)
    - Prepare difficult airway equipment (see 📖 p.26)
    - Laryngoscopy/intubation will be required (use uncut ETTs in case of later facial swelling)
    - Cricothyroidotomy or emergency tracheostomy is indicated in the event of failed intubation, or as the first-line technique

If patient is at risk of airway obstruction early intubation should be performed using an uncut ETT. Once **A**irway and **B**reathing are stabilized, continue **ABC** approach:
- Follow trauma/ATLS principles (📖 p.404).
- Assess any associated chest and lung burns (📖 pp.68 and 416):
    - Urgent management of circumferential burns (especially neck and chest) may be required
    - Raised COHb levels require an FiO_2 of 100% initially (📖 p.476)
    - Fluid resuscitate using a burns protocol

Further management

- Assess and treat other traumatic injuries.
- If intubated, consider ventilation and sedation on ICU for a number of days until airway inflammation has resolved; assess airway swelling (by laryngoscopy and/or cuff-leak test) before extubation.
- Consider transfer to burns unit (see 📖 p.419), anaesthetic assessment of airway risk may be required in unintubated patients.
- Treat inhalational injury (📖 p.68).
- Consider giving antibiotics and check tetanus status.

Pitfalls/difficult situations

- If in doubt intubate, as delay may make a difficult intubation impossible.
- Complete airway obstruction can occur in only a few hours.
- Hoarse voice is an early sign of laryngeal oedema.
- Trauma including chest, head and neck injuries are common.
- Using suxamethonium >48 hours after burn may cause hyperkalaemia.

Further reading

Cancio LC. Current concepts in the pathophysiology and treatment of inhalation injury. *Trauma* 2005; **7**: 19–35.
Hettiaratchy S, et al. Initial management of a major burn: I overview. *Br Med J* 2004; **328**: 1555–7.
Hilton PJ, et al. The immediate care of the burned patient. *BJA CEPD Rev* 2001; **1**(4): 113–16.

:☼: Airway infections

(See also 📖 p.332.)

Airway infections are associated with inflammation, extrinsic or intrinsic to the upper airway, which may cause obstruction (partial or complete). Complications include abscess rupture and airway soiling.

Causes

Extrinsic

- Pharyngeal, retropharyngeal, or peri-tonsillar abscess.
- Ludwig's angina (soft tissue infection of the floor of the mouth).
- Deep-neck infections.

Can be caused by streptococci or staphylococci, but may be polymicrobial and include anaerobic or Gram-negative organisms.

Intrinsic

- Diphtheria: airway inflammation and a greyish pseudo-membrane in the respiratory tract (caused by *Corynebacterium diphtheriae*).
- Epiglottitis: inflammation of epiglottis, vallecula, aryepiglottic folds, and arytenoids (commonly *Haemophilus* spp., but also *Streptococcus pneumoniae* and *Staphylococcus aureus*).

Risk factors for airway infections include:

- Poor dental hygiene.
- Recent sore throat, tonsillitis, pharyngitis, URTI.
- Recent oral/pharyngeal surgery/trauma.

Presentation and assessment

Depending on cause, may include:

- Tachypnoea, dyspnoea, hypoxia and cyanosis.
- Stridor.
- 'Hunched' posture; sitting forward, mouth open, tongue protruding.
- 'Muffled' or hoarse voice, painful swallowing, drooling.
- Neck swelling, cervical lymphadenopathy.
- Trismus, neck pain, neck stiffness.
- Fever and signs of systemic sepsis (see 📖 p.322)
- Diphtheria exotoxin may cause CNS symptoms or cardiac failure.
- Infection may spread causing: pneumonia, mediastinitis, pericarditis.

Investigations

- FBC (raised WCC).
- Blood cultures and throat swabs.[1]
- Laryngoscopy (indirect/fibreoptic) performed by a skilled operator.[1]
- CXR (if mediastinal/chest involvement suspected).
- Lateral soft tissue neck X-ray may demonstrate soft tissue swelling and 'thumb sign' and 'vallecula' signs in epiglottitis.
- CT or MRI of head and neck.

Differential diagnoses

- Airway foreign body or tumour.

---

1 Airway interventions in a patient with a partially obstructed airway can provoke complete airway obstruction.

Immediate management
- Humidified 100% O_2, pulse oximetry.
- Rapid assessment (note that manipulating airway or adjusting patient position may completely obstruct airway, particularly in children).

If patient is in extremis or obstruction is severe:
- Call for senior help (anaesthetic and ENT).
- Elective intubation is required, prior to complete airway obstruction.
- Prepare difficult airway equipment (see 📖 p.26) and equipment for inhalational induction (anaesthetic machine with sevoflurane).
- Consider transferring patient to an operating theatre or critical care area where required equipment is present, if this is quicker.
- Emergency surgical tracheostomy by a skilled surgeon is indicated in the event of a 'failed intubation', or as the first-line technique.
- If there is a need to 'buy' time waiting for senior help consider:
  - Heliox or nebulized adrenaline (5 mg/5 ml 1:1000 in a nebulizer).

In more stable patients:
- Transfer to critical care environment for close observation.
- The risk of airway obstruction may still mandate early intubation.

Once **A**irway and **B**reathing are stabilized, continue **ABC** approach:
- Take blood cultures and pharyngeal/epiglottic swabs.
- Obtain IV access and consider steroids (dexamethasone 8 mg IV).
- Empirical antibiotics will depend upon the type of infection (seek microbiological advice), but may include:
  - Epiglottitis: cefotaxime 1–2g IV 12-hourly
  - Deep-seated neck infections: clindamycin 600 mg IV 6-hourly, benzyl penicillin 600 mg IV 6-hourly, metronidazole 500 mg IV 8-hourly
  - For diphtheria: clarithromycin 500 mg IV 12-hourly, and possibly antitoxin (if strain is toxin producing)

For those patients in extremis, blood cultures and epiglottic swabs should not be obtained until airway is secured.

Further management
- Ventilation and sedation may be required for a number of days until inflammation has resolved .
- Surgical drainage of abscesses and collections may be required.
- Supportive measures on the ICU for septic patients (see 📖 p.322).
- Assess airway swelling (laryngoscopy/cuff-leak test) before extubation.

Pitfalls/difficult situations
- Delaying intubation may make a difficult intubation impossible.
- Failure to appreciate how rapidly these conditions can progress, normal to complete airway obstruction in only a few hours.

Further reading
Ames WA, et al. Adult epiglottitis: an under-recognized, life-threatening condition. *Br J Anaesth* 2000; **85**: 795–7.
Ng HL, et al. Acute epiglottitis in adults: a retrospective review of 106 patients in Hong Kong. *Emerg Med J* 2008; **25**: 253–5.

⚙ Airway foreign bodies

The most common foreign bodies are food boluses (including sweets and nuts), dentures, toys (in children), chewed items (e.g. pen tops), blood clots, and vomit. In adults objects are commonly lodged in the right main bronchus. In children, either bronchus may be obstructed. Larger objects may be lodged at the larynx or trachea.

Causes

Foreign bodies are commonly associated with:
- ↓consciousness: alcohol, overdose, CVA, head injury.
- Dementia.
- Children.

Presentation and assessment

- May be witnessed.
- May present as a cardiac arrest (see 📖 p.98).
- May present as sudden total or near-total airway obstruction where bag and mask ventilation is impossible.

Total or near-total obstruction
- Anxiety.
- Patient prefers sitting, standing, or leaning forward.
- Inability to speak, lump in throat, difficulty in swallowing.
- Stridor (inspiratory noise accompanying breathing) or noisy breathing.
- Choking, coughing, or drooling.
- Respiratory distress:
  - Tachypnoea and dyspnoea
  - Use of accessory muscles of respiration
  - Paradoxical breathing: indrawing chest and suprasternal recession
  - Unilateral, diminished or absent air entry
- Altered consciousness, hypoxia, cyanosis, bradycardia, and hypotension are pre-terminal signs.

Late presentation
- Classic triad: unilateral monophonic wheeze, cough, unilateral reduced breath sounds.
- Lobar pneumonia, abscess, or atelectasis unresponsive to treatment.

Investigations

- CXR, inspiratory/expiratory films (atelectasis on inspiration, hyperinflation on expiration).
- Neck X-ray, AP & lateral (although foreign bodies may be radiolucent).
- Fibreoptic endoscopy or direct laryngoscopy will aid diagnosis and allow interventions to restore airway patency (ENT or anaesthetic experience required).
- Consider chest CT (if the patient is stable enough).

Differential diagnoses

- Bronchospasm.
- Pneumonia.

Immediate management
- If patient is choking follow choking algorithm (Fig. 2.4), otherwise:
- 100% O_2, pulse oximetry.

If patient has suffered cardiac arrest follow BLS guidelines (p.98); remove obvious obstruction and commence CPR.
  If patient is in extremis or obstruction is severe:
- Call for senior help (anaesthetic and ENT).
- Prepare difficult airway equipment (see p.26) and equipment for inhalational induction (anaesthetic machine with sevoflurane).
- Consider transferring patient to an operating theatre or critical care area where required equipment is present, if this is quicker.
- Elective intubation may be needed before total airway obstruction:
  - Maintain spontaneous ventilation throughout anaesthesia
- Foreign body may be removed at laryngoscopy/rigid bronchoscopy.
- Surgical tracheostomy is indicated in the event of failed intubation.

In stable patients awake flexible bronchoscopy may be possible.

Once Airway and Breathing are stabilized, continue ABC approach
- Consider transfer to critical care environment for close observation.

Further management
- Consider antibiotics and dexamethasone.

Pitfalls/difficult situations
- There may be more than one foreign body.
- Rule out pneumothorax/pneumomediastinum.
- Airway oedema and bleeding can occur after removal of object.

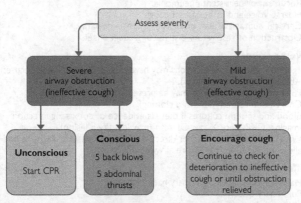

Fig. 2.4 Adult choking algorithm. UK Resuscitation Council guidelines 2010. Reproduced with kind permission from the Resuscitation Council (UK).

☠ Airway haemorrhage

Airway haemorrhage is an emergency that can cause airway obstruction, deterioration in gas exchange (due to flooding of alveoli with blood), or circulatory collapse.

Causes

- Following airway surgery or interventions (e.g. tonsillectomy).
- Following upper airway interventions, especially tracheostomy.
- Upper airway infection.
- Airway or neck trauma.
- Airway or neck tumours:
  - Smoker or previous history of cancer
- Coagulopathic or anticoagulated patients.
- Epistaxis may occasionally be so severe as to compromise the airway.

Presentation and assessment

- Anxiety.
- Haemoptysis, epistaxis, or spitting blood.
- Airway obstruction: stridor (inspiratory noise accompanying breathing), use of accessory muscles, paradoxical breathing.
- Alveolar soiling: cough, widespread crepitations, diminished air entry.
- Respiratory distress:
  - Tachypnoea and dyspnoea
  - Respiratory accessory muscle usage, diminished/absent air entry
  - Paradoxical breathing: indrawing chest and suprasternal recession
- Altered consciousness, hypoxia, cyanosis, and bradycardia, are pre-terminal signs.
- Signs of blood loss: pallor, tachycardia.

Where tumour is the cause, the following may also be present:
- Recurrent or persistent pneumonia.
- Hoarse voice and/or persistent cough.
- Cervical, supraclavicular, or axillary lymphadenopathy.
- Obstruction or respiratory distress of gradual onset.

Investigations

Diagnosis is clinical; investigations may have to wait until airway is secure:
- ABGs (hypoxia, hypercapnia).
- FBC, crossmatch (anaemia may be present).
- Coagulation screen (deranged clotting).
- Blood and sputum cultures if there is evidence of coexisting infection.
- Imaging: CXR, neck X-ray, CT scan (may identify a lesion).
- When possible endoscopy or direct laryngoscopy will aid diagnosis and allow interventions to restore airway patency.

Differential diagnoses

- Haemoptysis due to pulmonary haemorrhage.
- Pulmonary oedema.
- Upper airway infection.
- Foreign body.

Immediate management

- 100% O_2, pulse oximetry.
- For trauma patients: simultaneously assess C-spine and other associated trauma.
- Assess the degree of bleeding and extent of lung soiling, if severe:
  - Call for senior help (anaesthetic and surgical/ENT)
  - The first priority is to secure patency of airway
  - Airway obstruction will require immediate laryngoscopy, suctioning of the upper airway, and tracheal intubation
  - Two suction devices may be needed if bleeding is rapid
  - The aim should be to place the cuff of an ETT beyond the site of haemorrhage or insert a double lumen tube (DLT) if haemorrhage is pulmonary and unilateral in origin
  - Surgical airway (cricothyroidotomy or tracheostomy) may be needed if intubation fails
  - Surgical control of bleeding should then be attempted
  - Urgent fibreoptic bronchoscopy may be required to remove clots from lower airways
- Where bleeding is not severe, airway obstruction may still be a risk, especially if airway tumour is present.
  - Make as full an assessment as possible as detailed earlier in this list (and 📖 p.18); including CT scanning if the clinical situation allows
  - Airway manipulation may provoke complete obstruction

Once **A**irway and **B**reathing are stabilized, continue **ABC** approach:
- Establish IV access and restore circulatory volume with fluid/colloid.
- Blood and blood product transfusion may be required.

Further management

- Correct any coagulopathy that may be present.
- Fibreoptic laryngoscopy or bronchoscopy to assess the source of haemorrhage.
- Assessment by ENT surgeon and/or thoracic surgeon for more definitive management of bleeding.
- Sedate and ventilate in intensive care until haemorrhage is controlled or if oxygenation is poor despite a patent airway.
- Circulatory support including inotropes may be required.
- Antibiotics for prophylaxis or treatment of concurrent infection may be required.

Pitfalls/difficult situations

- Deterioration may be rapid.
- Don't use sedatives unless airway is secure.
- In extensive lung soiling, hypoxia may not be relieved by securing airway and ventilation; also watch for development of pneumonia or ARDS.

Further reading

Mason RA, et al. The obstructed airway in head and neck surgery. *Anaesthesia* 1999; **54**: 625–8.

:⚙: Endotracheal tube complications

Indications for intubation can be found on 📖 p.12; a description of how to perform rapid sequence intubations can be found on 📖 p.522; and what to do if unable to pass an ETT at the time of intubation (the failed intubation drill) can be found on 📖 p.27.

Other ETT complications include:
- Tube obstruction (malposition, cuff herniation, mucous plugging).
- Cuff leak.
- Aspiration of gastric contents.
- Accidental extubation.
- Laryngeal damage or tracheal ulceration.

Causes

Complications are more likely if:
- Patients are agitated, very mobile, or have abnormal anatomy.
- During transfer.
- There are large amounts of airway secretions.
- Aspiration is more likely where patients have:
  - Been intubated as an emergency, or by inexperienced operator
  - Had a full stomach at time of intubation, or intubation was delayed in a patient at risk of aspiration

Presentation and assessment

- Occluded, semi-occluded, or malpositioned ETT:
  - Hypoxia, cyanosis, diminished or unilateral air-entry
  - Difficulty ventilating with high airway pressures
  - Loss of capnograph trace
  - ETT position at lips has changed
- Cuff leak, audible leak on inspiration if ventilated:
  - Ventilator may alarm indicating a leak, low airway pressure, or low expiratory volumes
- Airway soiling with gastric contents:
  - Widespread crepitations, wheeze, or high airway pressures
  - Hypoxia
  - Gastric contents suctioned from airway

Investigations

Diagnosis is clinical; investigations may have to wait until airway is secure:
- ABGs (hypoxia, hypercapnia).
- Fibreoptic endoscopy (may reveal malpositioning, or airway soiling with gastric contents).
- CXR: to check ETT position (above carina).

Differential diagnoses

- Bronchospasm.
- Pneumothorax.
- Pneumonia.

Immediate management
(See Fig. 2.5 for ETT displacement algorithm.)
- 100% O_2, pulse oximetry.
- Assess degree of airway obstruction.
- Call for anaesthetic help.
- Check ETT position (*average* position at the lips for females is 20–22 cm, and 22–24 cm for males, but this varies with patient size):
  - If too far try withdrawing tube slowly, preferably under direct vision using a laryngoscope to avoid accidental extubation
- Try manually ventilating with Water's circuit, check ventilator tubing and connections.
- Pass suction catheter via ETT (removes secretions and checks patency of lumen).
- If patient is in extremis or obstruction is severe:
  - Try deflating cuff, if it has herniated the obstruction should relieve quickly
  - If this fails, consider laryngoscopy to check tube position (cuff should be just below cords)
- Consider removing ETT and re-intubating, this will require:
  - Increasing/commencing sedation
  - Muscle relaxants (suxamethonium, atracurium)
  - Suction immediately available
  - Consider changing ETT over bougie or airway exchange catheter
- In the event of accidental extubation:
  - Assist ventilation via bag and mask with airway adjuncts (oropharyngeal/nasal airways) if required
  - Consider re-intubation (sometimes not required as patient may achieve adequate ventilation breathing spontaneously without support or with non-invasive ventilation)
- In there is a cuff leak try further inflating cuff, if this fails or gradually deflates consider electively changing tracheal tube if patient stable.

If ever in doubt, oxygenate by any means possible, this may mean removing ETT and inserting an LMA or using bag and mask ventilation until help arrives.

Once **A**irway and **B**reathing are stabilized, continue **ABC** approach:
- Check to ensure adequate ventilation, if poor consider the possibility of a pneumothorax.
- In the event of airway soiling pass suction catheter.

Further management
- Continue ventilation in an ICU setting.
- If the patient has airway soiling:
  - Send tracheal aspirate samples to microbiology
  - Consider bronchodilators, chest physiotherapy, and regular suction

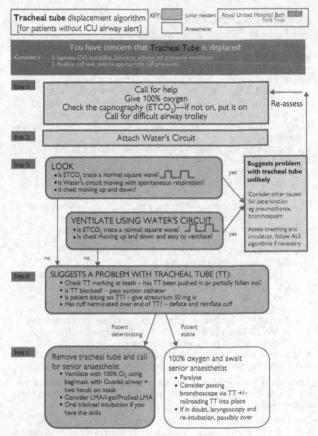

Fig. 2.5 ICU endotracheal tube displacement algorithm. Adapted from the reports and findings of the 4th National Audit Project of The Royal College of Anaesthetists 2011. Reproduced here with the permission of the Royal College of Anaesthetists.

Further reading

Cook TM, et al. Fourth National Audit Project. Major complications of airway management in the UK: results of the Fourth National Audit Project of the Royal College of Anaesthetists and the Difficult Airway Society. Part 2: intensive care and emergency departments. *Br J Anaesth* 2011; **106**: 632–42.

Tracheostomy complications

:☼: Tracheostomy complications

Complications can arise on first or on subsequent insertion of tracheostomy tubes, and can include:
- Aspiration of gastric contents.
- Bleeding.
- Surgical emphysema, pneumothorax, air embolism.
- Malpositioning (including para-tracheal tracheostomy placement)
- Infection.
- Tracheostomy occlusion (malposition, cuff herniation, mucous plug).
- Cuff leak, or accidental decannulation (removal).
- Mucosal erosion with tracheo-oesophageal fistula formation.

Causes

Complications are more likely if:
- The tracheostomy is performed as emergency procedure, or by inexperienced operator.
- The tracheostomy is performed in a patient who has:
  - A full stomach
  - Severe chest problems (FiO_2 >60% and/or PEEP >10 cmH_2O)
  - Coagulation abnormalities or platelet dysfunction
  - Large amounts of airway secretions
- Patients have abnormal anatomy, or are very mobile/agitated.

Presentation and assessment

- Occluded/semi-occluded airway:
  - Agitation
  - Hypoxia and cyanosis
  - Diminished air entry
  - Difficulty ventilating with high airway pressures
  - Loss of capnograph trace
- Malpositioning:
  - Difficulty ventilating with ↑airway pressures
  - Rapidly developing respiratory insufficiency and hypoxia
  - Pneumothorax, pneumomediastinum or subcutaneous emphysema
  - Loss of capnograph trace
- Airway soiling with gastric contents:
  - Widespread crepitations, wheeze or high airway pressures
  - Hypoxia
- Bleeding:
  - Obvious blood loss from or around tracheostomy
  - Presence of blood in airway
  - ↑airway pressure
  - Hypoxia
- Cuff leak:
  - Audible leak on inspiration if ventilated
  - Ventilator may alarm indicating a leak, low airway pressure, or low expiratory volumes
  - Able to talk past cuffed tube
- Infection: cellulitis, skin erosion, or frank pus.

Investigations
Diagnosis is clinical; investigations may have to wait until airway is secure
- ABGs (hypoxia, hypercapnia).
- FBC, coagulation studies (coagulopathy).
- Fibreoptic endoscopy (may reveal malpositioning, or airway soiling with blood or gastric contents).
- CXR (to check tracheostomy position, to exclude pneumothorax) (above carina).

Differential diagnoses
- Bronchospasm.
- Pneumothorax.

Immediate management
(See Fig. 2.6 for ICU tracheostomy tube displacement algorithm)
- 100% O_2, pulse oximetry, capnography.
- Apply O_2 to face *and* tracheostomy tube.
- Call for anaesthetic help and prepare difficult airway equipment (see ▢ p.26).
- Check tracheostomy position, attach Water's circuit:
  - Is Water's circuit and chest moving normally with respiration?
  - If yes: check ventilator tubing and connection
  - If *no*: hand ventilate cautiously; if no capnograph trace and difficult to bag consider malposition
  - Remove inner tube
  - Pass suction catheter to remove secretions and assess patency
  - Deflate cuff, if it has herniated the obstruction should relieve quickly

If patient is in extremis or obstruction is severe:
- Try deflating cuff.
- If this fails, *stop* ventilating through tracheostomy tube.
- Remove tracheostomy and apply occlusive dressing to neck.
- Ventilate using:
  - Bag and mask ventilation with adjuncts
  - Or insert LMA
  - Or re-intubate

In the event of accidental decannulation:
- Call for anaesthetic help.
- Attempt ventilation via a bag and mask using airway adjuncts (oropharyngeal/nasal airways) if required.
- If the tracheostomy was sited for upper respiratory tract obstruction attempt to resite the tracheostomy as soon as possible:
  - Some tracheostomy stomas if >7 days old will remain patent and ventilation may be assisted via the stoma
  - If tracheostomy >7 days old attempt to resite the tracheostomy as soon as possible
  - Use fibreoptic bronchoscope ± airway exchange catheter to re-insert tracheostomy under direct vision
  - If this is not possible consider endotracheal intubation

In the event of airway bleeding:
- Call for skilled help—senior anaesthetist and ENT.
- Assess degree of bleeding and extent of lung soiling.
- Fibreoptic laryngoscopy or bronchoscopy to assess the source of haemorrhage.
- If minor bleeding from tracheostomy site:
  - Apply direct pressure ± suture to obvious bleeding point. If still bleeding consider soaking a haemostatic dressing (e.g. Kaltostat®) in 1 in 80,000 adrenaline and pack bleeding site
- If major stoma bleeding:
  - Suction upper airway and tracheostomy to remove clots
  - Orally intubate, use uncut tube and ensure cuff is inflated below tracheostomy stoma
  - Achieve haemostasis of stoma using digital pressure, packing, or sutures
  - Arrange theatre for definitive haemostasis
  - Urgent endoscopy may be required to remove clots from airway and lungs
- If major bleeding occurs late it may be due to erosion of right brachiocephalic artery (usually preceded by insignificant sentinel bleed):
  - Bleeding can by massive and life threatening
  - 100% oxygen, call for senior help
  - Suction airway
  - Inflate tracheostomy cuff with up to 50 ml air to provide local tamponade
  - Apply digital pressure to root of neck in sternal notch
  - Commence IV fluid resuscitation, cross-match blood
  - Arrange an emergency theatre team, may also require vascular and cardiothoracic surgeons

If ever in doubt, secure airway using endotracheal intubation. Once **A**irway and **B**reathing are stabilized, continue **ABC** approach:
- Check to ensure adequate ventilation, if poor consider the possibility of pneumothorax.
- Urgent endoscopy may be required to remove clots from airway and lungs.
- Fluid/colloid/blood to restore circulatory volume.
- Correct any coagulopathy if there is airway bleeding.

Further management

If condition is stable and any severe airway obstruction has been relieved:
- Continue ventilation in an ICU setting.
- If obstruction only mild or after the airway is re-established using ETT:
  - Re-explore tracheostomy wound and re-insert tube, this can be difficult, particularly via recent (<7 days) percutaneous tracheostomy wounds, senior anaesthetic or ENT help may be required
  - Resiting over an endoscope may help to ensure correct positioning

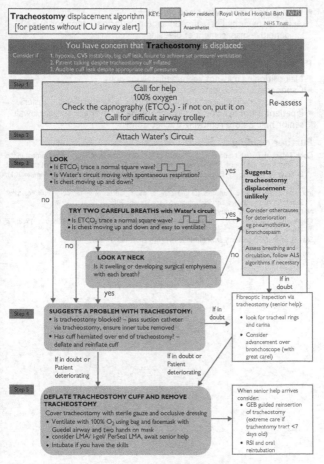

Fig. 2.6 ICU tracheostomy tube displacement algorithm. Adapted from the reports and findings of the 4th National Audit Project of The Royal College of Anaesthetists 2011. Reproduced here with the permission of the Royal College of Anaesthetists.

- If the patient has airway soiling or cellulitis:
  - Send wound or tracheal aspirate samples to microbiology
  - Use appropriate antibiotics
  - Consider bronchodilators, chest physiotherapy, and regular suction

- If the patient has airway bleeding:
  - Assessment by ENT surgeon and/or thoracic surgeon for more definitive management of bleeding
  - Circulatory support including inotropes may be required

Pitfalls/difficult situations

- Malpositioning may not be immediately obvious.
- Capnography is mandatory.
- Tracheostomy displacement often occurs during turns and transfers.
- If patient is not hypoxic, or has undergone recent neck surgery, await senior help before removing tracheostomy.

Further reading

Cook TM, et al. Fourth National Audit Project. Major complications of airway management in the UK: results of the Fourth National Audit Project of the Royal College of Anaesthetists and the Difficult Airway Society. Part 2: intensive care and emergency departments. *Br J Anaesth* 2011; **106**: 632–42.

Intensive Care Society. *Standards for the care of adult patients with temporary tracheostomy. Standards and guidelines.* London: Intensive Care Society, 2008.

National Tracheostomy Safety Project website: ⅋ <http://www.tracheostomy.org.uk>

Quigley RL. Tracheostomy, an overview. Management and complications. *Br J Clin Pract* 1988; **42**: 430–4.

Seay SJ, et al. Tracheostomy emergencies. *Am J Nurs* 2002; **102**: 59–63.

Chapter 3

Breathing

⚙️ Respiratory failure

Respiratory failure occurs when air transfer in and out of the lungs is reduced, or when gas exchange within the lungs fails (due to shunt, VQ mismatch, or poor gas diffusion), resulting in either:
• Type I respiratory failure—causing hypoxia.
• Type II respiratory failure—causing hypoxia and hypercapnia.

Type I respiratory failure typically has parenchymal causes. Type II respiratory failure occurs with mechanical/obstructive causes, or as a result of fatigue/↓consciousness alongside respiratory failure.

Definitions
• Hypoxia—PaO_2 <8 kPa or PaO_2 <11 kPa on FiO_2 ≥40%.
• Hypercapnia—$PaCO_2$ >6.3 kPa.

Blood gas values must be interpreted flexibly with regard to:
• Inspired oxygen concentration (FiO_2) required to avoid hypoxia.
• Respiratory distress in the presence of normal blood gases.
• Lack of symptoms of respiratory distress in patients with chronic lung conditions giving rise to abnormal blood gases.
• Intracardiac shunt.
• Pre-existing metabolic alkalosis leading to hypercapnia.

Causes
• Upper airway obstruction (see 📖 p.18).
• Lower airway obstruction:
  • Acute bronchoconstriction, asthma, anaphylaxis
  • COPD
  • Foreign body, mucous plugging, atelectasis
• Lung tissue damage/gas exchange failure:
  • Pneumonia
  • Lung contusion
  • ARDS
  • Pulmonary haemorrhage
  • Cardiogenic pulmonary oedema
  • Lung fibrosis
• Pulmonary circulatory compromise:
  • Pulmonary embolus
  • Pulmonary vascular disease
  • Heart failure
  • Excessively raised cardiac output
• Neuromuscular damage:
  • ↓level of consciousness (e.g. intracranial catastrophe or sedative agents)
  • Paralysis/weakness (e.g. spinal damage, tetanus, Guillain–Barré, myasthenia gravis)
• Mechanical compromise of lung tissue (e.g. pneumothorax, haemothorax, pleural effusion, flail chest, kyphoscoliosis, obesity or ascites).
• Inadequate mechanical ventilation.

Presentation and assessment

Respiratory failure may present with respiratory or cardiac arrest (📖 p.98).

Evidence of respiratory distress that may precede or accompany respiratory failure includes:
- Agitation, sense of impending doom.
- Sense of 'tight chest' or breathlessness in conscious patients.
- Inability to talk normally or in full sentences.
- Sweating, clamminess.
- Tachypnoea >25 breaths/minute.
- Dyspnoea, or laboured breathing, with use of accessory muscles.
- Gasping or 'pursed-lip' breathing.
- Sitting, or hunched posture.
- Cyanosis.
- Hypoxia, as evidenced by ABG or SpO_2 <92%.
- Hypercapnia: flapping tremor, warm peripheries and bounding pulse.
- Tachycardia (> 110 beats/minute).

Pre-terminal signs include:
- Bradycardia, arrhythmia, or hypotension.
- Silent chest on auscultation.
- Bradypnoea or exhaustion.
- Confusion or ↓level of consciousness.

In mechanically ventilated patients, evidence of respiratory failure may also be accompanied by:
- High, or low, ventilator pressure alarms.
- Low delivered tidal volume alarm, or low minute-volume alarm.
- Audible leak from ventilator circuit, or leak alarm.
- Inability to ventilate using self-inflating bag.
- Lack of chest movement.
- Lack of respiratory sounds on auscultation.

Other features associated with respiratory failure depend upon the cause, but may include:
- Cough.
- Pleuritic chest pain.
- Haemoptysis.
- Evidence of sepsis (pyrexia, rigors, purulent sputum).
- Reduced air-entry or altered percussion note associated with pneumothorax, consolidation, or effusion.
- Audible wheeze on external examination; or wheeze, rub, or bronchial breathing on auscultation.
- Reduced peak flow.
- Mediastinal deviation (tracheal deviation, altered apex).
- Raised JVP; evidence of cardiac failure (peripheral oedema, hepatic engorgement, cardiomegaly).

Investigations

In most cases clinical assessment will reveal evidence of respiratory distress. Investigations which may aid in assessing severity or establishing a diagnosis include:

- ABGs:
  - The PaO_2/FiO_2 ratio may be calculated to give a measure of the degree of respiratory failure (see 🕮 p.90)[1]
- FBC (↑ Hb in chronic hypoxia, ↓Hb in acute anaemia).
- U+Es (hyponatraemia in pneumonia, raised urea/creatinine in pneumonia, pulmonary-renal syndrome, heart failure).
- LFTs (deranged in heart failure, malignancy).
- Peak flow measurements, where appropriate (restrictive: lung fibrosis, obstructive: asthma, COPD).
- ECG (RV strain pattern in PE, severe lung disease).
- CXR (consolidation, collapse, alveolar/interstitial shadowing, pneumothorax).
- Chest ultrasound (pleural fluid, pneumothorax).

Further investigations may be required depending on cause or clinical progress:

- Coagulation studies (DIC in sepsis/trauma).
- CRP (↑ in sepsis/inflammation).
- D-dimers (↑ in PE, but of limited use in ICU as also ↑ by inflammation).
- Culture (blood, sputum).
- Atypical serology .
- Urine for legionella and pneumococcal antigen.
- Bronchoscopy or non-directed BAL (see 🕮 p.548).
- Echocardiogram (acute RV strain in PE; chronic RV strain in severe chronic lung disease; LV impairment in IHD).
- CT chest.
- CT pulmonary angiogram.

Differential diagnoses

Patients may appear to be in respiratory distress despite having adequately saturated arterial blood, in these cases it is important to consider:

- Anaemia (severe).
- Cytotoxic hypoxia (e.g. cyanide or carbon monoxide poisoning).
- Metabolic acidosis (with compensatory respiratory alkalosis: Kussmaul breathing).
- Hyperventilation, either hysterical or associated with disease (e.g. thyrotoxicosis or pain).

Also consider:

- Upper airway obstruction (see 🕮 p.18).
- Endotracheal tube/breathing system obstruction (see 🕮 pp.38 and 42).

---

1 Alternatively the alveolar arterial (A–a) O_2 gradient may be calculated: A–a difference = $(FiO_2 \times 94.8) - (PaCO_2 + PaO_2)$

Immediate management

If the patient is spontaneously breathing without ventilatory support:
- Ensure that the airway is patent (use adjuncts if necessary).
- Increase FiO_2 to maintain SpO_2 at 94–98% for most acutely ill patients, or 88–92% for those at risk of hypercapnic respiratory failure.
- Assist breathing with bag and mask if required.
- Consider escalating respiratory support in a stepwise progression (non-invasive CPAP or BIPAP may be indicated 🕮 p.53).
- Endotracheal intubation and mechanical ventilation may be required (see 🕮 pp.12 and 52).

If patient is already intubated and/or receiving ventilatory support (non-invasive or invasive) the following may be necessary:
- Increase FiO_2 to 100%.
- Check that the airway is patent; in intubated patients check the patency and position of the endotracheal or tracheostomy tube (check with a suction catheter if in doubt, see 🕮 pp.38 and 42).
- If already on a ventilator, ensure ventilation is possible; check equipment is working and not disconnected.
- If in doubt switch to self-inflating ambu-bag and manually ventilate.

Establish a probable diagnosis as soon as possible and treat as appropriate, especially any reversible causes such as: endobronchial intubation, pneumothorax, pulmonary oedema, secretions and mucous plugs, bronchospasm, and pleural effusions

Once **A**irway and **B**reathing are stabilized, continue **ABC** approach:
- Patients may require aggressive circulatory support.

Further management

- Titrate oxygen therapy and respiratory support to keep PaO_2 >8 kPa and $PaCO_2$ <6.3 kPa (and respiratory rate <30 breaths/minute if spontaneously breathing) where possible.
- If basic ventilatory support is not enough, consider additional manoeuvres for hypoxia (🕮 p.58) or hypercapnia (🕮 p.56).
- Consider invasive monitoring with serial ABG analysis.
- If mechanical ventilation is necessary, sedation (with or without muscle relaxation) will be required, at least initially (🕮 p.13).
- Follow a lung-protective ventilation strategy (🕮 p.53).

Pitfalls/difficult situations

- Double-check equipment as it may be faulty or not be delivering high enough O_2; switch to alternative equipment if in doubt.
- Cold limbs or poor skin perfusion may make SpO_2 readings unreliable or difficult to maintain.
- Chest X-ray interpretation can be difficult in supine patients; certain conditions such as anterior pneumothoraces or pleural effusions may require additional imaging (CT or US).
- The presence of a metabolic acidosis increases dyspnoea; do not ignore circulatory support and correction of acidosis.

Oxygen delivery devices

Devices which deliver variable concentrations (and *estimated* FiO_2):
- Nasal cannulae:[1]
  - At 2 L/minute O_2 flow: maximum $FiO_2 = 28\%$
  - At 4 L/minute O_2 flow: maximum $FiO_2 = 35\%$
  - At 6 L/minute O_2 flow: maximum $FiO_2 = 45\%$
- Non-Venturi masks (e.g. Hudson mask):
  - At 5 L/minute O_2 flow: maximum $FiO_2 = 35\%$
  - At 8 L/minute O_2 flow: maximum $FiO_2 = 55\%$
  - At 12 L/minute O_2 flow: maximum $FiO_2 = 65\%$
- Reservoir bag masks (non-rebreathing masks, trauma masks):
  - At 15 L/minute O_2 flow: maximum $FiO_2 = 80-90\%$

Devices which deliver fixed O_2 concentrations:
- All Venturi masks: 24–60% if O_2 flow rate is set according to instructions written on adapter (to change FiO_2, change adapter).
- Ventilator circuits: up to 100% O_2 as set.
- Oxylog portable ventilators:
  - Modern machines up to 100% O_2 as set
  - Older machines: if set to 'Airmix' 50–60%, if set to 'No airmix' 100%

[1] High-flow O_2 (at rates of >20 L/minute) can be delivered by some delivery devices which obtain near 100% humidification (e.g. Vapotherm™).

Indications for ventilatory support

Invasive ventilatory support should be considered where:
- Endotracheal intubation is required:
  - Airway protection
  - Secretion clearance
- Respiratory failure is present, or likely to occur:
  - Respiratory rate >30 breaths/minute, or apnoea/bradypnoea
  - Vital capacity <10–15 ml/kg
  - Hypercapnia with pH <7.35
  - PaO_2 <11 kPa on FiO_2 <40%
  - Fatigue, exhaustion, inadequate respiratory effort
  - ↓level of consciousness
  - Acute pulmonary oedema
- Cardiopulmonary support is required:
  - Following cardiac arrest
  - Postoperative support of certain high-risk patients
  - Severe shock or LVF
- Sedation, anaesthesia, and/or paralysis is required to:
  - Control intracranial pressure
  - Transfer critically ill patients
  - Control muscle spasms (e.g. tetanus)
  - Allow assessment or treatment, particularly in agitated or combative patients

Also see indications for endotracheal intubation (📖 p.12).

Respiratory failure, actual or incipient, as outlined here may also be considered as an indication for non-invasive ventilation, but it should be borne in mind that this will not provide any degree of airway protection (see 📖 'Non-invasive respiratory support', p.53.).

Lung protective mechanical ventilation[1]

Lung protective ventilation strategies help to reduce the development of ALI/ARDS by attempting to avoid barotrauma, volutrauma, and shearing forces in the ventilated lungs:

- Use tidal volumes of ~6 ml/kg ideal body weight (IBW).
- Keep maximum ventilatory pressure at <30 cmH$_2$O.
- Use adequate level of PEEP.
- Keep I:E ratio >1:1 where possible.
- Use assist-controlled ventilation where possible.
- Use the minimum required FiO2 to keep SpO$_2$ above 90% (or PaO$_2$ above 8 kPa).
- Allow CO$_2$ to rise if necessary (permissive hypercapnia).

Ideal body weight calculation

In morbidly obese patients IBW should be used to calculate appropriate tidal volumes.

Male: IBW (kg) = 50 + 2.3 × (height (inches) − 60)
Female: IBW (kg) = 45.5 + 2.3 × (height (inches) − 60)

Alternative means of estimating height are also available, see Fig. 17.29 on 📖 p.579.

[1] From *The New England Journal of Medicine*, The Acute Respiratory Distress Syndrome Network, 'Ventilation with lower tidal volumes as compared with traditional tidal volumes for acute lung injury and the acute respiratory distress syndrome', 342, 18, pp. 1301–1308. Copyright © 2000 Massachusetts Medical Society. Reprinted with permission from Massachusetts Medical Society.

Non-invasive respiratory support

Potential advantages

- ↓incidence of ventilator-associated pneumonia (VAP).
- No endotracheal intubation or tracheostomy required:
  - No risk of failure to intubate
  - No risk of long-term tracheal damage
- No sedation required:
  - Patient can communicate
  - Patients can often eat and drink

Indications

- Acute pulmonary oedema:
  - (Use CPAP or BIPAP[1] with PEEP of 10–15 cmH$_2$O)
- Obstructive sleep apnoea:
  - (Use CPAP or BIPAP with PEEP and inspiratory pressure adjusted to alleviate obstruction)

- COPD:
  - (Use CPAP or BIPAP with inspiratory pressure adjusted to ease work of breathing or avoid hypercapnic acidosis and PEEP adjusted to ~80% of intrinsic PEEP)
- Weaning from mechanical ventilation.
- Respiratory failure in immunocompromised patients at high risk of VAP (e.g. neutropaenic patients).
- Other causes of acute respiratory failure where there are no contraindications.

Contraindications[2]

- Risk of airway obstruction or inability to protect the airway.
- Facial abnormalities, trauma, or burns; or recent facial/airway surgery.
- Upper airway obstruction.
- Excessive secretions or vomiting; bowel obstruction.
- Very high oxygen requirement/life-threatening hypoxia.
- Severe acidaemia.
- Haemodynamic instability, arrhythmias, or severe comorbidity.
- Confusion, agitation, or patient refusal.
- Pneumothoraces (an intercostal drain should be inserted first).
- Upper GI surgery is a relative contraindication.

Complications

- Intolerance of mask (up to 25%).
- Airway may still become obstructed—especially if patient becomes obtunded, or if there is airway trauma.
- Skin damage.
- Gastric distension, vomiting and/or aspiration.

[1] Evidence supporting the efficacy of NIV is variable, as is the evidence for which mode to use (CPAP or BIPAP), see 🕮 Further reading and p.89.

[2] NIV may be used in the presence of contraindications provided there is a contingency plan for intubation or the decision not to proceed to invasive ventilation has previously been made.

Further reading

Baudouin S, et al. BTS Guidelines: Non-invasive ventilation in acute respiratory failure. *Thorax* 2002; **57**: 192–211.

O'Driscoll BR, et al. BTS guideline for emergency oxygen use in adult patients. *Thorax* 2008; **63**(SVI): vi1–vi68.

Levy MM. Pathophysiology of oxygen delivery in respiratory failure. *Chest* 2005; **128**(5 S2): 547S–553S.

Malarkkan N, et al. New aspects of ventilation in acute lung injury. *Anaesthesia* 2003; **58**: 647–67.

Riley B. Strategies for ventilatory support. *Br Med Bull* 1999; **55**(4): 806–20.

The Acute Respiratory Distress Syndrome Network. Ventilation with lower tidal volumes as compared with traditional tidal volumes for acute lung injury and the acute respiratory distress syndrome. *N Engl J Med* 2000; **342**: 1301–8.

① **Severe hypercapnia**

Hypercapnia is defined as a $PaCO_2$ >6.3 kPa. It can occur as a result of ↓clearance of CO_2 or, less commonly, as a result of ↑production.

Causes

↓ventilation—all causes of type II respiratory failure (see 📖 p.48), including:
- Acute severe bronchospasm.
- COPD—acute exacerbation.
- Airway obstruction—partial/chronic.
- Inadequate respiratory rate (e.g. head injury or overdose).
- Inadequate ventilation (e.g. neuromuscular disease or traumatic damage).
- Impaired gas exchange (e.g. ALI, ARDS, or infection).
- Inadequate mechanical ventilation.

↑production of CO_2:
- Severe sepsis/SIRS (e.g. major burn injury).
- Thyroid storm.
- Reperfusion event (e.g. following release from crush injury).
- Hyperpyrexias (e.g. malignant hyperpyrexia, neuroleptic malignant syndrome).
- Drug reaction (e.g. serotonin syndrome, ecstasy (MDMA) poisoning).

Equipment failure may also cause re-breathing of expired CO_2; this is associated with breathing circuits in anaesthetic rather than ICU practice.

Presentation and assessment
- Most commonly revealed by ABG analysis:
  - Hypercapnia results in a respiratory acidosis, which may be compensated for metabolically by retention of bicarbonate ions in chronic conditions (e.g. COPD)
- Where end-tidal CO_2 measurements are available these will be raised.
- Symptoms of hypercapnia include:
  - Agitation, sweating, flapping tremor
  - Respiratory distress: tachypnoea, dyspnoea
  - Tachycardia, bounding pulse, hypertension, vasodilatation
  - ↓consciousness level, narcosis

Investigations
- ABGs (to confirm diagnosis and estimate whether acute, acute-on-chronic, or chronic on basis of pH and bicarbonate ('Boston rules') see 📖 p.207).
- FBC, coagulation studies (possible raised WCC; DIC).
- U&Es (hyperkalaemia 2° to acidosis; AKI 2° to underlying cause, e.g. rhabdomyolysis).
- TFTs (↑ T4,T3 in thyroid storm).
- CK and urine myoglobin (where MH or reperfusion injury suspected).
- ECG (for signs of hyperkalaemia).

Immediate management

- Titrate FiO_2 to maintain SpO_2 94–98%—via reservoir mask if spontaneously breathing or ventilator if receiving respiratory support:
  - If spontaneously breathing and suspected of having hypercapnic respiratory failure caused by COPD then aim for 88–92%
- Treat any underlying cause of type II respiratory failure:
  - If hyperpyrexia is suspected (MH, neuroleptic malignant syndrome, serotonin syndrome, MDMA poisoning) see 📖 p.246
  - If thyroid storm is suspected see 📖 p.238.

If the patient is spontaneously breathing without ventilatory support:
- Secure airway and support ventilation if required.
- Consider NIV or endotracheal intubation and mechanical ventilation if the patient is tiring, or hypercapnia/oxygenation are worsening.

If patient is already intubated and/or receiving ventilatory support (non-invasive or invasive) the following may be necessary:
- Tolerate moderate hypercapnia ($PaCO_2$ <8 kPa) if it is not obviously compromising the patient.
- Alter ventilation parameters:[1]
  - Increase inspiratory pressure, inspiratory time, or tidal volume if ventilatory volumes are inadequate
  - Increase respiratory rate if minute volumes are inadequate despite good tidal volumes
  - Increase PEEP to maintain lung recruitment
- Progress to intubation/ventilation if NIV is ineffective; if intubated:
  - Try increasing sedation or use short-term muscle relaxation to allow greater tolerance of hypercapnia and to reduce CO_2 produced by the work of breathing
  - Consider advanced airway manoeuvres or oxygenation techniques (e.g. alveolar recruitment measures (📖 p.65); patient positioning: either positioning bad lung uppermost if lung pathology is unilateral, or prone position)

Once **A**irway and **B**reathing are stabilized, continue **ABC** approach.

[1] Follow a lung-protective strategy in intubated/ventilated patients where possible (📖 p.53).

Further management

- If acidaemia is severe with mixed metabolic/respiratory components consider starting renal replacement therapy or bicarbonate infusions.
- Aggressively treat hyperpyrexia with antipyretics and/or cooling measures (non-invasive or invasive).
- High-frequency oscillatory ventilation may aid CO_2 clearance, as may tracheal gas insufflation (TGI).
- Extracorporeal CO_2 removal ($ECCO_2R$) may be possible.

Pitfalls/difficult situations

- Avoid hypercapnia where possible in patients with head injuries.
- Where hypercapnia has been tolerated for a prolonged period, and metabolic compensation has occurred, avoid rapid correction as the relative hypocapnia may result in cerebral vasoconstriction.

:⚙: Complications of mechanical ventilation

Complications of mechanical ventilation that may require emergency treatment include:
- Failure to ventilate.
- Failure to oxygenate.
- Haemodynamic instability.
- Pneumothorax.
- Mucous plugging.

Other complications covered in more detail in other sections include:
- Hypercapnia (📖 p.56).
- Air trapping (📖 p.78).
- Ventilator-associated pneumonia (📖 pp.62 and 334).

Causes

Complications are more likely in:
- Agitated, undersedated, or very mobile patients.
- Patients with abnormal anatomy.
- Patients with severe respiratory diseases, especially severe pneumonia, ARDS, bronchospasm, trauma, and contusions.
- Patients with underlying chronic chest conditions.
- Patients requiring airway pressures >35 cmH$_2$O, or patients receiving high tidal volumes via mechanical ventilation.

Haemodynamic instability:
- May result from ↓venous return/cardiac output.
- Is made worse by coexisting dehydration, hypovolaemia, sepsis, cardiac ischaemia or failure.

Presentation and assessment

Difficulty in ventilating/oxygenating may present with:
- Hypoxia (SpO$_2$ <92%, or PaO$_2$ <8kPa), cyanosis.
- Increasing airway pressures.[1]
- High, or low-pressure, ventilator alarms.
- Evidence of low delivered tidal volume, or low minute-volume alarm.
- Audible leak from ventilator circuit, or leak alarm.
- Inability to ventilate using self-inflating ambu-bag.
- Lack of chest movement or respiratory sounds on auscultation.
- Hypercapnia.
- Dynamic hyperinflation (next inspiratory cycle starts before last expiratory cycle finished), see 📖 p.78.

Where the patient is conscious and/or spontaneously breathing alongside mechanical ventilatory support complications of ventilation may result in:
- Agitation, sweating, clamminess.
- Increasing respiratory distress, tachypnoea, dyspnoea.

---

1 Increasing airway pressures will occur if using volume-controlled ventilation; decreasing tidal volumes will occur with pressure-controlled ventilation.

Cardiovascular abnormalities may include:
• Cardiac arrest.
• Tachycardia, bradycardia, or arrhythmia.
• Hypotension.

Evidence of pneumothorax may include:
• Tracheal deviation away from affected side.
• Absent/diminished breath sounds on affected side.
• Hyper-resonant percussion note on affected side.
• Subcutaneous emphysema.
• Pneumothorax or pneumomediastinum on CXR.

Investigations
• ABGs (hypoxia, hypercapnia).
• FBC (↑WCC in infection).
• CXR (collapse, consolidation, pneumothorax, effusion).
• Bronchoscopy (ETT or bronchial obstruction: mucous plug, blood clot, foreign body, extrinsic compression, tumour).
• ECG if CVS instability (ischaemia, RV strain).
• Chest US (pneumothorax, effusion).
• CT chest (if considering anterior/loculated pneumothorax, effusion).

Differential diagnoses
• Where there is difficulty in ventilating always consider the possibility of an occluded or semi-occluded airway (see 📖 pp.38 and 42).

Indications for fibreoptic bronchoscopy in ventilated patients
• To obtain microbiological samples via suction or lavage, particularly if patients are immunocompromised or suspected of having atypical infections.
• To localize and control haemoptysis.
• Removal of secretions, blood clots, or foreign bodies allowing lung re-expansion.
• To examine for strictures, tumours, or tracheobronchial trauma
• To assess patency or position of ETT.
• To evaluate degree of tracheobronchial trauma following airway burns or smoke inhalation.

Relative contraindications include:
• Moderate/severe hypoxia or hypercapnia.
• Coagulopathy, SVC obstruction, or other risk of bleeding.
• Near-complete tracheal obstruction.
• Myocardial ischaemia, arrhythmias, or hypotension.

Immediate management

If there is difficulty in ventilating the patient:

- Increase FiO_2 to 100%, pulse oximetry, and capnography.
- Airway: check ETT or tracheostomy for position, patency, and presence of cuff leak; exchange of ETT/tracheostomy or re-intubation may be required (see 📖 pp.38 and 42).
- Check for equipment failure and disconnection; if in doubt switch to self-inflating bag and manually ventilate.
- Consider the possibility of the following (treat as appropriate):
  - Bronchospasm (bronchodilator therapy, reduce RR and lengthen I:E ratio; 📖 p.79)
  - Breathing against ('fighting') the ventilator (increase sedation/anxiolysis and consider instituting neuromuscular blockade)
  - Foreign body, mucous plugs, retained chest secretions, or major collapse of the lung tissue (📖 pp.34 and 65)
  - Pneumothorax (tension or non-tension), tension haemothorax, massive effusion (📖 pp.80 and 82)
  - ARDS (📖 p.90)
- Ventilation parameters may need adjusting:[1]
  - Increase inspiratory pressure, inspiratory time, or tidal volume if ventilatory volumes are inadequate
  - Increase respiratory rate if minute volumes are inadequate despite good tidal volumes
  - A trial of ↑ PEEP to find best lung compliance/maintain lung recruitment
  - Reduce rate and increase expiratory time if bronchospasm

Where there is haemodynamic instability:

- Treat hypotension using fluid and/or inotropes where required
- Consider the possibility of the following (treat as appropriate):
  - Hypovolaemia (📖 p.112)
  - Sepsis (📖 p.332)
  - Tension pneumothorax (📖 p.80)
  - Cardiac ischaemia, failure, or arrhythmia (📖 p.122).

Where there is hypoxia despite adequate ventilation:

- Increase FiO_2 to 100%; double check this value and switch to alternative supply if concerned.
- Consider the possibility of the following—treat as appropriate:
  - Endobronchial intubation (📖 p.26)
  - Pneumothorax (📖 p.80)
  - Pleural effusions (📖 p.82)
  - Mucous plugs or retained chest secretions (📖 p.65)
  - Acute pulmonary oedema (📖 p.86)
  - Pulmonary embolism (📖 p.92)
  - ARDS (📖 p.90)
  - Cardiac shunting/ASD
- Ventilation parameters may be altered as outlined earlier in box:[1]
  - Decreasing I:E ratios to 1:1.5, 1:1 (or even less, 2:1) may maximize inspiration and allow gas redistribution with lower pressures
  - Tolerate moderate hypercapnia

- Consider advanced airway manoeuvres or oxygenation techniques:
  - Alveolar recruitment measures (📖 p.65)
  - Bronchoscopy to aid diagnosis or remove secretions
  - If lung pathology is unilateral try positioning bad lung uppermost
  - Start a neuromuscular blocking agent infusion (e.g. atracurium)
  - Prone positioning
  - Inhaled nitric oxide or nebulized epoprostenol
  - High-frequency oscillatory ventilation (HFOV)
  - Extra corporeal membrane oxygenation (ECMO)

[1] Follow a lung-protective strategy where possible (📖 p.53).

Further management
- Identify and treat any coexisting/exacerbating infections.
- Where possible use assist-controlled or pressure-support ventilation.

Pitfalls/difficult situations
- Have a high index of suspicion for tension pneumothorax in patients with cardiovascular collapse.
- CXR interpretation can be difficult in supine patients; certain conditions such as anterior pneumothorax or pleural effusion may require additional imaging (CT or US).
- Obese patients may require much higher inspiratory pressures and levels of PEEP than expected.
- Insert prophylactic chest drains in patients with severe chest trauma who require ventilation.
- Minimize intravenous volume replacement in patients who have had major lung surgery.

Complications associated with HFOV
- Hypotension: very common at initiation of HFOV (may need aggressive fluid therapy and/or vasopressor support), can also be caused by pneumothorax/air-trapping.
- Blocked ETT or secretions (fall in PaO_2, reduced 'wiggle', rise in amplitude, rise in $PaCO_2$); may need suction, bronchoscopy and/or re-intubation.
- Pneumothorax (fall in PaO_2, unilateral 'wiggle', fall in amplitude, hypotension); will need intercostal drainage (📖 p.532).
- Air trapping/dynamic hyperinflation (gradual fall in PaO_2, hypotension and rise in CVP); try temporary disconnection, or reduce frequency and/or cycle volume.

Further reading
Bell D. Avoiding adverse outcomes when faced with 'difficulty with ventilation'. *Anaesthesia* 2003; **58**: 945–50.

Honeybourne D, et al. British Thoracic Society guidelines on diagnostic flexible bronchoscopy. *Thorax* 2001; **56**(S1): i1–i21.

Papazian L, et al. Neuromuscular blockers in early acute respiratory distress syndrome. *N Engl J Med* 2010; **363**: 1107–16.

☼ Severe pneumonia

(See also 📖 p.334.)

Severe community-acquired (CAP), hospital-acquired (HAP), or ventilator-associated pneumonia (VAP) are common causes, or complications of, critical illness.

Causes

Advancing age and any coexisting medical conditions (particularly heart disease, lung disease, immunocompromised patients—e.g. HIV, haematological malignancy, hepatic failure, drug use) increase the likelihood of severe pneumonia.

CAP:
* Common bacterial organisms include: S. pneumoniae, H. influenza.
* Common viruses: influenza A and B subtypes (e.g. H1N1).
* Less common organisms (often associated with COPD): S. aureus, M. catarrhalis, K. pneumonia, Pseudomonas.
* Atypical organisms: Legionella, Mycoplasma, Chlamydophila pneumoniae, Chlamydophila psittaci, Coxiella burnetti.

HAP and VAP:
* HAP is defined as pneumonia occurring >48 hours after hospital admission (or alternatively where there has been a previous admission within the past 7 days).
* VAP is defined as pneumonia that develops >48 hours after the institution of mechanical ventilation by means of an ETT or tracheostomy.
* In both cases aspiration, or micro-aspiration, of oral or gastric secretions is a common cause.
* Risk factors include: neurological injury, prolonged hospital stay, supine position, severe illness, immune system compromise, and mechanical ventilation.
* Common organisms include: S. pneumoniae, S. aureus, Pseudomonas, Acinetobacter, H. influenzae, and Gram-negative enterobacteriaceae (e.g. Klebsiella, E. coli, Enterobacter).

Where there is no response to treatment or the patient is immunocompromised consider less common causes:
* 'Unusual' organisms: TB, Pneumocystis jiroveci, Stenotrophomonas, Cryptococcus neoformans.
* Resistant species: MRSA, resistant Pseudomonas.
* Viral: varicella, CMV.
* Fungal: Candida spp., Aspergillus.

Presentation and assessment

* Agitation or malaise.
* Increasing respiratory distress, tachypnoea, dyspnoea.
* Cough, purulent sputum, haemoptysis.
* Pleuritic chest pain or abdominal pain.
* Rigors, pyrexia, sweating, clamminess.

- Hypoxia, hypercapnia.
- Pleural effusion.
- Tachycardia and/or hypotension.

Where the patient is mechanically ventilated the only indications may be:
- Worsening oxygenation.
- ↑sputum production.
- Indices of infection (pyrexia, WCC, CRP, culture results).
- CXR changes on routine films.

Investigations
- ABGs (hypoxia, respiratory/metabolic acidosis, or respiratory alkalosis).
- FBC (WCC may be high, >12, or low <4 × 10⁹/L; neutrophilia).
- U&Es (hyponatraemia caused by SIADH; ↑urea/creatinine).
- LFTs (non-specific abnormalities).
- Coagulation screen (↑INR, DIC).
- CRP (raised).
- CK (occasionally raised: *Legionella*, H1N1).
- CXR (new or progressive infiltrates, consolidation, or cavitation).
- ECG (ST changes for IHD, RV strain for PE—differential diagnoses).
- Culture of blood and sputum (possibly including AFB for TB).
- Urine for *Pneumococcal* antigen and *Legionella* antigen.
  Other investigations that may be of use include:
- Viral throat swab PCR (influenza, parainfluenza, respiratory syncytial virus, herpes, varicella, adenovirus).
- Bronchoscopy or non-directed BAL (if safe to do so) testing for:
  - Routine culture and sensitivity
  - Specific cultures (e.g. AFBs, fungus, *Legionella*)
  - Immunofluorescence (e.g. *Pneumocystis, Mycoplasma*)
  - Galactomannan (*Aspergillus*)
  - Viral PCR
- Pleural fluid (if present) for microscopy culture and pneumococcal antigen.
- Serum antigen serology (*Mycoplasma*).
- Echocardiogram if cardiac cause/complication suspected.
- CT chest.
- US chest (parapneumonic effusion).

Differential diagnoses
- Acute myocardial infarction/pulmonary oedema (ECG changes: ST segments, T waves; cold peripheries, fine bi-basal crackles).
- Pulmonary embolism (ECG changes: RV strain pattern; ECHO changes: RV dilatation/strain).
- Pneumothorax (CXR/US changes).
- Pneumonitis, vasculitis, sarcoidosis, or malignancy.

Hospital assessment of community-acquired pneumonia (using CURB65)
- Initial assessment suggestive of CAP: Yes/No.
- CXR evidence of consolidation: Yes/No.

If Yes to both assess **CURB65** score (1 point for each factor present):
- **C**onfusion: new mental confusion.
- **U**rea: >7 mmol/L.
- **R**espiratory rate: ≥30/minute.
- **B**lood pressure: systolic <90 mmHg or diastolic ≤60 mmHg.
- Age ≥**65** years
  - 0–1: low severity (risk of death <3%)
  - 2: moderate severity (risk of death 9%)
  - 3–5: high severity (risk of death 15–40%)

A CURB65 score of 4 or 5 indicates a strong likelihood of the need for critical care admission, other poor prognostic features include:
- Presence of any coexisting disease.
- Hypoxia (SaO_2 <92% or PaO_2 <8 kPa) regardless of FiO_2.

Patients with a high CURB65 score (3–5) should undergo the following:
- Blood cultures (minimum 20 ml).
- Sputum or other respiratory sample (e.g. BAL) for routine culture.
- Pleural fluid, if present, for microscopy, culture, and pneumococcal antigen detection.
- Pneumococcal urine antigen test.
- Investigations for legionella pneumonia:
  - Urine for legionella antigen
  - Sputum or other respiratory sample for legionella culture and direct immunofluorescence (if available)
- Investigations for atypical and viral pathogens:
  - If available, sputum or other respiratory sample for PCR or direct immunofluorescence for *Mycoplasma*, *Chlamydophila* spp, influenza A and B, parainfluenza, adenovirus, RSV, *P jiroveci* (if at risk)
  - Consider initial follow-up viral and 'atypical pathogen' serology

Reproduced from *Thorax*, Lim WS, et al., 'British Thoracic Society guidelines for the management of community acquired pneumonia in adults: update 2009', 64, sIII, pp. iii1–iii55, copyright 2009, with permission from BMJ Publishing Group Ltd.

Immediate management
- 100% O_2 initially, then titrate to SpO_2 or blood gas results.
- Consider urgent physiotherapy and/or tracheal suctioning:
  - Awake patients may require insertion of a nasopharyngeal airway to facilitate suction catheters to be passed into the trachea
- If the patient is spontaneously breathing but requires further support non-invasive ventilation may be used; but it probably does not reduce the need for endotracheal intubation and should only be used if there is facility to intubate (unless intubation is not appropriate).
- Consider intubation and mechanical ventilation[1] if patient tiring, oxygenation worsening, or if airway needs to be secured.

- If patient is already intubated/ventilated adjust ventilation to maintain SpO_2[1] (see 📖 p.60).

Once Airway and Breathing are stabilized, continue ABC approach. Antibiotics guided by local protocols should be commenced as soon as possible after cultures. Empirical treatment protocols may include:
- CAP: co-amoxiclav 1.2 g IV 8-hourly and clarithromycin 500 mg 12-hourly.
- HAP: piptazobactam 4.5 g IV 8-hourly ± linezolid 600 mg IV 12-hourly.
- If legionella is suspected, add levofloxacin IV 500 mg 12-hourly.

[1] Follow a lung-protective strategy where possible (📖 p.53).

Further management
- Apply the general measures for sepsis management (📖 p.322).
- Remember analgesia for chest pain where required.
- Consider invasive monitoring and serial blood gas analysis.
- If mucous plugging or atelectasis is a problem, consider:
  - Increase PEEP to improve lung recruitment
  - Recruitment manoeuvres—various techniques described including: stepwise increase in PEEP and Vt up to a maximum peak airway pressure of 35 cmH_2O which is maintained for approximately 5 minutes, then PEEP and Vt returned to previous settings
  - Fibreoptic bronchoscopy and bronchial toilet
  - Nebulized therapy: β_2-agonists (salbutamol 5 mg) to bronchodilate, or 0.9% saline (5–10 ml) to loosen secretions
  - Mucolytics, e.g. nebulized N-acetylcysteine (5–10 mg in 3 ml 0.9% saline) or oral/NG carbocisteine 750 mg 8-hourly
- Occasionally elective endotracheal or tracheostomy tube change may be required if secretions become encrusted and cause obstruction.

Pitfalls/difficult situations
- Pneumonia is more common in patients with chronic lung conditions which may require concurrent treatment.
- Malignancies or foreign bodies may give rise to pneumonia.
- Organisms found on tracheal aspirates may not be causative.
- Pneumonia can be caused by mixed organisms.
- Consider Legionella where there is evidence of other organ failure (especially renal) and/or a community outbreak.
- If necrotizing pneumonia caused by a PVL-producing strain of S. Aureus is suspected see 📖 p.356.

Further reading
Lim WS, et al. British Thoracic Society Guidelines for the management of community acquired pneumonia in adults: update 2009. Thorax 2009; 64(sIII): iii1–iii55.
Masterton RG, et al. Guidelines for the management of hospital-acquired pneumonia in the UK: Report of the Working Party on Hospital-Acquired Pneumonia of the British Society for Antimicrobial Chemotherapy. J Antimicrob Chemother 2008; 62: 5–34.
Stiller K. Physiotherapy in intensive care: towards an evidence-based practice. Chest 2000; 118(6): 1801–13.

☼ Aspiration

Aspiration presents either with acid inhalation leading to acid pneumonitis, or with the inhalation of particulate matter causing small airway obstruction and/or aspiration pneumonia.

Causes

Risk factors include:
- Neurological injury or ↓consciousness level.
- Difficulty swallowing (e.g. stroke and Parkinson's disease).
- Complicated endotracheal intubation, especially if the patient:
  - Was intubated as an emergency, or by an inexperienced operator
  - Was at risk of aspiration: full stomach, hiatus hernia, delayed gastric emptying, incompetent lower oesophageal sphincter
- General anaesthesia: aspiration can occur as an occult event.
- Mechanical ventilation.

Where there is pneumonia, common bacterial organisms include:
- Community-acquired: anaerobes and streptococci.
- Hospital-acquired: *S. pneumoniae*, *S. aureus*, *Pseudomonas*, *Acinetobacter*, *H. influenzae*, and Gram-negative enterobacteriaceae (e.g. *Klebsiella*, *E. coli*, *Enterobacter*).

Presentation and assessment

- Both pneumonia and pneumonitis may coexist and presentation may be acute/subacute, or delayed.
- Aspiration may be witnessed.
- Increasing respiratory distress, tachypnoea, dyspnoea.
- Cough and/or wheeze, particularly with acid pneumonitis.
- Rigors, pyrexia, sweating, and purulent sputum production.
- Tachycardia, hypotension, sepsis.
- Indices of infection (pyrexia, WCC, CRP, culture results).

Investigations

- ABGs (hypoxia).
- FBC (↑WCC).
- U&Es, CRP.
- CXR (new infiltrate, consolidation, collapse).
- Culture (blood and sputum).
- Bronchoscopy (if evidence of collapse on CXR).

Differential diagnoses

- Bronchospasm (generalized wheeze rather than localized).
- Acute pulmonary oedema (bi-basal crackles rather than unilateral).
- Endobronchial intubation (ETT position: at teeth/on CXR/on bronchoscopy).
- Mucous plugging, or foreign body inhalation (CXR/bronchoscopic appearance).
- Undiagnosed preoperative chest infection.

Immediate management
- 100% O_2 initially (humidified if possible); titrate to SpO_2/PaO_2
- Consider non-invasive respiratory support (contraindicated if aspiration $2°$ to reduced conscious level or ongoing aspiration risk).
- Endotracheal intubation and mechanical ventilation[1] are likely to be needed if the airway needs securing, the patient is tiring, or oxygenation is worsening.
- Bronchodilators should be prescribed if there is significant wheeze.

Acid pneumonitis treatment (mostly supportive in nature):
- Evidence does not support the use of prophylactic antibiotics or steroids.
- Patients with particulate aspirate matter may require rigid bronchoscopy to remove large obstructing pieces.

Aspiration pneumonia
- Antibiotic therapy guided by local protocols, culture results, and sensitivity is the basis of management; empirical treatment protocols may include:
  - Co-amoxiclav 1.2 g IV 8-hourly
- Consider fibreoptic bronchoscopy to collect lavage specimens for microbiological diagnosis and exclude obstructing neoplasms.

Once **A**irway and **B**reathing are stabilized, continue **ABC** approach.

[1] Follow a lung-protective strategy where possible (📖 p.53).

Further management
- Apply the general measures for sepsis management (📖 p.322).
- Consider invasive monitoring and serial blood gas analysis.

Pitfalls/difficult situations
- Complications of aspiration include: lung abscess formation, empyema, lobar collapse and ARDS.
- Use of a VAP prevention bundle in intubated patients is recommended (see 📖 p.383).

Further reading
Englehart T, et al. Pulmonary aspiration of gastric contents in anaesthesia. *Br J Anaesth* 1999; **83**: 453–60.

:⚙: Inhalational injury

Inhalational injury occurs following the inhalation of smoke particles or caustic chemicals, which cause tracheitis, bronchitis, bronchiolitis, and alveolitis. Systemic absorption of toxins also occurs, and both/either may lead to a severe SIRS and subsequent infectious complications. Inhalational injury increases the mortality from burns injury significantly.

Causes
- Commonly occurs in burns victims who have been trapped in an enclosed space.
- Can also occur with self-immolation.
- Inhalation of steam or hot/corrosive gases.
- It is associated with alcoholism, chronic ill health, psychiatric illness, trauma, and extremes of age.

Presentation and assessment
Significant inhalational injury is suggested by:
- Compatible history.
- Severe generalized burns, or burns associated with:
  - The face: oedema, blistering, peeling skin, singeing of facial hair
  - The neck: circumferential or anterior neck burns
  - The airway: airway oedema present, blistering/peeling of mucosal membranes, or presence of soot on mucous membranes
  - Airway injury requiring intubation (p.30)
- Loss of consciousness.
- Change in voice.
- Carbonaceous sputum.
- Respiratory distress.
  - Tachypnoea, dyspnoea, and/or wheeze/bronchospasm
  - Hypoxia (though SpO_2 may appear may appear misleadingly normal in presence of CO poisoning)
  - Cyanosis (though pink flush may also occur due to CO poisoning).

Investigations
- ABGs (hypoxia, metabolic acidosis).
- COHb (elevated levels of carboxyhaemoglobin in the blood make inhalational injury more likely. e.g. >15%).
- FBC (↑WBC).
- U&Es, LFTs.
- CXR (infiltration, consolidation, collapse).
- ECG (ischaemia is associated with CO poisoning).
- Bronchoscopy (the presence of soot within the bronchial tree confirms inhalational injury; mucous plugging is a common occurrence).

Differential diagnoses
- Carbon monoxide poisoning without inhalational injury.
- Facial burns without inhalational injury.
- Burns injury with associated COPD, ARDS, pneumonia, or PE.

Immediate management

- Give 100% oxygen:
  - Raised COHb levels will require 100% FiO_2 until COHb < 6%
- Consider intubation and mechanical ventilation[1] if patient is tiring, oxygenation is worsening, or if airway needs to be secured.
- Early endotracheal intubation is likely to be necessary where:
  - GCS ≤8 or rapidly decreasing
  - Burns are widespread (>30% BSA)
  - There are facial or airway burns
- Continue ventilation with 100% O_2 to minimize/reverse effects of carboxyhaemoglobin.

Once Airway and Breathing are stabilized, continue ABC approach:
- Support circulation with IV fluid as guided by burns fluid regimens (🕮 p.416).
- Any associated skin and airway burns should be managed appropriately (🕮 p.416).

[1] Follow a lung-protective strategy where possible (🕮 p.53)

Further management

- Supportive medical treatment includes nebulized bronchodilators.
- High-dose steroids are contraindicated, and as yet there is no evidence for the use of low-dose steroids.
- There is also no evidence to support the use of prophylactic antibiotics.
- Airway injuries are difficult to manage; where there is soot evident within the airways the following has been tried, although there is little evidence to support routine usage:
  - Bronchoscopic saline lavage and toilet of adherent soot should be performed on a daily basis until the trachea and bronchi are soot-free
  - BAL with $NaHCO_3$ 1.4%
  - Nebulized unfractionated heparin
  - Mucolytics, e.g. nebulized N-acetylcysteine or enteric carbocisteine

Pitfalls/difficult situations

- Airway protection: if in doubt intubate—delay may make a difficult intubation impossible.
- Both pulse oximetry and standard ABG analysis can give misleading results in the presence of significant carboxyhaemoglobin.
- Inhalation of the toxic components of smoke, e.g. cyanide, can have further serious metabolic consequences.
- The development of severe SIRS, ARDS, and pneumonia are common in burns patients.

Further reading

Mlcak RP, et al. Respiratory management of inhalational injury. Burns 2007; 33: 2–15.
Young CJ, et al. Smoke inhalation: diagnosis and treatment. J Clin Anesth (1989); 1(5): 377–86.

:☹: Asthma/severe bronchospasm

Acute wheeze, severe enough to cause respiratory and/or cardiovascular compromise.

Causes
- Known asthma/COPD.
- Eczema, hay fever, atopy.
- Trigger agent exposure in susceptible individuals (e.g. cigarette smoke and ozone).

Presentation and assessment

In conscious patients:
- Symptoms of asthma/bronchospasm include:
  - Sense of 'tight chest' or 'can't breathe'
  - Increasing respiratory distress associated with bilateral wheeze
- Severity of bronchospasm should be assessed as outlined as follows.

If patient is already intubated/ventilated, signs and symptoms include:
- Hypoxia (SpO_2 <92%, or PaO_2 <8 kPa), cyanosis.
- Increasing airway pressures or reduced tidal volume.[1]
- Dynamic hyperinflation (next inspiratory cycle starts before last expiratory cycle finished, see 🕮 p.78); may present as hypotension.

Assessment of asthma severity

Acute severe asthma, any one of:
- Inability to complete sentences in one breath.
- Heart rate ≥110/minute.
- Respiratory rate ≥25/minute.
- PEFR 33–50% of best or predicted.

Life-threatening asthma
- Any one of the following in a patient with severe asthma:
  - Poor respiratory effort
  - Silent chest
  - Cyanosis, SpO_2 <92% or PaO_2 <8 kPa
  - 'Normal' $PaCO_2$ (4.6–6.0 kPa)
  - PEFR <33% of best or predicted
  - Arrhythmia, hypotension
  - Altered conscious level, exhaustion

Near-fatal asthma
- Raised $PaCO_2$ and/or requiring mechanical ventilation with raised inflation pressures.[1]

[1] BTS/SIGN British Guideline on the Management of Asthma, May 2008, Revised January 2012.

---

1 Increasing airway pressures will occur if using volume-controlled ventilation; decreasing tidal volumes will occur with pressure-controlled ventilation.

Where COPD is suspected it may be appropriate to follow a slightly different treatment pathway (📖 p.74), although if in doubt, or if the patient is in extremis and further history is unavailable, then *treat as for acute bronchospasm* and review once the patient is stable.

Investigations
- ABGs (see comments on asthma severity).
- FBC (raised WCC with infection), U&Es.
- Blood and sputum cultures (possible infective cause).
- CXR (pneumothorax, foreign body, pneumonia or malpositioned ETT).
- Peak expiratory flow (PEFR) measurements (see comments on asthma severity and Fig. 17.27 on 📖 p.571):
  - PEFR measurements are often difficult to obtain in patients who are in extremis, and may detract from ongoing treatment

Differential diagnoses
- Anaphylaxis causing bronchospasm (history of exposure, urticarial rash, CVS collapse).
- Acute pulmonary oedema: 'cardiac wheeze' (history of cardiac pain, clammy peripheries, ischaemic ECG changes).
- Endobronchial intubation (ETT position at teeth, CXR).
- Breathing against ('fighting') the ventilator.
- Airway/ETT/breathing system obstruction or foreign body.
- Pneumothorax/tension pneumothorax (unilateral signs).
- Pulmonary embolism.

Immediate management
- Give 100% O_2, via reservoir mask if spontaneously breathing or ventilator if receiving respiratory support.
- Secure airway if required.
- Nebulized β_2-agonist (salbutamol 5 mg or terbutaline 10 mg) up to every 15 minutes using an oxygen-driven nebulizer, if the appropriate nebulizer is available use a continuous nebulization of β_2-agonist.
- Hydrocortisone 100 mg IV 6-hourly (or prednisolone 40 mg PO).
- Add nebulized ipratropium bromide 0.5 mg 4–6 hourly using an oxygen-driven nebulizer in severe/life-threatening asthma.

If condition continues to deteriorate despite treatment, further management may include:
- Magnesium sulphate IV infusion 2 g (8 mmol) over 20 minutes.
- Aminophylline 5 mg/kg IV loading dose over 20 minutes followed by an infusion of 0.5 mg/kg/hour (if patient is on regular theophyllines omit loading dose).
- Salbutamol 250 mcg IV over 10 minutes followed by an infusion of 5 mg salbutamol in 500 ml saline 0.9% at 1–3 ml/minute IV (5–30 μg/minute).
- Consider adrenaline 250–500 mcg SC if in extremis.
- If condition does not improve proceed to intubation/ventilation (see 📖 Further management, p.72).

Once **A**irway and **B**reathing are stabilized, continue **ABC** approach.

Further management

- If bronchospasm persists/recurs consider:
  - Repeated β_2-agonist nebulizers as in immediate management
  - Ipratropium bromide nebulizers: 500 mcg 6-hourly
  - Repeated magnesium sulphate infusion: 2 g over 20 minutes
  - Aminophylline or β_2-agonist infusions as in immediate management
- Non-invasive respiratory support has been used with non-invasive BIPAP set to IPAP with no EPAP (zero PEEP/CPAP). The evidence for this is poor and it should not be used outside of critical care areas with access to intubation/ventilation.
- In patients who require endotracheal intubation, or are already intubated, sedation (with or without muscle relaxation) may be difficult and may require the combination of several agents including:
  - Propofol (may obtund airway irritation)
  - Alfentanil, fentanyl, or remifentanil (morphine *may* exacerbate bronchospasm)
  - Midazolam
  - Ketamine (has bronchodilator activity, but should not be used without benzodiazepine cover)
  - The volatile agents isoflurane and sevoflurane (halothane may provoke cardiac arrhythmias) all have sedative and bronchodilator properties but require scavenging to be available
  - Neuromuscular blockade can be useful when trying to establish ventilatory support (vecuronium or rocuronium may be preferable to atracurium, as they cause less histamine release)
- Patients are often dehydrated and may require aggressive fluid resuscitation, especially after induction of anaesthesia for intubation.
- In ventilated patients—attempt to follow a lung-protective strategy aimed at avoiding lung damage or air trapping (see 📖 p.79), however:
  - Higher than 'normal' inflation pressures are often required to achieve adequate tidal volumes (5 ml/kg IBW)
  - Reducing the ventilator rate has a much greater effect on increasing the expiratory time than changing the I:E ratio
  - 'Permissive hypercapnia' is often required
- Identify and treat any coexisting/exacerbating infections; send appropriate blood and sputum cultures.
- Monitor oxygenation and arterial CO_2 with serial ABG analyses.
- Monitor serum potassium concentrations—many asthma treatments decrease serum potassium which may need supplementing.
- Continuation of steroid therapy, convert to oral prednisolone when appropriate:
  - Although there is thought to be no benefit to nebulized/inhaled steroids alongside parenteral steroids in the acute setting, it has been suggested that they should be started early as part of the ongoing management of asthma
- In patients where COPD is suspected, decrease oxygen after the initial resuscitation (provided the patient is stable) in order to avoid precipitating CO_2 retention (type II respiratory failure, see 📖 p.48).

- In patients where COPD is suspected or who are known to be CO_2 retainers (type II respiratory failure, see 🕮 p.48) titrate ventilation aiming for whatever the 'normal' levels of arterial O_2, SpO_2 and arterial CO_2 are for the patient (these may be recorded in the patient's notes or may have to be estimated according to the patient's exercise tolerance), see 🕮 p.75.

Indications for mechanical ventilation in asthma

Absolute:
- Apnoea.
- ↓consciousness.

Relative:
- Increasing hypercapnia.
- Exhaustion (normal or low respiratory rate).
- Drowsiness.
- Haemodynamic instability.
- Refractory hypoxia.

Endotracheal intubation should be performed semi-electively before acute decompensation occurs.

Pitfalls/difficult situations

- Be aware that a silent chest or bradycardia are pre-terminal events.
- It is often difficult to adequately ventilate severe asthmatics whilst avoiding using high inflation pressures.
- It is important to allow a long enough I:E ratio to prevent dynamic hyperinflation/air trapping.
- As bronchospasm improves remember to alter ventilator settings so as to avoid barotrauma/volutrauma.
- Tension pneumothorax is common in asthmatic patients.
- Various treatments have been tried for which there is no supporting evidence, or too little evidence to allow comment:
  - Heliox appears to offer no advantage (either when spontaneously breathing or when ventilated)
  - There is no evidence that nebulized adrenaline offers any advantage over regular β_2-agonists
  - Nebulized lidocaine has been used in refractory cases; there is currently insufficient evidence to support its routine usage
  - Leukotriene receptor antagonists have insufficient evidence to currently support their usage in the acute setting
  - There is no evidence to support the routine prescription of antibiotics in cases where there no signs of infection

Further reading

BTS/SIGN. *British guideline on the management of asthma, a national clinical guideline*. London: The British Thoracic Society/Scottish Intercollegiate Guidelines Network, 2008, revised 2011.

Papiris S, et al. Clinical review: severe asthma. *Crit Care* 2002; 6:30–44.

Stather DR, et al. Clinical review: Mechanical ventilation in severe asthma. *Crit Care* 2005; 9: 581–7.

☼ Exacerbation of COPD

Chronic obstructive pulmonary disease (COPD) includes diseases causing chronic airflow limitation (CAL) such as chronic bronchitis and emphysema. Patients may present as a result of gradual deterioration leading to type I or type II respiratory failure (📖 p.48), or may present with an acute exacerbation of their symptoms.

It is important to fully assess the severity of their underlying disease prior to any current exacerbation. It may be desirable to avoid endotracheal intubation, or inappropriate to treat the patient within a critical care environment. Any decision to limit treatment should be made by senior clinicians, involving the patient and/or their relatives where possible.

The patient may be in extremis, or further history unavailable. *If in doubt, treat as for acute bronchospasm* and review once the patient is stable.

Causes (of an acute exacerbation)
- Bacterial infection (e.g. *H. influenzae*, *H. parainfluenzae*, *S. pneumoniae*, *S. aureus*, *M. catarrhalis*, *K. pneumonia*, and *Pseudomonas*).
- Viral infection (e.g. influenza A and B, parainfluenza, rhinovirus, coronavirus).
- Trigger factors (e.g. air pollution, ozone, environmental conditions).
- Failure to comply with medication.
- Following anaesthesia or major surgery.
- Major systemic illness.
- Pneumothorax.
- Pulmonary embolism.
- Cardiac failure.

Presentation and assessment

Unlike acute bronchospasm indicators of hypoxia and respiratory distress may be chronic. Signs associated with acute deterioration may include:
- New sensation of 'tight chest', breathlessness, or inability to talk.
- ↑sputum purulence and/or volume.
- Worsening respiratory distress with or without bilateral wheeze.
- SpO_2 <90%, or PaO_2 <7 kPa .
- Tachypnoea or bradypnoea (>25 or <10 breaths/minute).
- Raised $PaCO_2$ (>6.3 kPa) with associated acidaemia (pH <7.35).
- Exhaustion, confusion or ↓level of consciousness.
- Tachycardia (>110 beats/minute), or bradycardia (<50 beats/minute).
- Arrhythmia or hypotension.
- Pyrexia.
- Worsening peripheral oedema (cor pulmonale).

If possible, assess the severity of the patient's airway disease when they are 'well', and the degree of reversibility of the current exacerbation:
- Exercise tolerance when well (see Table 3.1).
- Any previous history and investigations:
  - Pulmonary function tests
  - Normal SpO_2 on air

Table 3.1 Medical Research Council dyspnoea scale

Grade	Degree of breathlessness related to activities[1]
1	Not troubled by breathlessness except on strenuous exercise
2	Short of breath when hurrying or walking up a slight hill
3	Walks slower than contemporaries on level ground because of breathlessness, or has to stop for breath when walking at own pace
4	Stops for breath after walking about 100 m or after a few minutes on level ground
5	Too breathless to leave the house, or breathless when dressing or undressing

[1]Reproduced from British Medical Journal, C. M. Fletcher et al., 2, pp. 257–266, Copyright 1959, with permission from BMJ Publishing Group Ltd.

- • Previous CXRs and/or chest CT scans
- • History and examination may reveal any of the causes listed here as triggers for an acute exacerbation.

Investigations
(See also pneumonia investigations, 📖 pp.62 and 334.)
- • ABGs (pH <7.35, PaO_2 <7 kPa).
- • FBC (↑WCC may suggest bacterial infection).
- • CRP (raised CRP may suggest infection).
- • U&Es, LFTs.
- • Theophylline concentration (in patients using theophyllines).
- • Blood cultures, sputum cultures, nasopharyngeal viral swabs.
- • ECG (acute/chronic RV strain, coexisting ischaemia).
- • CXR (pneumonia, pneumothorax, foreign body).

Differential diagnoses
- • Acute severe bronchospasm due to:
  - • Acute asthma (normal lung function prior to episode)
  - • Anaphylaxis (precipitant, associated rash, hypotension)
- • Pneumonia (consolidation on CXR).
- • Mucous plugging.
- • Acute pulmonary oedema ('cardiac wheeze', other signs of acute LVF).
- • Endobronchial intubation (unilateral signs, position of ETT on CXR), or carinal irritation.
- • Breathing against ('fighting') the ventilator (observe respiratory pattern).
- • Airway/ETT/breathing system obstruction or foreign body (expiratory flow pattern on ventilator).
- • Pneumothorax/tension pneumothorax (unilateral signs, CXR changes).
- • Pulmonary embolism (acute RV strain on ECG/ECHO).

Immediate management

- High FiO_2 initially; then titrate to achieve an SpO_2 of 88–92% in patients with risk factors for, or a history of, hypercapnia:
  - Venturi masks allow close control of FiO_2 (📖 p.52)
  - Regular ABGs will be needed to identify development or worsening of hypercapnia
  - If pH and $PaCO_2$ remain normal, aim for an SaO_2 of 94–98% unless there is a history of previous hypercapnia requiring NIV
- Nebulized β_2-agonist (salbutamol 5 mg or terbutaline 10 mg) up to every 15 minutes.
- Ipratropium bromide nebulizers, may be added (500 mcg 6-hourly).
- Hydrocortisone 100–200 mg IV or prednisolone PO 30–40 mg.
- Consider aminophylline 250 mg IV (if not on regular theophyllines) and/or salbutamol 250 mcg IV over 10 minutes.

Non-invasive ventilation (NIV, 📖 p.53):
- NIV BIPAP should be considered in all patients with an acute exacerbation of COPD with $PaCO_2$ >6 kPa or pH <7 despite maximal treatment on controlled oxygen therapy for no more than 1 hour:
  - Mask NIV BIPAP using an inspiratory pressure (IPAP) 10–20 cmH_2O with 0–5 cmH_2O PEEP
  - Starting settings are typically IPAP 10 cmH_2O PEEP 5 cmH_2O
  - Pressures should be titrated to clinical effect and ABGs
- Where there is no hypercapnia, and NIV BIPAP is not available, NIV CPAP may improve gas exchange or reduce the work of breathing.
- NIV CPAP/BIPAP may obviate the need for invasive ventilation; may be used as a trial before, or a bridge to, endotracheal intubation; or may be the 'ceiling' of intervention.

If the patient fails to respond and there is any doubt as to the reversibility of the patient's condition then proceed to endotracheal intubation/ mechanical ventilation; *treat as for acute bronchospasm*.

Once **A**irway and **B**reathing are stabilized, continue **ABC** approach:
- Patients are often dehydrated and may require aggressive fluid resuscitation, especially after induction of anaesthesia for intubation.

Further management

- If NIV is successful it may need to be continued for 2–3 days in order to allow exacerbating factors to resolve.
- The decision to abandon NIV and proceed to intubation/ventilation can normally be made within the first 4 hours of treatment as improvements in ABGs and physiological signs should be evident within this time.
- Consider the use of respiratory stimulants such as doxapram where there is an absolute contraindication to NIV.
- Where there is evidence of infection, treat accordingly (see 📖 pp.62 and 334).
- ↑sputum production is common; physiotherapy, suctioning, and tracheostomy insertion may help.

Pitfalls/difficult situations

- It can be difficult to predict which patients won't benefit from endotracheal intubation and ventilation, with intensive care physicians sometimes unduly pessimistic.
- Bacterial or viral infection is thought to be a very common cause of acute exacerbation of COPD; where infection is suspected follow local guidelines regarding antibiotic choice (a reasonable empirical treatment might be co-amoxiclav 1.2 g IV 8-hourly).
- Chronic infection is common and organisms cultured in tracheal aspirates may not represent the cause of an acute exacerbation.
- The incidence of pulmonary embolism is thought to be high in patients with acute exacerbation of COPD; D-dimer tests are only useful in ruling out PE, where there is doubt leg vein Doppler and/or CTPA should be performed.
- Bullae may mimic the appearances of pneumothoraces.
- Coexisting cardiac disease is common in patients with COPD.
- Avoid 'normalizing' respiratory parameters in ventilated patients; if possible aim for any previously documented ABG values from when the patient was well.
- Where mechanical ventilation is considered inappropriate, NIV may still be beneficial, even in situations where it might normally be contraindicated (e.g. ↓level of consciousness).
- Patients with COPD who require intubation often take a long time weaning from mechanical ventilation.
- Consider early tracheostomy in intubated patients as it *may* assist weaning by allowing less sedation and ↓dead-space (hence less work of breathing).
- Many patients who have been intubated/ventilated and survived report that they would undergo treatment again, despite ongoing severe symptoms.

Further reading

Currie GP, et al. ABC of chronic obstructive pulmonary disease, acute exacerbations. *Br Med J* 2006; **333**: 87–9.

Celli BR, et al. Standards for the diagnosis and treatment of patients with COPD: a summary of the ATS/ERS position paper. *Eur Resp J* 2004; **23**: 932–46.

NICE. *Management of chronic obstructive pulmonary disease in adults in primary and secondary care (partial update)*. London: NICE, 2011.

O'Driscoll BR, et al. BTS guideline for emergency oxygen use in adult patients. *Thorax* 2008; **63**(SVI): vi1–vi68.

Roberts CM, et al. Non-invasive ventilation in chronic obstructive pulmonary disease: management of acute type 2 respiratory failure. *Clin Med* 2008; **8**(5): 517–21.

Wildman MJ, et al. Implications of prognostic pessimism in patients with chronic obstructive pulmonary disease (COPD) or asthma admitted to intensive care in the UK within the COPD and asthma outcome study (CAOS): multicentre observational cohort study. *Br Med J* 2007; **335**: 1132–5.

Wildman MJ, et al. Survival and quality of life for patients with COPD or asthma admitted to intensive care in a UK multi-centre cohort: the COPD and Asthma Outcome Study (CAOS). *Thorax* 2009; **64**(2): 128–32.

Air trapping

Air trapping occurs in ventilated patients when there is insufficient time for all the air to escape from the lungs during expiration. As a result, extra air accumulates within the lungs with each breath until the lungs become hyperinflated and respiratory and/or cardiovascular collapse occur. This phenomenon is also known as breath-stacking, ↑auto-peep, intrinsic PEEP (PEEPi), or dynamic hyperinflation (DHI).

Causes
- Only occurs in ventilated patients.
- Severe bronchospasm with long expiratory times; air trapping typically occurs when hyperventilation is used to maintain normocapnia.
- Inverse ratio ventilation where the inspiratory time on the ventilator is longer than expiratory times (used in conditions such as ARDS).
- Mechanical obstruction (e.g. by foreign body, sputum plug, or clot) leading to 'ball-valving'.
- Possibly more likely to occur in patients who are undersedated or breathing against ('fighting') the ventilator.
- Can occasionally occur in chest trauma.

Presentation and assessment
Not associated with spontaneous ventilation:
- Gradually increasing airway pressures will occur if using volume-controlled ventilation and decreasing tidal volumes will occur with pressure-controlled ventilation.
- Bilateral breath sounds with wheeze or a silent chest may be present.
- High auto-PEEP.
- Hypotension 2° to raised intrathoracic pressure.
- Sudden cardiovascular collapse or inability to ventilate; or PEA arrest.

Investigations
- Many ventilators have a facility for measuring PEEPi (auto-PEEP), a PEEPi above 15 cmH$_2$O should be considered high (temporary disconnection from ventilator will decrease PEEPi).
- Flow-time display of ventilator showing expiratory flow failing to return to baseline before next inspiration (see Fig. 3.1).
- CXR may show hyperinflation.

Differential diagnoses
- Tension pneumothorax (unilateral signs).
- Endobronchial intubation (unilateral signs, bronchoscopic findings).
- ETT /airway obstruction, or ventilator failure.

Immediate management
- Check ETT, ventilator, and ventilator tubing to exclude blockage or malfunction.
- In extremis or arrest: disconnect ventilator and allow chest to empty.

Once **A**irway and **B**reathing are stabilized, continue **ABC** approach.

Further management
- Treat bronchospasm (📖 p.70).
- Set ventilator settings as advised in Box 3.1.
- If already on appropriate ventilator setting consider:
  - Further decreasing minute ventilation (rate and/or tidal volume)
  - Increasing expiratory time further (IE ration >1:5)
  - Tolerating greater levels of hypercapnia
  - Further sedation and paralysis
  - Bronchoscopy to rule out foreign body, or sputum plug

Box 3.1 Ventilator management of bronchospasm
- Initially use manual ventilation with Water's circuit or self-inflating bag—until ventilator settings configured.
- Aim for tidal volumes of ~4–8 ml/kg IBW.
- Low respiratory rate (6–10 breaths/minute).
- Aim for a long I:E ratio (1:3 to 1:5).
- Aim for an inspiratory flow of approximately 80–100 L/minute.
- Aim for 'permissive hypercapnia' allowing $PaCO_2$ to rise to as much as 10 kPa; if pH falls too severely consider a bicarbonate infusion.
- Where ventilation is difficult consider heavy sedation or short-term neuromuscular blockade.
- Avoid PEEP if possible; if it is required to improve oxygenation then consider a trial of extrinsic PEEP set at 80% of calculated PEEPi.

Pitfalls/difficult situations
- Tension pneumothorax can occur alongside air trapping.

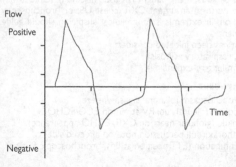

Fig. 3.1 Ventilator flow-time display for a patient with air trapping.

Further reading

Mehrishi S, et al. Intrinsic PEEP: an underreconized cause of pulseless electrical activity. *Hosp Physician* 2004; **40**(3) 30–6.
Stather DR, et al. Clinical review: mechanical ventilation in severe asthma. *Crit Care* 2005; **9**: 581–7.

☠ Tension pneumothorax

A tension pneumothorax (progressive accumulation of air in pleural cavity) leads to over-expansion of one side of the thorax, which in turn compresses the contralateral side and the great vessels.

Causes

- Chest trauma, especially where fractured ribs are present.
- Subclavian or internal jugular central line insertion.
- High ventilation pressures (especially severe asthma).
- Chronic lung disease.
- Following chest or upper abdominal surgery.

Presentation and assessment

- Patient may be in PEA cardiac arrest (see 📖 p.98).
- Sense of impending doom in the conscious patient.
- Respiratory distress: tachypnoea, dyspnoea, hypoxia, cyanosis.
- Cardiovascular compromise or complete cardiovascular collapse.
- Increasing airway pressures in the ventilated patient.[1]
- Tracheal deviation away from affected side.
- Absent/diminished breath sounds on affected side.
- Hyper-resonant percussion note on affected side.
- Distended external jugular veins.
- Surgical emphysema may be present.

It is important to have a high index of suspicion for tension pneumothorax in patients with cardiovascular collapse.

Investigations

The diagnosis of a tension/tensioning pneumothorax can be difficult, especially in ventilated patients. If the patient is cardiovascularly stable it may be appropriate to perform an urgent CXR, chest US, or bronchoscopy prior to intervention. In extremis, strong clinical suspicion should guide first line of treatment.

Once treatment has been initiated consider:
- ABGs (hypoxia, respiratory acidosis).
- CXR (to confirm lung re-expanding).

Differential diagnoses

- Severe acute bronchospasm (bilateral signs, wheeze).
- Pulmonary embolism (pleural rub, RV strain on ECG/ECHO).
- Cardiac tamponade (globular heart on CXR, ECHO appearance).
- Massive haemothorax (dull percussion note on affected side).
- Endobronchial intubation (ETT position at lips, bronchoscopic finding, CXR appearance).
- ETT/breathing system obstruction.
- Anaphylaxis.

---

1 Increasing airway pressures will occur if using volume-controlled ventilation; decreasing tidal volumes will occur with pressure-controlled ventilation.

Immediate management
- Give 100% O_2 via reservoir mask if spontaneously breathing or ventilator if receiving respiratory support.
- Secure airway if required.
- Needle decompression: large-bore cannula (14 gauge or larger), inserted through the anterior chest wall in the mid-clavicular line at the second intercostal space (at the level of the Angle of Louis). Insert just above top of third rib to avoid neurovascular bundle along lower edge of second rib.

Once **A**irway and **B**reathing are stabilized, continue **ABC** approach.

Further management
- Insertion of a formal chest drain should follow rapidly after initial decompression to avoid re-tensioning (see 📖 p.532).
- Where the patient is ventilated, a lung-protective strategy should be adopted when possible (see 📖 p.53).
- Check CXR for chest drain position and to confirm lung re-expansion.
- Consider ABG analysis to monitor changes in hypoxia.

Pitfalls/difficult situations
- Tension pneumothorax may be spontaneous, without apparent cause.
- Tension pneumothorax may be present without significant tracheal deviation.
- The external jugular veins may not be distended if there is associated hypovolaemia (trauma patients).
- Tensioning may recur despite the presence of a functioning chest drain, especially with positive pressure ventilation.
- A standard cannula may not be long enough to reach pleural cavity in obese or muscular patients.
- Bilateral tension pneumothoraces may occur causing absent bilateral chest sounds with equal percussion notes.
- Tension pneumothorax in an asthmatic patient may be difficult to diagnose, and treatment may not reduce airway pressures.

Further reading
American College of Surgeons Committee on Trauma. *ATLS guidelines*, 8th edn. Washington, DC: American College of Surgeons, 2008.

British Thoracic Society. Pleural disease guideline 2010. *Thorax* 2010; **65**(S1): ii8–ii13.

Britten S, et al. Needle thoracocentesis in tension pneumothorax: insufficient cannula length and potential failure. *Injury* 1996; **27**(5): 321–2.

Campbell-Smith TA, et al. Tension pneumothorax in the presence of bilateral intercostal chest drains. *Injury* 1998; **29**(7): 556–7.

Friend KD. Prehospital recognition of tension pneumothorax. *Injury* 2000; **4**(1): 75–7.

Laws D, et al. British Thoracic Society guidelines for the insertion of a chest drain. *Thorax* 2003; **58**(S2): ii53–ii59.

Leigh-Smith S, et al. Tension pneumothorax – time for a rethink? *Emerg Med J* 2005; **22**(1): 8–16.

Plewa MC, et al. Delayed tension pneumothorax complicating central venous catheterization and positive pressure ventilation. *Am J Emerg Med* 1995; **13**(5): 532–5.

:☻: Massive haemothorax

Massive haemothorax is defined as >1500 ml of blood in the chest cavity. Haemothorax often results from vascular damage at the time of the original injury/surgery, although other causes including rib fractures and infection may cause vascular damage some time after injury and so delay presentation.

Causes

- Penetrating chest injury.
- Blunt chest trauma, especially where fractured ribs are present.
- Subclavian or internal jugular central line insertion.
- Following chest or upper GI surgery.
- Following needle decompression/chest drain insertion.
- Minor chest trauma in anticoagulated patients.
- Abdominal haemorrhage with transdiaphragmatic communication.

Presentation and assessment

- Anxiety.
- Increasing respiratory distress:
  - Tachypnoea, dyspnoea
  - Hypoxia, cyanosis
- Stony dull percussion note on the affected side (although there may be an accompanying pneumothorax, percussion note may be raised where it overlies a pneumothorax).
- May be associated with signs of tension (see 🕮 p.80):
  - Increasing airway pressures in the ventilated patient[1]
  - Trachea deviated to the opposite side
  - Absent or diminished breath sounds on the affected side
- Signs of associated hypovolaemia may predominate (see 🕮 p.112):
  - Tachycardia
  - Hypotension
  - Oliguria
  - Delayed capillary refill
  - ↓level of consciousness.

Investigations

- ABGs (hypoxia, acidosis).
- Crossmatch blood.
- FBC (↓Hb).
- U&Es.
- Coagulation screen (coagulopathy may be present).
- CXR (may show evidence of tension with mediastinal shift, or pleural fluid/effusion).
- US, if available and time allows.
- Echocardiography (to exclude tamponade).

In extremis, strong clinical suspicion should guide first line treatment.

---

1 Increasing airway pressures will occur if using volume-controlled ventilation; decreasing tidal volumes will occur with pressure-controlled ventilation.

Differential diagnoses
- Pleural effusion (less CVS compromise, fluid aspiration findings).
- Chest consolidation (percussion note, ↑ bronchial breathing).
- Tension pneumothorax (hyper-resonant percussion note on affected side).
- Cardiac tamponade (raised JVP/CVP, globular heart on CXR, ECHO appearance).

Immediate management
- Give 100% O_2 via reservoir mask if spontaneously breathing or ventilator if receiving respiratory support.
- Secure airway; endotracheal intubation and ventilation are likely to be required in severe cases.
- Needle decompression may be required in extremis to treat any associated tension pneumothorax (📖 p.530).
- Insert large-bore IV cannula for fluid resuscitation; crossmatch blood.
- Insert chest drain; this may precipitate rapid blood loss in extreme cases (📖 p.532).
- Restore circulatory volume/blood transfusion.

Once **A**irway and **B**reathing are stabilized, continue **ABC** approach.

Further management
- Proceed to emergency thoracotomy if blood loss persists at >200 ml/hour for >2 hours.
- Check CXR, for position of chest drain and to confirm re-expansion of lung.
- Early fibrinolytics (e.g. tranexamic acid) may help decrease blood loss.
- Invasive monitoring may be required.

Pitfalls/difficult situations
- Haemothoraces may be bilateral.
- Signs of tension are not always present.
- Cardiovascular collapse may be severe, masking chest signs.
- Needle decompression cannulae may not be long enough in obese patients.
- A number of people may be required for successful resuscitation.

Further reading

American College of Surgeons Committee on Trauma. *ATLS guidelines*, 8th edn. Washington, DC: American College of Surgeons, 2008.

British Thoracic Society. Pleural disease guideline 2010. *Thorax* 2010; 65(S1): ii8–ii13.

CRASH-2 collaborators, et al. The importance of early treatment with tranexamic acid in bleeding trauma patients: an exploratory analysis of the CRASH-2 randomised controlled trial. *Lancet* 2011; 377(9771): 1096–101.

CRASH-2 trial collaborators, et al. Effects of tranexamic acid on death, vascular occlusive events, and blood transfusion in trauma patients with significant haemorrhage (CRASH-2): a randomised, placebo-controlled trial. *Lancet* 2010; 376(9734): 23–32.

Laws D, et al. British Thoracic Society guidelines for the insertion of a chest drain. *Thorax* 2003; 58(S2): ii53–ii59.

Mowery NT, et al. Practice management guidelines for management of hemothorax and occult pneumothorax. *J Trauma* 2011; 70(2): 510–18.

✛ Pulmonary haemorrhage

Haemoptysis most commonly presents as bloodstained sputum, or small amounts of fresh blood. Occasionally bronchial artery or vein rupture can occur, or bleeding can be so widespread, that haemorrhage is massive and life threatening (as it may obstruct the airway, disrupt gas exchange, or lead to hypovolaemia).

Causes

Minor haemoptysis
- Pneumonia.
- Pulmonary embolism.
- Cancer.
- Suction catheter trauma.

Major haemoptysis
- Severe infection (e.g. TB, bronchiectasis, angio-invasive fungal infections).
- Arterio-venous malformations.
- Vasculitides (e.g. RA, Wegener's granulomatosis, microscopic polyangiitis, systemic lupus erythematosus (SLE), Goodpasture's syndrome, Henoch–Schönlein purpura (HSP) and idiopathic haemosiderosis).
- Severe coagulopathy.
- Pulmonary artery flow catheters can cause pulmonary artery rupture.

Trauma more often causes haemothorax than pulmonary haemorrhage.

Presentation and assessment
- Frank blood or bloody sputum.
- Increasing respiratory distress:
  - Tachypnoea, dyspnoea
  - Hypoxia, cyanosis
- Signs of associated hypovolaemia (see 📖 p.112):
  - Tachycardia, hypotension, oliguria, delayed capillary refill.

Signs of respiratory distress and hypoxia are likely to occur before signs of hypovolaemia.

Investigations
- ABGs (hypoxia, acidosis).
- CXR (alveolar shadowing, consolidation, collapse).
- FBC (↓Hb).
- Coagulation screen (DIC).
- U&Es (rheumatological causes may have associated renal compromise).
- Vasculitis screen (e.g. autoantibodies, ANCA, ANA, rheumatoid factor, immunoglobulins, complement, anti-GBM antibodies).
- Blood and sputum cultures.
- Urine microscopy (for red cell casts suggestive of glomerulonephritis).
- Bronchoscopy/BAL if appropriate.
- CT chest.
- Echocardiography (infective endocarditis, mitral stenosis).

Differential diagnoses
- Cardiogenic pulmonary oedema (pink frothy sputum, ↑JVP/CVP).
- Oropharyngeal bleeding or epistaxis (clinical/bronchoscopic findings).
- Airway infection (purulent blood-stained sputum).
- Foreign body (CXR/bronchoscopic findings).

Immediate management
- Give 100% O_2 via reservoir mask if spontaneously breathing or by ventilator if receiving respiratory support.
- Secure airway if required; endotracheal intubation may be required in the event of massive haemoptysis:
  - If the bleeding source is one-sided rather than diffuse it may be possible to isolate that side using a double-lumen endotracheal tube (DLT)
  - As a temporary measure consider managing the patient with the bleeding side lowermost
- Once ventilated:
  - Increasing PEEP (>10 cmH_2O if tolerated) may aid lung recruitment and decrease bleeding
  - Repeated recruitment manoeuvres may be required (□ p.65)
- Depending upon likely diagnosis:
  - Urgent bronchoscopy may be required to identify and treat bleeding lesions
  - Urgent pulmonary angiography may be required to identify and treat bleeding lesions.

Once Airway and Breathing are stabilized, continue ABC approach:
- If haemorrhage is severe blood replacement may be required.
- Replace clotting products/platelets where indicated.

Further management
- Exclude oropharyngeal bleeding.
- Blood clots can cause large casts to form obstructing the bronchial tree; these may require bronchoscopy to remove.
- Diagnosis-specific treatments may be available:
  - Immunomodulatory therapy for rheumatological conditions
  - Antibiotics for infections
  - Bronchial artery embolization
- Fibrinolytics (e.g. tranexamic acid) may help decrease blood loss.

Pitfalls/difficult situations
- Conscious patients will often swallow blood, blood loss is often higher than can be seen by examining collecting bowls.
- Epistaxis and oropharyngeal trauma can cause copious bleeding to occur; careful examination is required (in unconscious patients intubation and tracheal suction will confirm haemoptysis).

Further reading
Hakanson E, et al. Management of life-threatening haemoptysis. Br J Anaesth 2002; 88(2): 291–5.

:☻: **Pulmonary oedema**

Cardiogenic pulmonary oedema is characterized by accumulation of excessive fluid in the lung leading to respiratory distress and impaired gas exchange. It results from ↑hydrostatic pressure within the pulmonary capillaries, usually as a consequence of acute LV failure. It may be worsened by, or occur earlier, if there is ↑capillary permeability in conditions such as SIRS/sepsis.

Pulmonary oedema may also be associated with other diseases that are not primarily cardiac in origin.

Causes

- Acute LV myocardial ischaemia or infarction.
- Acute decompensation of longstanding cardiac failure.
- Arrhythmia or tachycardia.
- Valvular heart disease (mitral, aortic).
- Cardiomyopathy.
- Cardiac tamponade.
- Myocarditis.
- Severe sepsis (2° to circulating myocardial depressant factors).
- Atrial myxoma (causing pulmonary venous outflow obstruction).
- Drugs/toxins (e.g. chemotherapy agents, cocaine).

In patients with normal LV function, cardiogenic pulmonary oedema is occasionally seen as a result of gross volume overload or severe high output states:
- Fluid balance/volume overload (e.g. iatrogenic, renal artery stenosis, CKD).
- Systemic disease causing high-output cardiac failure (e.g. severe anaemia, hyperthyroidism).

Other non-cardiac causes of pulmonary oedema include:
- Altitude sickness.
- Negative pressure pulmonary oedema:
  - Laryngospasm (see 🕮 p.18)
  - Acute decompression of pneumothorax
- Neurogenic pulmonary oedema (see 🕮 p.152).
- Pulmonary embolism.
- Drugs/toxins (e.g. chlorine, ammonia, or smoke inhalation; chemotherapy agents, cocaine, heroin).
- ARDS (see 🕮 p.90).

Pulmonary oedema can be caused by many factors at the same time, e.g. infection may lead to ARDS and also provoke cardiac failure.

Presentation and assessment

- Anxiety, cold/clammy peripheries.
- Patients often prefer sitting, standing, or leaning forward (orthopnoea).
- Increasing respiratory distress: tachypnoea, dyspnoea, hypoxia, cyanosis.
- Cough and/or frothy pink sputum.
- Bilateral crackles on auscultation and/or wheeze (cardiac asthma).
- Tachycardia, palpitations gallop rhythm.
- Raised JVP (worsened if there is concomitant RV dysfunction).

- Enlarged and tender liver, ascites and oedema of dependent areas (e.g. legs and sacrum) may be present with associated RV failure.
- Fluid balance charts may reveal increasingly positive cumulative balance, oliguria, or volumes of fluid administered which are large in relation to patient weight or disease.
- There may be evidence of ↓cardiac output: tachycardia and/or hypotension, oliguria, prolonged capillary refill, ↓level of consciousness.
- There may be ↓lung compliance causing increasing airway pressures in the ventilated patient (increasing airway pressures will occur if using volume-controlled ventilation, decreasing tidal volumes will occur with pressure-controlled ventilation).
- There may be a high CVP (>15 cmH$_2$O) or PCWP (>18 mmHg).

Investigations

- ABGs (may show hypoxia with or without hypercapnia).
- FBC (rule out severe anaemia, deranged WCC in severe sepsis).
- U&Es (associated AKI, hypo-/hypernatraemia, hypokalaemia).
- LFTs (associated hepatic congestion).
- Cardiac enzymes (↑troponin).
- Serum glucose (hyperglycaemia).
- Serum urate (gout may coexist).
- CRP (to identify evidence of infection).
- TFTs (hyper-/hypothyroidism).
- ECG (tachycardia, arrhythmias, evidence of ischaemia, infarction, LV hypertrophy).
- CXR (enlarged heart size, vascular redistribution, septal (Kerley B) lines, peri-hilar (bat's wing distribution) shadowing, pleural effusion).
- Echocardiography (LV dysfunction, valve disease or regional wall motion abnormality may be present).

Differential diagnoses

- Non-cardiogenic pulmonary oedema (normal ECHO or PAOP, ALI/ARDS picture, see 🕮 p.90).
- Bronchopneumonia (purulent sputum, pyrexia, ↑WCC).
- Pulmonary embolism (unilateral signs, frank haemoptysis, ECG/ECHO findings).
- Bronchospasm (history, normal ECG/ECHO).
- Anaphylaxis (precipitant, associated rash, hypotension).
- Pulmonary haemorrhage (frank haemoptysis).

Immediate management

- 100% O$_2$, pulse oximetry.
- Rapid assessment of the likely cause is essential, the most likely cause of *de novo* pulmonary oedema is cardiac failure, cardiac arrhythmia, or acute ischaemia/infarction.

If the patient is spontaneously breathing without ventilatory support:
- Give 100% O$_2$ via reservoir mask.
- Assist the patient into an upright/sitting position.

- Consider commencing non-invasive ventilatory support: CPAP or BIPAP with a PEEP of up to 5–15 cmH$_2$O (p.53).
- In extremis, consider assisting ventilation using by bag-and-mask.
- Endotracheal intubation/mechanical ventilation may be required (but care should be taken as induction of anaesthesia can precipitate cardiovascular collapse).

If patient is already intubated and/or receiving ventilatory support (non-invasive or invasive) the following may be necessary:
- Increase FiO$_2$ to maintain adequate O$_2$ saturation of 94–98%.
- Consider adjusting patient;s position to be more upright.
- Increase PEEP to recruit lung (be aware that PEEP may decrease cardiac output).

Other treatments for all patients:
- Morphine IV 2–10 mg (or diamorphine 2–5 mg), as a vasodilator and anxiolytic (titrate to level of anxiety and level of consciousness).
- Furosemide IV 20–40 mg and then double the dose if there is no response within 60 minutes.
- GTN IV infusion if the patient is normo- or hypertensive (1 mg/ml at 0–15 ml/hour); titrate to effect, avoiding hypotension.
- Consider dobutamine IV infusion if these measures fail or if the patient is hypotensive.
- If in extremis, consider venesecting 200–400 ml of blood whilst preparing other treatments (this can removed into a blood transfusion donor bag so that it may be transfused back to the patient later).
- If the patient is hypotensive (systolic <85mmHg) or has evidence of low cardiac output consider:
  - Dobutamine, or low-dose adrenaline, IV infusion
  - Intra-aortic balloon pump insertion
- Consider initiating treatment for the following causes simultaneously:
  - Arrhythmias (pp.132 and 138): anti-arrhythmics or cardioversion (digoxin, due to a positive inotropic effect, *may* be beneficial in pulmonary oedema complicated by fast AF)
  - Acute ischaemia (p.126): aspirin 300 mg PO, antianginal measures (including analgesia and nitrates as already mentioend), consider heparinization/anticoagulation
  - Acute MI (p.128): aspirin 300 mg PO, thrombolysis, or emergency angioplasty
  - Fluid overload: consider dialysis or haemofiltration to remove excess fluid

Further management
- Even if acute pulmonary oedema resolves rapidly, consider transfer to a critical care environment (HDU, CCU) for close observation.
- Further investigation or history taking may reveal acute trigger factors such as a change in medication or acute infection.
- Consider monitoring fluid balance and/or inserting a urinary catheter:
  - Restriction of fluid intake may be required

- Indications for considering ventilation include: persistent hypoxia; persistent arrhythmias; failure of listed measures.
- Further, preventative treatment may be considered including regular diuretics, ACE inhibitors, digoxin or antiarrhythmics.
- Obtain a cardiology opinion as further investigation/treatment may be required (e.g. ACE inhibitors, angiotensin antagonists, β-blockers, spironolactone, angiography).

Pitfalls/difficult situations

- X-ray features of cardiogenic pulmonary oedema overlap with ARDS.
- Early institution of CPAP non-invasive ventilation may help prevent tracheal intubation and ventilation;
  - The evidence for NIV is mixed, with little evidence for ↓mortality or requirement for endotracheal intubation, but good evidence of improved oxygenation
  - The evidence does not appear to identify which modality is better (NIPPV/NI BIPAP or CPAP), although to date there is more evidence for the use of CPAP
- The use of supplementary oxygen in patients with coronary syndromes *in the absence of hypoxia* is controversial; all guidelines recommend O_2 in the presence of hypoxia.
- Inotropic support of cardiogenic shock is controversial, although dobutamine is still recommended, it may not improve mortality:
  - Alternatives to dobutamine include levosimendan and milrinone
  - Noradrenaline is only indicated if heart failure is complicated by sepsis, or hypotension is resistant to other therapies
- Weaning from ventilator may be complicated by recurrence of pulmonary oedema.

Further reading

Agarwal R, et al. Non-invasive ventilation in acute cardiogenic pulmonary oedema. *Postgrad Med J* 2005; **81**: 637–43.

Baudouin S, et al. BTS Guidelines: non-invasive ventilation in acute respiratory failure. *Thorax* 2002; **57**: 192–211.

Cabello JB, et al. Oxygen therapy for acute myocardial infarction. *Cochrane Database Syst Rev* 2010; **6**: CD007160. DOI: 10.1002/14651858.CD007160.pub2.

Dickstein K, et al. ESC Guidelines for the diagnosis and treatment of acute and chronic heart fasilure 2008. *Eur Heart J* 2008; **29**: 2388–442.

Gray A, et al Noninvasive ventilation in acute cardiogenic pulmonary edema (3CPO trial). *N Engl J Med* 2008; **359**: 142–51.

Mariani J, et al. Noninvasive ventilation in acute cardiogenic pulmonary edema: a meta-analysis of randomized controlled trials. *J Cardiac Fail* 2011; **17**(10): 850–9.

Peter JV, et al. Effect of non-invasive ventilation (NIPPV) on mortality in patients with acute cardiogenic pulmonary oedema: a meta-analysis. *Lancet* 2006; **367**:1155–63.

Weng C-L, et al. Meta-analysis: non-invasive ventilation in acute cardiogenic pulmonary edema. *Ann Int Med* 2010; **152**: 590–600.

⊙ **Acute respiratory distress syndrome**

ARDS can be triggered by direct insults to the lung, or by the pulmonary component of a systemic inflammatory response. ARDS is a subset of acute lung injury (ALI) requiring higher levels of O_2 support. In the early stages it is caused by ↑ capillary permeability, in the later stages fibrosis predominates.

Definition of ARDS
- Acute onset (<24 hours) with known trigger/cause.
- High oxygen requirement: PaO_2/FiO_2 ≤26.7 kPa (200 mmHg).
- Reduced lung compliance.
- No left atrial hypertension; PAOP (if measured) ≤18 mmHg.
- CXR features consistent with ARDS: bilateral infiltrates.

The definition of ALI is as listed but with PaO_2/FiO_2 ≤40 kPa (300 mmHg).

Causes
- Pulmonary: ventilator-induced lung injury (barotrauma, volutrauma, high FiO_2); pneumonia; aspiration, near drowning, or inhalational injury; lung contusion; fat embolism, or anaphylactoid syndrome of pregnancy (📖 pp. 62, 66, 68, 92, 414, 438).
- Extrapulmonary: sepsis from any extrapulmonary cause; or SIRS-inducing conditions (e.g. multiple trauma/burns, pancreatitis, after cardiac bypass); transfusion related acute lung injury (TRALI).

Presentation and assessment
- Increasing respiratory distress, tachypnoea, dyspnoea, hypoxia (SpO_2 <92%, or PaO_2 <8 kPa), cyanosis, hypercapnia.
- The patient is often already mechanically ventilated, with worsening oxygenation and/or increasing hypercapnia, decreasing lung compliance, bilateral chest infiltrates on CXR.

Investigations
- ABGs (hypoxia, hypercapnia).
- FBC (↑WBC in SIRS/sepsis), U&Es, LFTs, CRP (↑ in SIRS/sepsis).
- CXR (bilateral infiltrates, absent Kerley's lines, air bronchogram, normal heart size, and no upper lobe blood diversion).
- ECG, ECHO (evidence of RV strain; exclude AMI/LVF).
- Chest US or CT chest (to exclude pneumothoraces/effusions).
- Fibreoptic bronchoscopy (for BAL, and to exclude airway obstruction).
- PAFC catheter insertion is not indicated, but if *in situ* then PAOP should be ≤18 mmHg.

Differential diagnoses
- Cardiogenic pulmonary oedema or intracardiac shunt.
- Endobronchial intubation, equipment failure, or disconnection.
- Pneumothorax, pleural effusions, pneumonia, PE.
- Bronchospasm, or breathing against ('fighting') the ventilator.
- Foreign body, mucous plugs, or major collapse of the lung tissue.

Immediate management

- After initial resuscitation and stabilization of ABC.
- Identify and treat the underlying cause where possible.
- Increase sedation and/or add muscle relaxation to aid ventilation.
- Increase inspiratory pressure, aiming to keep peak inspiratory pressure ≤35 cmH_2O and/or plateau pressure ≤30 cmH_2O.
- Increase PEEP to maintain lung recruitment.
- Maintain a tidal volume of 4–6 ml/kg IBW.
- Decrease or even invert I:E ratios (avoiding dynamic hyperinflation).
- Accept higher-than-normal CO_2 levels as long as the pH ≥ 7.3, 'permissive hypercapnia'.
- Accept lower-than-normal levels of oxygenation aiming for a PaO_2 ≥8 kPa and SaO_2 ≥90% (80–85% may be considered acceptable in extreme cases, 'permissive hypoxia').
- Consider advanced airway manoeuvres or oxygenation techniques if FiO_2 remains >0.6:
  - Alveolar recruitment manoeuvres (🕮 p.65)
  - Consider positioning the patient prone, or if lung pathology is worse on one side try positioning bad lung uppermost
  - Inhaled nitric oxide or nebulized prostacyclin
  - High frequency oscillatory ventilation and/or ECMO
- Cardiovascular optimization with may improve gas exchange and oxygen delivery, *but* positive fluid balance is likely to worsen lung compliance and oxygenation.

Further management

- In some centres steroids are given, once ARDS has been established for 7 days, as a means of minimizing lung fibrosis.
- Maintaining a neutral, or negative, fluid balance and judicious use of diuretics may improve oxygenation.

Pitfalls/difficult situations

- Barotrauma is common; pneumothoraces may be occult.
- In ARDS, weaning from mechanical ventilation is often prolonged.

Further reading

Fan E, et al. Ventilatory management of acute lung injury and acute respiratory distress syndrome. *JAMA* 2005; **294**(22): 2889–96.

Hudson L, et al. Epidemiology of acute lung injury and ARDS. *Chest* 1999; **116**(S1): 74S–82S

Moran I, et al. Recruitment manoeuvres in acute lung injury/acute respiratory distress syndrome. *Eur Resp J* 2003; **42**: 37s–42s.

Noah MA, et al. Referral to an extracorporeal membrane oxygenation center and mortality among patients with severe 2009 influenza A(H1N1). *JAMA* 2011; **306**(15): 1659–68.

Papazian L, et al. Neuromuscular blockers in early acute respiratory distress syndrome. *N Engl J Med* 2010; **363**: 1107–116.

Ritacca FV, et al. Clinical review: high-frequency oscillatory ventilation in adults – a review of the literature and practical applications. *Crit Care* 2003; **7**(5): 385–90.

Taccone P, et al. Prone positioning in patients with moderate and severe acute respiratory distress syndrome: a randomized controlled trial. *JAMA* 2009; **302**(18): 1977–84.

:☹: Pulmonary embolism/fat embolism

PE is the mechanical obstruction of the pulmonary arterial system by embolus resulting in cardiovascular and/or respiratory compromise.

PE is classified into 2 main groups:

- Non-massive PE: where patients are haemodynamically stable:
  - Submassive PE is a subgroup of patients who have echocardiographic signs of right ventricular strain; this group has a poorer prognosis and may benefit from more aggressive treatment
- Massive PE: where the patient is shocked or hypotensive (a systolic BP <90 mmHg or a pressure drop of 40 mmHg for >15 minutes not caused by new-onset arrhythmia, hypovolaemia or sepsis).

Fat embolism syndrome (FES) occurs when fat is embolized into the systemic circulation, typically following orthopaedic injury. Classical features of FES include cardiorespiratory effects as well as other multisystem complications. The diagnosis is often one of exclusion.

Causes

Pulmonary embolism
- Current DVT or previous thromboembolic disease.
- Major surgery, especially involving:
  - Major abdominal/pelvic surgery
  - Hip/knee replacement
  - Postoperative intensive care
- Obstetrics (including postpartum), especially involving:
  - Late pregnancy
  - Caesarean section
- Lower limb problems (e.g. fractures, varicose veins).
- Malignancy, especially involving:
  - Abdominal/pelvic/renal disease
  - Advanced/metastatic disease
- Reduced mobility (e.g. caused by major medical illness, hospitalization, institutional care).
- Congenital or acquired pro-thrombotic disorders (e.g. factor V Leiden deficiency, HIT, DIC).

Fat embolism syndrome
- Orthopaedic trauma/surgery, especially involving pelvis or long-bones.
- Also reported following pancreatitis, burns, liposuction, sickle cell crisis, and parenteral lipid infusion.

Presentation and assessment

- May present as PEA cardiac arrest.
- Dyspnoea, tachypnoea, hypoxia, hypercapnia.
- Pleural rub and/or wheeze can sometimes be heard.
- Pleuritic chest pain, cough, or haemoptysis.

- Syncope, hypotension, tachycardia, cardiovascular collapse.
- Right ventricular gallop, accentuated second heart sound, RV heave.
- Raised JVP.
- Clinical evidence of a DVT.

Fat embolism syndrome commonly presents 12–36 hours following injury and may also present with:
- Anaemia and coagulopathy.
- Neurological sequelae: delirium, seizures, coma.
- Dermatological changes: reddish-brown non-palpable petechiae, suconjunctival and oral haemorrhages.
- Renal dysfunction.

Investigations

- ABGs (hypoxia, acidosis, ↑A–a gradient, or may be normal).
- FBC, U&Es (FES is associated with anaemia, thrombocytopaenia).
- Coagulation studies, fibrinogen (FES is associated with low fibrinogen).
- D-dimer (when negative in the low-risk patient excludes PE, a negative result in the high-risk patient does not exclude PE; nearly all ICU patients are high risk).
- ECG (tachycardia, right bundle branch block, right axis deviation, T-wave inversion, prominent R in V1, ST elevation or depression, right heart strain, rarely S1 Q3 T3 pattern).
- CXR (may show focal oligaemia, infarct/consolidation, raised hemi-diaphragm, pleural effusion, or be normal).
- ECHO (investigation of choice in unstable patients; high RV and PA pressures, TR, RV dilatation/dysfunction, septal shift).
- CT pulmonary angiogram (investigation of choice in the stable patient).
- Ventilation perfusion (VQ) scan (good negative predictive value but hard to interpret when other abnormalities present on CXR).
- Pulmonary angiogram (may identify filling defects).

Differential diagnoses

- Acute myocardial infarction (ECG changes, ECHO findings).
- Cardiac tamponade (muffled heart sounds, ECHO findings).
- Aortic dissection ('quality' of pain, CXR findings, unequal peripheral pulses).
- Anaphylaxis (precipitant, associated rash, hypotension).
- Acute severe bronchospasm (prior history, bilateral wheeze) .
- Pneumonia (pyrexia, purulent sputum, consolidation on CXR).
- Pneumothorax/tension pneumothorax (unilateral reduced breath sounds, CXR).
- FES may also be confused with DIC or thrombotic thrombocytopenic purpura.

Immediate management

- Give 100% O_2, via reservoir mask if spontaneously breathing.
- Secure airway if required, only intubate if cardiorespiratory arrest imminent: mechanical ventilation can make hypotension worse.

Once **A**irway and **B**reathing are stabilized, continue **ABC** approach:
- Support circulation with IV fluid bolus and inotropes/vasopressors.
- Consider arterial line/central venous line before commencing thrombolysis or heparin.
- Arrange routine and definitive investigations.

For PE

- If the patient is unstable consider an urgent ECHO and thrombolysis.
  - Thrombolysis: alteplase 100 mg over 90 minutes IV, or 50 mg rtPA IV bolus on clinical suspicion alone if cardiorespiratory arrest is imminent followed by full heparinization (contraindications to thrombolysis are on 🕮 p.130)
  - Alternative thrombolysis: urokinase 4400 iu/kg over 10 minutes, followed by 4400 iu/kg/hour for 12 hours
- If the patient is stable arrange an urgent CTPA, heparinize without thrombolysis:
  - LMWH (e.g. enoxaparin 1.5 mg/kg daily)
  - Heparinization with unfractionated heparin (for patients with renal failure or at high risk of bleeding): loading dose of 80 iu/kg (not required in a thrombolysed patient), commence 18 iu/kg/hour as a continuous infusion (titrate the dose against APTT, aiming to maintain a value 1.5–2.5 × the normal range)
  - APTT should be measured 4–6 hours after starting treatment to ensure adequate anticoagulation and exclude over-anticoagulation
  - APTT 6–10 hours after every change of dose and thereafter daily

Further management

- Morphine for chest pain.
- Consider surgical embolectomy if hypotension persists for >1 hour despite medical therapy or if there are contraindications to thrombolysis or anticoagulation.
- Consider IVC filter placement in patients with recurrence despite adequate anticoagulation or where anticoagulation is contraindicated.
- Commence oral anticoagulation with warfarin when PE has been reliably confirmed, target: INR 2.0–3.0, stop heparin when levels are therapeutic.
- When managing FES the correction of coagulopathy may be required.
- FES may require the early fixation of fractures.

Pitfalls/difficult situations

- Thrombolytic therapy is equally effective via a peripheral vein or pulmonary artery catheter.
- Intubation and ventilation can worsen cardiovascular compromise.
- Where diagnosis is unclear strongly consider anticoagulation if there are no contraindications.

- Where haemodynamic compromise is present failure to thrombolyse may greatly increase mortality .
- Right ventricular dysfunction with normotension: opinions are divided as to whether thrombolysis is appropriate, seek expert help.
- In pregnancy if thrombolysis is required seek expert help:
  - Unfractionated heparin can easily be reversed and is favoured in late pregnancy; warfarin is contraindicated during pregnancy
- Cancer: high risk of recurrence but also high risk of bleeding.
- ARDS may result from FES.

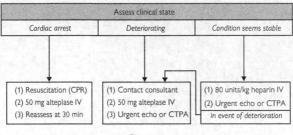

Comments

1. Massive PE is highly likely if:
   - collapse/hypotension, and
   - unexplained hypoxia, and
   - engorged neck venis, and
   - right ventricular gallop (often)

2. In stable patients where massive PE has been confirmed, iv dose of alteplase is 100 mg in 90 min (i.e. accelerated myocardial infarction regimen).

3. Thrombolysis is followed by unfractionated heparin after 3 hours, preferably weight adjusted.

4. A few untis have facilities for clot fragmentation via pulmonary artery catheter. Elsewhere, contraindications to thrombolysis should be ignored in life threatening PE.

5. "Blue light" patients with out-of-hospital cardiac arrest due to PE rarely recover.

Fig. 3.2 Management of probable massive pulmonary embolism. Reproduced from *Thorax*, British Thoracic Society guidelines for the management of suspected acute pulmonary embolism, Jan. Copyright 2003, with permission from BMJ Publishing Group Ltd.

Further reading

BTS guidelines for the management of suspected acute pulmonary embolism. *Thorax* 2003; **58**: 470–84.

Jaff MR, et al. Management of massive and submassive pulmonary embolism, iliofemoral deep vein thrombosis, and chronic thromboembolic pulmonary hypertension: a scientific statement from the American Heart Association. *Circulation* 2011; **123**: 1788–830.

Kearon C. Diagnosis of pulmonary embolism. *Can Med Assoc J* 2003; **168**(2): 183–94.

Mellor A, et al. Fat embolism. *Anaesthesia* 2001; **56**(2): 145–54.

Torbicki A, et al. Guidelines on diagnosis and management of acute pulmonary embolism. *Eur Heart J* 2008; **29**: 2276–315.

Wood KE. Major pulmonary embolism: review of a pathophysiologic approach to the golden hour of hemodynamically significant pulmonary embolism. *Chest* 2002; **121**(3): 877–905.

Circulation

☹: Cardiac arrest

Critical care teams are often involved in the resuscitation of in-hospital cardiac arrests, and in the aftercare of successfully resuscitated patients.

Unexpected cardiac arrests in the ICU are relatively uncommon and they are often preceded by prolonged attempts to resuscitate or support failing organs. If CPR is required, follow BLS/ALS guidelines (📖 pp.100 and 101).

Causes

Cardiac arrests are often cardiogenic in origin, and are more common in patients with a history of ischaemic heart disease. Hypoxia, hypovolaemia/hypoperfusion, neurologic or metabolic causes are all common in critical care settings. Potentially reversible causes include:

- Hypoxia.
- Hypovolaemia.
- Hypo/hyperkalaemia (and other metabolic disorders).
- Hypothermia.
- Hypoglycaemia.
- Tension pneumothorax.
- Tamponade, cardiac.
- Toxins.
- Thrombosis (coronary or pulmonary).
- Severe acidaemia.

Presentation and assessment

- Periods of physiological deterioration often precede within-hospital arrests.
- 1/3 of in-hospital cardiac arrests present with pulseless electrical activity (PEA), 1/3 with asystole, and 1/3 with ventricular fibrillation/pulseless ventricular tachycardia (VF/VT).
- Features requiring immediate assessment include:
  - Sudden loss of consciousness
  - Impalpable pulse, or loss of arterial pressure trace
  - Obvious apnoea, or terminal gasping
  - ECG trace of VT, VF, asystole, profound bradycardia or tachycardia
  - Sudden loss of end-tidal CO_2 trace

Investigations

Investigations that may affect an ongoing cardiac arrest include:

- U&Es (to identify hypo/hyperkalaemia):
  - The fastest way of measure this is often via a blood gas analyser using an arterial *or* venous sample
- Finger-prick blood glucose (hyperglycaemia).
- ABGs (to identify profound acidaemia).
- Echocardiography (tamponade, hypovolaemia, right ventricular hypertension in PE, regional wall motion abnormality, aortic dissection).

Differential diagnoses

- Equipment failure (ECG electrode failure or damped arterial trace).
- Any cause of syncope or severe hypotension.

Immediate management
- Adopt a **SAFE** approach (**S**hout for help, **A**pproach with caution, **F**ree from danger, **E**valuate ABC); don gloves/PPE as appropriate.
- Assess the patient: check for a response 'shake and shout':
  - If unresponsive call for help, position the patient on their back and open the airway (chin lift or jaw thrust)
  - Assess the breathing for up to 10 seconds (if ventilated confirm tube connections and tidal volume delivery)
  - At the same time manually confirm that the pulse is absent; do not rely on arterial pressure trace alone
- If the patient has no signs of life, or is pulseless, or if there is any doubt, then commence CPR.
- Ensure that the cardiac arrest team has been summoned (dial 2222).
- ALS algorithms (Figs 4.1 and 4.2; 📖 pp.100 and 101) should be followed; do not delay defibrillation if appropriate.
- Obtain information about the patient as soon as possible from notes, staff or relatives as this may help identify underlying cause and will clarify the resuscitation status of the patient.
  - *Where doubt exists as about the patient's resuscitation status CPR should be commenced*

Within the ICU/HDU
- If a monitored cardiac VF/VT arrest is witnessed deliver 3 'stacked' shocks, commencing CPR for 2 minutes immediately after the third.
- Check the airway, and if in doubt about ETT or tracheostomy consider re-intubating or reverting to bag-and-mask ventilation.
- If mechanically ventilated, turn the ventilator O_2 to 100% and do not disconnect ventilator tubing during defibrillation:
  - Minimizing PEEP, if possible, may aid defibrillation
  - If CPR prevents the ventilator from working, switch to a self-inflating bag; this can also be left connected during defibrillation
- Arterial pressure traces can be used to guide CPR; aim for a diastolic pressure >40 mmHg.
- Drugs:
  - Whilst waiting for adrenaline bolus to be available consider increasing adrenaline/noradrenaline infusion rates
  - Central IV administration is usually the best route for drug delivery and is often available in ICU patients
- Other treatments:
  - If hypovolaemia is suspected IV fluids may be rapidly infused
  - Thrombolysis (📖 p.94): where PE is strongly suspected consider giving a thrombolytic immediately
  - Needle thoracocentesis/pericardiocentesis: for tension pneumothorax or cardiac tamponade (📖 pp. 546, 530, 146, and 80)
  - Open-chest cardiac compression should be considered following cardiothoracic surgery or chest trauma
- Echocardiography during the arrest may identify reversible causes.

In postoperative cardiac surgery patients follow the CALS algorithm (see 📖 p.395).

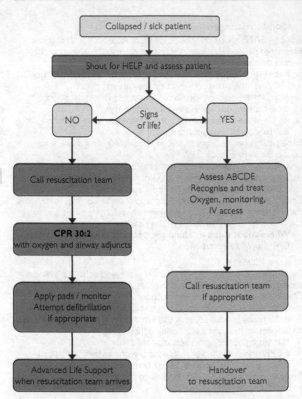

Fig. 4.1 In-hospital resuscitation algorithm. UK Resuscitation Council guidelines 2010. Reproduced with the kind permission from the Resuscitation Council (UK).

Further management

Following the return of spontaneous circulation (ROSC):
- ICU/HDU/CCU admission: it may be necessary to admit patients to a critical care setting for management of their underlying condition or post-arrest stabilization/treatments.
  - Any decision not to admit the patient following ROSC should be made by senior clinicians, where possible with the involvement of the patient's relatives (and in light of the patient's views, if known)
  - Transfer to a critical care environment is unlikely to be beneficial unless there is a period of cardiovascular stability

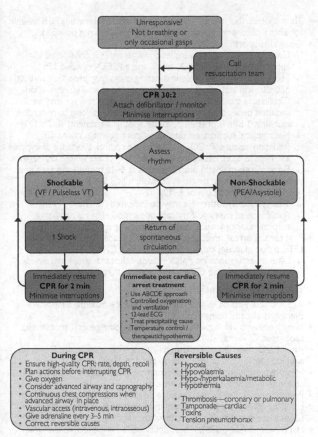

Fig. 4.2 Adult advanced life support algorithm. UK Resuscitation Council guidelines 2010. Reproduced with the kind permission from the Resuscitation Council (UK).

- Surgical intervention: on occasion urgent surgery is required following ROSC (e.g. following trauma or ruptured ectopic pregnancy); surgical advice must be sought, and a decision taken as to whether to transport to theatre or operate within the current environment.
- Angiography: where there is evidence of an acute ischaemic event it may be necessary to perform urgent angiography/coronary intervention; obtain an urgent cardiological opinion.

- Thrombolysis: this may be necessary if a massive/submassive PE is evident (or after a coronary occlusion where angiography is not possible).
- General support:
  - Continued mechanical ventilation: where this is considered appropriate aim for a SaO_2 >94% and a $PaCO_2$ of 4.5–5 kPa
  - Sedation: if required use short-acting drugs (e.g. propofol) so that neurological status can be rapidly assessed after discontinuation
  - Circulatory support: inotropic support or fluid therapy may be required depending on the underlying disease or degree of cardiac stunning; if LVF is present consider specific treatments (📖 p.122)
  - Neurological support: employ measures to combat raised ICP (sedation, seizure, $PaCO_2$ and glycaemic control; avoidance of hypoxia and hypotension; raising the bed-head to improve venous drainage)
  - Electrolytes: maintain blood glucose at 6–10 mmol/L; correct any hypomagnesaemia; maintain potassium at 3.5–4.5 mmol/L
  - Maintain haemoglobin of 8–10g/dL
  - Therapeutic hypothermia may be indicated (see Box 4.1)
  - Avoidance of pyrexia: if therapeutic hypothermia is not being employed, antipyretics, or surface cooling, may be necessary
- Post cardiac arrest investigations should include: ABGs, FBC, U&Es, LFTs, blood glucose, cardiac enzymes, ECG, CXR.
  - Later investigations may also include echocardiography to assess cardiac damage and CT head to assess neurological damage

Pitfalls/difficult situations

- ALS is unlikely to be successful in cases where maximal supportive therapy is already being provided.
- In patients who are hypothermic, or undergoing general anaesthesia, prolonged CPR may still be successful.
- After CVC insertion, chest trauma or chest surgery do not forget to exclude tension pneumothorax or tamponade.
- Hypo/hyperkalaemia and hypo/hypermagnesaemia are relatively common in critical care environments.
- Pregnancy (📖 p.429): use a wedge or tilt to decrease aortocaval compression where possible, urgently arrange for obstetric help (Caesarean section may facilitate resuscitation and save the fetus).
- Hypothermia (📖 p.250): if first defibrillation is ineffective withhold further attempts until temperature is >30°C; actively re-warm.
- Drowning or trauma (📖 pp. 404 and 414): consider the possibility of cervical spine trauma, and drug or alcohol intoxication.
- Prognostication of neurological recovery after a cardiac arrest is difficult; absence of pupillary and corneal reflexes at 72 hours (or 72 hours after cooling) is associated with a poor outcome.

Box 4.1 Therapeutic hypothermia

Therapeutic hypothermia may improve the long-term neurological outcomes after cardiac arrest:
- Indications include comatose patients (GCS <9) with ROSC after a VF/VT out-of-hospital arrest with short 'down-times'.
- It may also be beneficial for other types of arrest in other settings.

Relative contraindications include:
- Hypothermic patients.
- Cardiovascularly unstable patients (including inotrope-dependent shock, septic shock, major haemorrhage).
- Pregnancy.
- Coagulopathy.

Technique:
- Rapid induction of cooling (e.g. an infusion of 20–30 ml/kg 0.9% saline or Hartmann's).
- Continued induction/maintenance using:
  - Peripheral cooling using exposure, tepid sponging and fans
  - Cooling blankets and mattresses
  - Cold IV fluid maintenance infusions
  - Use of intravascular cooling systems (i.e. CoolGard™)
  - Trans-nasal evaporative cooling (e.g. RhinoChill™)
  - Haemofiltration or cardiac bypass using cold fluids
- Shivering may be controlled by deepening sedation and the use of neuromuscular blocking drugs (e.g. atracurium).
- Monitor core body temperature, aiming for 32–34°C for 24–36 hours before rewarming at a rate of 0.25–0.5°C/hour.
- Intravascular volume and electrolytes may require correction during cooling/rewarming.

Further reading

Choi HA, et al. Prevention of shivering during therapeutic temperature modulation: the Columbia anti-shivering protocol. *Neurocrit Care* 2011; **14**(3): 389–94.

Nadkarni, VM, et al. First documented rhythm and clinical outcome from in-hospital cardiac arrest among children and adults. *JAMA* 2006; **295**(1): 50–7.

Resuscitation Council (UK). *Advanced life support*, 6th edn. London: Resuscitation Council (UK) (2011)

Intensive Care Society. *Standards for the management of patients after cardiac arrest*. London: Intensive Care Society, 2008.

Holzer M. Targeted temperature management for comatose survivors of cardiac arrest. *N Engl J Med* 2010; **363**: 1256–64.

☼ Hypotension and shock

Hypotension is defined as systolic BP <90 mmHg and/or MAP <60 mmHg.
    Shock is defined as underperfusion of multiorgan systems. Clinical signs include tachycardia, hypotension, oliguria, and altered mental status.

Causes

Cardiogenic shock

(See causes listed on 🕮 p.122.)

Hypovolaemic shock: loss of intravascular volume

- Haemorrhage (e.g. trauma, aortic dissection, postoperative bleeding).
- GI loss of fluids (e.g. vomiting, diarrhoea, high-output stoma).
- Renal loss of fluids (e.g. diabetes insipidus, excessive diuretics).
- Fluid redistribution (e.g. burns, trauma, major surgery, sepsis, posture).

Distributive shock: venous dilation or obstruction

- Overdose of sedatives or vasodilators.
- Spinal/epidural anaesthesia or analgesia.
- Autonomic neuropathy (e.g. spinal cord lesion/trauma, Guillain–Barré).
- Anaphylaxis.
- Major vein compression (e.g. tumour, pregnancy, ascites, extensive intra-abdominal surgery).

Obstructive shock: impairing ventricular filling

- Cardiac tamponade (e.g. pericardial bleeding, pericardial effusion).
- Constrictive pericarditis.
- ↑intrathoracic pressure (e.g. tension pneumothorax, massive pleural effusion, mechanical ventilation).
- PE.

Miscellaneous causes

- Hepatic failure.
- Thyrotoxicosis.
- Myxoedema coma.
- Adrenal insufficiency.
- Poisoning (e.g. cyanide, carbon monoxide).

Presentation and assessment

Shock may be associated with a low cardiac output, or a compensatory high cardiac output; presentation depends on the 1° cause.

General presentation
- Anxiety and sweating.
- Tachypnoea, dyspnoea; Kussmaul's breathing (if hypoperfusion causes reduced tissue perfusion and a metabolic acidosis).
- Hypoxia, cyanosis.
- Hypotension: systolic BP <90 mmHg (or >30mmHg *below* normal resting pressure); or MAP <60 mmHg.
- Tachycardia (bradycardia may be a pre-terminal sign, or be associated with a arrhythmia).
  - Arrhythmias (e.g. AF, atrial flutter, VT, complete heart block)
- Cardiac hypoperfusion: angina, or ECG evidence of ischaemia.

- Renal hypoperfusion: oliguria/anuria, raised urea and creatinine.
- Neurological hypoperfusion: confusion, syncope, ↓GCS.

In low-output shock expect:
- Cold peripheries, poor peripheral perfusion and delayed capillary refill.
- Thready pulse with reduced pulse pressure.
- ↓cardiac output (cardiac index <2.2 L/minute/m² with adequate preload).
- ↑systemic vascular resistance.
- In hypovolaemic shock JVP/CVP is ↓; there may be evidence of fluid or blood loss, or venous pooling.
- In cardiogenic shock JVP/CVP may be ↑; S3 may be present:
  - Examination of the lungs may show evidence of pulmonary oedema
  - CXR and ECG are often abnormal with evidence of pulmonary oedema, enlarged heart, and/or arrhythmia

In high-output shock expect:
- Bounding pulse with wide pulse pressure.
- Strong apical cardiac impulse.
- Normal or ↑ cardiac output.
- ↓systemic vascular resistance.
- Depending on the degree of skin perfusion peripheries may or may not be warm; capillary refill may be brisk or reduced.
- Pyrexia and raised WCC where there is associated sepsis.

If the presentation does not fit a pattern, mixed shock should be considered (e.g. sepsis with myocardial dysfunction).

Investigations
- ABGs (metabolic acidosis, hypoxia, compensatory hypocapnia).
- FBC (anaemia with haemorrhage, raised WCC with infection).
- Coagulation screen (deranged with haemorrhage or DIC).
- U&Es (AKI), serum calcium, magnesium, phosphate.
- Serum glucose (hypo/hyperglycaemia).
- LFTs (deranged with ischaemia or liver failure).
- Cardiac enzymes (if cardiac ischaemia suspected).
- Blood, urine, sputum culture (if infection suspected).
- 12-lead ECG (cardiac ischaemia, arrhythmias).
- CXR (evidence of infection, cardiomegaly, pulmonary oedema).
- Echocardiography (cardiac tamponade, hypovolaemia, RV hypertension in PE, regional wall motion abnormality, aortic dissection).
- Cardiac output monitoring (pulmonary artery catheterization, TOD, or pulse contour analysis may assist in differentiating between low cardiac output or low SVR states).
- US and/or CT scan of chest, abdomen, pelvis (if occult haemorrhage is suspected).

Differential diagnoses
- Damped arterial pressure traces or poorly fitting BP cuffs can giving spurious readings, if in doubt re-check manually.
- Mild 'hypotension' may be a normal finding in fit healthy individuals.

Immediate management
- Give 100% O_2
- The airway may be compromised due to impaired conscious level:
  - Intubate the trachea as appropriate
  - If this is impossible (i.e. in a remote location) the patient can be placed in the recovery position (depending on other injuries)
- Ensure breathing/ventilation is adequate:
  - In severe shock ventilatory support (non-invasive or invasive) may be needed to optimize oxygenation, especially in fatigued patients
  - If pulmonary oedema is present treat appropriately (🕮 p.86)
- Assess hypotension: questions which need to be answered include:
  - Is this BP low for this patient? What is their normal BP? Is there evidence of, or potential for, impaired cerebral perfusion, cardiac ischaemia, oliguria?
- Treat any identifiable underlying cause requiring immediate attention:
  - Tension pneumothorax (🕮 p.80)
  - Cardiac tamponade (🕮 p.146)
  - Arrhythmias (🕮 pp.132 and 138)
  - Major haemorrhage (🕮 p.112)
  - Anaphylaxis (🕮 p.110)
- Take a focused clinical history, carefully examine the patient, and review notes/charts where possible; identify the likely cause.

Hypovolaemia or haemorrhage (🕮 p.112):
- Fluid resuscitate and treat underlying cause or proceed to surgery.
- Ensure IV access (typically 2 large-bore cannulae).
- Initial resuscitation is usually in the form of crystalloids/colloids or warmed blood in the case of haemorrhage, given rapidly until there are signs of adequate filling (restoration of MAP, neurological function, urine output; normalization of tachycardia).
- In haemorrhage awaiting source control (e.g. ruptured AAA, penetrating trauma) limited resuscitation targets may be necessary: palpable radial pulse, systolic BP ≤80 mmHg ('permissive hypotension').
- Inotropes/vasopressors can be used but may mask hypovolaemia.

Vasodilatation (🕮 p.108): treat underlying cause and commence fluid resuscitation, with/without vasopressor therapy:
- Response to fluid bolus may be predicted by ↑ cardiac output or CVP (if monitored) after straight leg raising (45° for 4 minutes).

Cardiogenic failure (🕮 p.122):
- Record 12-lead ECG and compare to previous ECGs, assessing for evidence of myocardial infarction/ischaemia (🕮 p.126).
- Aggressive fluid therapy is not recommended in cardiogenic shock, although up to 500 ml can be given initially.

Inotropes/vasoactive agents: noradrenaline or adrenaline may be indicated in septic shock. In the case of a mixed picture adrenaline or dopamine may be started until a clearer diagnosis is possible. Dobutamine has been used in cardiogenic shock, but may not improve outcome.

Further management

- Admit patients with refractory hypotension (unresponsive to moderate fluid resuscitation) into a suitable critical care facility.
- Continue respiratory support until cardiovascular stability is achieved.
- Arterial and/or central venous cannulation are likely to be needed.
- Monitoring may be needed to obtain information about:
  - Ventricular filling (e.g. CVP, echocardiography, pulmonary artery catheterization)
  - Cardiac output and SVR (e.g. echocardiography, oesophageal Doppler, pulse contour analysis, pulmonary artery catheterization)
- Optimize preload using crystalloids, colloids (or blood if required).
- Consider optimizing cardiac contractility using inotropes (e.g. adrenaline, dobutamine).
- Optimize SVR using vasoconstrictors (noradrenaline) or vasodilators (glyceryl trinitrate).
- Correct any electrolyte imbalance and severe metabolic acidosis (renal replacement therapy may become necessary).
- If there is no response to volume replacement, consider the possibility of spinal shock (🕮 p.409) or adrenal insufficiency (🕮 p.236).
- See Table 4.1 for drugs used to treat hypotension.

Interpretation of CVC variables

Central venous pressure (CVP)

- There is no 'normal' or 'average' CVP number, the measurement is determined by venous return and right ventricular compliance.
- CVP measurement should be regarded as a trend.
- It is conventional to volume load an under-resuscitated patient to a target CVP of approximately:
  - 8–10 mmHg in non-ventilated patients
  - 12–16 mmHg in ventilated patients
- *But* CVP monitoring is dynamic, i.e. patients should be volume-loaded until a rise in CVP (or cardiac output) is sustained:
  - Repeated fluid challenges are likely to be required in shocked patients with low intravascular volume with compensatory vasoconstriction (initial rises in CVP or cardiac output are often transient)
  - Vasodilatory challenges (e.g. general anaesthesia) will cause the CVP to fall
- Complete heart block, AF, tricuspid stenosis, and tricuspid regurgitation will lead to difficulty in interpreting CVP readings.

Central venous O_2 saturations ($ScvO_2$)

- $ScvO_2$ may be measured on blood drawn from a CVC (mixed venous blood, $S\bar{v}O_2$, must be drawn from a PAFC).
- Low values (<65%) are associated with a worse outcome in trauma, severe sepsis, myocardial infarction, and cardiac failure.
- $ScvO_2$ is affected by O_2 content, O_2 consumption, and cardiac output.
- $ScvO_2$ may be 'artificially' high in the presence of a significant shunt.
- It is conventional to resuscitate patients to a target $ScvO_2$ of >70%.
- Monitoring should be dynamic to ensure that any rise is sustained.

Causes of deranged systemic vascular resistance

↑*systemic vascular resistance*
- Hypothermia.
- Vasoconstriction, or vasoconstrictive drugs (e.g. noradrenaline).
- Sympathetic stimulation.

↓*systemic vascular resistance*
- Sepsis.
- Hyperthermia.
- Hyperthyroidism.
- A–V shunts.
- Liver failure.
- Vasodilators.
- Spinal/epidural block or spinal shock.

Flow rates of different gauge cannulae[1]

- 14 G (orange) 250–360 ml/minute
- 16 G (grey) 130–220 ml/minute
- 18 G (green) 75–120 ml/minute
- 20 G (pink) 40–80 ml/minute
- 22 G (blue)

[1] At 10 kPa via 110-cm tubing (internal diameter 4mm); source: This information was published in *Anaesthesia and Intensive Care A-Z: An Encyclopedia of Principles and Practice*, Yentis S, Hirsch N, Smith G, fourth edition, copyright Elsevier 2009.

Pitfalls/difficult situations

- A MAP of 65 mmHg in a young fit patient (e.g. due to an epidural) may cause no tissue hypoperfusion, whereas in patients with vascular disease it may lead to myocardial ischaemia (coronary blood occurs mainly in diastole), cerebral ischaemia, or acute pre-renal failure.
- Overlapping aetiologies and mixed pictures occur (e.g. sepsis with myocardial failure).
- ↑CVP and lack of response to inotropes in suspected cardiogenic shock could be due to cardiac tamponade, pulmonary hypertension/embolism, or right ventricular infarction; use of echocardiography, or a right heart catheter (or radiological examination for PE) may assist in making the diagnosis.

Further reading

Antonelli M, et al. Hemodynamic monitoring in shock and implications for management: international consensus conference. *Intensive Care Med* 2007; **33**: 575–59.

Dellinger RP, et al. Surviving Sepsis Campaign: international guidelines for management of severe sepsis and septic shock. *Crit Care Med* 2008; **36**: 296–327.

Jackson K, et al. The role of hypotensive resuscitation in the management of trauma. *J Intensive Care Soc* 2009; **10**(2): 109–14.

Maizel J, et al. Diagnosis of central hypovolemia by using passive leg raising. *Intensive Care Med* 2007; **33**: 1133–8.

Pinsky MR. Hemodynamic evaluation and monitoring in the ICU. *Chest* 2007; **132**: 2020–9.

Rady MY. Bench-to-bedside review: Resuscitation in the emergency department. *Crit Care* 2005; **9**: 170–6.

Table 4.1 Drugs used to treat hypotension

Drug	Dose	Comments
Adrenaline / Epinephrine	0.5–1 mg IM in anaphylaxis 0.5–1 mg IV/IO in cardiac arrest 0.05–3 µg/kg/minute IV infusion	β- and α-agonist; increases myocardial contractility, heart rate, and SVR Agent of choice in anaphylaxis, cardiac arrest, and severe hypotension of undiagnosed cause Can cause increases in serum lactate
Noradrenaline/ Norepinephrine	0.05–3 µg/kg/minute IV infusion	Predominantly α-agonist: (increases SVR); agent of choice in high-output and/or septic shock Should be used with caution in hypovolemic shock and cardiogenic shock
Dopamine	0.5–10 µg/kg/minute IV infusion	<5 µg/kg/minute, predominantly dopaminergic effects: increases renal/splanchnic perfusion 5–10 µg/kg/minute, mainly β and some α-agonism: increases heart rate, contractility and SVR Often used as first-line agent for moderate hypotension until the cause is established
Dobutamine	0.5–10 µg/kg/minute IV infusion	Predominantly β-agonistic: increases heart rate and myocardial contractility, and reduces systemic vascular resistance by dilating vascular supply to the muscles Often used to treat cardiogenic shock Can worsen hypotension if given in hypovolaemia
Metaraminol	Bolus 0.5 mg over 2–3 minutes	Used to increase systemic vascular resistance in high-output failure; boluses can be repeated until IV infusion of vasopressor is established
Phenylephrine	Bolus 0.1mg–0.5mg over 2–3 minutes	Same as metaraminol
Vasopressin	0.01–0.04 units/minutes IV infusion	Used to increase SVR in severe refractory septic shock No evidence of superiority over noradrenaline
Terlipressin	1ng IV 8-hourly	Same as vasopressin

:☹: Anaphylaxis

Anaphylaxis is a severe, life-threatening, hypersensitivity reaction.

Causes

- Insect bites (especially wasp and bee stings).
- Foods and food additives (especially peanuts, fish, eggs).
- Drugs and IV infusions, especially:
  - Antibiotics and vaccines
  - Colloids and blood products
  - IV contrast media
  - Pabrinex, parenteral vitamin K
  - Anaesthetic induction agents, neuromuscular blocking drugs
- Latex allergy.
- Idiopathic (no readily identifiable cause).

Presentation and assessment

Any combination of:

- Cardiovascular collapse (75% of cases): cardiac arrest; or tachycardia, hypotension, and other signs of shock (🕮 p.104).
- Bronchospasm (40%): wheeze, cough, and/or accompanying desaturation, tachypnoea and dyspnoea.
- Angioedema (12%): leading to laryngeal oedema and/or airway obstruction/stridor.
- Cutaneous signs (72%): erythema, cutaneous rash, urticaria.

Investigations

- Take blood samples for mast cell tryptase level:
  - As soon as possible after treatment of initial reaction, *and*
  - 1 hour after the reaction, *and* 6–24 hours after the reaction
- ABGs (metabolic and/or respiratory acidosis).
- FBC.
- Clotting studies, fibrinogen (deranged with associated DIC).
- U&Es, LFTs, magnesium.
- CXR (to exclude differentials).

Tryptase samples should be stored at −20°C until it can be analysed. Concentrations peak at 1 hour, and concentrations of >20 ng/ml suggest anaphylaxis. A negative test does not exclude anaphylaxis. An immunologist may advise further tests after recovery.

Differential diagnoses

- Airway/ETT obstruction, or endobronchial intubation.
- Tension pneumothorax/haemothorax.
- Air embolus/amniotic fluid embolus/fat embolus.
- Severe bronchospasm/asthma.
- Distributive shock (e.g. sepsis/neuraxial blockade/spinal cord injury).
- Localized cutaneous reactions (e.g. type IV allergy: T cell mediated 6–48 hours after allergen exposure).
- Hereditary angioneurotic oedema.
- Thyroid crisis or carcinoid syndrome.

Immediate management

- Stop trigger agents and call for help.
- Give 100% O_2
- Secure the airway and ensure breathing/ventilation is adequate; early endotracheal intubation may be required, especially in angio-oedema.
- If already intubated exclude airway/breathing system obstruction.
- Lie patient flat with legs elevated.
- Give adrenaline (epinephrine): either IM or IV
  - IM dose 0.5–1 mg (0.5–1 ml of 1:1000) up to every 10 minutes
  - IV dose 50–100 mcg (0.5–1 ml of 1:10 000) over 1 minute, and repeat as necessary (only give if you are familiar with IV adrenaline usage)
  - Continuous ECG monitoring is advisable whilst giving adrenaline
- Ensure IV access and commence rapid infusion of crystalloid.
- Adrenaline infusions may be required.
- If bronchospasm persists give: salbutamol 250 mcg slow IV or 2.5–5 mg via nebulizer; with/without magnesium sulphate 8 mmol IV (2g) and/or aminophylline 250 mg IV slowly (up to 5 mg/kg) if not already on theophylline.

Second-line therapies (when time allows):
- Give chlorphenamine 10 mg IV slowly (ranitidine 50 mg IV may be given as well, but is of unknown benefit).
- Give hydrocortisone 200 mg IV, then 100 mg IV 6-hourly.

Further management

- If hypotension persists/relapses (5% of cases) start inotrope infusions.
- Deflate the ETT cuff prior to extubation in order to ascertain a leak (to gauge the degree of airway oedema).
- Refer the patient to an immunologist; include copies of the notes, drug chart, and a full description of the reaction chronology.
- Serum IgE and skin-prick tests will be required.
- Report anaphylactic reactions on a CSM 'yellow card'.
- If this was a 'wrong blood' reaction, send all products back to the lab and involve a haematologist.

Pitfalls/difficult situations

- Monitor for a 2° deterioration or biphasic response.
- Watch for the development of ARDS or DIC (may manifest hours later).
- Myocardial infarction and arrhythmias can occur, especially if there is pre-existing ischaemic heart disease, or if hypoxia/acidosis is present.
- Stridor may be mistaken for bronchospasm, and vice versa.
- Do not forget that colloids and latex can cause anaphylaxis:
  - Latex anaphylaxis may present up to 30–60 minutes after an event due to delayed airborne exposure or mucous membrane contact.

Further reading

Association of Anaesthetists of Great Britain and Ireland. Suspected anaphylactic reactions associated with anaesthesia. *Anaesthesia* 2009; **64**: 199–211.

NICE. *Anaphylaxis: assessment to confirm an anaphylactic episode and the decision to refer after emergency treatment for a suspected anaphylactic episode.* London: NICE, 2011.

✪ Haemorrhagic shock

Haemorrhagic shock occurs when loss of intravascular blood leads to hypotension and underperfusion of organs. Initially the body responds to hypovolaemia by peripheral vasoconstriction and tachycardia. Oliguria (urine <0.5 ml/kg/hour), and signs of organ failure (e.g. dyspnoea, myocardial failure, drowsiness) appear later.

Causes

- Trauma.
- GI bleeding.
- Surgery or postoperative/post-procedure bleeding.
- Bleeding in response to trivial trauma, associated with:
  - Coagulation factor abnormality (e.g. haemophilia)
  - Thrombocytopaenia
  - Splenomegaly
- Other occult bleeding (thoracic, intra-abdominal or retroperitoneal; e.g. ruptured aortic aneurysm or ruptured ectopic pregnancy).

Presentation and assessment

- There may be a bleeding site, or blood in postoperative drains.
- Certain mechanisms of trauma can cause occult bleeding (📖 p.411).
- Certain patients are more likely to have a coagulopathy (📖 p.302):
  - Patients receiving anticoagulant therapy
  - Patients with a history of congenital disease (may carry a card)
  - Patients being treated for haematological malignancy

In healthy individuals the physiological response to haemorrhage varies according to the volume of blood lost.

≤15% (0.75 L[1]) loss of total blood volume (TBV) results in:
- Slight tachycardia and mild peripheral vasoconstriction (mildly ↑diastolic BP and narrowed pulse pressure).
- Thirst may occur as accompanying symptom.

15–30% (0.75–1.5 L[1]) TBV loss:
- Pulse rate increases to 100–120/minute (see 📖 Pitfalls/difficult situations).
- Vasoconstriction with clearly raised diastolic BP, narrowed pulse pressure and delayed capillary refill (>2 seconds).
- Oliguria.
- Patient may be anxious.

30–40% (1.5–2 L[1]) TBV loss:
- Systolic hypotension develops; pulse becomes thready.
- Dyspnoea develops.
- Agitation ensues.

>40% (≥2 L[1]) TBV loss:
- Severe hypotension.
- Anuria.
- Ashen complexion.
- Drowsiness or unconsciousness.

1 Assuming a with total blood volume of about 5 L (70–80 ml/kg).

Investigations

Blood crossmatch samples should be taken, other investigations include:
- Diagnostic (to identify the bleeding source):
  - Plain radiographs (especially of pelvis and chest following trauma)
  - Abdominal US (may identify free blood, ruptured ectopic pregnancy, or aortic aneurysm)
  - CT scan, of pelvis, abdomen, or chest according to clinical indication
  - Diagnostic peritoneal lavage
  - Endoscopy (for suspected GI bleeding)
  - Angiography (may be diagnostic and/or potentially therapeutic)
  - Radio-labelled bleeding scan (may be considered if source unclear)
  - β-HCG, urine or blood (may aid in the diagnosis of ectopic pregnancy)
- To monitor progress and identify the development of complications:
  - ABGs (metabolic acidosis)
  - FBC (anaemia, thrombocytopaenia); near-patient testing may be available, e.g. Haemacue®
  - Coagulation studies, including fibrinogen (↑ PT/APTT, ↓fibrinogen in DIC); near-patient testing may be available, e.g. ROTEM®
  - U&Es, LFTs, ECG (tachycardia, possible ischaemia)

Differential diagnoses

Any cause of shock must be considered, particularly:
- Other causes of shock associated with trauma (e.g. tension pneumothorax, cardiac tamponade, cardiac contusion, spinal cord lesion).
- Hypovolaemic shock 2° to fluid losses other than blood:
  - Profound dehydration (e.g. DKA, vomiting, diarrhoea, diuresis)
  - Massive 'third-space' losses (e.g. profound ileus, sepsis, major burn)
- Cardiogenic shock; left or right ventricular failure (e.g. myocardial infarction, aortic stenosis, hypertrophic cardiomyopathy, PE).
- Distributive shock (e.g. sepsis, anaphylaxis, neuraxial blockade).

Immediate management

- Give 100% O_2 initially, then titrate SpO_2 to 94–98%.
- In cases of trauma ensure cervical spine protection.
- Secure the airway and ensure breathing/ventilation is adequate; endotracheal intubation may be required.
- Assess the degree of blood loss and control haemorrhage if possible:
  - Compression/elevation of external bleeding sites, or use of a tourniquet in life-threatening haemorrhage from a limb
  - The patient may require immediate life-saving surgery (e.g. ectopic pregnancy, ruptured spleen)
  - Stabilize fractures
  - Consider endoscopic or interventional radiological procedures
  - Reverse the effects of any anticoagulants if they are present (e.g. using vitamin K IV, or prothrombin complex IV)
  - Administering tranexamic acid IV 1 g and vitamin K IV 10 mg may promote haemostasis in major haemorrhage

- Commence circulatory support in shocked patients:
  - Head-down tilt (Trendelenburg) may be required
  - Insert large-bore (14 G) IV cannulae into both antecubital fossa
  - In difficult cases the use of femoral veins, external jugular veins may be required; or an IV cutdown at the ankle or antecubital fossa (📖 p. 540) or insert IO access
  - Take a sample for blood crossmatching when inserting cannulae
  - Start restoring intravascular volume (📖 p.116)
  - Commence blood transfusion[1] alongside crystalloids/colloids as soon as possible if bleeding is >30%TBV, >1.5 L, or Hb <8 g/dl with ongoing haemorrhage
  - O-negative or type-specific blood may be required in severe haemorrhage whilst waiting for crossmatched blood
- In haemorrhage awaiting source control (e.g. ruptured AAA, penetrating trauma) limited resuscitation targets may be necessary: palpable radial pulse, systolic BP ≤80 mmHg ('permissive hypotension').
- Use inotropes/vasopressors with caution (they may mask under-resuscitation).
- Where there is massive blood loss (≥6 units of blood or ≥30% TBV lost) involve haematologists for guidance on appropriate blood and component therapy; common protocols include the following:
  - FFP (12 ml/kg; or approximately 2 bags) if PT or APTT >1.5 × normal, or if more than 4–6 units of stored blood is transfused
  - Platelets (0.5–1 units/10 kg body weight; or 1–2 adult doses) if the count is <50 × 10^9/L
  - Cryoprecipitate (1 pack/10 kg body weight) if fibrinogen <0.8 g/L
  - Repeat coagulation studies every 2 hours, or after every 4–6 units of packed red cells
- Consider using recombinant factor VIIa.
- Cell-salvage may be available in some settings.

[1] Adhere strictly to the cross checking procedures for blood replacement.

Further management
- Many centres now have 'major haemorrhage packs' consisting of various quantities of packed red cells, fresh frozen plasma, cryoprecipitate, and platelets for use in the event of massive transfusion requirements.
- Look for and treat complications of massive blood transfusion (e.g. hypothermia, hypocalcaemia, hyperkalaemia, coagulation factor depletion, thrombocytopaenia, metabolic acidosis).
- Some or all of the following monitoring is likely to be needed:
  - CVC to assess intravascular fluid status
  - Urinary catheterization to allow urine output measurements
  - Arterial line insertion for invasive BP measurements
  - CO monitoring to assess cardiac contractility and vascular resistance
- Inotropic support may be required, but this should be discontinued as soon as volume replacement and the control of bleeding allows; adrenaline or noradrenaline are the initial agents of choice.

Major haemorrhage protocol

Once severe haemorrhagic shock has been identified contact consultant-in-charge, switchboard, haematologist/blood bank; provide the following information:

- The contact name and telephone number for doctor in charge
- Location of patient and any *known* patient details:
  - Name, Date-of-Birth, Gender
  - Identification no., Estimated weight, ABO/Rh group
  - Type and volume of blood components required
- Send pre-transfusion screening sample for group and antibody screen, and FBC and coagulation studies.
- Send request forms for any blood products (including O-negative)
- Red cells needed immediately?
  - Use emergency O-negative from designated fridge or blood bank
- Red cells needed in 15 minutes?
  - ABO/RhD group-specific available within 15 minutes of receiving sample; retrospective full crossmatch carried within 30 minutes
- Red cells needed in 45 minutes?
  - Full crossmatch performed and blood released within 45 minutes of receiving sample; *if patient has a historic sample and a group and screen on current sample, blood may be available immediately*
- Platelets, FFP, cryoprecipitate needed?
  - Consider adjuvant therapy with antifibrinolytic (e.g. tranexamic acid) or recombinant factor VIIa (NB this is an unlicensed indication)
  - Anticipate platelet count $<50 \times 10^9$/L after 1.5–2 × blood volume replacement, aim for $>100 \times 10^9$/L for multiple/CNS trauma; $>75 \times 10^9$/L for other situations
  - Anticipate coagulation factor deficiency after blood loss of 1–1.5 × blood volume; aim for PT and APTT <1.5 × normal and fibrinogen >1.0 g/L; allow for 30 minutes thawing time and give 12–15 ml/kg (1 litre/4 units for an adult). If FFP required before laboratory results available; take sample for PT, APTT, fibrinogen before transfusion
  - Cryoprecipitate may be needed to replace fibrinogen and FVIII, aim for fibrinogen >1.0 g/L; allow for 30 minutes thawing time and give 2 × 5 donation pools for mid-sized adults

Use crystalloids/colloids alongside blood products as required using wide-bore venous access to maintain normal BP and urine output >0.5ml/kg/hour. Use blood warmers where possible.

Identify/control source of bleeding where possible (may require surgical, endoscopic or radiological intervention); use cell salvage if possible/appropriate. In patients with cardiac or large vessel injury volume replacement may need to be restricted, discuss with the surgical team.

Treat any underlying causes of DIC where possible.

Check FBC, PT, APTT, fibrinogen, biochemical profile, blood gases; and repeat every 4 hours, or after FFP or 1/3 blood volume replacement.

Pitfalls/difficult situations

- Lack of clinical improvement despite apparently adequate resuscitation may indicate continuing bleeding, or suggest another form of shock.
- Elevated CVP may indicate the pneumothorax, cardiac tamponade, or cardiac contusion; these can also occur alongside major haemorrhage.
- Where concealed bleeding is suspected enlist the help of surgeons, radiologists, and GI endoscopists (endoscopic cautery, sclerotherapy, or open surgery may be required to stop bleeding).
- Long-bone fractures can be a source of significant occult blood loss.
- Wound drains can become blocked or displaced leading to underestimation of blood loss.
- Tachycardia does not always develop:
  - Up to 10% of patients with intra-abdominal bleeding respond with bradycardia, or fail to develop tachycardia
  - Elderly patients and those on β-blockers do not develop tachycardia and may develop hypotension at relatively lesser blood loss
- Patients with cardiac illness or severe coexisting morbidity do not compensate well for hypovolaemia; athletes, children, and pregnant women may initially compensate well for blood loss.

Fluids suitable for use in haemorrhage

- Crystalloids: 0.9% saline,[1] Hartmann's solution[2]
  - Often used as first-line fluid until diagnosis becomes clear
  - Only approximately 1/3 of the volume remains intravascular, 3L of crystalloid are needed to replace every litre of blood lost
  - Consider colloids/blood if the requirement is >2L
- Colloids: gelatins, starches,[3] human albumin solution (HAS).
  - Remain intravascular for 4–6 hours, therefore blood volume can be replaced on a 'one-for-one' basis
  - Can cause coagulopathies if more than 1.5L is given
- Blood,[4] if blood loss is >30%TBV, >1.5 l or Hb <8 g/dl:
  - If a massive blood transfusion is required (≥6 units of blood), look for and prevent coagulopathies and problems related to massive blood transfusion

[1] Also known as normal saline

[2] Also known as compound sodium lactate (CSL); Ringer's lactate is equivalent

[3] See 🕮 p. 261 for a description of some of the gelatin and starch containing fluids available

[4] Blood for transfusion is likely to be packed red cells (PRC), rather than whole blood

---

Further reading

Association of Anaesthetists of Great Britain and Ireland. *Blood transfusion and the anaesthetist: blood component therapy.* London: AAGBI, 2005.

Association of Anaesthetists of Great Britain and Ireland. *Blood transfusion and the anaesthetist: management of massive haemorrhage.* AAGBI, 2010.

Jackson K, et al. The role of hypotensive resuscitation in the management of trauma. *J Intensive Care Soc* 2009; **10**(2): 109–14.

McClelland DBL, et al. *Handbook of transfusion medicine,* 4th edn. London: United Kingdom Blood Services, 2007.

Rossaint R, et al. Management of bleeding following major trauma: an updated European guideline. *Crit Care* 2010; **14**: R52.

Table 4.2 Coagulants/antifibrinolytics

	Administration	Compatibility	Indication	Dosing
Fresh frozen plasma (FFP)	Use a 170–μm filter Use within 2 hours	Use ABO-compatible plasma	Deficiencies of factors II, V, VII, IX, X, and XI; reversal of warfarin; massive transfusion; antithrombin III deficiency	INR or APTTR > 1.5× normal, infuse 15 ml/kg
Cryoprecipitate (CPT)	Use a 170–μm filter		Haemophilia A; von Willebrand disease; Factor XIII deficiency; following massive transfusion	Infuse 10–15 units of if fibrinogen < 0.8 g/L
Platelet concentrate (PC)	Use a 170–μm filter Shelf life 5 days	ABO-incompatible platelets safe	Thrombocytopaenia or platelet abnormality & bleeding; bleeding prophylaxis in severe thrombocytopaenia; following massive transfusion	If platelets < 50 × 10⁹/L infuse 1unit/10 kg body weight
Vitamin K			Antagonism of warfarin; hepatic coagulopathies	1–10mg IM or slow IV bolus
Factor VIIa			Licensed: haemophilia A or B with inhibitors to Factor VIII or Factor IX; congenital FVII deficiency Unlicensed: massive blood transfusion, trauma	100micrograms/kg repeated at 1–2 hourly intervals if required
Protamine			Reversal of unfractionated heparin	1 mg slow IV, neutralizes 80–100 units of heparin
Tranexamic acid			Menorrhagia; haemophilia (prior to surgery); cardiac surgery, to minimize blood loss; minimize surgical blood loss; reversal of thrombolytic therapy	10–20mg/kg slow IV injection two to four times daily

☼ Septic shock

(See also sepsis, 📖 p.322.)

Severe infection may cause profound vasodilatation with/without myo-cardial depression. The resulting hypoperfusion results in organ damage.

A definition of sepsis may be found on 📖 p.322. Septic shock is defined as sepsis-induced hypotension despite fluid resuscitation, with perfusion abnormalities.

Causes

Most infections have the potential to cause septic shock, and variations will occur according to individual hospital case mix. Sepsis is more commonly caused by Gram-positive than Gram-negative bacterial infections. Fungal (up to 5–10%) and viral infections may also be responsible.

Common sites of infection:
- Respiratory (~38%).
- 1° bacteraemia (~15%).
- Wound/soft tissue (~9%).
- Abdominal (~9%).
- Genitourinary (~9%).
- Device related (~5%).
- Endocarditis (~1.5%).
- CNS (~1.5%).
- Other/unidentified (~12%).

Predisposing factors include:
- Extremes of age.
- Major surgery.
- Loss of tissue coverage (e.g. burns or trauma).
- Chronic disease (e.g. heart failure, COPD, diabetes, CKD).
- Immunocompromise (e.g. HIV, chemotherapy, haematological malignancy, neutropaenia, malnutrition, alcoholism and/or hepatic failure).
- Implants or indwelling vascular access.

Presentation and assessment

- Anxiety and sweating.
- Tachypnoea, dyspnoea, hypoxia, cyanosis.
- Cardiovascular findings may include:
  - Hypotension (systolic BP <90 mmHg, or >30 mmHg below normal resting systolic pressure, or MAP <60 mmHg)
  - Tachycardia (bradycardia may occur as a pre-terminal sign)
  - Arrhythmias (particularly AF, atrial flutter or SVT)
  - There may be evidence of ischaemia/angina
  - ↓JVP/CVP
- Cardiac output (CO) monitoring may reveal:
  - ↑CO (or relatively ↓ in severe sepsis)
  - Reduced systemic vascular resistance (SVR)
- Renal: oliguria, raised urea and creatinine, AKI.
- Neurological: syncope, ↓consciousness or confusion.
- Skin: peripheries may initially be warm and well perfused, even flushed; later poor peripheral perfusion may occur.

There may be evidence of infection:
- Pyrexia (or relative hypothermia) or rigors.
- High or low WCC, or raised CRP.
- Obvious abscesses, frank pus in wounds, wound drains or in urine.
- Examination of devices and lines which have been inserted may reveal evidence of inflammation around entry site (e.g. joint prosthesis, central venous catheters, epidural catheters).
- Other symptoms vary according to the system(s) affected: respiratory (📖 p.334), abdominal (📖 p.346), wound/soft tissue (📖 p.342), genitourinary (📖 p.344), endocarditis (📖 p.338), CNS (📖 p.340).

Investigations
- ABGs (metabolic acidosis).
- Lactate, arterial or venous (raised with hypoperfusion).
- FBC (high or low WCC, thrombocytopaenia).
- Clotting screen, fibrinogen (raised PT/APTT and low fibrinogen in DIC).
- U&Es (raised urea/creatinine in AKI).
- LFTs, serum magnesium, calcium, and phosphate (all may be deranged).
- Blood glucose (hypo- or hyperglycaemia).
- CRP/ESR; procalcitonin may be available in some centres (all may be raised).
- Full septic screen (this should include 2–3 blood cultures, including blood from indwelling lines and a peripheral stab; urine and sputum culture).
- ECG (if arrhythmia or ischaemia suspected).
- CXR (if a respiratory source suspected).
- Echocardiography, TTE or TOE (if endocarditis suspected or to assess LV function).
- Other investigations aimed at locating a septic focus may include:
  - CT abdomen, pelvis, chest, or head
  - Lumbar puncture (see 📖 p.554)
  - Wound swabs, throat swabs, or speculum exam and vaginal swabs
  - Nasopharyngeal viral swabs (for viral PCR)
  - BAL (e.g. for culture, viral/PCP PCR, fungal culture, AFBs, immunofluorescence)
  - Stool (for culture, toxin detection, or ova/cysts/parasite detection)
  - Serum, urine, or other fluid, for antigen testing (e.g. urine *Legionella* antigen testing)

Differential diagnoses
Any cause of shock must be considered, particularly:
- Cardiogenic shock; left or right ventricular failure (e.g. myocardial infarction, aortic stenosis, hypertrophic cardiomyopathy, PE).
- Distributive shock (e.g. sepsis, anaphylaxis, neuraxial blockade).
- Haemorrhagic shock.
- Hypovolaemic shock 2° to fluid losses other than blood:
  - Profound dehydration (e.g. DKA, vomiting, diarrhoea, diuresis)
  - Massive 'third-space' losses (e.g. ileus, sepsis, major burn)

Immediate management

- Give 100% O_2 initially, then titrate to SpO_2 94–98%.
- Secure the airway; endotracheal intubation may be required.
- Ensure breathing/ventilation is adequate:
  - Fatigue may lead to respiratory failure; NIV may be of benefit
  - In severe shock, endotracheal intubation and full ventilatory support may be needed
- Ensure adequate IV access: typically 2 large-bore (≥16 G) cannulae.
- Take all appropriate cultures: ensure 1–2 percutaneous blood culture samples; also sample blood from each intravascular catheter.
- Commence appropriate antibiotics, ideally within the first hour:
  - For suggested empirical antibiotics see: respiratory (🕮 p.334), abdominal (🕮 p.346), wound/soft tissue (🕮 p.342), genitourinary (🕮 p.344), endocarditis (🕮 p.338), CNS (🕮 p.340), neutropaenic sepsis (🕮 p.309).
- Commence circulatory support in patients with hypotension or elevated serum lactate.
- Treat any identifiable underlying cause, make a full survey for likely sources of infection, take a focused clinical history, and review notes and charts where possible.
- Perform arterial and/or central venous cannulation for monitoring.
- Resuscitate with crystalloids/colloids, aiming for:
  - CVP 8–12 mmHg (or 12–16 mmHg in ventilated patients)
  - MAP ≥65 mmHg (higher in the elderly or chronically hypertensive)
  - Urine output ≥0.5 ml/kg/hour
  - Central venous or mixed venous oxygen saturations ≥70%
- Consider red blood cell transfusion to achieve a haematocrit ≥30% if venous oxygen saturation <70% despite a CVP of 8–12 mmHg.
- Consider dobutamine up to 20 mcg/kg/minute if venous oxygen saturation <70%, or if cardiac output is low despite fluid resuscitation.
- Vasopressor therapy with noradrenaline 0.05–3 µg/kg/minute or dopamine 0.5–10 µg/kg/minute (via a central catheter) is indicated if fluid challenges fail to restore adequate BP and organ perfusion, or until fluid resuscitation restores adequate perfusion.
- Remove intravascular access devices if they are suspected of harbouring infection, after establishing other vascular access.
- If required, arrange surgery to remove any focus of infection.

Further management

(See 🕮 p.322.)
- Admit the patient into a suitable critical care facility.
- Consider instituting monitoring to obtain information about:
  - Ventricular filling/function: echocardiography
  - Cardiac output and systemic vascular resistance: transoesophageal Doppler, pulse contour analysis, pulmonary artery catheter
- Correct any electrolyte imbalances.
- Consider treating pyrexia using antipyretics and/or peripheral cooling.
- Vasopressin 0.01–0.04 units/minute may be added for refractory shock.
- Reassess antimicrobial regimen within 72 hours and adjust according to culture results.

Treat or prevent complications
- Respiratory:
  - ALI/ARDS: use a lung protective ventilation strategy (📖 p.53)
  - Ventilator-associated pneumonia precautions (📖 p.383)
  - Use a weaning protocol
- Renal:
  - There is no place for 'renal dose' dopamine
  - Severe metabolic acidosis may require renal replacement therapy (CVVH or IHD); or bicarbonate therapy (if pH ≤7.15)
- Haematology:
  - Do not use erythropoietin to treat sepsis-related anaemia
  - Do not use FFP to correct laboratory clotting abnormalities unless there is active bleeding or invasive procedures are planned
  - Correct fibrinogen in DIC if there is active bleeding, or a high risk of bleeding
  - Minimize blood product usage by following a restrictive transfusion policy (📖 p.299—aim for ≥7.0 g/dl where there is no bleeding or coronary artery disease) and for platelets (📖 p.304 – transfuse if <10 × 10⁹/L, or if 10–30 × 10⁹/L and there is a bleeding risk, or if <50 × 10⁹/L and surgery or invasive procedures are planned)
  - Do not use antithrombin therapy

Pitfalls/difficult situations
- Mixed pictures of shock often occur as sepsis may coexist with other diseases such as cardiac failure.
- New infections are common in patients already admitted to critical care and are often picked up via routine blood sampling (e.g. raised WCC) or on X-rays performed for other reasons.
- A low threshold should be maintained for suspecting vascular access catheters as a source of bacteraemia.
- Organisms are often not isolated from culture (in up to 40% of cases).
- The use of steroids is controversial; if used, a typical regimen might be hydrocortisone 50 mg IV 6-hourly for 3–7 days, (with/without fludrocortisone 50 mcg PO daily).
- Activated protein C is no longer recommended.

Further reading
Angus DC, et al. Epidemiology of severe sepsis in the United States: analysis of incidence, outcome, and associated costs of care. *Crit Care Med* 2001; **29**(7):1303–10.

Chu YF, et al. Stress-related mucosal disease in the critically ill patient: Risk factors and strategies to prevent stress-related bleeding in the intensive care unit. *W J Emerg Med* 2010; **1**(1): 32–6.

Dellinger RP, et al. Surviving Sepsis Campaign: International guidelines for management of severe sepsis and septic shock. *Crit Care Med* 2008; **36**: 296–327.

Rivers E, et al. Early goal-directed therapy in the treatment of severe sepsis and septic shock. *N Engl J Med* 2001; **345**(19): 1368–77.

Rivers E. The outcome of patients presenting to the emergency department with severe sepsis or septic shock. *Crit Care* 2006; **10**(4): 154.

Sprung CL, et al. Hydrocortisone therapy for patients with septic shock (CORTICUS). *N Engl J Med* 2008; **358**: 111–24.

Surviving Sepsis Campaign ® website: ✍ <http://www.survivingsepsis.org>.

The NICE-SUGAR Study Investigators. Intensive versus conventional glucose control in critically ill patients. *N Engl J Med* 2009; **360**: 1283–97.

:❂: Cardiogenic shock

Cardiogenic shock occurs when cardiac output falls acutely and fails to provide adequate organ perfusion. The commonest cause is myocardial stunning following myocardial infarction, ischaemia, or reperfusion.

Causes

Left ventricular failure
- Pump failure:
  - Myocardial ischaemia/infarction/reperfusion
  - Acute dilated cardiomyopathy (e.g. peripartum, post-viral, sepsis)
  - Stress cardiomyopathies (e.g. takotsubo syndrome)
  - Myocarditis (e.g. viral)
  - Myocardial contusion (following chest/abdominal trauma)
- Outflow obstruction:
  - Aortic stenosis or coarctation
  - Malignant hypertension
  - Hypertrophic obstructive cardiomyopathy
- Valve abnormalities (mitral, aortic).

Right ventricular failure
- Pump failure (e.g. myocardial ischaemia/infarction/reperfusion).
- Outflow obstruction:
  - Acute pulmonary hypertension (caused by hypoxia, acidosis, PEEP, ARDS, vasculitis, extremes of lung volume, vasopressors)
  - Pulmonary embolism (air, thrombus, amniotic fluid, tumour, fat)
- Valve abnormalities (tricuspid, pulmonary).

Causes of valve dysfunction include
- Native valves: infective endocarditis, perforation, rupture, prolapse, papillary muscle dysfunction, thrombosis.
- Prosthetic valves: thrombosis, disintegration.

Global direct myocardial depression (negative inotropy)
- Metabolic (e.g. hypoxia, acidosis, hypocalcaemia, hypophosphataemia, hypothyroidism).
- Drugs (e.g. β-blockers, calcium-channel blockers, alcohol, IV or volatile anaesthetic agents, local anaesthetic toxicity).
- Sepsis.
- Hypothermia.

Arrhythmias
- Severe bradycardia or tachycardia.
- Loss of atrial contribution to ventricular filling in acute atrial fibrillation may provoke cardiogenic failure if there is underlying cardiac disease.

High output states
- Hyperthermia, hyperthyroidism, MH, NMS.
- Severe anaemia.
- Heart disease and pregnancy.
- Large arteriovenous shunts.
- Severe Paget's disease.
- Beri-beri (thiamine deficiency).

Presentation and assessment

Acute cardiogenic shock is often associated with acute cardiogenic pulmonary oedema (🕮 p.86). In situations where it is not, or where pulmonary
oedema has been treated, the predominant symptoms are of hypoperfusion of vital organs, and fluid maldistribution.

Signs and symptoms may include:
- Anxiety and sweating.
- Chest pain (rarely present).
- Tachypnoea, dyspnoea, respiratory distress, cyanosis, hypoxia.
- Pulmonary oedema (if present):
  - Patient may prefer sitting, or leaning forward (orthopnoea)
  - Cough and/or frothy pink sputum
  - Bilateral crackles/wheeze; ↑IPPV inflation pressures
- Poor perfusion may result in pallor or mottled skin, cold peripheries:
  - Prolonged capillary refill (>2 seconds)
  - Dizziness, syncope, agitation, confusion, ↓consciousness
  - Oliguria, acidaemia
- Cardiovascular findings may include:
  - Hypotension (systolic BP <90 mmHg, or >30 mmHg below normal
    resting pressure, or MAP <60 mmHg)
  - Tachycardia (bradycardia may precipitate cardiogenic shock, or be a
    pre-terminal sign associated with it)
  - Raised JVP (>4 cm from sternal angle) or CVP (>15 cmH$_2$O)
  - Gallop rhythm; S3 heart sound may be present
  - Enlarged and tender liver, ascites, sacral/leg oedema
- Cardiac output monitoring or PAFC catheterization may demonstrate:
  - ↓cardiac output (cardiac index < 2L/minute/m^2)
  - PAOP may be ↑ (>18 mmHg)
  - ↑systemic vascular resistance.

Investigations

- ABGs (hypoxia, metabolic acidosis).
- FBC (to exclude anaemia, raised WCC in sepsis).
- U&Es, (AKI).
- LFTs, blood glucose, serum magnesium, calcium, and phosphate.
- TFTs (hypo/hyperthyroidism); cardiac enzymes (if infarct suspected).
- Urine/blood βHCG (to exclude pregnancy/eclampsia).
- Blood cultures, viral serology (if infective endocarditis or myocarditis
  suspected).
- ECG (tachycardia, arrhythmias, A–V dissociation, ischaemia/MI, LVH).
- CXR (enlarged heart size, evidence of pulmonary oedema).
- Echocardiography, TTE/TOE (LV/RV systolic or diastolic dysfunction,
  regional wall motion abnormalities, valve disease, chamber dimensions,
  contractility, filling status).

Differential diagnoses

- Any cause of hypotension (e.g. tension pneumothorax, cardiac
  tamponade, aortic dissection, sepsis, haemorrhagic shock,
  anaphylaxis).

- Pulmonary oedema not of cardiac origin (e.g. fluid overload, neurogenic or negative pressure pulmonary oedema, inhalation injury, ARDS).

Immediate management

- Give 100% O_2 initially, then titrate to SpO_2 94–98%.
- Secure the airway and ensure breathing/ventilation is adequate; NIV or endotracheal intubation and ventilation may be required.
- Ensure IV access.
- In cardiogenic shock following cardiac surgery always consider the possibility of bleeding or cardiac tamponade (see 🕮 pp.146 and 394).
- If possible obtain bedside TTE/TOE to assist in diagnosis/treatment.
- Record 12-lead ECG and compare with previous ECGs:
  - Treat any arrhythmias (🕮 pp.132 and 138)
  - Where there is evidence of myocardial infarction follow appropriate reperfusion strategies
  - Where angioplasty, revascularization surgery or valvular dysfunction are involved discuss with a cardiologist
  - Where there is evidence of myocardial ischaemia follow the appropriate treatment protocol (🕮 p.126), avoiding any measures which will worsen hypotension (e.g. vasodilators, β-blockade, aggressive sedation)
- Treat pulmonary oedema with appropriate therapy (🕮 p.86):
  - NIV with PEEP of up to 15 cmH_2O is likely to improve oxygenation
  - Use diuretics and therapies which may worsen hypotension with extreme caution and invasive monitoring
- Arterial and central venous cannulation should be performed early by an experienced operator, avoiding the subclavian route if thrombolysis or anticoagulation have been used.
- Fluid administration may be required where there is evidence of right heart dysfunction (e.g. acute PE, inferior MI) or coexisting hypovolaemia (e.g. sepsis, trauma):
  - If CVP is low (<5 cmH_2O) or PAOP is low (<15 mmHg) small fluid boluses (100–200 ml) may be given according to response; aim for a well-filled left ventricle on echocardiography or a PAOP of 15–20 mmHg
- Correct any electrolyte imbalance.
- Inotropes may be considered if hypotension persists despite the above measures; titrate according to organ response/perfusion, or aim for a systolic BP >90 mmHg, and MAP >65 mmHg:
  - Dobutamine 0.5–20 mcg/kg/minute IV infusion is the first line inotrope in treating pump failure in cardiogenic shock,[1] and can be given via peripheral or central access (dobutamine occasionally worsens hypotension, especially if hypovolaemia present)
  - Adrenaline 0.05–3 mcg/kg/minute IV infusion may be used (but may increase heart rate, SVR, myocardial oxygen demand, and promote arrhythmias)

- Dopamine 0.5–10 mcg/kg/minute IV infusion may be used (can have the same effects as adrenaline, particularly at higher doses)
- Milrinone or enoximone may be considered in refractory cardiogenic shock of reversible origin
- IABP counterpulsation should be considered for patients with refractory cardiogenic shock, especially where it can be used as a bridge to further treatment (e.g. 1° PCI, CABG), or recovery from myocardial stunning.
- CPB may be initiated if there is a surgically correctible cause of cardiogenic shock.

[1] When using inotropes in patients with cardiogenic shock following cardiac surgery follow the advice of cardiac anaesthetists and cardiac surgeons.

Further management
- Perform serial ECGs and monitor cardiac enzymes for evidence of an evolving myocardial infarct.
- In certain circumstances (e.g. cardiac failure 2° to viral myocarditis, or peripartum cardiomyopathy) cardiac surgeons may be able to offer insertion of a LVAD as a bridge to recovery or cardiac transplantation.
- Once stable, consider long-term cardiac failure therapies (obtain cardiology advice):
  - Available therapies may include diuretics (including spironolactone), ACE inhibitors or ARAs, β-blockers, digoxin
  - Pacing or cardiac resynchronization therapy (biventricular pacing) may be considered
- Monitor/treat complications associated with hypotension (e.g. AKI).

Pitfalls/difficult situations
- Cardiogenic shock often occurs in combination with other diseases such a sepsis, providing a mixed diagnostic picture.
- Early revascularization is particularly important in patients with myocardial infarction complicated by cardiogenic shock; minimize delays to reperfusion.
- The use of inotropes in cardiogenic shock is controversial; there is little evidence that outcomes are improved.
- HOCM may require acute beta-blockade: obtain specialist advice early.

Further reading
Chockalingam A, et al. Acute left ventricular dysfunction in the critically ill. *Chest* 2010; 138: 198–207.

Dickstein K, et al. ESC Guidelines for the diagnosis and treatment of acute and chronic heart failure 2008. *Eur Heart J* 2008; **29**: 2388–442.

Ratib K, et al. *Emergency cardiology*, 2nd edn. London: Hodder Arnold, 2010.

Royse C, et al. *Pocket guide to perioperative and critical care echocardiography*. Sydney: McGraw Hill, 2006.

Young R, et al. Current concepts in the management of heart failure. *Crit Care Resuscit* 2004; **6**: 31–53.

⚙️ Acute coronary syndromes

Myocardial ischaemia occurs when myocardial oxygen demand exceeds myocardial oxygen supply. Untreated, it causes myocardial dysfunction, and can progress to infarction and acute cardiac failure (cardiogenic shock, pulmonary oedema). Ischaemia is a potent cause of arrhythmias. Ischaemia and infarction present initially in similar ways and are termed acute coronary syndromes (ACS).

MI occurs when acute ischaemic injury results in irreversible necrosis of cardiac muscle.

The 12-lead ECG offers an early tool to identify the 2 subtypes of MI, with different early treatment algorithms: ST elevation MI (STEMI), and non-ST elevation MI (NSTEMI). ECG is the essential early investigation.

Causes

Ischaemia/angina/unstable angina
- ↓supply:
  - Coronary artery disease (coronary atheroma)
  - Prinzmetal's angina, or drug-induced coronary vasoconstriction
  - ↓arterial oxygen content (e.g. hypoxia or anaemia)
  - ↓coronary perfusion pressure (CPP = DAP – LVEDP) due to hypotension or raised LV wall tension (hypertrophy, dilatation)
  - Tachycardia (reduced diastolic time)
  - Vasodilator drugs ('coronary steal')
  - Fixed cardiac output states (valve disease, HOCM).
- ↑demand:
  - Sustained tachycardia, arrhythmias, hypertension, shivering
  - Sympathetic stimulation (pain, agitation, laryngoscopy, procedures or interventions without inadequate sedation)
  - Hyperdynamic states (e.g. pregnancy, anaemia, sepsis, inotropes, hyperthyroidism)
  - Ventricular hypertrophy (e.g. associated with AS, hypertension, coarctation)

Myocardial infarction
- Likely single-vessel involvement:
  - Coronary artery thrombosis
  - Atherosclerotic plaque rupture and coronary artery thrombosis
  - Sustained stress or drug-induced coronary artery spasm
  - Single coronary artery dissection (e.g. pregnancy, pre-eclampsia)
- Single- or multi-vessel involvement:
  - Aortic dissection (type A), may involve both LCA and RCA
  - After CABG (intracoronary air, thrombosis, or vessel kinking)
  - Following cardiac arrest, or other causes of sustained severe hypotension
  - Malignant hypertension
  - Vasculitis (e.g. Takayasu's, Kawasaki's, giant cell arteritis)

There is a continuum from ischaemia to infarction.

Myocardial infarction definitions
- Detection of a rise and fall in cardiac biomarkers (preferably troponin) above 99th centile of the upper normal reference limit (URL), together with evidence of myocardial ischaemia *with at least one of the following*:
  - Symptoms of ischaemia
  - ECG changes indicative of new ischaemia (new S-T changes or new LBBB)
  - Development of pathological Q waves in the ECG
  - Imaging evidence of new loss of viable myocardium, or new regional wall motion abnormality
- Cardiac biomarker rise and fall following PCI (troponin >3 × URL).
- Cardiac biomarker rise and fall following CABG (troponin >5 × URL), or new Q waves.
- Pathological findings of acute MI.

Presentation and assessment
- Agitation, feeling of impending doom.
- Central crushing chest pain often radiating to the left arm or jaw:
  - 'Silent' ischaemia/infarction (i.e. with no pain) may occur, especially in diabetic patients, elderly patients, or patients with epidurals or other forms of analgesia
- Epigastric pain or vomiting.
- Pallor and sweating.
- Syncope or acute confusional states.
- Tachycardia, bradycardia, palpitations, ventricular arrhythmias:
  - ECG changes may be present (true analysis should be done using a 12-lead ECG, as single-lead analysis may be misleading)
- Hypertension or hypotension/cardiogenic shock, and/or oliguria.
- Pulmonary oedema (may present as difficulty ventilating patients).

Ischaemia/infarction may occur concurrently with other diseases, typically: pneumonia, stroke, DKA

Investigations
- ABGs (hypoxia, metabolic acidosis).
- FBC (exclude severe anaemia).
- Clotting screen, and D-dimer (to rule out low-probability PEs).
- U&Es, LFTs, blood glucose.
- Serum magnesium, calcium, and phosphate.
- TFTs.
- Serum lipids, serum amylase.
- Serial cardiac enzymes, particularly CK MB and troponin I/T (6–12 hours after onset of chest pain, depending on sensitivity).
- Serial 12-lead ECGs (compare with old ECGs where possible).
- Echocardiography, TTE/TOE (may demonstrate regional wall motion abnormalities, valvular disease, LV/RV impairment).
- CXR (cardiac size, pulmonary oedema, pneumonia).

ECG changes associated with acute coronary syndromes

STEMI (requires acute treatments, and immediate reperfusion therapy):
- ST elevation >2 mm contiguous chest leads V1–V6.
- ST elevation >1 mm contiguous limb leads I, aVL, II, III, aVF, aVR.
- New LBBB.
- 'True posterior' MI changes.

NSTEMI (requires acute treatments, and symptoms control, with risk stratification for investigation or reperfusion therapies):
- The ECG may be normal.
- T wave inversion, or hyperacute T waves.
- ST depression, or borderline ST elevation.
- Tachycardia or bradycardia.
- Arrhythmias.

Differential diagnoses
- Cardiovascular: pericarditis, aortic dissection.
- Respiratory: pneumothorax, PE, pneumonia.
- GI: gastro-oesophageal reflux, oesophageal spasm or rupture, acute pancreatitis, peptic ulcer disease, biliary tract pathology.
- Musculoskeletal pain.

ECG changes may be associated with other conditions:
- Pre-existing or rate-related bundle branch block.
- Pericarditis (saddle-shaped ST segments).
- Old LV aneurysm (may result in persistent ST elevation).
- Normal 'high take-off' or single rhythm strip ST elevation.
- Brugada syndrome (inherited condition with ST elevation leads V1–3 and right bundle branch block).
- Cardiac contusion.
- Digoxin toxicity.
- Electrolyte abnormalities (e.g. hyperkalaemia).
- Subarachnoid haemorrhage.

Immediate management
- Give 100% O_2 only if required, titrate to SpO_2 94–98%.
- Secure the airway and ensure breathing/ventilation is adequate (endotracheal intubation is unlikely to be required unless cardiogenic shock or cardiac arrest occur).
- Ensure IV access and commence ECG monitoring.
- Record 12-lead ECG (compare with previous ECGs).
- Treat tachyarrhythmias or bradyarrhythmias (📖 pp.132 and 138).
- Where there is evidence of ongoing ischaemia:
  - Give aspirin 300 mg (chewed, via NGT, or PR)
  - For pain administer cardio-stable analgesia (e.g. diamorphine IV 2.5–5 mg, or morphine IV 5–10 mg), with an accompanying anti-emetic (e.g. ondansetron 4 mg IV)

- In sedated/ventilated patients sedation may be carefully bolused
- Sublingual or buccal GTN, or a GTN infusion may be used to relieve angina pain
- Where there is no evidence of heart failure, hypotension, pulmonary oedema or bradycardia metoprolol IV 5–15 mg IV (or 50–100 mg PO) may be administered
- Stop/reduce any vasopressor/inotropic drugs if they are possible triggers (if this is possible without provoking severe hypotension).
- If severe anaemia is present give blood (with diuretic cover if required); aim for an Hb concentration of 7–9 g/dl.

ST elevation MI
- Give clopidogrel[1] 300 mg PO/NG (then 75mg daily), or prasugrel[1] 60 mg PO/NG (then 10 mg daily).
- Arrange early transfer to a cardiac catheter suite for 1° PCI.
- If 1° PCI is not available within 2 hours:
  - Proceed to thrombolysis provided there are no contraindication (e.g. reteplase (r-PA) 10 units IV followed by a further 10 units IV after 30 minutes)
  - Give unfractionated heparin 5000 units IV alongside thrombolysis
  - Record serial ECGs
  - If thrombolysis fails to resolve ST segments (≥50%) or pain at 90 minutes, arrange transfer to cardiac catheter suite for rescue PCI
- Angiography may reveal vessel disease, or depressed LV function, or other angiographic findings which suggest CABG may be more beneficial with PCI.

Non-ST elevation MI or unstable angina
- Give clopidogrel[1] 300 mg PO/NG (then 75 mg daily) if there is ECG evidence of ischaemia or a raised troponin concentration.
- Give LMWH (e.g. enoxaparin 1 mg/kg SC 12-hourly); alternatively other selective factor Xa inhibitors may be used (e.g. fondaparinux 2.5 mg SC daily):
  - In patients with renal failure, or after recent surgery (or at high risk of needing surgery), it may be safer to use unfractionated heparin infusions initially
- A GTN infusion, may be used: 50 mg/50 ml IV starting at 3 ml/hour, titrating to effect.
- Obtain a cardiological opinion, in patients with medium- to high-risk disease or recurrent symptoms:
  - Proceed to early angiography
  - Consider GP2b3a inhibitor infusion

In cardiovascularly unstable patients with ACS
- If hypovolaemic, cautiously administer 250–500 ml crystalloid/colloid.
- Consider inserting an arterial line, CVC, and/or cardiac output monitoring devices.
- IABP counter-pulsation may be used in patients with ongoing symptoms, as a bridge to reperfusion therapies.

[1] Relative contraindications include: planned/recent surgery, bleeding, stomach ulceration.

Relative contraindications to thrombolysis
- CPR for >10 minutes.
- Pancreatitis.
- Pregnancy.
- Severe hypertension (>180/110 mmHg); this may be managed by:
  - Treating pain (e.g. using IV diamorphine/morphine/fentanyl)
  - Increasing sedation (in ventilated patients)
  - Commencing an IV GTN infusion
  - Titrating 1–5 mg metoprolol IV

Absolute contraindications to thrombolysis
- Aortic dissection suspected.
- Active GI bleeding within the past 2 weeks.
- Major surgery or trauma in previous 6 weeks.
- Puncture of a non-compressible vessel or organ biopsy within the past 2 weeks.
- Previous haemorrhagic stroke.
- Ischaemic stroke within the previous 3 months.
- History of intracranial lesion.
- Anticoagulation with an INR >2; or known bleeding disorder.
- Recent central neuraxial blockade (e.g. within the past 12 hours).

Further management
- Admit to a CCU, HDU, or ICU dependent on airway/breathing status.
- Check serial ECGs and cardiac enzymes (including troponin at 12 hours); ECGs may identify an evolving STEMI, elevated troponin indicates an NSTEMI or STEMI.
  - Observe for new ST-segment and T-wave changes or left bundle branch block (initial ECG may be normal in 10–20% cases of MI)
  - Observe for the formation of pathological Q waves (hours to days)
  - Where thrombolysis has been performed repeat the 12-lead ECG after thrombolysis to ensure > 50% resolution of ST changes; if it does not, rescue angioplasty should be considered
- Monitor for complications of MI (murmurs, arrhythmias, heart failure, pericardial effusion) and its treatment (GI haemorrhage).
- Further chest pains, dynamic ECG changes, new heart failure, or valvular dysfunction should prompt cardiology consultation; further antiplatelet and/or anticoagulant therapy, or emergency coronary intervention may be indicated:
  - GP2b3a inhibitor infusion (e.g. eptifibatide, tirofiban, abciximab)
  - Calcium channel antagonist for continuing angina
  - Coronary reperfusion therapies (e.g. angioplasty and/or coronary stenting, or surgical coronary artery bypass grafting)
- Continue/commence ACS medical therapies:
  - Aspirin and clopidogrel/prasugrel, β-blockers, ACE inhibitor, statins
  - LMWH/fondaparinux (this may be discontinued at day 8 after successful revascularization)
  - Once stabilized on other therapies wean GTN; if it is required for >24 hours allow 'nitrate free' periods to reduce nitrate tolerance

- Be vigilant to the further complications of bradycardia and heart block, tachyarrhythmias, LVF, pericarditis, DVT and PE, cardiac tamponade, MR, VSD, Dressler's syndrome, and LV aneurysm.
- If the patient requires CABG, clopidogrel/heparins/GP2b3a inhibitors should be stopped prior to surgery—be guided by cardiologist/cardiac surgeon/cardiac anaesthetist.
- Consider TTE/TOE post infarction to assess LV function/valve status.
- Avoid hyperglycaemia, maintain blood glucose <11 mmol/L.
- Maintain serum potassium 3.5–4.5 mmol/L.

Pitfalls/difficult situations

- Ventilated/sedated patients may not manifest the usual symptoms or signs of acute MI; arrhythmias, ST segment changes, or T wave inversions on ECG monitor may be the first signs.
- If β-blockade is contraindicated (asthma, LVF, bradycardia) consider a rate-limiting calcium channel blocker (e.g. diltiazem).
- Acute aortic dissection can present with myocardial ischaemia or infarction, through involvement of coronary arteries:
  - Platelet antagonism/anticoagulation must be avoided if suspected
  - CT aortogram or TOE are the diagnostic investigations of choice
- The risk of fatal haemorrhage is high if surgery is required for an ICU patient who has received GP2b3a inhibitors or clopidogrel.
- Where possible, invasive lines should be inserted prior to systemic anticoagulation and antiplatelet therapy.
  - Where this is not possible it CVC insertion should be performed by an experienced operator, avoiding the subclavian route
  - Coronary reperfusion should not be delayed due to anticoagulation
- If coronary artery spasm is likely, vasodilatation with nitrates or alternatives, with analgesia and anxiolysis, may be all that is required (serial ECGs are still required; cardiac enzymes should be checked).
- Antiplatelet/anticoagulant medication increases the risk of GI bleeds.
- Cardiac failure is common and cardiogenic shock can be difficult to recognize in the patient with pre-existing septic shock.

Further reading

Goyal A, et al. Serum potassium levels and mortality in acute myocardial infarction. *JAMA* 2012; **307**(2): 157–64.

Hoenig MR, et al. Early invasive versus conservative strategies for unstable angina and non-ST elevation myocardial infarction in the stent era. *Cochrane Database Syst Rev* 2010; **3**: CD004815.

Keeley EC, et al. Primary coronary intervention for acute myocardial infarction. *JAMA* 2004; **291**: 736–9.

Management of acute myocardial infarction in patients presenting with persistent ST-segment elevation. *Eur Heart J* 2008; **29**: 2909–45.

NICE. *Unstable angina and NSTEMI. The early management of unstable angina and non-ST elevation myocardial infarction.* London: NICE, 2010.

Patel MR, et al. ACCF/SCAI/STS/AATS/AHA/ASNC 2009 appropriateness criteria for coronary revascularization. *Circulation* 2009; **119**: 1330–52.

SIGN. *Acute coronary syndromes: A national guideline.* Edinburgh: SIGN, 2007.

Thygesen K, et al. Universal definition of myocardial infarction. *Circulation* 2007; **116**: 2634–53.

Zimetbaum PJ, et al. Use of the electrocardiogram in acute myocardial infarction. *N Engl J Med* 2003; **348**: 933–40.

:⚙: Bradycardia

Bradycardia is defined as a heart rate <60 beats/minute. *Excessive brady-cardia* of <40 beats/minute is likely to be pathological, symptomatic, and potentially harmful. In patients with poor cardiac/respiratory reserve even moderate bradyarrhythmias may cause symptoms.

Bradycardia may also be relative. Heart rate should be appropriate to circumstances (e.g. sepsis or haemorrhage would normally be expected to cause tachycardia).

Causes

Sinus bradycardia
- May be normal (physiological), especially in sleep, resting healthy young adults, athletes, sedated patients.
- Vagal stimulation (e.g. laryngoscopy, lung recruitment manoeuvres, ocular pressure, peritoneal stretching, vagino-cervical stimulation).
- Neuraxial blockade (e.g. spinal or epidural analgesia).
- Hypothermia.
- Head injury, or raised ICP.
- Pre-terminal sign associated with hypoxia, shock, or cardiac injury.
- Drugs (e.g. β-blockers, calcium channel antagonists, remifentanil, propofol, metaraminol, noradrenaline, phenylephrine, ergometrine, suxamethonium, neostigmine).
- Hypothyroidism.
- Myocardial ischaemia or infarction.
- Bradycardia/tachycardia syndrome.

Heart block
- Myocardial ischaemia/infarction (particularly inferior infarcts).
- Following cardiac surgery (especially valve replacement or CABG).
- Electrolyte abnormalities, especially hyperkalaemia.
- Drugs (e.g. β-blockers, calcium channel antagonists, digoxin, neostigmine, local anaesthetic toxicity).
- Cardiac contusion.
- Myocarditis/infection (e.g. Lyme disease).
- Amyloid or sarcoid infiltration.
- Idiopathic or congenital (with or without structural abnormality).

Presentation and assessment

Asymptomatic
- Physiological bradycardia may be asymptomatic.
- Occasionally second-degree heart block, or complete heart block, is found as an incidental finding.
- In anaesthetized or sedated patients evidence of symptoms such as angina or myocardial ischaemia may be hard to identify.

Symptomatic
- Anxiety and sweating.
- Tachypnoea, dyspnoea, hypoxia, cyanosis.
- The patient may have chest pain/angina, or ischaemia on an ECG.
- Hypotension (systolic BP <90 mmHg).

- Poor perfusion may result in:
  - Cold peripheries, prolonged capillary refill (>2 seconds)
  - Dizziness, syncope, ↓consciousness
  - Oliguria
- If heart failure is present:
  - Raised JVP (>4cm from sternal angle) or CVP (>15 cmH₂O)
  - Cannon 'a' waves may be seen in ventricular tachycardia (these are a sign of AV dissociation and are also seen in asymptomatic individuals in the absence of heart failure)
  - Gallop rhythm, S3 may be present
  - Enlarged and tender liver, ascites and oedema of dependent areas (e.g. legs or sacrum) may be present
- Haemodynamic measurements may reveal ↓cardiac output and ↑systemic vascular resistance.
- If pulmonary oedema is present:
  - Patient may prefer sitting, or leaning forward (orthopnoea)
  - Cough and/or frothy pink sputum; bilateral crackles and/or wheeze
  - There may be difficulty ventilating patients on IPPV

Investigations

In symptomatic individuals, or if heart block is second degree or worse:
- 12-lead ECG with a rhythm strip.
- ABGs (hypoxia, metabolic acidosis).
- FBC, U&Es (hyperkalaemia, hypokalaemia).
- LFTs, TFTs, serum magnesium and calcium .
- Cardiac enzymes.
- CXR (pulmonary oedema, cardiac size).
- Consider echocardiography once stable, and heart rate improved.

Types of heart block
- First degree: PR interval >0.2 seconds (does not require treatment).
- Second degree:
  - Mobitz type I (Wenkebach): PR interval gradually lengthens with each beat until there is an absent QRS following a P wave; the cycle then repeats
  - Mobitz type II: PR interval remains the same, intermittently there is failure of AV conduction and no QRS follows a P wave
- Complete heart block: there is complete dissociation between P waves and QRS complexes; where the ventricle establishes its own 'escape' rhythm the QRS complexes are wide (>0.12 seconds) and the heart rate is typically 20–40 beats/minute (occasionally a nodal escape rhythm is established and QRS complexes may be narrow with heart rate around 50–60 beats/minute).

Differential diagnoses
- Equipment failure, electrical interference (e.g. shavers, diathermy).
- Any cause of shock, heart failure, or a terminal bradycardia (e.g. bronchospasm, head injury, tension pneumothorax).
- PEA if cardiac arrest occurs.

Immediate management (see also Fig. 4.3)
- Give 100% O_2 initially, then titrate to SpO_2 94–98%.
- Secure the airway and ensure breathing/ventilation is adequate.
- Confirm bradycardia by palpating pulse.
- Obtain IV access and attach cardiac monitoring or pacing defibrillator.
- Record 12-lead ECG with a rhythm strip.
- Correct any immediately reversible cause (e.g. warming, electrolytes).
- Temporary pacing wires are often left *in situ* following cardiac surgery; pacing via these is first-line therapy.

If there are no adverse features and risk of asystole is low:
- Observe, monitor, reverse obvious causes, seek cardiologist advice.

If there are adverse features or risk of asystole is high:
- Give atropine 500 mcg IV, repeat as necessary to a maximum of 3 mg:
  - Glycopyrronium bromide 200–600 mcg IV may be used as an alternative.
- If this is ineffective commence other chemical treatments whilst arranging transvenous pacing:
  - Adrenaline infusion 2–10 mcg/minute IV, titrate to response, *or*
  - Isoprenaline 1–10 mcg/minute IV, *or*
  - Dopamine dose 5–20 mcg/kg/minute IV, *or*
  - Aminophylline 0.5 mg/kg/hour IV, *or*
  - Transcutaneous/external pacing
- Transvenous pacing should be performed by a cardiologist as soon as possible for those patients dependent on chemical/external pacing.

Transcutaneous/external pacing:
- Use a defibrillator with transcutaneous pacing function.
- Attach pads to dry skin (sternum/apex, or anterior/posterior).
- Choose *fixed* mode (consider *demand*, if available, once stable).
- Set the rate for 60–90/minute.
- Increase the *output* (in mA) until *capture* occurs: pacing spikes are seen and QRS complexes are triggered by them.
- Ensure there is *mechanical capture* (a pulse present with QRS complexes), otherwise treat for PEA.
- Muscle twitching is normal; analgesia may be required if there is pain.

Specific treatments:
- Glucagon 1–5 mg IV (slow), or 1–7.5 mg/hour, may be used if bradyarrhythmia is caused by β-blockers or calcium channel blockers.
- Calcium chloride 10 ml 10% IV for calcium channel blocker overdose.
- Administer sodium bicarbonate 50 ml 8.4% solution IV for tricyclic antidepressant overdose.
- Give digoxin-specific antibody fragments if digoxin toxicity is present.
- If LA toxicity thought likely give Intralipid® solution 1.5 ml/kg 20% solution, followed by infusion of 15 ml/kg/hour (see 📖 p.493).

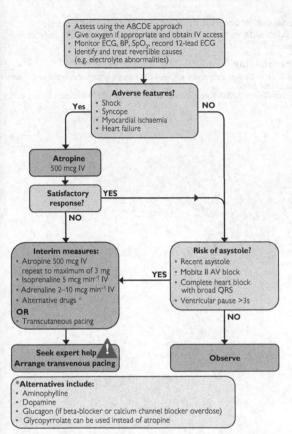

- Assess using the ABCDE approach
- Give oxygen if appropriate and obtain IV access
- Monitor ECG, BP, SpO₂, record 12-lead ECG
- Identify and treat reversible causes
  (e.g. electrolyte abnormalities)

Adverse features?
- Shock
- Syncope
- Myocardial ischaemia
- Heart failure

Yes   NO

Atropine
500 mcg IV

Satisfactory response?   YES

NO

Interim measures:
- Atropine 500 mcg IV repeat to maximum of 3 mg
- Isoprenaline 5 mcg min⁻¹ IV
- Adrenaline 2–10 mcg min⁻¹ IV
- Alternative drugs *

OR
- Transcutaneous pacing

Risk of asystole?
- Recent asystole
- Mobitz II AV block
- Complete heart block with broad QRS
- Ventricular pause >3s

YES

NO

Seek expert help
Arrange transvenous pacing

Observe

*Alternatives include:
- Aminophylline
- Dopamine
- Glucagon (if beta-blocker or calcium channel blocker overdose)
- Glycopyrrolate can be used instead of atropine

Fig. 4.3 Adult bradycardia algorithm. UK Resuscitation Council guidelines 2010. Reproduced with the kind permission from the Resuscitation Council (UK).

Further management
- Look for any other coexisting conditions, especially if signs and symptoms fail to respond to correction of heart rate.
- Monitor for an evolving infarct with cardiac enzymes and serial ECGs.

Pitfalls/difficult situations
- Complete heart block only rarely responds to drug therapy.
- Treat bradyarrhythmias in cardiac arrests as PEA (📖 p.101), pacing should be considered for complete heart block but not asystole.

- Agonal rhythm occurs in dying patients, characterized by slow, irregular, wide ventricular complexes, progressing through PEA to asystole.

Further reading

Durham D, et al. Cardiac arrhythmias: diagnosis and management: the bradycardias. *Crit Care Resusc* 2002; 4: 54–60.
Resuscitation Council (UK). *Advanced life support*, 6th edn. London: Resuscitation Council (UK), 2011.

☼ Tachycardia

Tachycardia is defined as a heart rate >100 beats/minute. It is more likely to be pathological, and patients more likely to be compromised, at rates >150 beats/minute. Patients with pre-existing cardiac disease may be compromised to a greater extent, even at lower heart rates.

Tachycardias can be sinus or tachyarrhythmias. The latter can be either broad complex or narrow complex (QRS), regular or irregular.

Types of tachyarrhythmias
- Sinus tachycardia may occur (not strictly a cardiac arrhythmia).
- Narrow complex 'supraventricular'[1] tachyarrhythmia (QRS <0.12 seconds):
  - Ectopic atrial tachycardia or multifocal atrial tachycardia
  - Atrial fibrillation with fast ventricular response rate ('fast AF')
  - Atrial flutter
  - Re-entrant tachycardia: AV nodal (AVNRT); atrioventricular (AVRT)
- Broad complex tachyarrhythmia (QRS >0.12 seconds):
  - Ventricular tachycardia (monomorphic)
  - Torsade de pointes (polymorphic VT)
  - Any cause of narrow complex tachycardia with aberrant conduction (e.g. SVT with bundle branch block, pre-excited AF)

[1] The term supraventricular tachycardia (SVT) can represent any cause of narrow complex tachycardia, though in practice it most commonly refers to re-entrant tachycardia or ectopic atrial tachycardia.

Causes

Sinus tachycardia may be a physiological response to:
- Pain, anxiety, inadequate sedation, awareness (paralysed patients).
- Sepsis and systemic inflammatory response, pyrexia.
- Anaemia, hypovolaemia, haemorrhage, hypoxia, hypercapnia, PE.
- Tension pneumothorax, tamponade.
- Thyrotoxicosis.
- Drug therapy (e.g. inotropes, pancuronium, salbutamol, aminophylline).
- Drug intoxication (e.g. cocaine, ecstasy, amphetamines, TCAs, SSRIs).
- Drug withdrawal (e.g. alcohol, opiate, benzodiazepines).

Tachyarrhythmias (1° cardiac: atrial or ventricular origin):
- 1° cardiac disease: ischaemic heart disease, cardiomyopathy, valve disease, abnormal conduction (long QT syndrome: torsade de pointes).
- Hypoxia, hypercapnia, acidaemia, hypovolaemia, shock, sepsis.
- Electrolyte abnormalities, especially potassium and magnesium.
- Thyrotoxicosis.
- Extremes of temperature (hypothermia, hyperpyrexia).
- Pulmonary artery catheterization or CVC line placement.
- During or after cardiac surgery, revascularization, or defibrillation.
- Drug therapy (e.g. inotropes, salbutamol, aminophylline).

- Drug toxicity (e.g. alcohol, cocaine, ecstasy, amphetamines, TCAs, SSRIs, local anaesthetic toxicity); drug interactions (e.g. tricyclics, macrolide antibiotics, antifungals, antipsychotics: torsade de pointes).

Presentation and assessment

Patients may be asymptomatic, present in cardiac arrest, or have:
- Anxiety and sweating.
- Palpitations, chest pain, and/or ischaemia on ECG.
- Tachypnoea, dyspnoea, hypoxia, cyanosis.
- Hypotension (systolic BP <90 mmHg) *or* hypertension.
- Poor perfusion may result in:
  - Cold peripheries and prolonged capillary refill (>2 seconds)
  - Dizziness, syncope, ↓consciousness
  - Oliguria
- If heart failure is present:
  - Raised JVP (>4 cm from sternal angle) or CVP (>15 cmH₂O)
  - Cannon 'a' waves may be seen in ventricular tachycardia (these are a sign of AV dissociation and are also seen in asymptomatic individuals in the absence of heart failure)
  - Gallop rhythm, S3 may be present
  - Enlarged and tender liver, ascites and oedema of dependent areas (e.g. legs or sacrum) may be present
- Haemodynamic measurements may reveal ↓cardiac output and ↑systemic vascular resistance.
- If pulmonary oedema is present:
  - Patient may prefer sitting, or leaning forward (orthopnoea)
  - Cough and/or frothy pink sputum
  - Bilateral crackles and/or wheeze
  - There may be difficulty ventilating patients on IPPV.

Investigations

- 12-lead ECG with rhythm strip (determine QRS width and regularity; compare with old ECGs).
- ABGs (hypoxia, hypercapnia, metabolic acidosis).
- FBC (anaemia).
- U&Es, (hyperkalaemia, hypokalaemia).
- LFTs, TFTs, serum magnesium, calcium, phosphate, glucose.
- D-dimer (may rule out PE in low probability cases).
- Cardiac enzymes/troponin, after 12 hours (can be raised following tachyarrhythmias, but persistent ECG/echocardiography changes may suggest MI as cause).
- CXR (pulmonary oedema, pneumothorax, pneumonia, cardiac size).
- Consider echocardiography once stable and heart rate controlled (structural heart disease, signs of infarction, and functional assessment).

Differential diagnoses

- Interference from equipment or patient (e.g. CVVH, shivering, tremor).
- Any cause of sudden hypotension (e.g. haemorrhage or anaphylaxis).
- Sinus tachycardia as a response to trauma, or sepsis, is often mistaken for SVT. SVT is more likely if: onset is sudden, rate is very high, rhythm is irregular, rhythm responds to treatment.

Immediate management

- Stop any triggers (e.g. drugs or procedures).
- *Check pulse*; if a central pulse is absent treat as:
  - Narrow complex tachycardia: PEA (📖 p. 101)
  - Broad complex tachycardia: VF/pulseless VT (📖 p. 101)
- Give 100% O_2, secure the airway, ensure breathing/ventilation is adequate; endotracheal intubation may be required.
- Obtain IV access and attach cardiac monitoring.
- Record 12-lead ECG with a rhythm strip.
- Correct reversible cause (e.g. electrolyte imbalance, hypoxia).
- If it is a sinus tachycardia treat the cause, do not cardiovert.

If (non-sinus) tachyarrhythmia is present

(See also Fig. 4.4.)

If the patient has any of the following adverse features
  - Significant hypotension (systolic BP <90 mmHg)
  - Heart failure
  - Chest pain or ischaemia on ECG
  - Reduced consciousness level or syncope
- Proceed to urgent *synchronized* DC cardioversion[1] with 200–360 J;[2]
  - If AF or atrial flutter consider giving heparin 5000–10,000 units IV
  - Perform 3 successive attempts at DC cardioversion[1] (fixed or escalating energy); if this fails to restore sinus rhythm then give amiodarone 300mg IV and repeat DC cardioversion attempt.

If the patient has no adverse features present
  - Analyse the 12-lead ECG (QRS width, regularity of complexes); look for evidence of accessory pathway[2] treat accordingly

Regular narrow complex tachycardia (QRS <0.12 seconds).
- Exclude sinus tachycardia.
- Use vagal manoeuvres (Valsalva, carotid sinus massage, lung recruitment manoeuvres).
- If this fails try a bolus of adenosine 6 mg IV continuously monitoring ECG; effect may be delayed for up to 30 seconds.
  - Two further boluses of adenosine 12 mg may be given if required
- If adenosine is contraindicated, or fails to terminate the tachyarrhythmia, verapamil 2.5–5 mg IV may be given.
- If drugs fail a synchronized DC cardioversion[1] may be administered.

Irregular narrow complex tachycardia[2] (QRS <0.12 seconds):
- ('Fast AF', atrial flutter with variable AV block).
- Attempt rhythm control if the onset is known to be <48 hours ago:
  - This may be achieved by chemical cardioversion (amiodarone IV or flecainide IV) or synchronized DC cardioversion[1]
- If onset is unknown or >48 hours ago rate control may be achieved by β-blockade (e.g. metoprolol IV 1–5 mg; or esmolol 0.5 mg/kg followed by an esmolol infusion).
  - Diltiazem or digoxin[2] may be used if β-blockade is contraindicated (e.g. by heart failure, or asthma)

Regular broad complex tachycardia (QRS >0.12 seconds) (monophasic or polymorphic VT or SVT with aberrant conduction):
- If it is VT give amiodarone IV 300 mg over 1 hour (followed by 900 mg over next 24 hours), or
  - *Synchronized* DC cardioversion,[1] *or*
  - β-blocker IV, overdrive pacing
- If it is polymorphic VT or torsade de pointes: (axis of VT is continuously changing; can degenerate into VF)
  - Give magnesium sulphate 2 g IV (8 mmol) over 10 minutes
  - Correct serum potassium
  - Give amiodarone IV 300 mg over 1 hour (followed by 900 mg over next 24 hours), or
  - DC cardioversion[1] (*synchronized* shock should be attempted, but may not be possible; an unsynchronized shock may be necessary)
  - Consider overdrive pacing in resistant cases
  - Occurs with long QT syndrome: stop all drugs which prolong the QT interval
- If it is SVT with aberrant conduction, treat as SVT (see earlier in this box).
- If it is unclear whether it is VT or SVT with aberrancy then:
  - Try vagal manoeuvres or adenosine IV (may terminate SVT or slow rhythm; will have no effect on VT)
  - If in doubt treat broad complex tachycardia as VT.

Irregular broad complex tachycardia (QRS >0.12 seconds):
- Treat as AF.[2]

[1] Where possible perform cardioversion under sedation or anaesthesia. Energy levels vary with manufacturers (typically 200–360 J monophasic or 150 J biphasic); if in doubt use the highest available energy for first and subsequent shocks

[2] If there is evidence of AF with pre-excitation (e.g. WPW syndrome) avoid AV node blocking drugs (e.g. adenosine, digoxin, diltiazem, verapamil, β-blockers); amiodarone or DC cardioversion are safe

Further management
- Monitor for an evolving infarct with cardiac enzymes and serial ECGs.
- Consider referral to cardiologist for all tachyarrhythmias which are complex or do not respond to treatment.
- In stable AF or atrial flutter >48 hours old where rate control has been achieved, consider anticoagulation and/or TOE to identify any atrial thrombus before proceeding to elective cardioversion.
- Look for any other coexisting conditions, especially if signs and symptoms fail to respond to correction of heart rate.
- CVC position is a common cause of arrhythmias: confirm the position with a CXR, aiming for above the carina.
- Consider obtaining an ECHO where structural heart disease or myocardial damage is suspected.
- New AF is a common postoperative occurrence and may respond to fluid loading and magnesium bolus (as for torsade de pointes but over 20–30 minutes); magnesium may cause flushing and hypotension.

Pitfalls/difficult situations

- The *emergency* treatment of tachyarrhythmias with patient compromise is *electricity*: *synchronized* DC cardioversion × 3 attempts 200–360 J.
- Any pulseless tachyarrhythmia besides VF/VT is treated as PEA.
- Many critical care patients are already sedated/anaesthetized, proceeding directly to cardioversion may be more appropriate than drug therapy; where cardioversion has failed, consider repeating after normalization of electrolytes, or after treatment with amiodarone.
- Sinus tachycardia is very common; at heart rates above 140 beats/minute the ECG rhythm may be difficult to interpret (consider increasing recording speed to 50 mm/second to identify P-QRS-T).

Cardiac drugs

Adenosine:
- 6 mg IV as rapid bolus, followed by saline flush, if no response try two 12-mg boluses.
- Side effects: flushing, chest tightness/bronchospasm, choking, nausea, bradycardia.
- Contraindications: asthma, sick sinus syndrome, second- or third-degree heart block, AF or atrial flutter and pre-excitation syndromes, in heart transplant recipients.

Amiodarone, loading dose 5 mg/kg IV (~300 mg) over 15–30 minutes, (in 100 ml 5% glucose, via CVC if possible), maintenance dose 15 mg/kg (~900 mg) over 24 hours.

Digoxin, loading dose 0.75–1.0 mg IV over 1–2 hours (in 100 ml 5% glucose), maintenance dose of 0.0625–0.25 mg/day:
- Adjust according to age, renal function, and drug interactions.
- Contraindicated in AF or atrial flutter and pre-excitation syndromes.

Esmolol loading dose 500 µg/kg IV over 1 minute, then 50–200 µg/kg/minute.

Magnesium IV replacement infusion 20 mmol (5 g) over 1–2 hours (in 100 ml 5% dextrose) via a central line:
- Aim for a plasma concentration of 1.4–1.8 mmol/L.
- In torsade de pointes consider giving 8 mmol (2g) in 100 ml 5% glucose IV over 2–5 minutes followed by an infusion of 2–4 mmol/hour (0.5–1 g/hour).

Potassium IV 40 mmol over 1–4 hours (in 10 ml 5% glucose) via a central line:
- Aim for plasma concentration of 4.0–5.0 mmol/L.

Verapamil IV 2.5–5 mg over 1 minute:
- Avoid with re-entry tachycardia.
- May cause profound hypotension if given to misdiagnosed VT or in hypotensive patients (or patients with LV dysfunction).
- May cause profound bradycardia in combination with β-blockade.

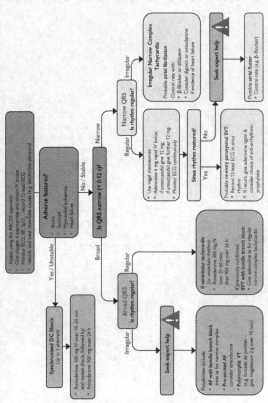

Fig. 4.4 Adult tachycardia (with pulse) algorithm. UK Resuscitation Council guidelines 2010. Reproduced with the kind permission from the Resuscitation Council (UK).

Further reading

Blomström-Lundqvist C, et al. ACC/AHA/ESC guidelines for the management of patients with supraventricular arrhythmias – executive summary. *Eur Heart J* 2003; **24**: 1857–97.

Camm JA, et al. Guidelines for the management of atrial fibrillation. *Eur Heart J* 2010; **31**: 2369–429.

Resuscitation Council (UK). *Advanced life support*, 6th edn. London: Resuscitation Council (UK), 2011.

Zipes DP, et al. ACC/AHA/ESC 2006 Guidelines for the management of patients with ventricular arrhythmias and the prevention of sudden death – executive summary. *Eur Heart J* 2006; **27**: 2099–140.

☺ Cardiac tamponade

Tamponade occurs when blood/fluid accumulates in the pericardium and impairs cardiac output. The rapid accumulation of 100–200 ml may cause acute tamponade; up to 1000 ml may build up in chronic tamponade.

Causes

Acute
- Blunt or penetrating thoracic trauma.
- Recent cardiac surgery/catheterization/pacing, or CVC insertion.
- Dissecting aortic aneurysm, or cardiac rupture after an acute MI.
- Coagulopathy (e.g. thrombocytopaenia/uraemia/anticoagulation).

Chronic
- Metastatic disease; or following radiotherapy.
- Pericarditis (idiopathic, uraemia, or connective tissue disorders/SLE).
- Infection (e.g. bacterial, viral, fungal, TB, HIV).
- Hypothyroidism.

Presentation and assessment
- May present as cardiac arrest.
- Anxiety, restlessness, and/or palpitations.
- Respiratory distress: tachypnoea, dyspnoea and cyanosis.
- Dizziness, syncope, ↓consciousness.
- Chest pain which is relieved by sitting upright and leaning forwards.
- Tachycardia, hypotension, peripheral oedema or poor perfusion.
- Raised JVP/CVP; especially with a prominent 'x' descent and loss of 'y' descent (Kussmaul's sign).
- ↓pulse pressure, pulsus paradoxus, loss of radial pulse on inspiration.
- Muffled heart sounds or a pericardial rub.
- Elevated and equalized ventricular filling pressures (CVP/PAOP).

Investigations
- ABGs (metabolic acidosis).
- FBC (↑WCC in pericarditis, thrombocytopaenia).
- Coagulation screen (deranged in anticoagulation).
- U&Es (uraemia, AKI); LFTs (deranged if hepatic congestion present).
- ECG (low voltage with electrical alternans or T-wave changes).
- Echocardiography, TTE or TOE (visible pericardial fluid, small ventricles with impaired filling, diastolic collapse of right ventricle).
- CXR (widened mediastinum or globular heart); CT/MRI chest.
- PAFC/TOD (low cardiac output, high SVR, and high PCWP).
- Cytology and culture of pericardial fluid.

Differential diagnoses
- Sudden cardiovascular collapse (e.g. tension pneumothorax, pulmonary embolus, anaphylaxis, air trapping in acute severe asthma).
- ↓cardiac output (e.g. cardiogenic shock, myocardial failure, myocardial infarction, constrictive/restrictive pericarditis).
- Volume overload; SVC obstruction.

Immediate management
- Give 100% O_2 initially, then titrate to SpO_2 of 94–98%.
- Secure the airway and ensure breathing is adequate; endotracheal intubation and ventilation may be required.
- Ensure adequate IV access and administer an IV fluid challenge.
- Commence inotropic support if patient remains shocked.
- Under no circumstances remove any penetrating foreign body.
- Monitor the patient's ECG.

Imminent/actual cardiac arrest
- Commence basic/advanced life support.
- Perform emergency pericardiocentesis (📖 p. 546).

Post cardiac surgery
(See 📖 p. 394.)
- Clear any obstruction to chest drains.
- Call for surgical help, alert theatres, obtain wire cutters.
- Administer anaesthesia prior to chest opening using the most cardiostable induction agents/analgesics (be prepared to open chest immediately post induction).
- Intubate and ventilate (if patient is not already).
- If cardiac arrest occurs, reopen chest immediately.
- Ensure blood and clotting factors are available/requested.

Other situations
- Arrange urgent ECHO to confirm tamponade.
- Proceed to immediate ECHO-guided pericardiocentesis if:
  - ECHO shows >1.5 cm fluid plus diastolic collapse
- Seek cardiology advice if:
  - ECHO shows <1.5 cm fluid plus diastolic collapse
  - ECHO shows >1.5 cm fluid but no collapse
  - ECHO shows effusion with dilated LV

Further management
- Avoid bradycardia, maintain filling pressures and sympathetic tone
- Correct metabolic acidosis.
- IPPV may worsen hypotension and tamponade.
- Antibiotic prophylaxis will be needed if the chest has been opened.
- Follow-up cytology and culture of pericardial fluid.

Pitfalls/difficult situations
- An indwelling pericardiocentesis catheter, or creation of a pericardial window or pericardectomy may be required in some patients.
- Pulmonary oedema may occur after drainage of tamponade.
- Low pressure tamponade can occur; in these cases JVP is not elevated, RAP is normal, and the patient may respond to IV fluids.
- Ensure wire cutters are available for cardiac surgery patients.
- Echocardiography is the investigation of choice to diagnose tamponade.

Further reading
Bodson L, et al. Cardiac tamponade. *Curr Opin Crit Care* 2011; **17**(5): 416–24.
Spodick DH Current concepts: Acute cardiac tamponade. *N Engl J Med* 2003; **349**: 684–90.

☼ Hypertensive crises

Moderate hypertension is a common finding in critical care patients and rarely needs aggressive management.

Hypertensive crises (or emergencies) with end-organ dysfunction require urgent IV treatment to prevent associated morbidity/mortality.

Causes

Hypertension may be as a result of:
- 1° hypertension (no identifiable underlying cause).
- 2° hypertension:
  - Drugs (e.g. cocaine, sympathomimetics)
  - Renal/renovascular disease
  - Endocrine (e.g. phaeochromocytoma or Cushing's syndrome)
  - Coarctation
  - Pregnancy, pre-eclampsia/eclampsia
- Reactive hypertension (pain, anxiety, hypercapnia).

Severely elevated blood pressure equates to: systolic >180 mmHg, or diastolic >110 mmHg (sometimes referred to as hypertensive urgencies). Hypertensive crisis occurs when hypertension causes acute end-organ dysfunction (see 📖 Presentation and assessment).

Presentation and assessment

End-organ dysfunction includes:
- Neurological dysfunction (headache, blurred vision, papilloedema, fundal haemorrhages, encephalopathy, limb weakness).
- ACS, acute myocardial infarction.
- Aortic dissection.
- Pulmonary oedema.
- Acute kidney injury.
- Microangiopathic haemolytic anaemia.
- Pregnant patients: pre-eclampsia/eclampsia, or HELLP syndrome (see 📖 pp. 432 and 436).

Critically ill patients with a BP of >220 mmHg systolic or >130 mmHg diastolic should be reviewed to exclude end-organ damage.

Investigations

- ABGs (metabolic acidosis).
- FBC, coagulation screen, fibrinogen (MAHA, DIC).
- U&Es (raised urea/creatinine/hyperkalaemia).
- LFTs, TFTs (hyperthyroidism), blood glucose (hyperglycaemia).
- Urine dipstick (haematuria and/or proteinuria).
- Urine/blood βHCG (to exclude pregnancy/eclampsia).
- ECG (cardiac ischaemia, LVH), CXR (pulmonary oedema).
- CT head (to rule out other causes of encephalopathy).
- Renal US/Doppler, renal angiography (CT or MRI).

Differential diagnoses

- Coincidental hypertension (e.g. alongside MI, or encephalitis).

Immediate management
- Ensure airway, breathing, and circulation are stabilized.
- Treat any underlying cause, in particular:
  - Ensure adequate analgesia and/or adequate sedation/anaesthesia, particularly where neuromuscular blockade is being used
  - Follow the protocols for suspected phaeochromocytoma (📖 p.244), thyroid storm (📖 p.238), or pre-eclampsia (📖 p.432)
- If hypertensive crisis is present (with end-organ damage) reduce MAP by 10–20% MAP (greater reductions may cause complications):
  - Insert an arterial line for continuous BP measurement
  - Use short-acting IV drug infusions to achieve initial BP control to allow rapid discontinuation if necessary

Drug choices:
- Glyceryl trinitrate (GTN) 0.5–20 mg/hour IV, titrated to effect (venodilator, half-life 3 minutes; side effects: tachycardia, headache, and tolerance).
- Sodium nitroprusside (SNP) 0.25–10 mcg/kg/minute IV titrated to effect (vasodilator, half-life 2 minutes, side effects include tachycardia and cyanide toxicity, giving sets need to be protected from sunlight).
- Esmolol hydrochloride 500 mcg/kg/minute IV for 1 minute, followed by 50–300 mcg/kg/minute IV titrated to effect (β-blocker, half-life 8 minutes, side effects include bradycardia and bronchospasm).
- Labetalol hydrochloride 20 mg IV over 2 minutes, followed by an infusion at 2 mg/minute until a satisfactory response is obtained; maximum dose 300 mg (combined alpha1 and non-selective β-blocker, half-life 4 hours, side effects include bradycardia and bronchospasm, caution in impaired hepatic function).
- Hydralazine 5–10 mg by slow IV bolus, repeated after 15 minutes, followed by an infusion at 5–15 mg/hour (arteriolar vasodilator, half-life 2–4 hours, less tritratable).

Hypertension should not be aggressively treated when it occurs as a response to raised intracranial pressure i.e. following head injury.

Further management
- Once BP control is achieved consider longer-term antihypertensive therapy, e.g. ACE inhibitors, β-blockers, diuretics.

Pitfalls/difficult situations
- Sublingual nifedipine should be avoided for the treatment of severe hypertension as it may cause precipitous drops in BP.
- Hypertension as a consequence of acute neurological events is difficult to manage; treatment depends upon the underlying pathology.
- Combinations of drugs may be more effective (e.g. β-blocker and vasodilator), and alternative drugs infusions include phentolamine or fenoldapam; diuretics are not recommended.

• Mild hypoperfusion may cause ischaemia in patients with cerebrovascular or carotid disease; *treatment should be aimed at reducing MAP by a maximum of 20%.*

Further reading

Cherney D, et al. Management of patients with hypertensive urgencies and emergencies. *J Gen Intern Med* 2002; **17**: 937–45.

Marik P, et al. Hypertensive crises: challenges and management. *Chest* 2007; **131**; 1949–62.

Perez MI, et al. Pharmacological interventions for hypertensive emergencies. *Cochrane Database Syst Rev* 2008; **1**: CD003653. DOI: 10.1002/14651858.CD003653.pub3.

Santhi R, et al. Hypertension in the critically ill patient. *Critical Care Resusc* 2003; **5**(1): 24–42.

Chapter 5

Neurology

:Ö: **Decreased consciousness**

↓consciousness occurs in many diseases requiring admission to intensive care, and is often a cause for admission in its own right. Changes in neurological state may be related to intracranial pathology, or may occur in response to respiratory, circulatory, or metabolic disorders.

The immediate management of ↓consciousness should aim to protect the airway, ensure adequate respiration, prevent BP fluctuations, and maintain adequate oxygen delivery to the brain.

Causes

Physiological derangement
- Hypoxia.
- Hypercapnia.
- Hypotension.
- Hypothermia/hyperthermia.
- Hypoglycaemia/hyperglycaemia.
- Other metabolic derangement (e.g. hyponatraemia/hypernatraemia, hypocalcaemia, hypermagnesaemia, hyper-osmolar states).
- Endocrine disease (e.g. hypothyroidism/hyperthyroidism, Addison's disease).
- Hepatic failure, renal failure.

Intracranial damage
- Diffuse brain injury.
- Extradural haemorrhage, subdural haemorrhage, intracerebral bleed.
- Stroke/ischaemia.
- Tumour/other intracerebral mass.
- Cerebral oedema.

Seizures
- Status epilepticus, post-ictal states.

Infections
- Meningitis, encephalitis, intracranial abscess.
- Systemic sepsis.

Drugs and toxins
- Alcohol, sedatives, illicit drugs.

Presentation and assessment

Level of consciousness should be quantified using the Glasgow coma score (GCS) or AVPU systems (rather than poorly defined terms such as unconscious, semi-conscious, obtunded, comatose).

GCS assesses eye, verbal and motor responses and has a maximum score of 15 (fully conscious) and a minimum score of 3 (deeply unconscious/comatose). A GCS <8 equates to 'unconsciousness' (in the AVPU scale P is taken as the cut-off).

Glasgow coma score[1]

- Best motor response (out of 6):
  - Obeys commands 6
  - Localizes to pain 5
  - Withdraws to pain (normal flexion to pain) 4
  - Abnormal flexion to pain 3
  - Extends to pain 2
  - No response to pain 1
- Best verbal response (out of 5):
  - Appropriate orientated response 5
  - Confused speech 4
  - Inappropriate/non-conversational speech 3
  - Incomprehensible sounds 2
  - No speech 1
- Best eye response (out of 4):
  - Spontaneous eye opening 4
  - Eyes open to speech 3
  - Eyes open to pain 2
  - Eye remain closed 1

Minimum score = 3 Maximum score = 15

Painful stimuli should not result in skin damage or marking, alternatives include supraorbital pressure, jaw thrust manoeuvre, nail bed pressure, and sternal rub.

Record each individual component of the GCS or why they might not be possible (e.g. patient intubated).

[1]Reprinted from *The Lancet*, 304, 7872, Teasdale and Jennett, 'Assessment of coma and impaired consciousness: a practical scale', pp. 81–84, Copyright 1974, with permission from Elsevier.

AVPU scale

An alternative to the GCS, which is particularly useful in children, in which there are 4 levels of alertness:
- A—alert
- V—responds to voice
- P—responds to pain
- U—unresponsive.

- Transient loss of consciousness, or changes in consciousness are also important, particularly following head injuries.
- Obtain a contemporaneous history if possible (e.g. from patient, relatives or ambulance crew):
  - Mechanism of injury (particularly in trauma cases, 📖 p.178)
  - Any history of headaches, amnesia, limb weakness, seizures, vomiting, slurred speech
  - Any past or current medical history
  - Any medications (especially anticoagulants) or illicit drug use
  - Previous neurosurgery

Other indicators of altered neurological state may include:
- Drowsiness, agitation, incoherence.

- Incontinence.
- Headache, amnesia.
- Vomiting.
- Seizures.
- Evidence of meningism (painful neck flexion or straight-leg raising—often lost if GCS ≤5) may indicate meningitis or encephalitis.
- Evidence of head or neck trauma, especially evidence of vault or base-of-skull fracture (see 📖 p.179).
- Focal neurological signs and symptoms including:
  - Loss or change in sensation (anaesthesia or paraesthesia) or power
  - Gait or balance problems
  - Problems speaking or understanding speech
  - Problems reading or writing
  - Abnormal peripheral or central reflexes (including lack of gag/cough reflex)
  - Abnormal plantar responses
  - Visual changes (e.g. blurred or double vision, or loss of visual field)
- Eye examination may reveal:
  - Pupil signs: abnormal size, difference in size, reactivity, accommodation, deviation, or movements
  - Fundoscopy (if possible): haemorrhages, papilloedema
- Raised ICP (>20 mmHg) where monitored.

Other signs and symptoms may include:
- Airway: grunting, snoring, or complete obstruction may occur (airway obstruction may cause, or be caused by, loss of consciousness).
- Respiratory:
  - Hypoventilation is a late sign unless associated with narcotic/drug overdose
  - Hyperventilation and/or Kussmaul's breathing may indicate a metabolic acidosis (e.g. DKA)
  - Cheyne–Stokes is associated with brainstem events or raised ICP
  - Tachypnoea causing a respiratory alkalosis may sometimes occur
  - Neurogenic pulmonary oedema
- Cardiovascular changes:
  - Tachycardia or hypotension may occur if there is associated trauma (especially spinal)
  - Bradycardia is often a late or pre-terminal sign
  - Hypertension may be associated with pain or agitation, or may be associated with severe neurological injury (more likely in patients who are deeply unconscious)
  - Cushing's response of hypertension combined with bradycardia is a late sign indicative of severe intracranial hypertension
  - ECG changes: ischaemic changes can occur in association with subarachnoid or intracerebral bleeding; cardiac ischaemic events or arrhythmias (Stokes–Adams attacks) can cause ↓consciousness; chronic AF is associated with thromboembolic events
- Renal: incontinence, polyuria.

Investigations
- ABGs (for hypoxia, hypercapnia, acidaemia and anion gap).
- FBC, coagulation screen (particularly in anticoagulated patients, or where acute liver failure is possible).
- U&Es (especially to look for hyponatraemia or AKI, LFTs, CK).
- Serum glucose, with urinalysis for ketones if indicated (may identify hypo-, hyperglycaemia, or HHS/HONK).
- Plasma osmolality (may help identify ethanol, methanol, or ethylene glycol poisoning).
- Crossmatch blood (if there is trauma or risk of bleeding).
- Blood alcohol levels and/or urine toxicology (for illicit drugs).
- Blood, urine, and sputum cultures where infection is a possible cause.
- ECG (tachyarrhythmia or bradyarrhythmia).
- CXR (malignancy or pneumonia may be present).
- Lumbar puncture (usually after CT head, see 📖 p.574).
- CT head (and possible also neck, see 📖 Criteria for the request for CT scan of the head and also p.182).
- MRI head (investigation of choice for suspected brainstem lesions).
- In patients with associated trauma also consider: C-spine X-rays, other trauma X-rays (e.g. pelvis or long bones), skull or facial X-rays.
- CFAM/EEG may be indicated if status epilepticus is suspected.

Criteria for the request for CT scan of the head
Immediate CT head scan for a head injury with any of the following:
- GCS <13 on initial assessment in the emergency department.
- GCS <15 at 2 hours after the injury on assessment in the emergency department.
- Suspected open or depressed skull fracture.
- Any sign of basal skull fracture (haemotympanum, 'panda' eyes, cerebrospinal fluid leakage from the ear or nose, Battle's sign).
- Post-traumatic seizure.
- Focal neurological deficit.
- >1 episode of vomiting.
- Coagulopathy and any amnesia/loss of consciousness.

Other possible head trauma indications
- Amnesia for events >30 minutes before a head injury.
- Amnesia or loss of consciousness in the elderly or those with a coagulopathy (e.g. patients on warfarin).
- Any injury with a suspicious mechanism (e.g. fall from height or ejection from a car).

Other indications
- Any prolonged, unexplained episode of ↓consciousness or focal neurology.
- History suggestive of subarachnoid haemorrhage, meningitis, encephalitis, or intracranial abscess.
- Suspected stroke or other central neurological deficit.
- Status epilepticus.
- Raised ICP (if measured) resistant to treatment.

Immediate management
- Give 100% O_2, supporting airway/breathing/circulation as required .
- Use cervical spine precautions if trauma is suspected/possible.
- Obtain a contemporaneous history if possible (e.g. from relatives or ambulance crew):
  - An 'AMPLE' history should be obtained as a minimum (📖 p.2)
- Roughly assess neurological state (e.g. conscious and talking, or unconscious):
  - Simultaneously treat neurological complications which may interfere with ABC (e.g. seizures)
- Complete basic ABC 1° survey before formally assessing neurological state.

Airway
- The airway may be compromised due to impaired conscious level:
  - Intubate the trachea as appropriate
  - If this is impossible (i.e. in a remote location) the patient may be placed in the recovery position (depending on the risk posed by other injuries)
- If endotracheal intubation is required a rapid sequence intubation will be required to minimize the risk of aspiration.
- The stress response to endotracheal intubation should be avoided if possible, by using induction agents/short-acting opiates.
- Rapid sequence endotracheal intubation should be considered if:
  - GCS ≤8, or rapidly deteriorating
  - There is risk of aspiration of vomit or blood
  - There is a lack of gag reflex
  - There is facial or neck trauma putting the airway at risk
  - There is hypoxia (SaO_2 <94%, PaO_2 <9 kPa on air, <13 kPa on oxygen), hypercapnia ($PaCO_2$ >6 kPa) or marked tachypnoea
  - Short-term deliberate hyperventilation is required
  - There is ongoing seizure activity
  - The patient is unlikely to remain still for investigations (e.g. CT)
  - The patient is agitated and combative but requiring treatment

Breathing
- Ensure breathing/ventilation is adequate:
  - Ventilatory support may be needed to optimize oxygenation, avoid hypoxia, and/or control hypercapnia
  - Avoid hyperventilation and hypocapnia unless required for short periods to treat raised ICP
  - If acute pulmonary oedema is present treat with appropriate therapies (📖 p.86).

Circulation
- Establish IV access.
- Avoid hypotension, where possible aim for a BP which would be near normal for the patient.
- Resuscitate with fluids and/or inotropes where required.

Neurology
- Formally assess neurological status, including:
  - GCS (see 📖 p.153)
  - Eye examination; including pupil size and reactivity and fundoscopy if possible
  - Evidence of trauma, especially evidence of vault or base-of-skull fracture
  - Plantar reflexes
- Re-assess GCS after stabilizing airway, breathing, and circulation, and continue to re-assess consciousness and neurological state at regular intervals.

Other
- Exclude and treat hypoglycaemia.
- Exclude blockage of V-P shunt (if present).
- Urgent CT scan may be required for diagnosis and appropriate management (prevent hypoxia, hypercapnia, hypotension, and hypertension throughout).
- Raised ICP may be treated with hypertonic saline or mannitol until more definitive measures are employed (see 📖 p.186).
- Treat seizures as per protocol (📖 p.160).
- Check electrolytes.
- Consider the possibility of unexpected overdose (see 📖 pp. 448 and 472); trials of naloxone or flumazenil may be appropriate.

Further management
- Worsening neurological state due to respiratory, cardiac, or metabolic disorders will often respond to successful management of the 1° precipitating disorder.

Neurosurgical referral
- Where ↓level of consciousness is suspected, or proven, to be neurosurgically treatable then referral is indicated.

Indications for neurosurgical referral
- Fractured skull with impaired consciousness, focal neurology, fits or other neurology.
- Compound skull fractures, depressed skull fractures, or fracture to the base of skull.
- Head injury with coma (GCS <9), deteriorating consciousness, neurological disturbance, which continue after resuscitation.
- Head injury with confusion or neurological disturbance lasting >8 hours.
- Evidence of intracranial haemorrhage (subarachnoid, subdural, extradural, or intracerebral) or mass lesion seen on CT.

Ventilation
- Hypoxia should be avoided, as should hypo- or hypercapnia; an SaO_2 >94%, PaO_2 >13 kPa, and $PaCO_2$ 4.0–4.5 kPa should be maintained.

- Pulmonary oedema may require the addition of PEEP (although caution may be required as high levels of PEEP may increase ICP).
- Aspiration and chest infections are common in patients with ↓consciousness and should be actively sought/treated.
- Head-up positioning may decrease the risk of aspiration and improve cerebral venous drainage.

Cardiovascular

- Hypotension should be avoided; a MAP >90 mmHg should be sufficient initially:
  - MAP may be guided later by ICP (allowing calculation of CPP) or other measurements (see 📖 p.186)
- Fluid resuscitation (avoiding hypotonic fluids) is often sufficient, although inotropes may be needed.

Sedation

- Sedation will be required in most cases where patients are intubated and ventilated.
- Sedatives with rapid offset (e.g. propofol) are useful initially as they can be discontinued and the level of consciousness rapidly reassessed.
- Muscle relaxants may be required initially for endotracheal intubation, or for short periods during transfer or CT scanning; however, they run the risk of masking seizure activity:
  - Where neuromuscular blockade is used consider concurrent sedative infusions with anticonvulsive prophylaxis (e.g. propofol or midazolam), or CFAM/EEG monitoring.

Metabolic

- Hyper- or hypoglycaemia should be avoided.
- Hyper- or hyponatraemia should be corrected (see 📖 pp. 208 and 210).
- Pyrexia should be avoided; the place of mild/moderate hypothermia for severe neurological injuries is unclear, but is practised by some hospitals (mild/moderate hypothermia following cardiac arrest *is* indicated, see guidelines, 📖 p. 103).

Pitfalls/difficult situations

Hypoglycaemia is a common treatable cause; every patient with ↓consciousness should have a finger-prick blood sugar test.

- Drug or alcohol use is frequently associated with other causes of diminished consciousness; a high suspicion of metabolic derangement or head injury/intracranial haemorrhage is essential in these patients.
- Diminished consciousness is common in patients sedated in intensive care for prolonged periods, or where there has been renal or hepatic dysfunction leading to a prolonged washout period of sedative medications; a low threshold for suspecting metabolic derangement, intracranial haemorrhage/ischaemia is advisable.
- Alcoholic and coagulopathic patients are at ↑ risk of intracranial haemorrhage even after relatively minor trauma.
- Transfer to CT or MRI is hazardous (particularly MRI where monitoring and ventilators need to be 'magnet compatible'); scans should only be attempted once patients are stable.

- In some cases general surgical interventions (e.g. for major internal haemorrhage) may take precedence over investigating or treating neurological problems.

Further reading

Bateman DE. Neurological assessment of coma. *J Neurol Neurosurg Psychiatry* 2001; **71**(SI): i13–i17.

Holzer M. Targeted temperature management for comatose survivors of cardiac arrest. *N Engl J Med* 2010; **363**: 1256–64.

Mayer S, et al. Critical care management of increased intracranial pressure. *J Intensive Care Med* 2002; **17**: 55–1767.

Moppett IK. Traumatic brain injury: assessment, resuscitation and early management. *Br J Anaesth* 2007; **99**(1): 18–31.

NICE. Head injury. *Triage, assessment, investigation and early management of head injury in infants, children and adults.* London: NICE, 2007.

Sanap MN, et al. Neurologic complications of critical illness: Part I. Altered states of consciousness and metabolic encephalopathies. *Crit Care Resusc* 2002; **4**(2): 119–32.

Scottish Intercollegiate Guidelines Network. *Early management of patients with a head injury: a national clinical guideline.* Edinburgh: Scottish Intercollegiate Guidelines Network, 2009.

Sydenham E, et al. Hypothermia for traumatic head injury (review). *Cochrane Database Syst Rev* 2009; **2**: CD001048. DOI: 10.1002/14651858.CD001048.pub4

Varon J, et al. Therapeutic hypothermia: past, present, and future. *Chest* 2008; **133**: 1267–74.

:☹: Seizures and status epilepticus

Seizures require intensive care management if they are prolonged, are associated with underlying disease, or cause severe physiological disturbance. Prolonged seizure activity carries a significant mortality. Any seizure lasting >5 minutes should be treated as an emergency.

A working definition of status epilepticus is: a seizure lasting >10 minutes, or repeated seizure activity without full consciousness between seizures, or failure to respond to 2 first-line treatments.

Causes

- Hypoxia.
- Brain injury (e.g. traumatic brain injury, intracranial tumour, haemorrhagic or ischaemic stroke, TTP).
- Metabolic/electrolyte abnormalities (e.g. hypoglycaemia, hyperglycaemia, uraemia; sodium, calcium, or magnesium derangement).
- Eclampsia (📖 p. 432).
- Infection (e.g. meningitis, encephalitis, brain abscess).
- Drug associated: drug withdrawal (especially alcohol), drug overdose, or illicit drug use (particularly cocaine).
- In patients known to have epilepsy, seizures may be triggered by:
  - Head trauma, alcohol, intercurrent infection
  - Subtherapeutic blood levels of antiepileptic medications

Presentation and assessment

Seizures are most commonly generalized convulsive, with:
- Loss of consciousness.
- Tonic–clonic muscle movements (these may become very subtle when prolonged seizure activity leads to exhaustion).
- Subtle eye movements (sometimes the only sign).
- Teeth clenching, tongue biting, and/or urinary incontinence.
- Physiological response to seizure:
  - Sweating and/or hyperthermia
  - Tachypnoea (airway obstruction may occur; hypoxia is associated airway obstruction and with prolonged fits)
  - Tachycardia and hypertension
  - Organ failure: rhabdomyolysis, AKI, DIC

Non-convulsive episodes are difficult to characterize, but may involve:
- Impaired consciousness (defined as absence or complex seizures, and can range from lack of awareness to stupor).
- Partial seizures: features may include focal twitching, facial tics, autonomic symptoms, and/or hallucinations (gustatory, acoustic, sensory, or visual), automatic behaviour (e.g. chewing, lip-smacking).

Investigations

- ABGs (hypoxia, metabolic acidosis, raised lactate).
- FBC, CRP (meningitis/encephalitis or intercurrent infection).
- Serum glucose.
- U&Es, LFTs, serum magnesium and calcium.
- CK (raised after prolonged fits).

- Urine/blood βHCG (to exclude pregnancy/eclampsia).
- Blood and/or urine toxicology screen (for alcohol or illicit drugs).
- Serum anticonvulsant drug levels (in patients with known epilepsy).
- CXR (to exclude malignancy, infection, or aspiration).
- Head CT/MRI (if seizures are prolonged, or have no obvious precipitant; or if focal neurology, papilloedema, or head injury are present).
- Lumbar puncture (if infection is possible/likely).
- Blood, urine, and sputum cultures (if infection is likely).
- EEG as advised by neurologists.

Differential diagnoses
- Any disease causing spasms (e.g. rigors, myoclonic jerks, dystonia).
- Any disease causing syncope or agitation (see 📖 pp.152 and 192).
- Psychogenic seizures, also known as pseudoseizures (see 📖 Pitfalls/ difficult situations).

Immediate management
- Give 100% O_2, monitor SpO_2.
- Airway may be compromised due to seizure activity:
  - Maintain airway until fit is terminated, adjuncts may be required (consider nasal airways where there is marked jaw clenching)
  - Consider placing the patient in recovery position
- Ensure breathing/ventilation is adequate (in some cases bag and mask support of ventilation may be needed).
- Assess/monitor circulation and obtain IV access:
  - Fluid resuscitation may be needed to restore BP
- Rapidly assess consciousness level and confirm presence of seizure.
- Obtain a brief history.
- Administer *first-line* antiseizure therapy: lorazepam IV 4 mg bolus:
  - Use diazepam IV (or rectally) 10 mg if lorazepam unavailable
  - Alternatively: midazolam 10 mg to buccal mucosa, or 200 mcg/kg intranasally (unlicensed alternative to lorazepam)
  - Within ICU a 2–4-mg bolus of midazolam may be used as first-line therapy if an infusion is already running
- If there is no response after 5 minutes dose can be repeated (with monitoring of pulse oximetry and respiration).
Further seizure assessment and control:
- Perform finger-prick blood sugar test, if hypoglycaemic, give 50 ml of 50% glucose IV or 500 ml 10% glucose (the need for hypoglycaemia correction outweighs the risk of exacerbating cerebral ischaemia).
- If alcoholism, or malnourishment, is suspected give thiamine 250 mg (Pabrinex® 2 ampoules) IV over 10 minutes.
- In women of child-bearing age perform a pregnancy test: if eclampsia is suspected follow protocol (📖 p.432, magnesium sulphate, loading dose: 20 mmol/4g IV over 3–5 minutes, followed by maintenance infusion of 5–10 mmol/hour).

- If seizure activity persists despite initial therapy commence **second-line** therapy: phenytoin (in 0.9% saline) 18 mg/kg IV infusion at a rate not exceeding 50 mg/minute; ECG monitoring is required:
  - Alternatively use fosphenytoin, 15mg(P.E.[1])/kg IV infusion (maximum rate 100–150mg(P.E.[1])/minute); ECG monitoring required
  - In patients known to be on regular phenytoin avoid loading dose but consider using maintenance dose.

If seizure activity persists 20 minutes from first presentation (or if the patient is severely hypoxic, acidotic or hypotensive *at any time*):

- Induce general anaesthesia using thiopental or propofol, as a rapid sequence intubation with suxamethonium (or rocuronium *if serum potassium is high*).
- Sedate with propofol or midazolam infusions (both may be required).
- Avoid further muscle relaxant infusions unless absolutely necessary (may mask further seizures).
- EEG monitoring must be used if muscle relaxant infusions are used (e.g. atracurium infusions).
- If seizures persist discuss diagnosis and treatment with neurology:
  - Possible treatments include: levetiracetam (500–1000 mg IV), sodium valproate (800 mg IV over 3–5 minutes), lacosamide (50 mg IV BD over 15–60 minutes), or the addition of thiopental 1–5 mg/kg/hour IV or phenobarbital 5–12 mg/kg IV (maximum rate 100 mg/minute); follow-up doses of antiepileptics should be discussed with a neurologist
  - EEG/CFAM monitoring should be organized, aiming for a burst suppression pattern

[1]Phenytoin equivalents (P.E.) are used for fosphenytoin: fosphenytoin 1.5 mg = phenytoin 1 mg.

Further management

- Perform a head CT if required (📖 p.155).
- Ensure that a full neurological assessment has been carried out and discuss the case with a neurologist.
- Maintain $PaCO_2$ 4.5–5 kPa, PaO_2 ≥10 kPa, temperature ≤37°C, Hb ≥10 g/dl, glucose 6–10 mmol/L, serum Na 135–140 mmol/L, where possible.
- If ICP monitoring in place, maintain ICP <20 mmHg, CPP >65 mmHg.
- Where there is evidence of hypotension commence fluid resuscitation with inotropic support if required.
- Other complications which may require treatment include: cerebral oedema (📖 p.186), neurogenic pulmonary oedema (📖 p.86), aspiration (📖 p.66), lactic acidosis (📖 p.204), electrolyte disturbances, rhabdomyolysis and acute renal failure (📖 p.268), DIC (📖 p.306).

Pitfalls/difficult situations

- If seizure control is achieved reassess airway as the sedative effects of treatment may require endotracheal intubation/ventilation.
- Many drugs lower the fit threshold (e.g. flumazenil and antipsychotics).

- Status epilepticus is not common in epileptics; always consider other causes of seizures such as infections.
- Psychogenic seizures may be superficially similar to convulsive status epilepticus; the diagnosis is supported by the absence of hypoxia or acidosis, and if suspected a neurology opinion should be sought.
- Where tumour or vasculitis are present consider dexamethasone.
- Valproate may be preferred as second-line therapy for absence states.

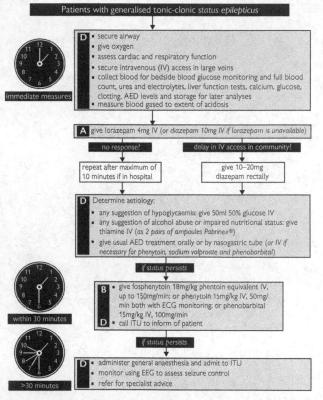

Fig. 5.1 Algorithm for the management of status epilepticus, SIGN (2003). Reproduced with permission from Scottish Intercollegiate Guidelines Network.

Further reading

Costello DJ, et al. Treatment of acute seizures and status epilepticus. *J Intensive Care Med* 2007; **22**: 319–47.

Meierkord H, et al. EFNS guideline on the management of status epilepticus in adults. *Eur J Neurol* 2010; **17**: 348–55.

Maganti R, et al. Nonconvulsive status epilepticus. *Epilepsy Behav* 2008; **12**: 572–86.

NICE. *The epilepsies: the diagnosis and management of the epilepsies in adults and children in primary and secondary care*. London: NICE, 2012.

Rossetti AO, et al. Management of refractory status epilepticus in adults: still more questions than answers. *Lancet Neurol* 2011; **10**: 922–30.

Scottish Intercollegiate Guidelines Network. *Diagnosis and management of epilepsy in adults. A national clinical guideline*. Edinburgh: SIGN, 2003.

① Stroke/thromboembolic stroke

A stroke (sometimes called a cerebrovascular accident, CVA, or occasionally a 'brain attack') is defined as an acute focal neurological deficit caused by cerebrovascular disease that lasts >24 hours or causes death. If the focal neurological deficit lasts <24 hours the diagnosis is a transient ischaemic attack (TIA).

Cerebral infarction is caused either by thromboembolic disorders (85%) or by haemorrhage (10% intracerebral haemorrhage, see 📖 p.172; 5% subarachnoid haemorrhage, 📖 p.174; subarachnoid and intracerebral haemorrhages may also be caused by head injury, see 📖 p.178).

Causes

The incidence of stroke increases with age. Causes include:
Emboli:
- Platelet aggregates from ruptured atherosclerotic plaques.
- Left atrial or ventricular thrombus 2° to atrial fibrillation, poor ventricular function, or myocardial infarction.
- Paradoxical emboli (venous emboli entering the arterial circulation via patent foramen ovale, ASD, or VSD).
- Prosthetic heart valves; indwelling lines/prosthesis.
- Infective endocarditis.
- Following carotid or cardiac surgery.
- As a complication of endovascular coiling of SAH (see 📖 p.174).
Thrombosis:
- Rupture of atherosclerotic lesions (risk factors for atherosclerosis include age, male sex, family history, smoking, diabetes, hypertension, and hyperlipidaemia).
- Vasculitis.
- Cerebral venous thrombosis (caused by hypercoagulable states like dehydration, polycythaemia, thrombocythaemia, OCP medication, protein S/C deficiency, factor V Leiden deficiency).
Other:
- Vertebral or carotid dissection (spontaneous or post traumatic).
- Vessel occlusion by tumour/abscess.
- Carotid occlusion (post strangulation).
- Systemic hypotension (e.g. post cardiac arrest).
Patients who have had TIAs are at high risk of stroke, especially if:
- They have had 2 or more TIAs within 1 week.
- They have an 'ABCD' (**A**ge, **B**lood pressure, **C**linical features, **D**uration) score of ≥4.

• Age ≥60	1 point
• BP ≥140/90 mmHg	1 point
• Speech disturbance *without* weakness	1 point
• TIA lasting 10–59 minutes	1 point
• Diabetes present	1 point
• Unilateral weakness	2 points
• TIA lasting ≥60 minutes	2 points

Presentation and assessment

Strokes are atraumatic, but *may result in associated trauma* (e.g. by causing falls). They result in rapid focal or global neurological deterioration. Other signs and symptoms may include
- Airway: grunting, snoring or complete obstruction .
- Respiratory: Cheyne–Stokes breathing, tachypnoea, bradypnoea (hypoventilation is a late sign):
  - Neurogenic pulmonary oedema may sometimes occur
- Cardiovascular changes: tachycardia and/or hypertension (hypertension associated with bradycardia is a late or pre-terminal sign):
  - ECG changes: ischaemic changes can occur in association with stroke (especially subarachnoid or intracerebral bleeding); AF is associated with thromboembolic events
- Renal: incontinence.
- Neurological: agitation, diminished consciousness:
  - Common presentations: a commonly used system combining anatomical and clinical systems for classifying strokes is the Oxford acute stroke classification system (📖 p.169)
  - Atypical presentations: seizures, falls, or personality change
  - Thrombotic stroke often presents with evolving neurology, whilst embolic stroke presents with sudden onset, rapidly developing neurology

Investigations
- ABGs (in case of hypoxia or metabolic acidosis).
- FBC.
- Coagulation screen (in case of coagulopathy).
- U&Es, LFTs, serum calcium.
- Serum glucose (hypo/hyperglycaemia).
- Serum lipids.
- ECG (ischaemia, AF).
- Head CT scan (to clarify diagnosis, extent of cerebral damage, differentiate infarct from haemorrhage and exclude hydrocephalus).
- Carotid Doppler studies (to identify carotid stenosis of >70%).
- ECHO (the source of any emboli may be cardiac).
- Other investigation that may be of benefit include:
  - CRP, ESR
  - Thrombophilia screen
  - Auto-antibody screen
  - Plasma electrophoresis
  - Blood cultures
  - Syphilis screen

Differential diagnoses
- Migraine.
- Hypoglycaemia.
- Partial epileptic seizures, or following seizures (post-ictal states).
- Space-occupying lesions (e.g. tumour, abscess or subdural haematoma).
- Demyelinating disease.
- Cerebral venous thrombosis.

Immediate management
- Titrate O_2 to achieve SpO_2 >94% (O_2 may not be required).
- Airway may be compromised due to impaired conscious level, place patient in recovery position or intubate trachea as appropriate.
  - Few stroke patients benefit from invasive ventilatory support but some might if gag reflex is absent, the GCS is <8, and the diagnosis is unclear before further investigation is undertaken (or there is evidence of other illness, e.g. pneumonia)
- Ensure breathing/ventilation is adequate.
- Assess circulation and obtain IV access; commence fluid resuscitation where hypotension is present.
- Hypertension is common and should not be corrected unless:
  - Thrombolysis is required and BP is ≥185/110 mmHg
  - Hypertensive encephalopathy, nephropathy, or cardiac failure/MI are suspected
  - Aortic dissection is present
  - Pre-eclampsia/eclampsia is present
- Assess and monitor consciousness level.
- Perform a rapid, detailed neurological assessment (with fundoscopy).
- An urgent CT is required if:
  - There are indications for thrombolysis or early anticoagulation
  - There is evidence of trauma
  - The patient is anticoagulated or has a known bleeding tendency
  - There is rapidly progressive, inconsistent, poorly localized, or fluctuating neurology; or brainstem symptoms
  - The patient has a ↓level of consciousness (GCS <13)
  - Papilloedema, fever, or meningism are present
  - The patient had a severe headache at onset of neurology
- Aspirin 300 mg (oral, or if dysphagic rectally or via NGT) should be given once a diagnosis of haemorrhage has been excluded (unless thrombolysis is used, then it should be withheld for 24 hours):
  - Aspirin should also be given to patients with >1 TIA in a week, or an 'ABCD' score ≥4
- Thrombolysis with t-PA of ischaemic strokes must be considered.
- Neurosurgical intervention may be needed in patients with hydrocephalus or a large infarcted area of the middle cerebral artery (MCA) territory causing oedema (a 'malignant' stroke):
  - Decompressive craniectomy for 'malignant' stroke is indicated in patients aged ≤60 years with: clinical deficits suggestive of infarction in the territory of the MCA with a National Institutes of Health Stroke Scale (NIHSS) score above 15; a decrease in the level of consciousness to give a score of 1 or more on item 1a of the NIHSS; signs on CT scan of an infarct of at least 50% of MCA territory, with or without additional infarction in the territory of the anterior or posterior cerebral artery on the same side, or infarct volume greater than 145 cm³ as shown on diffusion-weighted MRI

Further management

• If not already performed, brain imaging should be undertaken within 24 hours where possible.
• Ensure adequate hydration and nutrition (often NG feeding is required until a swallowing assessment can be performed).
• Aspirin (50–300 mg) should be continued until an alternative antiplatelet therapy is started.
• Prior statin therapy should be continued.
• Anticoagulation is controversial; heart lesions are the only definite indication for full anticoagulation.
• Lowering BP may extend the infarct; it is unclear at what point a high BP requires may benefit from treatment:
  • Consider using short-acting agents to reduce BP slowly if ≥220/110 mmHg
• Ensure adequate analgesia and DVT prophylaxis.
• Maintain blood glucose 4–10 mmol/L.
• Investigate and treat fever aggressively (aspiration is a common cause of infection).
• Aggressive physiotherapy and transfer to a specialist stroke unit are associated with better outcomes.
• Consider initiating treatment aimed at modifying cardiovascular risk factors.

Pitfalls/difficult situations

• Strokes in young patients should always raise the suspicion of 'atypical' causes (e.g. procoagulant disorders such as vasculitis).
• Up to 5% of patients presenting with stroke have underlying space-occupying lesions (e.g. tumour, abscess, or subdural haematoma)
• Where there is any history of scalp tenderness always consider temporal arteritis and measure ESR.
• Careful BP monitoring is important following carotid endarterectomy as strokes are associated with hyper-/hypotension.
• Haemorrhagic transformation of ischaemic strokes may occur (with or without thrombolysis).
• Strokes after cardiac surgery or cardiac bypass present diagnostic and therapeutic challenges, especially as these patients are often extensively anticoagulated.
• Cerebral oedema caused by a 'malignant' MCA territory infarct commonly occurs on day 2–5.

The Oxford acute stroke classification system[1]

TACS[2] (total anterior circulation syndrome): 15% of strokes, mortality ≈60%; *all* of the following:
• Hemiparesis with/without hemisensory loss.
• Homonymous hemianopia and higher cerebral dysfunction (e.g. dysphasia, visuospatial dysfunction neglect).

PACS[2] (partial anterior circulation syndrome): 30% of strokes, mortality ≈16%; one of:

- Any *two* TACS features (see earlier list).
- Higher cerebral dysfunction.
- Isolated motor and/or sensory deficit in one limb or in the face.

LACS[2] (lacunar syndrome): 20% of strokes, mortality ≈11%; any of:
- Pure motor or sensory stroke (involving two of face, arm, or leg).
- Ataxic hemiparesis.
- Dysarthria or 'clumsy hand' syndrome.

POCS[2] (posterior circulation syndrome): 20% of strokes, mortality ≈19%; any of:
- Bilateral motor sensory and sensory signs.
- Cerebellar signs, unless accompanied by ipsilateral motor deficit.
- Disorder of conjugate eye movement.
- Ipsilateral cranial nerve palsy with contralateral motor and/or sensory deficit.
- Isolated homonymous visual field deficit.

[1] Reprinted from The Lancet, 337, 8756, J. Bamford et al., 'Classification and natural history of clinically identifiable subtypes of cerebral infarction', pp. 1521–1526.
[2] The final letter may be changed to denote the type of stroke: S for syndrome, I for infarct, H for haemorrhage (i.e. TACS, TACI, or TACH).

Thrombolysis with alteplase[1]

Consider giving alteplase for treatment of acute ischaemic stroke if indicated by exclusion of intracranial haemorrhage. Alteplase must be used in full accordance with its marketing authorization, which states:
- Use within 3 hours of symptom onset.
- Treatment must be by a physician specialized in neurological care.

Alteplase should be administered only within in a stroke service with:
- Staff trained in delivering thrombolysis and in monitoring for any associated complications, including level 1 and level 2 nursing care staff trained in acute stroke and thrombolysis.
- Immediate access to imaging and re-imaging, and staff trained to interpret the images.
- Staff in A&E who are trained and supported can administer thrombolysis (in accordance with its marketing authorization) if patients are managed within a specialist acute stroke service.
- Consider BP reduction to 185/110 mmHg or lower in people who are candidates for thrombolysis.

[1] National Institute for Health and Clinical Excellence (2008) Adapted from 'CG 68 Stroke: diagnosis and initial management of acute stroke and transient ischaemic attack (TIA) Quick Reference Guide'. London: NICE. Available from Ⓜ www.nice.org.uk. Reproduced with permission.

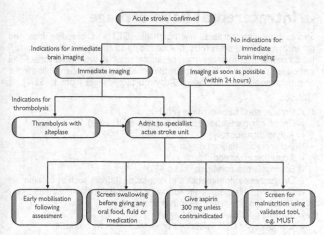

Fig. 5.2 Emergency management of patients with acute stroke. Adapted from NICE. *Stroke: diagnosis and initial management of acute stroke and transient ischaemic attack (TIA)*. London: NICE, 2008.

Further reading

AHA. Adult stroke. *Circulation* 2005; **112**: 111–20.

Lukovits TG, et al. Critical care of patients with acute ischemic and hemorrhagic stroke: update on recent evidence and international guidelines. *Chest* 2011; **139**: 694–700.

NICE. *Stroke: diagnosis and initial management of acute stroke and transient ischaemic attack (TIA)*. London: NICE, 2008.

Sandset EC, et al. The angiotensin-receptor blocker candesartan for treatment of acute stroke (SCAST): a randomised, placebo-controlled, double-blind trial. *Lancet* 2011; **377**: 741–50.

SIGN. *Management of patients with stroke or TIA: assessment, investigation, immediate management and secondary prevention: a national clinical guideline*. Edinburgh: SIGN, 2008.

Wardlow JM, et al. Thrombolysis for acute ischaemic stroke (review). *Cochrane Database Syst Rev* 2009; **4**: CD000213. DOI: 10.1002/14651858.CD000213.pub2.

Vahedi K, et al. Early decompressive surgery in malignant infarction of the middle cerebral artery: a pooled analysis of three randomised controlled trials. *Lancet Neurol* 2007; **6**: 215–22.

van der Worp B, et al. Acute ischaemic stroke. *N Engl J Med* 2007; **357**: 572–9.

① Intracerebral haemorrhage

Spontaneous intracerebral haemorrhage (SICH) is bleeding into the parenchyma of the brain (possibly extending to the subarachnoid space). Intracerebral haemorrhage may be supratentorial or infratentorial. The associated mortality is higher than that of either thromboembolic stroke or subarachnoid haemorrhage (30-day mortality ranges from 35–52%.).

Causes

- 1° intracerebral haemorrhage (PICH):
  - Chronic hypertension (commonest overall cause)
  - Amyloid angiopathy
- 2° intracerebral haemorrhage:
  - Acute hypertension
  - Eclampsia/pre-eclampsia (📖 p.432)
  - Drugs: sympathomimetics and recreational drugs such as cocaine
  - Coagulopathies, especially following thrombolysis and warfarin use
  - Aneurysms and arteriovenous malformations
  - Tumours; following neurosurgery
  - Complicating CNS infections or venous sinus thrombosis
  - Haemorrhagic transformation of thromboembolic stroke.

Presentation and assessment

The presentation of intracerebral haemorrhage overlaps with that of ischaemic/thromboembolic stroke (📖 p.166):

- Supratentorial haemorrhages cause sensory/motor deficits, aphasia, neglect, gaze deviation, and hemianopia.
- Infratentorial haemorrhages cause brainstem dysfunction, cranial nerve defects, ataxia, and nystagmus.
- The following are also common:
  - Headache, nausea, and vomiting
  - Elevated BP (up to 90% of patients)
  - Seizures (up to 10% of patients)
  - Signs and symptoms of hydrocephalus/raised ICP (📖 p.186).

Investigations

(See also 📖 p.167.)

- FBC, coagulation studies (in case of thrombocytopaenia/coagulopathy).
- βHCG (to exclude pregnancy).
- Urine toxicology.
- CT scan of brain, angiography, or MRI (especially if: no pre-existing hypertension, young patients, atypical appearance; i.e. tumour or aneurysm, is suspected).

Differential diagnoses

(See 📖 p.167.)

Immediate management

- Give 100% O_2 initially, then titrate to achieve SpO_2 >94%.
- Airway may be compromised due to impaired conscious level, place the patient in recovery position or intubate trachea as appropriate.

- Ensure breathing/ventilation is adequate:
  - Avoid hypercapnia
  - Avoid hyperventilation and hypocapnia unless required for short periods (<20 minutes) to treat raised ICP
  - Treat pulmonary oedema appropriately (📖 p.86)
- Assess circulation and obtain IV access:
  - If there is evidence of hypotension, commence fluid resuscitation
  - Treat severe hypertension only (BP ≥ 220/110 mmHg), aiming to reduce BP slowly and by ≤20%
- Assess and monitor consciousness level.
- Perform a rapid, detailed neurological assessment with fundoscopy.
- Treat seizures as per protocol (📖 p.160).
- Keep normothermic.
- Consider mannitol 0.5–1 g/kg (approx. 200–400 ml 20% solution) if intracranial mass effect is likely.
- Organize an urgent head CT if haemorrhagic stroke is suspected.
- Check for coagulopathies and reverse if possible.
- Neurosurgical evacuation is more likely to be indicated where:
  - There is cerebellar clot >3 cm, or occluding the 4th ventricle
  - A supratentorial haemorrhage of 20–80 ml volume causes GCS >4 and <13, with midline shift and/or raised ICP, especially if it involves the non-dominant hemisphere.

Further management

(Also follow guidance on 📖 p.169.)
- Avoid hypotonic fluids if possible.
- Administer prophylactic antiepileptic medication if indicated.
- These patients have a high risk for VTE, use mechanical means initially and seek expert advice regarding pharmacological prophylaxis.
- ICP monitoring may be commenced, maintain CPP >60 mmHg where appropriate.
- Manage intracranial hypertension as appropriate (📖 p.186).
- Maintain blood glucose at 6–10 mmol/L.

Pitfalls/difficult situations

(See 📖 p.169.)
- It is difficult to clinically distinguish between ischaemic stroke and ICH, early CT scan will show ICH, but may not show ischaemic strokes.
- Neurosurgery is unlikely to benefit those patients who have: GCS <5, GCS >12 with small haemorrhages, brainstem haemorrhage, significant comorbidity (or who are elderly).
- Up to 5% of patients have a recurrent ICH, risk factors for recurrence include: uncontrolled hypertension, lobar location of initial ICH, older age, ongoing anticoagulation, apolipoprotein E epsilon 2 or epsilon 4 alleles, large number of microbleeds on MRI.

Further reading

Hemphill JC et al. The ICH score: a simple, reliable grading scale for intracerebral haemorrhage. *Stroke* 2001; **32**(4): 891–7.

Mendelow AD, et al. Surgical treatment of intracerebral haemorrhage. *Curr Opin Crit Care* 2007; **13**(2): 169–74.

Morgernstern LB, et al. Guidelines for the management of spontaneous intracerebral haemorrhage AHA/ASA Guideline. *Stroke*. 2010; **41**(9): 2108–29.

:⚙: Subarachnoid haemorrhage

Subarachnoid haemorrhage (SAH) is bleeding into the subarachnoid space and not into the brain parenchyma itself. It accounts for up to 7% of strokes with an incidence of 6–8:100,000. 50% of patients with SAH will die, 12% before reaching hospital. 20% will have multiple aneurysms.

Causes

Risk factors for spontaneous (non-traumatic) SAH include:
- Hypertension/malignant hypertension.
- Diabetes and/or hyperlipidaemia.
- Smoking.
- Migraine.
- Drug abuse (particularly cocaine).
- Family history (first-degree relatives have a 2–5-fold increase of risk).
- Female to male ratio is 2:1; black/Afro-Caribbean > white/Caucasian.
- Associated with syndromes (Marfan's, Ehlers–Danlos, Klinefelter's).
- Associated with polycystic kidney disease and coarctation of the aorta.

Saccular (berry) aneurysms account for 80% (often occurring at cerebral vessel junctions); the larger the aneurysm, the higher the risk of rupture. Other causes include:
- Non-aneurysmal perimesencephalic haemorrhage.
- Arterial dissection; cerebral or dural arteriovenous malformations; vascular lesions of the spinal cord; cerebral venous thrombosis .
- Mycotic aneurysms.
- Sickle cell disease.
- Pituitary apoplexy.
- Cerebral amyloid.

Presentation and assessment

Patients can present with symptoms ranging from 'the worst headache in my life' to coma. Patients needing critical care commonly present with:
- Airway/respiratory: grunting, snoring, or obstruction; Cheyne–Stokes breathing, tachypnoea, bradypnoea (hypoventilation occurs late):
  - Neurogenic pulmonary oedema may sometimes occur
- Cardiovascular changes: tachycardia and/or hypertension (hypertension associated with bradycardia is a late or pre-terminal sign):
  - ECG changes associated with ischaemia can occur

Neurological signs and symptoms may include:
- Headache (SAH accounts for ~8% of headaches presenting to A&E):
  - Classically a sudden-onset (peaks within minutes), worst-ever, 'thunderclap' headache, often occipital (as if 'hit from behind')
  - Any severe headache may be suspicious, particularly in patients who do not usually suffer headaches
  - Some patients describe recent minor headaches (sentinel bleeds)
- Meningism: nausea and vomiting, photophobia, neck stiffness.
- Diminished consciousness, or loss of consciousness.
- Focal neurological signs and/or seizures.
- Signs of raised ICP may be present (see 📖 p.186).

> **World Federation of Neurological Surgeons (WFNS) grading of subarachnoid haemorrhage[1]**
>
> | | | |
> |---|---|---|
> | I | GCS 15 | Conscious with/without meningism |
> | | | No motor deficit |
> | II | GCS 14–13 | Drowsy with no significant neurological deficit |
> | | | No motor deficit |
> | III | GCS 14–13 | Drowsy with neurological deficit |
> | | | Motor deficit present or absent |
> | IV | GCS 12–7 | Deteriorating patient |
> | | | Major neurological deficit |
> | | | Motor deficit present or absent |
> | V | GCS 3–6 | Moribund patient with extensor rigidity |
> | | | Failing vital centres |
> | | | Motor deficit present or absent. |
>
> The grade, extent of haemorrhage on CT scan, combined with patient age can be used to estimate prognosis.
>
> Other grading scales include Hunt and Hess, and the Fisher scale (radiological scale).
>
> [1] Reproduced from *Journal of Neurology, Neurosurgery and Psychiatry*, G.M. Teasdale, 51, 11, pp. 1457, copyright 1988, with permission from BMJ Publishing Group Ltd.

Investigations

- ABGs (to exclude hypoxia and hypercapnia).
- FBC, coagulation studies.
- U&Es (salt wasting can be present), LFTs.
- Serum glucose, serum magnesium (hypomagnesaemia is common).
- ECG (arrhythmias, ischaemia, and infarcts are common).
- CXR (may identify pulmonary oedema).
- Initial CT head (to clarify diagnosis, extent of cerebral damage, differentiate infarct from haemorrhage and exclude hydrocephalus); CT scans done within the first 24 hours have a sensitivity of 95–98%:
  - CT angiogram can identify aneurysm and is the gold standard in centres where this service is available
  - Initially negative angiography should be repeated as up to 24% of vascular lesions are identified on repeat angiography
- LP if CT head is negative (may identify xanthochromia):
  - Sequential collection of CSF with RBC count shows no reduction in RBC in all 3–4 bottles collected (not always reliable)
  - Xanthochromia may not be present until at least 6–12 hours after episode (as blood has to lyse in CSF)
  - Opening pressure protein and glucose should also be measured
  - CSF should also be examined to exclude meningitis (📖 p.574).

Differential diagnoses

- Meningitis, encephalitis (the major differential diagnosis).
- Migraine, cluster and thunderclap headaches.
- Postdural puncture headache.
- Subdural/extradural haemorrhage; ischaemic stroke, intracerebral haemorrhage; acute hydrocephalus.
- Temporal arteritis.

Immediate management

- Give 100% O_2 initially, then titrate to achieve SpO_2 >94%.
- Airway/breathing may be compromised due to impaired conscious level, this may require endotracheal intubation/mechanical ventilation:
  - Avoid hypercapnia (maintain $PaCO_2$ 4.5–5 kPa)
  - Avoid hyperventilation/hypocapnia unless required for short periods (<20 minutes) to treat raised ICP
  - If pulmonary oedema is present treat appropriately (📖 p.86)
- Assess circulation and obtain IV access:
  - If there is evidence of hypotension, commence fluid resuscitation; avoid hypotonic solutions where possible
  - Only severe hypertension should be treated (BP ≥220/110 mmHg); aim to reduce BP slowly by ≤ 20% reduction (use β-blockers or calcium antagonists to avoid effects on cerebral vessel calibre; glyceryl trinitrate/nitroprusside are contraindicated)
- Assess and monitor consciousness level.
- Perform rapid, detailed neurological assessment with fundoscopy.
- Treat seizures as per protocol (📖 p.160); prophylactic anticonvulsants may be required, along with CFAM if sedated and ventilated.
- Ensure adequate pain relief and antiemesis (provide laxative cover).
- Nurse in a darkened, quiet environment and monitor for any change in neurological status, deterioration may warrant a repeat CT scan.
- Early transfer to a neurological/neurosurgical centre is recommended.
- Surgical or radiological management may be possible: the aneurysm may be clipped or 'coiled' (endovascular intervention).
- Referral information should include time from onset of headache, age, comorbidities, GCS, and neurological deficit.

Further management

Treatment of neurosurgical complications

- Re-bleeding: there is a 4% risk of re-bleed in the first 24 hours and a 1.5% risk every day for the next 4 weeks; each re-bleed may require intubation and ventilation and carries a 60% risk of death; early endovascular or open surgical securing of the aneurysm is the preferred therapy.
- Medical therapy to prevent re-bleed includes antifibrinolytics for <72 hours (except in patients with a history of thromboembolic disease); these should be discontinued ≥2 hours before securing the aneurysm.
- Seizures occur in up to 5% of cases after surgical/endovascular intervention; treat with anticonvulsants (e.g. levetiracetam 500 mg IV 12-hourly for 3–7 days; phenytoin is not recommended as initial therapy).
- Acute hydrocephalus may develop (signs may include a drop in GCS, sluggish pupils, bilaterally downward deviating eyes):
  - If hydrocephalus is suspected perform a CT (an extraventricular drain may be required, although this may provoke more bleeding)
- Regular neurological assessments are required to identify diffuse or focal neurological deficit caused by delayed cerebral ischaemia (also known as vasospasm), found in 30% of patients 4–14 days after SAH:
  - If suspected, digital subtraction angiography (gold standard) or CT angiography should be performed

- In sedated patients continuous EEG, transcranial Doppler or PBO_2 monitoring is indicated to assess the need for angiography
- Oral nimodipine 60 mg 4-hourly for 21 days reduces ischaemia (IV nimodipine may be used, but with care to avoid hypotension)
- Statin therapy is controversial; continue if started premorbidly
- Clinical and angiographic evidence of ischaemia, with no other identifiable cause, should prompt the cautious, stepwise use of vasoactive treatments (vasopressors ± inotropes)
- In unsecured aneurysms hypertensive therapy should be cautious
- Patients unresponsive to vasopressors/inotropes should be considered for physiological doses of hydrocortisone and fludrocortisone
- 'Triple H' therapy (Haemodilution, Hypervolaemia and Hypertension) is no longer recommended
- If neurological symptoms do not resolve within 6–12 hours despite maximal medical therapy, consider transluminal angioplasty
- Cerebral salt wasting (diagnosed by serum sodium and ↑urinary sodium) may need sodium or magnesium replacement.
- Persistent negative fluid balance, despite adequate IV and enteral fluids, may require hydrocortisone and/or fludrocortisone treatment.

Treatment of medical complications (40% of patients have medical complications, accounting for 23% of deaths)

- LV impairment/cardiogenic shock, arrhythmias, or neurogenic pulmonary oedema may occur; treatment of pulmonary oedema with PEEP or vasodilators must be balanced against detrimental effects on CPP.
- Serial ECGs, cardiac enzymes and cardiac ECHO may be indicated; cardiac output monitoring may be required in unstable patients.
- The avoidance of IV or PO hypotonic solutions where possible means careful monitoring of U&Es is required.
- Provide early enteral/NG feeding, with ulcer prophylaxis if indicated.
- Thromboprophylaxis with antiembolic stockings or boots is recommended; depending upon neurosurgical advice, LMWH thromboprophylaxis may be instituted 24 hours after securing the aneurysm.
- Avoid pyrexia, especially if ischaemia is suspected; antipyretics are first-line therapy, but surface cooling may be used if required.
- Avoid hyper/hypoglycaemia; maintain blood glucose of 4–11 mmol/L.
- Anaemia occurs frequently in these patients as a result of multiple blood samples obtained, aim for a haemoglobin of 8–10 g/dl.

Pitfalls/difficult situations

- <50% of patients have the classic headache.
- Traumatic SAH or spontaneous SAH which then causes a fall may be associated with other injuries, including cervical spine injuries.
- Lumbar puncture is indicated if the CT scan is negative and SAH is suspected; or if another diagnosis (e.g. meningoencephalitis) is likely.

Further reading

Al-Shahi R, et al. Subarachnoid haemorrhage. Br Med J 2006; **333**: 235–40.
Diringer MN, et al. Critical care management of patients following aneurysmal subarachnoid hemorrhage: recommendations from the Neurocritical Care Society's multidisciplinary consensus conference. Neurocrit Care 2011; **15**(2): 211–40.

⊕ Traumatic brain injury

Traumatic brain injury (TBI) occurs with an incidence of approximately 450 per 100,000/year, and accounts for about 20% of deaths in males aged 5–35 in the UK.

- Head injuries can be classified according to decrease in consciousness:
  - Mild: GCS 14–15
  - Moderate: GCS 9–13
  - Severe: GCS 3–8
- TBI can also be classified as penetrating and blunt, diffuse, or focal:
  - Diffuse injuries include: diffuse axonal injury and traumatic sub-arachnoid injury
  - Focal injuries include: subdural haematoma, extradural haematoma and intracerebral haematoma

The 1° injury is the initial injury causing the insult; the management of TBI aims to prevent further neurological damage (2° brain injury) and optimize the penumbra (the area around the initial insult, which is compromised).

Causes

- Any high-impact injury, especially involving head, spine, or chest.
- A low-impact injury, such as a fall, in a patient who is anticoagulated.
- Head injuries are associated with drug- and alcohol-related injuries.

2° injuries may be caused by factors that can be managed medically or neurosurgically:

- Systemic hypotension or hypertension.
- Hypoxia, hypercapnia/hypocapnia.
- Hypoglycaemia/hyperglycaemia.
- Anaemia.
- Hyponatraemia.
- Hyperthermia.
- Coagulopathy.
- Sepsis/infection (both systemic or intracranial).
- Seizures.
- Cerebral vasospasm or conversely cerebral hyperaemia.
- Intracranial swelling or mass-effect (extradural/subdural/intracerebral haematomas; cerebral oedema).

Presentation and assessment

Identifying the mechanism of injury will help identify high-velocity/high-risk cases, e.g.:

- Pedestrian versus car; car versus car; motor bicycle accident (MBA).
- Ejection from car; turned-over car.
- Fall >1 m (or 5 stairs); fall from a horse.

Presentation can be subtle or obvious, signs and symptoms may include:

- Headache, amnesia, nausea, and vomiting.
- Diminished consciousness, or loss of consciousness, which may be delayed, especially where trauma leads to a progressive bleed:
  - Airway: grunting, snoring, or complete obstruction
  - Respiratory: Cheyne–Stokes breathing, tachypnoea, bradypnoea (hypoventilation is a late sign); neurogenic pulmonary oedema

- Cushing's triad (hypertension, bradycardia and irregular respiration) are late signs
- Focal neurological signs (e.g. problems understanding speech, speaking, reading or writing, loss of sensation, loss of balance, weakness, problems walking, visual changes, abnormal reflexes).
- Seizures and/or incontinence.

Localized injuries may be evident:

- Bruising, swelling, depressed skull fracture, epistaxis.
- Skull fracture or base-of-skull (BOS) fracture (see 📖 Signs of base-of-skull fracture).

Signs of base-of-skull fracture

- CSF rhinorrhoea.
- CSF otorrhoea.
- 'Raccoon' eyes (bilateral periorbital haematoma).
- Mastoid bruising or tenderness (Battle's sign).
- Tympanic blood (on examination with an otoscope).
- Epistaxis.
- New unilateral deafness.

- Penetrating head or eye injury.

Always look for associated injuries, especially:

- Haemorrhage: tachycardia and/or hypotension are likely.
- Spinal, chest, abdomen, or long-bone injuries.

Investigations

- ABGs (monitor PaO_2, $PaCO_2$, and degree of acidaemia).
- Crossmatch blood.
- FBC, coagulation studies (to identify ↓Hb or coagulopathic patients).
- Serum glucose.
- U&Es, serum osmolality (where osmolality >320 mmol/L and Na >150mmol/L, hypertonic saline and mannitol are contraindicated).
- LFTs.
- Consider blood alcohol levels and other drug levels where appropriate (e.g. paracetamol and salicylate).
- ECG (ischaemic changes may be present).
- Trauma X-rays (C-spine, CXR, pelvis).
- CT scan head and neck (see indications 📖 p.155): ideally should be done within 10 minutes of arrival in hospital and be reported within 1 hour.

Differential diagnoses

- Stroke.
- Meningitis, encephalitis.
- Subarachnoid haemorrhage.
- Intoxication (alcohol or drugs); overdose.

Immediate management

• Give 100% O_2 and support airway, breathing, and circulation as required (see rest of box), maintain SaO_2 >94%.
• Use spinal precautions including hard collar, sand bags, and strapping (and in-line manual stabilization for intubation).
• Obtain a contemporaneous history if possible (e.g. from relatives or ambulance crew); an 'AMPLE' history (🔲 p.2) should be obtained as a minimum.
• Roughly assess neurological state (e.g. conscious and talking, level of consciousness, or lateralizing signs) and simultaneously treat neurological complications which may interfere with ABC (e.g. seizures).
• Complete basic ABC 1° survey before formally assessing neurological state.

Airway

• Airway may be compromised due to impaired conscious level, intubate the trachea as appropriate (placement of the patient in the recovery position is likely to be contraindicated by the need for spinal precautions).
• If endotracheal intubation is needed a rapid sequence intubation will be required to minimize the risk of aspiration; the hard collar will need to be undone, and manual in-line stabilization used in its place.
• Rapid sequence endotracheal intubation should be considered if:
  • GCS ≤8 (severe head injury), or rapidly deteriorating
  • There is risk of aspiration of vomit or blood
  • There is facial or neck trauma putting the airway at risk
  • There is evidence of hypoxia (SaO_2 <90%), hypercapnia ($PaCO_2$ >5 kPa) or marked tachypnoea
  • Short-term deliberate hyperventilation is required
  • There is ongoing seizure activity
  • The patient is unlikely to remain still for investigations (e.g. CT)
  • The patient is agitated and combative but requiring treatment
• Endotracheal intubation may be required to manage thoracic trauma resulting in respiratory compromise (see 🔲 p.80, 82 and 410).
• Any stress response to endotracheal intubation should be avoided if possible; IV induction and sedation will help avoid rises in ICP, and opioids should be given as part of the induction:
  • Muscle relaxants may be required for stabilization or transfer, but may mask seizures.

Breathing

• Ensure breathing/ventilation is adequate:
  • Ventilatory support may be needed to optimize oxygenation, avoid hypoxia aiming for a PaO_2 >10 kPa
  • Avoid hypercapnia (aim for $PaCO_2$ 4.5–5 kPa)
  • Avoid hyperventilation and hypocapnia unless required for short periods (<20 minutes) to treat raised ICP
  • If acute pulmonary oedema is present treat with appropriate therapies (🔲 p.86)
• Exclude/treat pneumothorax or haemothorax.

Circulation
- Establish IV access.
- Avoid hypotension, where possible aim for a BP which would be near normal for the patient (or a MAP >90 mmHg, whichever is higher).
- Resuscitate with fluids and blood as required, use normal saline preferentially and avoid hypotonic fluids (dextrose containing fluids); inotropes may be required after normovolaemia is established.

Neurology
- Further useful history may include:
  - History of significant period of amnesia, or loss of consciousness
  - Mechanism of injury in trauma cases
- Formally assess neurological status, including:
  - GCS (see 📖 p.153)
  - Eye examination including pupil size and reactivity, and fundoscopy if possible
  - Evidence of vault or base-of-skull fracture (otoscopy is required)
  - Plantar reflexes
- Reassess GCS once airway, breathing, and circulation have been stabilized, and continue to regularly reassess consciousness and neurological state.

Other
- Exclude and treat hypoglycaemia and hypothermia.
- Urgent CT scan may be required for diagnosis and appropriate management (prevent hypoxia, hypercapnia, hypotension, and hypertension throughout):
  - Patients should be stabilized for transfer prior to CT scan
- Raised ICP may be treated with mannitol (0.5–1 g/kg IV) or hypertonic saline (if serum sodium is <155 mmol/L and serum osmolality is <320 mmol/L), until more definitive measures are employed (see 📖 p. 186)
- Treat seizures as per protocol (📖 p.160).
- Aggressively correct any coagulopathy; thrombolysis is a cause of coagulopathies in trauma, early tranexamic acid treatment may help.
- Check electrolytes.
- Treat other causes of ↓consciousness, including respiratory or cardiovascular compromise (e.g. intra-abdominal bleeding).

Isolated head injury
- Patients with moderate to severe head injuries require CT scans and admission for observation.
- Some patients with mild head injuries might also require CT scans (see indications for CT 📖 p.155), or admission (see 📖 p.182).

In all cases neurosurgical advice should be sought where appropriate (see indications for neurosurgical referral, 📖 p.157).
- Subdural and extradural haematomas should be surgically evacuated.
- Head injuries may require active ICP monitoring via an intracranial pressure transducer (a 'bolt').

Indications for admission for observation

- Any head injury requiring CT (see 📖 p.155).
- Moderate to severe headache.
- Persistent vomiting.
- History of loss of consciousness or amnesia.
- Head trauma associated with coagulopathy (e.g. patient on warfarin).
- Alcohol/drug intoxication.
- Suspicion of non-accidental injury—patient is likely to remain at risk if discharged.
- No companion at home.

Spinal investigations for unconscious patients on ICU where spinal fractures could not be cleared clinically[1] prior to endotracheal intubation[2]

- Multiplane helical (spiral) CT of the entire cervical spine down to and including the T4/T5 disc space. *Or* (if no helical CT available) scanning of the craniocervical junction and the cervicothoracic junction (if not seen on plain radiographs) and any suspicious areas of the C-spine:
  - Lateral and AP cervical radiographs are not considered sufficient where CT scanning is available
  - In cases of polytrauma a CT scan from vertex to pelvis is recommended, followed by image reconstruction to review the spine
- Thoracolumbar AP and lateral radiographs, (unless spinal reconstructions from helical CT of chest/abdomen available, if so omit).
- Ideally a musculoskeletal consultant radiologist should radiographically clear the spine.

If *all* of these points are satisfied, and there are no external signs of injury, the spine may be regarded as stable and uninjured. Close observation during mobilization is essential, but will be limited in this group of patients.

[1] Criteria for clinically clearing the spine are (1) GCS score 15 and appropriate responses; (2) absence of intoxicants, alcohol, or sedation/opioid analgesics; (3) no midline spinal tenderness, no deformity or steps, and no neurological deficit referable to a spinal injury (e.g. abnormal tone, power or reflexes); (4) no significant distracting injury e.g. extremity fracture.

[2] Adapted from Morris C, Guha A, Farquhar I, Evaluation for spinal injuries among unconscious victims of blunt polytrauma: a management guideline for intensive care, 2005, with permission from the Intensive Care Society, 🔗 http://www.ics.ac.uk/professional/standards_and_guidelines/evaluation_of_spinal_injuries_in_unconscious_victims_of_blunt_polytrauma_guidance_for_critical_care_2005

Further management

TBI patients should be discussed with your regional neurosurgical centre (this is time-critical if the patient has a lesion such as an epidural or acute subdural haematoma).

The treatment of TBI outside a neurosurgical centre has been shown to increase mortality.

Ventilation
- Avoid hypoxia, maintain PaO_2 >10 kPa and $PaCO_2$ 4.5–5 kPa.
- Pulmonary oedema may require the addition of PEEP:
  - Very high intrathoracic pressure should be avoided where possible
- Aspiration events and chest infections are common in patients with ↓consciousness and should be actively sought/treated.
- Head-up positioning may decrease aspiration events and improve cerebral venous drainage; until spinal injuries have been excluded this can be achieved by tilting the whole bed 15° head up.

Cardiovascular
- Hypotension should be avoided:
  - An initial MAP >90 mmHg should ensure an acceptable CPP
  - Later MAP may be guided by ICP or other measurements (maintaining CPP of >60–65 mmHg)
  - Fluid resuscitation aiming for euvolaemia (avoiding albumin, and hypotonic fluids where possible) may be sufficient, though inotropes may be needed
- Monitor urine output.

Neurological
- If not intubated/ventilated, perform regular neurological observations:
  - If intubated and ventilated then pupillary reflexes should be observed and it would be prudent for an ICP bolt to be inserted
- Sedatives with rapid offset such as propofol may initially be advisable as it will allow level of consciousness to be easily reassessed.
- Heavy sedation may be required to avoid coughing and gagging on the ETT (which might raise ICP); occasionally thiopental coma will be used as a final attempt at medical management of high ICP.
- Muscle relaxants may be required for the initial intubation, stabilization, or transfer, but may mask fitting:
  - Where muscle relaxants are used consider concurrent antiepileptic sedative infusions (such as propofol or midazolam) and/or loading with anticonvulsants
  - In uncontrolled intracranial hypertension where patients are receiving muscle relaxants, CFAM should be used and burst suppression of 10% should be achieved
- A 15–30° head-up tilt will aid cerebral venous drainage (where spinal precautions are in place the whole bed may be tilted).
- Where ICP is measured it should be kept ≤20 mmHg (see p.186):
  - Cerebral perfusion pressure (CPP) should be maintained at ≥60–65 mmHg (CPP = MAP − ICP)
  - Hypothermia of no less than 35°C can be used to control severe intracranial pressure
  - Hypertonic saline has been used as a means to increase serum sodium and treat resistant high ICP
  - Some neurosurgical centres will perform decompressive craniectomy on patients who fail medical therapy (this is currently controversial and awaiting the outcome from further studies)
- Transcranial Doppler (TCD) monitoring may identify vasospasm.

- Consider seizure prophylaxis using phenytoin 15 mg/kg bolus then 300 mg daily IV/NG.
- Where seizures are witnessed or suspected, treat aggressively with antiepileptic drugs such as phenytoin.
- Further head CTs may be indicated if there is any change in GCS, pupil, or neurological signs.
- Polyuria may indicate hypothalamic injury causing diabetes insipidus (incidence 40%); or the use of osmotic diuretics.

Indications for considering ICP measurement

- Severe head injury (GCS <9 after resuscitation) and an abnormal CT scan (haematomas, contusions, oedema, or compressed basal cisterns).
- Severe head injury (GCS <9 after resuscitation) and a normal CT scan, but 2 of the following:
  - Age >40 years
  - Systolic BP <90 mmHg
  - Decerebrate posturing
- May be considered for moderate or mild head injuries (GCS >8) where sedation or anaesthesia are required for other indications.

ICP measurement should be continued until ICP is normal and not requiring treatment for 3 days.

Trauma

- A tertiary survey looking for occult traumatic injuries should be performed on all head injured patients with diminished GCS once they are stable.
- Spinal precautions (hard-collar, sandbags, strapping, supine positioning, and logrolls) should be in place for all intubated head injury patients in the initial stages:
  - The spine should be cleared as soon as possible according to the Intensive Care Society guidelines to allow better patient management, in particular removal of the hard collar which is likely to impair venous drainage of the head
- Where there is abdominal trauma intra-abdominal pressures (IAP) should be measured and high pressures avoided in order to avoid rises in CVP and ICP.

General

- Maintain haemoglobin of 8–10 g/dl.
- Maintain blood glucose between 6–10 mmol/L.
- Pyrexia should be avoided; antipyretics, or even surface cooling, may be necessary to maintain normothermia.
- Compression stockings should be the first-line DVT prophylaxis where there is a risk of bleeding; optimal timing of starting LMWH thromboprophylaxis is controversial.
- Feeding (via NG if possible) should be instituted in intubated patients as soon as appropriate, accompanied by commencement of aperients:

- If a base of skull fracture is suspected, insert an orogastric tube, do not insert a nasogastric tube
- Infections, particularly chest infections, are common following head injuries and should be treated aggressively.
- A high proportion of patients with TBI will develop electrolyte disturbances, which need to be diagnosed early and carefully managed; hypo- and hypernatraemia should be corrected (see 📖 pp.208 and 210), maintaining a serum sodium of >135 mmol/L.

Pitfalls/difficult situations

- There may be a lucid interval between the initial head injury and the development of an intracranial haematoma; close monitoring is advisable for 4–6 hours after serious injuries.
- In some cases general surgical interventions (e.g. for major internal haemorrhage) may take precedence over investigating or treating neurological problems.

Indicators of poor prognosis

- GCS 3–7.
- Fixed, dilated pupils.
- Hypotension (systolic < 90 mmHg).
- Age >60 years.
- CT scan findings:
  - Blood in the basal cisterns
  - Traumatic SAH
  - Midline shift
  - Intracerebral mass lesions

Data from the Brain Trauma Foundation guidelines, 'Early Indicators of Prognosis in Severe Traumatic Brain Injury'. ♫ https://www.braintrauma.org/pdf/protected/prognosis_guidelines.pdf

---

Further reading

Brain Trauma Foundation website: ♫<https://www.braintrauma.org/coma-guidelines/>.

Cooper DJ, et al. Decompressive craniectomy in diffuse traumatic brain injury. *N Engl J Med* 2011; **364**: 1493–502.

Girling K. Management of head injury in the intensive-care unit. *Cont Educ Anaesth Crit Care Pain* 2004; **4**(2): 52–6.

NICE. *Head injury. Triage, assessment, investigation and early management of head injury in infants, children and adults.* London: NICE, 2007.

Leal-Noval SR, et al. Optimal hemoglobin concentration in patients with subarachnoid hemorrhage, acute ischemic stroke and traumatic brain injury. *Curr Opin Crit Care* 2008; **14**(2): 156–62.

Morris C, et al. *Evaluation for spinal injuries among unconscious victims of blunt polytrauma: A management guideline for intensive care.* London: Intensive Care Society, 2005.

SAFE study Investigators. Saline or albumin for fluid resuscitation in patients with traumatic brain injury. *N Engl J Med* 2007; **357**: 874–84.

Vergouwen MDI, et al. Venous thromboembolism prophylaxis and treatment in patients with acute stroke and traumatic brain injury. *Curr Opin Crit Care* 2008; **14**(2):149–55.

☼ Raised intracranial pressure

ICP is the pressure of the brain parenchyma, CSF, and blood (venous and arterial) inside a rigid skull. Normal ICP is 0–10 mmHg. Raised ICP occurs when compensatory mechanisms to reduce ICP fail, and is defined as ≥20 mmHg for >5 minutes.

Management aims to maintain CPP ≥60 mmHg. CPP = MAP – ICP.

Causes[1]

- Space-occupying lesions, including neoplasm, abscess, or haematomas.
- Vasogenic cerebral oedema: TBI, infection, hepatic encephalopathy, eclampsia, hypertensive encephalopathy, sinus thrombosis, altitude cerebral oedema.
- Cytotoxic oedema: post-cardiac arrest, acute hyponatraemia.
- Interstitial oedema: hydrocephalus.
- Idiopathic intracranial hypertension.

Certain patients are at higher risk of developing raised ICP: following TBI; following neurosurgery (especially where haemostasis is poor); younger patients (compared with older patients).

Presentation and assessment

Within the ICU, raised ICP is most often identified as a result of ICP monitoring, or intraventricular drain, showing

- ↑pressures, or abnormal waveforms (normal ICP waves resemble arterial pressure waveforms, waveforms affected by raised ICP often have the highest peak *after* the dicrotic notch).

Clinical signs and symptoms of raised ICP are those associated with ↓consciousness (🕮 p.152) and any underlying cause, e.g. head injury (🕮 p.178), SAH (🕮 p.174), stroke (🕮 p.166). They may include:

- Listlessness, irritability, headache, vomiting.
- Pupils: unequal, sluggish or divergent; papilloedema on fundoscopy.
- Seizures or focal neurological signs.
- Hypertension, bradycardia; Cheyne–Stokes respiration.

Investigations

- ABGs (to assess $PaCO_2$), FBC, coagulation studies.
- U&Es, LFTs; serum osmolality and glucose.
- Core temperature.
- CT head is essential if raised ICP is suspected in an unmonitored patient; consider CT head if there is an acute rise in monitored ICP.

Differential diagnoses

- Where no monitoring is present: SAH, meningitis/encephalitis, migraine, stroke.
- Where ICP monitoring is present: incorrect calibration of probe.

---

[1] ICP monitoring is most frequently done for TBI. Management algorithms for other conditions are often extrapolated from evidence for TBI.

Immediate management:

In new patients with suspected raised ICP identify/treat the acute cause:

- Give 100% O_2; support airway, breathing, and circulation as required.
- Patients with raised ICP may need intubation/ventilation prior to CT.

Where ICP is shown to be raised in an already intubated ICU patient:

- Check transducers for errors if ICP is monitored.
- Ensure adequate analgesia (also ensuring urinary catheter is patent) and sedation; consider neuromuscular blockade after sedation.
- Tilt patient up to 30° head up; ensure neck veins not obstructed.
- Maintain $PaCO_2$ 4.5–5 kPa and PaO_2 ≥10 kPa; monitor ABG/ETCO₂
- Aim for a CPP ≥60 mmHg using inotropes/vasopressors (after achieving euvolaemia) ensuring a MAP of ≥80–90 mmHg.
- Avoid treating hypertension unless MAP >130 mmHg; use short-acting antihypertensives (e.g. esmolol) aiming for ≤20% reduction.
- Give mannitol 20%, 0.5–1 g/kg over 15 minutes (repeat up to 4-hourly; stop if plasma osmolality ≥320 mOsmol/L or sodium >155 mmol/L).
- Keep core temperature ≤37°C with surface cooling and paracetamol.

If ICP fails to reduce or continues to increase the following may help:

- Repeat CT head to identify new treatable case.
- Hypertonic saline infusion, further mannitol, or furosemide 20–40 mg.
- Thiopentone 75-mg boluses, or a thiopentone infusion.
- Inducing moderate hypothermia (34–35°C).
- Moderate hyperventilation to $PaCO_2$ <4 kPa as a temporary measure (<20 minutes), ideally with accompanying SjO_2/PBO₂ monitoring, as a bridge to definitive therapy such as neurosurgery.

Further management

- In patients who have a raised ICP in the absence of a TBI, definitive treatment is aimed at treating the cause of the raised ICP.
- In patients with brain tumours consider dexamethasone 16 mg IV.
- Treat seizures aggressively with anticonvulsants IV (these can be difficult to diagnosis if paralysed; EEG/CFAM monitoring may be helpful).
- Neurosurgical treatment: may include removal of new haematoma, decompressive craniectomy, CSF drainage, or lobectomy.
- Consider SjO_2/PBO₂ or TCD monitoring.

Pitfalls/difficult situations

- Ventricular drains can block very easily and pressure transducer accuracy can drift, use only as a guide; clinically assess the patient.
- Therapy which reduces ICP can reduce CPP if autoregulation is lost.
- Fluid overload can 'leak' across the BBB and increase cerebral oedema.
- Correct electrolyte abnormalities over 24–36 hours.

Further reading

Brain Trauma Foundation website: ℘ <https://www.braintrauma.org/coma-guidelines>

Mayer S, et al. Critical care management of increased intracranial pressure. *J Intensive Care Med* 2002; **17**: 55–67

NICE. *Head injury. Triage, assessment, investigation and early management of head injury in infants, children and adults.* London: NICE, 2007.

☢ **Meningitis and encephalitis**

(See also 📖 pp.340 and 348.)

Meningitis is a life-threatening inflammation of the meninges and CSF surrounding the brain and spinal cord. Encephalitis is inflammation of the brain parenchyma. Both carry a significant risk in terms of both mortality and morbidity. Rapid diagnosis and aggressive treatment is essential.

Meningitis is diagnosed following identification of pathogens and white cells in CSF obtained by lumbar puncture.

Causes

Risk factors for infectious meningitis include:
- Head injury, neurosurgery.
- Ear and/or sinus infection.
- Immunocompromised patients, including those with diabetes, chronic renal failure, or on immunosuppressant drugs (particularly steroids).

Infectious causes:
- Bacteria: *Streptococcus pneumoniae*, especially in asplenic patients, *Haemophilus influenzae*, *Neisseria meningitides*, *Listeria monocytogenes*).
- Viruses: herpes simplex virus, coxsackie enteroviruses.
- Nosocomial bacteria: *Escherichia coli*, *Pseudomonas*, *Klebsiella*, *Acinetobacter*.
- In the immunocompromised: TB, fungal infections (e.g. *Cryptococcus*)
- Following neurosurgery: *Staphylococcus aureus* and *S. epidermis*.

Non-infectious causes include SAH, malignant infiltration (lymphoma/leukaemia), and autoimmune processes.

Presentation and assessment

- Neurological/meningeal signs and symptoms:
  - Headache and/or neck stiffness (not always found with encephalitis)
  - Altered mental state or ↓consciousness
  - Photophobia
  - Vomiting
  - Cranial nerve lesions and/or focal neurological signs
  - Seizures
  - Papilloedema (an unreliable sign that can be difficult to detect; it may be absent or present late)
- Signs of infection (e.g. tachycardia, tachypnoea, pyrexia and/or rigors):
  - Evidence of severe sepsis (e.g. hypotension, cardiovascular collapse, DIC, ARDS)
  - Rash
- Airway and cardiorespiratory signs and symptoms associated with ↓consciousness (📖 p.152) may also be present.
- Intracerebral abscess may be associated with meningitis (see 📖 p. 340).

Classical symptoms and signs are not always present, especially in immunosuppressed or elderly patients where behavioural changes and/or low-grade fever may be the only signs. A high index of suspicion is the key to quick and effective management.

Viral meningitis should be considered in cases of reduced consciousness:
• Personality/behavioural changes are associated with HSV infection.
• May be associated with a history of exotic travel.
• A vesicular rash may be present.
• Viral meningitis is often self-limiting.

Meningococcal septicaemia may occur with meningococcal meningitis in ~70% of cases, (see 🕮 p.348):
• *Meningococcal* infection can to occur in clusters, especially where there is close contact (e.g. new university students, pilgrimages).
• Prodromal symptoms are non-specific and flu-like.
• A characteristic purpuric non-blanching rash can occur, which may initially appear erythematous.

Investigations
• ABGs.
• FBC, coagulation screen, G&S.
• U&Es, LFTs, serum osmolality.
• Serum glucose.
• CT head and/or MRI (serial CT scan may be required according to neurological status).
• LP (see 🕮 p.574; opening pressure, CSF for urgent Gram stain and microscopy, PCR, protein, glucose with paired serum sample).[1]
• Blood cultures, and serum PCR (or antigen tests) for *N. meningitides*.
• Throat/nasopharyngeal swabs (both for culture and PCR).
• Rash scrapings or skin pustule aspirates (for culture/PCR).
• Serial blood cultures or microbiological samples may be required.
• Blood serology may be indicated for mumps, HSV or HIV (especially if *Cryptococcus* or *Toxoplasmosis* is present).
Don't delay giving antibiotics to get microbiology samples.

Differential diagnoses
Differential diagnoses for meningitis include causes of severe headache and/or ↓consciousness:
• Migraine.
• SAH (exclude with CT scan).
• Causes of raised ICP (see 🕮 p.186).

Causes of aseptic meningitis (i.e. no organism found in LP samples):
• Viral meningitis (HSV, EBV, varicella zoster, CMV, geographically limited viruses, e.g. Murray Valley encephalitis).
• Partly treated bacterial meningitis.
• Bacterial meningitis due to TB, syphilis, Lyme disease, rickettsiae.
• Fungal meningitis (*Candida*, *Cryptococcus*, *Histoplasma*, *Coccidioides*).
• Protozoal meningitis (cerebral malaria, Toxoplasma).
• Non-infective meningitis (lymphoma/leukaemia, vasculitis).

1 Depending on CT/MRI results LP may be contraindicated, ensure platelets >50 × 10⁹/L, and INR <1.3.

Immediate management

- Give 100% O_2 initially, then titrate to achieve SpO_2 94–98%.
- Airway may be compromised due to impaired conscious level; support the airway or intubate the trachea if required:
  - Place the patient in recovery position if necessary
  - Keep patients nil by mouth initially as they are at risk of requiring intubation/ventilation
- Ensure breathing/ventilation is adequate.
- Indications for intubation and ventilation include:
  - GCS <10 or airway compromise
  - Respiratory insufficiency (PaO_2 <8 kPa or $PaCO_2$ >6.5 kPa)
  - Marked seizure activity
- Assess circulation:
  - Obtain IV access
  - Commence fluid resuscitation, with inotropic support if required
- Assess and monitor consciousness level.
- Perform a rapid, detailed neurological assessment.
- Treat seizures as per protocol (📖 p.160).

If you suspect bacterial meningitis do not delay treatment. Give antibiotics even if already given by GP/admitting physician.

Meningitis treatment

- Give 3rd-generation cephalosporin (e.g. ceftriaxone 2 g IV 12-hourly); local guidelines vary according to patterns of resistance:
  - If the patient is known to have severe penicillin allergy give chloramphenicol 12.5 mg/kg IV 6-hourly
- Start dexamethasone 10 mg IV 6-hourly for 4 days with first dose of antibiotic.
- Perform a CT scan prior to LP to exclude raised ICP and other causes of meningitis.
- Perform LP (see 📖 p.554):
  - Measure opening pressure (often elevated)
  - Take three 0.5 ml CSF samples for urgent Gram stain, microscopy, and culture; PCR and protein
  - Take 0.5 ml in glucose bottle for CSF glucose (and send a corresponding plasma sample)
  - See 📖 p.574 for interpretation of results
- Perform blood cultures (at least 2) and throat swab.
- If there are vasculitic lesions send scrapings (if skin pustules present send aspirations) for culture/PCR.
- If abscess is suspected add metronidazole IV 500 mg 8-hourly.
- If viral meningitis is suspected add aciclovir IV 10 mg/kg 8-hourly.
- If following neurosurgery add flucloxacillin IV 2g 6-hourly (vancomycin IV 500 mg 6-hourly if MRSA suspected).
- In elderly or immunocompromised patients consider adding amoxicillin IV 1 g 6-hourly.
- In the immunocompromised add gentamicin IV 5 mg/kg daily and liposomal amphotericin B IV (dose depends upon formulation) and aciclovir IV 10 mg/kg 8-hourly.

Further management

- Admission to a critical care facility may be required for further monitoring of neurological state and treatment of complications including:
  - Seizure activity resistant to anticonvulsants
  - ↓level of consciousness, especially where airway is at risk
  - Sepsis or SIRS requiring vasopressors or mechanical ventilation
- Report notifiable diseases (📖 p.380).
- Rarely, meningococcal meningitis prophylaxis for staff is required (e.g. after mouth-to-mouth resuscitation); discuss with microbiology (dose: oral ciprofloxacin 500mg, single dose).
- Reconsider antibiotic treatment once the Gram stain result is available; re-culture CSF if clinical improvement is slow.
- A travel history may help in cases of aseptic meningitis involving unusual organisms (rickettsiae, viral causes, *Histoplasma*, *Coccidioides*, cerebral malaria).
- Complications may include:
  - Meningococcal septicaemia: shock (likely to require inotropes), coagulopathy, renal failure, ARDS, adrenal insufficiency
  - Intracranial abscesses/hydrocephalus require neurosurgical referral
  - Raised ICP (see 📖 p.186)
  - Seizures: treat aggressively according to protocol (📖 p.160)
  - SIADH or cerebral salt wasting may occur; check fluid balance and electrolytes regularly
  - Infections: concurrent pneumonia is common requiring aggressive treatment; skin vesicles are likely to get infected
  - Other complications: venous sinus thrombosis, cerebral infarcts
- New focal neurology will require a repeat CT head.

Pitfalls/difficult situations

- Administration of antibiotic therapy prior to admission and LP may prevent the identification of a causative organism.
- CSF analysis does not always add clarity to the diagnosis as a CSF pleocytosis has a number of causes including partially treated bacterial meningitis, TB, Lyme disease, sarcoidosis, and Behçet's.
- LP is contraindicated if ICP is raised (📖 p.186) or abscess is suspected; if there is any doubt await the results of a CT head first.
- Herpes simplex meningoencephalitis may present with personality and behavioural changes; if there is any suspicion start acyclovir.
- If SAH has been excluded, the next most common cause, and the most life threatening, is infection which should be treated aggressively.
- In the immunosuppressed and elderly, behavioural changes and low-grade fever may be the only presenting signs.

Further reading

Heyderman RS, et al. Early management of suspected bacterial meningitis and meningococcal septicaemia in adults. *J Infect* 2003; **46**: 75–7.

Stephens DS, et al. Epidemic meningitis, meningococcaemia and Neisseria meningitidis. *Lancet* 2007; **369**: 2196–210.

Tunkel AR, et al. Practice guidelines for the management of bacterial meningitis. *Clin Infect Dis* 2004; **39**: 1267–84.

Van de Beek.D, et al. Community acquired bacterial meningitis in adults. *N Engl Med J* 2006; **354**: 44–53.

☼: **Agitation/confusion/aggression**

Agitation and confusion is commonly found in the critically ill, and may lead to difficulty in treating or investigating the patient's illness; or it may result in aggression directed towards staff or the patient's relatives.

Causes

Risk factors for agitation, aggression, and delirium include:
- **H**ypoxia or hypercapnia.
- **E**lderly patients.
- **A**cidaemia.
- **D**rug interactions and/or side effects.
- **W**ithdrawal states (especially alcohol).
- **A**nalgesia (inadequate analgesia, or urinary retention, or constipation).
- **T**ired (sleep deprivation).
- **C**erebral illnesses (e.g. Alzheimer's disease, post-ictal states, stroke).
- **H**ypotension.
- **E**ndocrine or metabolic derangement.
- **R**are causes (e.g. heavy metal poisoning).
- **S**epsis/infections.

Metabolic abnormalities may include hypo/hyperglycaemia, uraemia, liver failure (hepatic encephalopathy), hyper/hyponatraemia, hypercalcaemia.

Drugs related to agitation and delirium include alcohol (e.g. acute intoxication or acute withdrawal), illicit drugs (e.g. opioids or hallucinogens), benzodiazepines, antidepressants, steroids, dopamine, anticholinergics.

Presentation and assessment

Levels of agitation or aggression commonly fluctuate over the course of the day (often worse at night) and may present in a variety of ways:
- Fidgeting and interfering with invasive lines or monitoring.
- Shouting or calling out.
- Inattention.
- Disorganized thinking (e.g. confused responses to simple statements, inability to follow moderately complex commands, overfocusing on certain subjects disorientation in time, place, or person).
- Withdrawn behaviour or paranoia.
- Cardiorespiratory (where agitation is associated with physiological compromise): hyperventilation, tachycardia, and hypertension.

Sedation/agitation and delirium can be assessed using scoring mechanisms (e.g. the Richmond Agitation Sedation Scale, RASS, see 📖 p.13, and the Confusion Assessment Method of the ICU, CAM-ICU). Scoring of sedation and delirium is part of the daily assessment of ICU patients.

Investigations

- ABGs (to exclude hypoxia, hypercapnia, and acidaemia).
- FBC, CRP (to identify evidence of infection).
- U&Es, LFTs, serum glucose, calcium, magnesium.
- CXR (if chest infection likely).
- CT head and/or LP (if there is focal or other neurological abnormality).

Immediate management
- Titrate O_2 to achieve an SpO_2 >94%.
- Support airway, breathing, and circulation as required.
- Perform a brief neurological assessment.
- Diagnose and treat any underlying cause:
  - Check electrolytes, blood sugar, catheter patency
- Reassure confused patients of their surroundings and who you are.
- Avoid confrontation with aggressive patients.
- Antipsychotic or sedative medication should only be used if the patient is a risk to themselves or others:
  - Haloperidol 1–2 mg IV/IM every 2–4 hours (decrease dose in the elderly; in extreme agitation up to 15 mg may be required)
  - Alternatively olanzapine 2.5–5 mg PO/SL/IM once daily may be used (if dementia is present risk of stroke may be ↑)
  - Chlorpromazine 12.5 mg IV (slow) may be used as an alternative
  - Clonidine or dexmedetomidine infusions may be used as an alternative within critical care
  - Monitor airway and ECG if high doses are used
- Avoid benzodiazepines in delirium unless required to treat specific states (e.g. alcohol withdrawal), or required for rescue therapy:
  - Lorazepam 1–2 mg IV/IM or midazolam 2.5–5 mg IV/IM
- Where patients refuse treatment, make an early assessment of mental capacity.

Further management
- Attentive medical/nursing care may alleviate the need for medication:
  - Avoid too many nursing staff changes if possible
  - Involve family and relatives where possible; have familiar objects from the patient's home in the room
  - Remind patients of the day, time, location; provide a clock/calendar
  - Create a day/night cycle; minimize excess noise at night
  - Provide patients with their glasses, hearing aid, and dentures
  - Provide an interpreter if required.

Pitfalls/difficult situations
- In some critical care units, physical restraints may be used in place of, or in combination with, chemical treatments—do not use these unless you are familiar with indications, technique, and complications.
- Delirium may present with agitated behaviour or with hypoactive (e.g. withdrawn, quiet, paranoid) behaviour.
- Overt aggression or violence from mentally capable patients is unacceptable, consider involving security or police.

Further reading
Borthwick M, et al. *Detection, prevention and treatment of delirium in critically ill patients.* London: United Kingdom Clinical Pharmacy Association (2006.

Girard TD, et al. Feasibility, efficacy, and safety of antipsychotics for intensive care unit delirium: the MIND randomized, placebo- controlled trial. *Crit Care Med* 2010; **38**: 428–37.

Honiden S, et al. Managing the agitated patient in the ICU: sedation, analgesia, and neuromuscular blockade. *J Intensive Care Med* 2010; **25**: 187–204.

:☉: Alcohol withdrawal

Withdrawal from alcohol is common in the hospital setting, and is often unnoticed in the early stages. It can range from cravings with mild physical symptoms, to delirium and life-threatening autonomic dysfunction.

Causes

Identifying patients with a history of high alcohol intake will allow the use of anti-withdrawal prophylaxis. Patients may suffer from alcohol withdrawal if they have previously had a high alcohol intake and have:
• Voluntarily stopped or reduced their alcohol intake.
• Become incapacitated or otherwise unable to ingest alcohol.

Presentation and assessment

Symptoms commonly occur 24–72 hours after cessation of (or reduction in) prolonged and heavy alcohol use. Peak intensity occurs 24 hours after onset, and may last for 5–7 days with a fluctuating course.

Scoring systems for withdrawal are available (e.g. Clinical Institute withdrawal assessment of alcohol scale, CIWA-Ar). Signs/symptoms include:
• Autonomic hyperactivity (e.g. sweating, tachycardia, hypertension, pyrexia, mydriasis).
• Insomnia.
• ↑hand tremor.
• Nausea and vomiting (with or without anorexia).
• Anxiety.
• Psychomotor agitation.
• Transient visual, tactile, or auditory hallucinations or illusions.
• Seizures (2% of cases, more common if there is hypoglycaemia, hypomagnesaemia, hypokalaemia, or a past history of epilepsy).
Delirium (delirium tremens, DTs) may occur involving:
• Disturbance of consciousness, with inattentiveness.
• Altered cognition (e.g. amnesia, disorientation, language disturbance).

Investigations

• ABGs (to exclude hypoxia, hypercapnia, and acidaemia).
• FBC, CRP (thrombocytopaenia, macrocytic anaemia, infection).
• U&Es, LFTs, coagulation studies (hepatic dysfunction, coagulopathy).
• Serum glucose, magnesium, calcium, phosphate, CK.
• Serum amylase or lipase (exclude pancreatitis).
• Sepsis screen (blood, urine and sputum cultures if infection suspected).
• ECG (if other causes of tachycardia suspected).
• CT head and/or LP (if there is focal or other neurological abnormality).
• Urine toxicology (if other drug use is suspected).

Differential diagnoses

• Sepsis (especially meningitis/encephalitis).
• Metabolic disturbance (e.g. hypoglycaemia, hyperthyroidism).
• Other drug toxicity/poisoning (e.g. anticholinergics, CO poisoning, cocaine, amphetamines, neuroleptic malignant syndrome).
• Non-organic cause (e.g. schizophrenia).

Immediate management
- Titrate O_2 to achieve an SpO_2 of 94–98%.
- Support airway, breathing, and circulation as required.
- Airway may become compromised due to seizure activity or sedatives given as treatment:
  - Keep patients nil by mouth initially
- Perform a rapid, detailed neurological assessment.

Withdrawal treatment
- Benzodiazepines are the mainstay of delirium and seizure treatment.
- Chlordiazepoxide 20 mg 6-hourly PO (reduce by 25% every 2 days over 8 days); extra doses may be required up to 200 mg/day (reduce doses in the elderly or patients with severe liver impairment).
- Alternatively IV lorazepam 1–4 mg IV every 5–15 minutes, or IM 1–40 mg every 30–60 minutes (or IV diazepam at appropriate doses).
- Seizures should be treated initially with benzodiazepines (then as per protocol, 🔲 p.160, *but excluding the use of phenytoin*).
- Haloperidol IM/IV 0.5–5 mg every 30–60 minutes may be added for severe agitation (but may lower the threshold for seizures).
- Where withdrawal is unintentional and/or complicating other critical illness consider giving alcohol.
- If autonomic instability or agitation is severe use sedative infusions of propofol, benzodiazepines or barbiturates (with airway protection).
- Correction of hypomagnesaemia may be of benefit.
- β-blockers (especially propranolol, are not recommended).
- Commence fluid resuscitation with inotropic support if required.

Further management
- Supplemental vitamin therapy (may be given orally unless coma, delirium or Wernicke–Korsakoff syndrome is likely):
  - Thiamine 300 mg PO daily, ascorbic acid 100 mg PO daily
  - Pabrinex® 1–2 pairs IV 12-hourly for up to 7 days should be used
- Avoid glucose containing solutions until after thiamine administration.
- Consider treatment with vitamin K if PT is prolonged.
- Phosphate and magnesium electrolyte replacement may be required.

Pitfalls/difficult situations
- Chlordiazepoxide has a long half-life and may accumulate in liver failure, causing prolonged sedation.
- Wernicke–Korsakoff syndrome may cause ocular abnormalities (diplopia, nystagmus, VI nerve palsy and conjugate gaze defects) and confusion, amnesia, confabulation, hypotension, hypothermia, and coma.

Further reading

DeBellis R, et al. Management of delirium tremens. *J Intens Care Med* 2005; **20**: 164–73.
Lingford-Hughes AR, et al. Evidence-based guidelines for the pharmacological management of substance misuse, addiction and comorbidity. *J Psychopharmacol* 2004; **18**(3): 293–335.
Mayo-Smith MF, et al. Management of alcohol withdrawal delirium. *Arch Internal Med* 2004; **164**: 1405–12.
RCP. *Alcohol use disorders: diagnosis and clinical management of alcohol-related physical complications.* London: Royal College of Physicians, National Clinical Guidelines Centre, 2010.

① **Neuromuscular weakness and paralysis**

There are many causes of weakness or paralysis occurring in critically ill patients, either as a cause of intensive care admission, or occurring during admission. A systematic approach is required.

Causes

Central problems
- Stroke.
- Space-occupying lesions to brain or spinal cord.
- Trauma to brain or spinal cord.
- Multiple sclerosis.

Anterior horn cell disease
- Motor neuron disease.
- Poliomyelitis.

Peripheral nerve conduction
- Guillain–Barré syndrome.
- Critical illness polyneuropathy (and/or critical illness myopathy).
- Autoimmune diseases.
- Metabolic disorders (diabetes, porphyria, thyroid, liver or renal failure).
- Nutritional deficiencies.
- Toxins/poisons (including alcohol), or drugs (isoniazid, vincristine).
- Sarcoid or malignancy.

Neuromuscular junction
- Myasthenia gravis.
- Eaton–Lambert syndrome.
- Botulism.
- Muscle relaxant effects (including suxamethonium apnoea).
- Venoms.

Muscle problems
- Endocrine myopathies.
- Electrolyte disturbances (including periodic paralysis).
- Polymyositis.
- Acute rhabdomyolysis.
- Congenital abnormalities (including the muscular dystrophies).
- Critical illness myopathy (and/or critical illness polyneuropathy).

Presentation and assessment
- The exact presentation will depend on the cause:
- A full history and neurological examination is required.
- Difficulty weaning from the ventilator may be the first sign.
- Critical illness myopathy/polyneuropathy are associated with systemic inflammation, high-dose steroids, hyperglycaemia, and immobility.

Investigations
- ABGs, FBC, U&Es, LFTs, CRP.
- Serum CK, magnesium, phosphate, and calcium.

- Serum B$_{12}$, folate, and iron.
- Autoimmune screen.
- Nerve conduction studies and/or muscle biopsy.
- LP.
- Blood, sputum, and/or wound cultures (if infection suspected).
- Imaging of brain and spinal cord (MRI may be more useful than CT).
- PFTs.

Immediate management

In patients who are not intubated/ventilated:
- Titrate O$_2$ to achieve SpO$_2$ 94–98%.
- Support airway, breathing, and circulation as required.
- If the protective reflexes of the upper airway become obtunded, early intubation must be considered.
- Assess adequacy of ventilation by measuring FVC and FEV$_1$:
  - Support ventilation if FVC <15 ml/kg, or FVC <predicted TV, or aspiration occurs; repeat PFTs 4-hourly
- Endotracheal intubation and mechanical ventilation is likely to be more appropriate than non-invasive ventilation because of the lack of airway protective reflexes and the likely length of treatment.
- Fluid resuscitation or inotropes may be required, particularly in trauma or spinal shock.
- Correct calcium, magnesium, potassium, and phosphate.

Further management

- Further investigation is necessary to identify the cause of weakness .
- A tracheostomy may facilitate prolonged mechanical ventilation.
- Autonomic disruption causing cardiovascular instability, gastric stasis and urinary retention can occur with many causes.
- Impaired swallowing may be present requiring NG, NJ, or PEG feeding.
- Treatments aimed at reducing complications of neuromuscular weakness or paralysis include:
  - Respiratory infections: regular physiotherapy and tracheal toilet
  - DVT/PE prophylaxis: antiembolic stockings/devices or LMWH
  - Skin damage, joint contractures: pressure area care, and physiotherapy are required
  - Bowel care may be needed

Pitfalls/difficult situations

- Recovery of function may take months.
- The use of suxamethonium may cause hyperkalaemia in patients suffering from prolonged immobility.

Further reading

Maramattom BV, et al. Acute neuromuscular weakness in the intensive care unit. *Crit Care Med* 2006; **34**(11): 2835–41.

Sanap MN, et al. Neurologic complications of critical illness: Part II. Polyneuropathies and myopathies. *Crit Care Resusc* 2002; **4**: 133–40.

Schweickert WD, et al. ICU-acquired weakness. *Chest* 2007; **131**(5): 1541–9.

① Guillain–Barré syndrome

Guillain–Barré syndrome (GBS, also far less commonly known as Landry and Strohl syndrome) is an ascending acute inflammatory demyelinating polyradiculoneuropathy (AIDP). Remyelination occurs in most patients although about 25% of patients require intensive care, and 5% die.

Several subtypes of GBS exist, including a purely acute motor axonal neuropathy (AMAN), acute mixed sensorimotor axonal neuropathy (AMSAN), and a cranial form (Miller Fisher variant, which may overlap with other subtypes). A chronic, related condition also exists: chronic, inflammatory demyelinating polyneuropathy (CIDP).

Causes

GBS is more common in men and appears to be an autoimmune-mediated, cross-reactivity to infection. 2/3 of cases have had recent infections:
- Bacterial infection, including *Campylobacter jejuni* (associated with outbreaks), *Mycoplasma pneumonia*, and *Haemophilus influenza*.
- Viral infections EBV, CMV, HIV (and possibly other viruses such as influenza, and influenza-like illnesses).
- Immunization: rabies vaccine has been implicated; other current vaccines have little evidence of association (current influenza vaccines appear to have no association with GBS).
- Haematopoietic stem cell transplantation is also associated with GBS.

Presentation and assessment

GBS typically occurs 7–10 days after a precipitating event and develops over 2–3 weeks, signs and symptoms include:
- Ascending symmetrical (usually) motor weakness/paralysis:
  - May result in poor respiratory function, inability to clear secretions, and respiratory distress
- Absent or reduced reflexes.
- Minimal sensory loss in most cases (paraesthesia or pain may occur).
- Cranial nerve involvement (with Miller Fisher variant, or other variations): ophthalmoplegia, ataxia, facial palsy, bulbar palsy.
- Autonomic dysfunction may occur:
  - Arrhythmias (tachycardias, bradycardias, and asystole may occur)
  - BP instability (hyper/hypotension)
  - Gut and bladder paralysis

Investigations

(See also 📖 p.196.)
- FBC, U&Es, coagulation screen, CRP, ESR.
- Auto-antibody screen (in particular antinuclear factor).
- ECG, CXR.
- PFTs.
- LP (CSF protein >0.5 g/L, cell count normal; although protein may be normal initially).
- Nerve conduction studies (↓conduction velocities).
- Nerve biopsy.
- Serum antibody testing for GM1, GD1a, and GQ1b.
- Stool culture for *C jejuni* (and possibly poliovirus).

- Serology for *C jejuni*, *M. pneumoniae*, EBV, CMV.
- Possibly HIV testing.
- Possibly urine porphobilinogen.

Differential diagnoses
(See also 🕮 p.196.)

- Brainstem stroke or encephalitis, acute transverse myelitis, or spinal cord injury (especially epidural abscess or haematoma).
- Other infections (e.g. botulism, polio, tick paralysis, diphtheritic neuropathy, AIDS or CMV polyradiculoneuropathy).
- Metabolic (e.g. porphyria, hypokalaemia, hypophosphataemia, rhabdomyolysis).
- Drugs/toxins (e.g. heavy metal/arsenic exposure).
- Critical illness polyneuropathy.

Immediate management

- Give 100% O_2 initially and then titrate to achieve SpO_2 94–98%.
- Support airway, breathing, and circulation as required.
- If the protective reflexes of the upper airway become obtunded, early intubation must be considered.
- Assess adequacy of ventilation by measuring FVC and FEV_1:
  - Support ventilation if FVC <15 ml/kg, or FVC <predicted TV, or aspiration occurs; repeat PFTs 4-hourly
- Cardiovascular monitoring required if autonomic disturbance present.
- Tachycardias or bradycardias may need treatment with short-acting agents; expect exaggerated responses to vasoactive medications.

Guillain–Barré syndrome treatment

- Human immunoglobulin (gammaglobulin, IVIG) 0.4 g/kg/day IV for 5 days.
- Alternatively plasmapheresis (or plasma exchange) may be used, 4–6 exchanges over 8–10 days (exchange of total 250 ml/kg).

Further management
(See also 🕮 p.197.)

- Supportive care and treatment of the complications of paralysis are required.
- Ventilation is likely to be prolonged.
- SIADH may occur (monitoring of U&Es is advised).
- Analgesics are required for muscle, joint and soft tissue pain.

Pitfalls/difficult situations

- Steroids may make outcome worse.
- Suxamethonium may provoke arrhythmias.
- About 10% of patients develop a chronic relapsing form of GBS whilst 15% are left with residual neurological disability.

Further reading
Hadden RDM, et al. Preceding infections, immune factors and outcome in Guillain-Barré syndrome. *Neurology* 2001; **56**: 758–65.
Hughes RAC, et al. Guillain Barré syndrome. *Lancet* 2005; **366**: 1653–66.

ⓘ Myasthenia gravis

Myasthenia gravis is an autoimmune disease affecting the postsynaptic acetylcholine receptors (AChR) in the neuromuscular junction. Up to 90% of patients are seropositive for AChR antibodies, and in seronegative patients MuSK antibodies may be present. Patients may develop myasthenic or cholinergic crises requiring intensive care.

Causes

- Myasthenic crises may be precipitated by:
  - Trauma, infections, or pregnancy
  - Drugs (e.g. muscle relaxants, sedatives, aminoglycosides, antimalarials, antihistamines, lithium, phenytoin, carbamazepine; antiarrhythmics such as β-blockers, lidocaine, procainamide, quinidine)
- Cholinergic crises can occur after excess anticholinergic administration.

Presentation and assessment

Myasthenia gravis affects mostly women aged 20–40 or men over 50 (often associated with thymoma), and typically presents with gradual onset fatigable muscle weakness. The most commonly affected sites include extra-ocular (ptosis, diplopia), bulbar (dysphagia, aspiration), neck, and shoulder muscles. The symptoms may fluctuate in intensity, but there is no sensory loss or pain, and reflexes are normal.

Myasthenia gravis can present as a myasthenic crises involving:
- Fatigue when the patient is asked to perform repetitive shoulder or upward gaze eye movements; ptosis may be present.
- Severe weakness with respiratory insufficiency (hypoxia, hypercapnia, or deranged PFTs).
- Dysphagia and/or dysphonia; inability to swallow oral secretions, or protect the airway.
- Pyrexia and/or tachycardia if infection is the precipitant.

Cholinergic crises may present with profound muscle weakness causing respiratory failure and bulbar palsy:
- Associated with hypersalivation, lacrimation, vomiting, miosis, sweating.

Investigations

(See also 📖 p.196.)
- Edrophonium test (also known as a Tensilon® test).
- Electromyography.
- AChR or MuSK antibodies.
- TFTs (hyper/hypothyroidism).
- FBC CRP, blood/sputum/urine culture (if infection is likely).
- CXR (aspiration, or bronchial carcinoma/Eaton–Lambert syndrome).
- CT/MRI chest (may be considered later to identify thymoma).
- PFTs.

Differential diagnoses

(See also 📖 p.196.)
- Eaton–Lambert syndrome (muscle weakness improves with exercise).
- Drug related (e.g. penicillamine-induced myasthenia, suxamethonium apnoea; organophosphate/nerve-agent poisoning for cholinergic crises).
- Botulism.

Immediate management

- Give 100% O_2 initially and then titrate to achieve SpO_2 94–98%.
- Support airway, breathing, and circulation as required.
- If the protective reflexes of the upper airway become obtunded early intubation must be considered.
- Assess adequacy of ventilation by measuring FVC and FEV_1:
  - Support ventilation if FVC <15 ml/kg, or FVC <predicted TV, or failure to expectorate secretions occurs
  - Repeat PFTs 4-hourly
- Cardiovascular monitoring should be applied.
- If the diagnosis is unclear perform an edrophonium test:
  - Give edrophonium 2 mg IV and wait for 30–60 seconds
  - Observe for cholinergic symptoms (have atropine available)
  - Give further 8 mg IV edrophonium
  - Improvement in muscle function should occur within 5–10 minutes
  - Stop if cholinergic symptoms occur/worsen

Myasthenic crisis (responds to edrophonium)

- Discontinue possible medication triggers and treat infections.
- Commence acetylcholinesterase inhibitor treatment (e.g. pyridostigmine or neostigmine).
- Where respiratory failure is present consider human immunoglobulin or plasmapheresis treatment.
- In severe cases immunosuppressants may be required (e.g. methotrexate or azathioprine).
- Steroids may be required, but may exacerbate the illness in the acute stages (use as directed by a neurologist).

Cholinergic crisis (does not respond to edrophonium)

- Withdraw anticholinesterase medication.
- Control cholinergic symptoms with atropine 1 mg IV every 30 minutes (up to 8 mg).

Further management

(See also 📖 p.197.)

- Supportive care and treatment of the complications of paralysis.

Pitfalls/difficult situations

- Where possible avoid muscle relaxants.
- Respiratory infections are common.
- Dysphagia is common and NG feeding may be required.
- Thymectomy may reduce symptoms of myasthenia, put careful postoperative management within critical care may be required.
- If patients with known severe myasthenia gravis require mechanical ventilation for other diseases plasma exchange or immunosuppressive therapy may aid weaning.

Further reading

Chaudhuri A, et al. Myasthenic crisis. *Quart J Med* 2009; **102**: 97–107.
Jani-Acsadi A, et al. Myasthenic crisis: guidelines for prevention and treatment. *J Neurol Sci* 2007; **261**: 127–33.

Metabolic, endocrine, and environmental injury

☼ Metabolic acidosis

Metabolic acidosis is defined as pH <7.36 associated with low bicarbonate (<23 mmol/L). $PaCO_2$ is usually ↓ (respiratory compensation). ↑$PaCO_2$ along with reduced levels of bicarbonate would suggest mixed metabolic and respiratory acidoses (see 📖 p.207).

Base excess (BE), or alternatively base deficit, is commonly used as a means of isolating the metabolic component of an acidaemia or alkalaemia if there is a mixed respiratory/metabolic picture. BE is an estimation of the amount of acid or base that is required to correct blood pH to 7.4, given a $PaCO_2$ level of 5.32 kPa at 37°C. The normal range is +2 to −2; a BE more negative than −5 indicates a significant metabolic acidosis.

Normally commonly measured cations (Na^+ and K^+) exceed the measurable anions (Cl^- and HCO_3^-); this is known as the anion gap (normal 7–12 mmol/L). When the anion gap is ↑ this can indicate the accumulation of unmeasurable acid.

Acidaemia is the term classically used to describe the *state* of having acidified blood; acidosis refers to the process causing acid production.

Causes

See Table 6.1.

Presentation and assessment

The main presentation will be of the presenting illness or precipitating cause of metabolic acidosis (i.e. heart failure), in addition the following may also be present:

- Respiratory signs and symptoms:
  - Tachypnoea, dyspnoea
  - Gasping or sighing breathing (Kussmaul's breathing)
  - $PaCO_2$ is often <3.5 kPa due to compensatory hyperventilation
  - Bradypnoea is a late or pre-terminal sign
- Cardiovascular changes:
  - ↓myocardial contractility, vasodilatation, haemodynamic instability, ↓responsiveness to inotropes
  - ECG: ↑incidence of arrhythmias
  - Bradycardia is often a late or pre-terminal sign
- Neurological symptoms: agitation, confusion, coma.
- GI: impaired perfusion of gut, poor gut motility.
- Renal: where hypoperfusion or renal failure is present, oliguria or anuria may be present.

Investigations

- ABGs (low pH, low bicarbonate, negative base excess, hypocapnia):
  - Venous gases may be used where metabolic acidosis alone (i.e. no hypoxia or hypercapnia) is suspected; venous pH is slightly lower than arterial pH
- Serum lactate (raised lactate causes metabolic acidosis, see Table 6.1).
- Serum osmolality and osmolar gap (both raised if alcohols ingested).
- FBC (↑ /↓WCC in sepsis, thrombocytopaenia if DIC is present; severe anaemia may be a cause of metabolic acidosis).

Table 6.1 Causes of metabolic acidosis

Normal anion gap (<12 mmol/L)	Raised anion gap (>12 mmol/L)	
	Normal serum osmolality (osmolal gap < 10mOsm/kg H$_2$O)	Raised serum osmolality (osmolal gap > 10 mOsm/kg H$_2$O)

• Carbonic anhydrase inhibition, aceta-zolamide
 	
• GI loss:
  • Diarrhoea
  • Small bowel/biliary fistula
 	
• Hyperalimentation
 	
• Hyperchloraemic acidosis (commonly after aggressive saline resuscitation)
 	
• Diuretics
 	
• Renal tubular acidosis
 	
• Ureteroentrostomy
	• Diabetic ketoacidosis
	
	• Drugs and poisons:
	  • Salicylates
	  • Tricyclic antidepressants
	  • Toluene exposure (glue sniffing)
	
	• Infections
	
	• Lactic acidosis with tissue hypoperfusion:
	  • Shock/prolonged hypotension; sepsis
	  • Hypoxia
	  • Anaemia/blood loss
	  • Hypothermia, hyperthermia
	
	• Lactic acidosis without tissue hypoperfusion:
	  • Metformin and phenformin
	  • Hepatic or renal failure
	  • Pancreatitis
	  • Malignancy
	  • Glucose 6 phosphate dehydrogenase deficiency
	  • Renal failure
	
	• Rhabdomyolysis
		• Any form of alcohol ingestion:
		  • Ethanol
		  • Methanol
		  • Ethylene glycol
		  • Isopropyl alcohol
		  • Paraldehyde

- Coagulation screen (↑PT/APTT, ↓fibrinogen in sepsis/DIC).
- U&Es, serum chloride, and anion gap:
  - Urea/creatinine (AKI may be a 1° cause of acidosis, or 2° to the underlying cause of the acidosis)
  - Potassium (hyperkalaemia may occur as a result of acidosis, or be caused by AKI)
  - Anion gap (will help categorize the acidosis, see 📖 Table 6.1 and p.207)
- Serum magnesium, phosphate, and calcium.
- Serum glucose (to exclude DKA).

- LFTs (deranged in hepatic failure).
- Serum amylase (↑ in pancreatitis).
- Blood, urine, and sputum cultures (if infection suspected).
- Urine sample/dipstick for ketones (DKA), protein (underlying renal disease), or myoglobin (myoglobinuria is associated with rhabdomyolysis, trauma, burns and drug side effects; it can be a cause of AKI).
- Serum or capillary ketones may be tested (some dipstick tests do not detect βHBA, the predominant ketone body in DKA).
- ECG (MI/LVF/CCF, effects of hyperkalaemia).
- CXR (pneumonia, PE, LVF).
- Further imaging (e.g. abdominal US or CT scan) and investigations may be indicated by history and examination.

Differential diagnoses

- 1° respiratory alkalosis with metabolic compensation.

Immediate management

- Give O_2 and support airway, breathing, and circulation as required.
- The 1° concern should be to treat the underlying cause.
- Provide organ system support as indicated:
  - Ventilatory support may be required (see directions given later in box)
  - Fluid resuscitation and/or inotropic/vasopressor support may be required
  - Treat arrhythmias if these cause haemodynamic compromise
- Control of acidaemia:
  - Maintain respiratory compensation; avoid sedatives in awake patients
  - If mechanical ventilation is required temporarily maintain a supra-normal minute volume
  - Resistant or profound cases of metabolic acidosis may require renal replacement therapy (see indications, 📖 p.266); a degree of cardiovascular stability will be required for successful haemofiltration to be performed
  - Consider 50–100 mmol of $NaHCO_3$ 8.4% IV (or equivalent) if pH <7.1 and haemodynamic instability is present (mild acidaemia of Ph ~7.2 may be protective); $NaHCO_3$ therapy is controversial and probably requires the ability to hyperventilate, with any beneficial effects of therapy depending on the cause of the acidosis
  - 50–100 mmol of $NaHCO_3$ 8.4% IV may be the drug of choice in acidaemia complicated by hyperkalaemia or tricyclic overdose

Further management

- Invasive monitoring may be required.
- Monitor ABGs and electrolytes; correct any electrolyte abnormalities.

- If infection is suspected identify the source and initiate source control and empirical antibiotic therapy.
- Specific treatment for poisoning may be required (see 📖 pp.448–94) or diabetic ketoacidosis (📖 p.228).

Pitfalls/difficult situations

- The cause may not be immediately apparent, especially in poisoning.
- Consider gut ischaemia in patients with unexplained lactic acidosis.
- Inotropes and antiarrhythmic drugs may be less effective if pH is <7.15.
- Hyperkalaemia often accompanies metabolic acidosis; *hypokalaemia* may develop on treating the acidosis.
- Be prepared to treat severe arrhythmias

Anion gap and osmolal gap:
- Anion gap = $(Na^+ + K^+) - (Cl^- + HCO_3^-)$
  - Anion gap calculations involve 4 measured ions, so the margin of error is much higher than that of a single electrolyte determination; lab errors can result in a low anion gap
  - Albumin is the major unmeasured anion and contributes almost the whole of the value of the anion gap; every 1 g decrease in albumin will decrease anion gap by 2.5–3 mmol
  - Low albumin is common in ICU patients and will lower the anion gap so that what should give rise to a raised anion gap (i.e. lactic acidosis) may result in a normal anion gap
- Osmolal gap = (*measured* serum osmolality – *calculated* osmolality).
- *Calculated* osmolality = $(2 \times Na^+)$ + glucose + urea [all in mmol/L].

The 'Boston rules':
A practical approach to identifying 'appropriate' respiratory compensation is as follows:
- 'Expected' $PaCO_2$ *should be approximately* $1+(HCO_3^-/5)$; for example, for an HCO_3^- of 8 mmol/L *should* result in a $PaCO_2$ of approximately 2.6 kPa as a result of respiratory compensation (higher values indicate inadequate compensation or mixed respiratory/metabolic acidosis; lower values indicate metabolic alkalosis).

Similar 'rules' can be applied to other aspects of acid–base physiology:
- Primary *acute* respiratory acidosis: HCO_3^- increases by 1 mmol/L for every 1.3 kPa increase in $PaCO_2$
- Primary *chronic* respiratory acidosis: HCO_3^- increases by 4 mmol/L for every 1.3 kPa increase in $PaCO_2$
- Primary metabolic alkalosis: $PaCO_2 = (HCO_3^-/11) + 2.6 \pm 0.65$.

Further reading

Gunnerson KJ. Clinical review: the meaning of acid-base abnormalities in the intensive care unit part 1 – epidemiology. *Crit Care* 2005; **9**: 573–80.

Kaplan LJ, et al. Clinical review: the meaning of acid-base abnormalities in the intensive care unit part 2. *Crit Care* 2005; **9**: 198–203.

Sirker AA, et al. Acid-base physiology: the 'traditional' and the 'modern' approaches. *Anaesthesia* 2002; **57**(4): 348–56.

:☼: Hypernatraemia

- Mild: 145–150 mmol/L.
- Moderate: 151–160 mmol/L.
- Severe: >160 mmol/L.

Sodium is the major extracellular cation, so hypernatraemia is always accompanied by hyperosmolality.

Causes

Hypovolaemic (associated with low extracellular volume; water loss greater than sodium loss):
- Extrarenal losses: diarrhoea, vomiting, fistulas, significant burns.
- Renal losses: osmotic diuretics, diuretics, post-obstructive diuresis, intrinsic renal disease, uncontrolled diabetes mellitus.
- Adipsic: 2° to ↓thirst (may be behavioural or 2° to head injury and hypothalamic damage).

Hypervolaemic (associated with high extracellular volume; sodium gains greater than water gains):
- Administration of high concentration sodium bicarbonate, or of hypertonic saline.
- Conn's syndrome: hypertension, hypokalaemia, alkalaemia.
- Cushing's syndrome.

Euvolaemic
- Diabetes insipidus (nephrogenic or cranial); intracellular and interstitial water loss predominates, <10% is intravascular.
- Any increase in insensible losses: hyperventilation, fever.

Presentation and assessment

Patients may be asymptomatic, or have signs and symptoms, such as:
- General: weakness, malaise, ↓skin turgor.
- Neurological: irritability, confusion, delirium, brisk tendon reflexes, muscle twitches, spasticity, seizures, coma, intracranial haemorrhage.
- Cardiovascular: hypovolaemic states, resting or postural hypotension; hypervolaemic states; added S3 heart sound, oedema.
- GI: diarrhoea, vomiting excessive drain/fistula output.
- Renal: polyuria, polydipsia, massive diuresis.

Investigations

- U&Es, serum glucose (to exclude hyperglycaemic osmotic diuresis).
- Urinary sodium, coupled urinary and plasma osmolalities.
- Consider head CT/MRI, (intracranial haemorrhage, dural sinus thrombosis or pathological cause of central hypernatraemia).
- Consider a water deprivation test (urine osmolality does not increase in line with serum hyperosmolality in either type of DI).
- ADH stimulation test (if nephrogenic DI is present urine osmolality does not increase after ADH or desmopressin administration).

Differential diagnoses

- Hyperosmolar hyperglycaemic state.

Immediate management

- Give O_2 and support airway, breathing, and circulation as required.

Sodium correction: depends on rate of onset of symptoms

- If hyperacute (<12 hours) rapid correction can be attempted.
- Chronic hypernatraemia: correction should be attempted over 24–72 hours to minimize the risk of cerebral oedema, aim to lower plasma sodium at a rate of <2 mmol/hour (maximum 10 mmol/L/day).

Guide treatment according to cause

- Hypovolaemic:
  - If possible, encourage oral fluids or NG water
  - If hypotensive give fluids, monitoring serum sodium; choice of fluid depends upon the degree of hypovolaemia and hypernatraemia and the speed of correction which occurs (hypotonic solutions, 0.45% saline or 5% glucose IV, may be used; 0.9% saline is relatively hypotonic in severe hypernatraemia)
- Hypervolaemic:
  - Stop any high sodium-containing infusions/feed
  - Consider furosemide 20 mg IV or spironolactone 50 mg PO
  - Oral/NG water or hypotonic IV solutions may be appropriate, depending upon the degree of hypervolaemia or hypernatraemia
  - Haemofiltration with low sodium dialysate may be considered if patient is severely fluid overloaded or already on CVVH
- Euvolaemic:
  - Encourage oral/NG water intake
  - Hypotonic IV fluids (may need large volumes)
  - Where DI is present replace urinary losses and give desmopressin IV/SC/IM 1–2 mcg 12-hourly; or via intranasal spray 10 mcg 12-hourly

Further management

- Investigate any causes and treat appropriately.
- Minimize sodium intake (e.g. colloids, feed, or sodium bicarbonate).
- Maintain a strict input/output chart, including all drain losses.
- Monitor electrolytes frequently, initially 1–2-hourly, then ~4 hourly.

Pitfalls/difficult situations

- In liver failure keep sodium >145 mmol/L to avoid cerebral oedema.

Urine osmolality states	
Osmolality	*Likely cause*
• High	Extrarenal hypotonic fluid losses, salt overload
• Low	Diabetes insipidus
• Normal	Diuretics or salt wasting

Further reading

Adrogue HJ, et al. Hypernatraemia. *N Engl J Med* 2000; **342**(20): 1493–9.
Reynolds RM, et al. Disorders of sodium balance. *Br Med J* 2006; **332**(7543): 702–5.

☼ Hyponatraemia

- Mild: 125–134 mmol/L
- Moderate: 120–124 mmol/L
- Severe: <120 mmol/L.

Causes

Hypovolaemic (associated with loss of sodium and water)
- Renal losses (urinary sodium >20 mmol/L): diuretics, DKA, Addison's, sodium losing nephropathies, diuretic phase of AKI.
- Extrarenal (urinary sodium <20 mmol/L): diarrhoea, vomiting, fistula/drain losses, burns, small bowel obstruction, pancreatitis.

Hypervolaemic (urinary sodium usually >20 mmol/L; associated with total body water rise greater than sodium rise; oedema may be present)
- Iatrogenic: TUR syndrome (🕮 p.396); excess water administration.
- Cardiovascular: CCF (urinary sodium <20 mmol/L).
- Respiratory: pneumonia, TB, lung abscess, cystic fibrosis, vasculitis.
- Neurological: trauma, CVA, SAH, malignancy, vasculitis, infection.
- GI: cirrhosis with ascites.
- Renal: severe renal failure, nephrotic syndrome.
- Drugs: opiates, haloperidol, amitriptyline, vasopressin, carbamazepine, oxytocin, chlorpropamide, thiazides, ecstasy overdose.
- Endocrine: severe myxoedema, psychogenic polydipsia.
- Malignancy: lung (small cell), pancreatic, lymphoma, prostatic.

Euvolaemic (associated with a slight increase in total body water, minimal oedema, urinary sodium >20 mmol/L, urine osmolality >100 mosmol/kg, serum osmolality <270 mosmol/kg)
- General: following surgical stress response, HIV.
- Endocrine: glucocorticoid deficiency, hypothyroidism, SIADH.

Presentation and assessment

Signs and symptoms depend on rate and magnitude of the decrease:
- General: change in skin turgor, weakness, incontinence.
- Neurological:
  - Sodium ~120 mmol/L: headache, confusion, restlessness, irritability
  - Sodium ~110 mmol/L: ataxia, hallucinations, seizures, coma, fixed unilateral dilated pupil, decorticate or decerebrate posturing
- Cardiovascular: hypertension, CCF, elevated CVP/JVP, added S3 heart sound, oedema, bradycardia.
- Respiratory: hypoventilation or respiratory arrest associated with coma.
- GI: anorexia, nausea and vomiting.

Investigations

- U&Es (renal failure).
- TFTs (hypothyroidism).
- Random cortisol, ACTH stimulation test (Addison's).
- Urinary sodium level, coupled urinary and plasma osmolalities.
- CXR (pneumonia, TB, lung abscess, cystic fibrosis, vasculitis).
- Head CT (trauma, CVA, SAH, malignancy, vasculitis, infection).

Differential diagnoses
- Sampling error: sample taken from near a hypotonic IV infusion.
- Artificially low sodium due to hyperlipidaemia or hyperglycaemia.

Immediate management
- Give O_2 and support airway, breathing, and circulation as required.

Sodium correction, depends on rate of onset of symptoms
- In chronic hyponatraemia: correction should not exceed 1–2 mmol/L/hour until life-threatening complications resolve, and 0.5 mmol/L/hour once serum sodium reaches 120mmol/L.
- Acute hyponatraemia: allows faster correction, but no greater than 20 mmol/L/day is advised.
- Fluid resuscitation/sodium replacement can be with hypertonic or isotonic fluid, depending upon the degree of hyponatraemia and hypovolaemia:
  - Monitor serum sodium levels frequently, initially hourly
- In hypervolaemia with oedema:
  - If symptomatic give furosemide (20 mg IV PRN) with/without mannitol (100–500 ml 20% over 20 minutes; caution in severe hypervolaemia)
  - Replace urinary sodium losses with hypertonic saline as previously described
- If asymptomatic, fluid restrict to 1–1.5 L/day; persistent hyponatraemia in this circumstance points to SIADH.
- If in established renal failure, dialysis may be necessary.
- Monitor plasma potassium and magnesium concentrations as they may alter dramatically.

Further management
- Use isotonic solutions for drug reconstitution and PN.
- Correct other electrolyte abnormalities (hyponatraemia may intensify the cardiac effects of hyperkalaemia).
- Correct adrenal insufficiency or hypothyroidism.

Pitfalls/difficult situations
- Rapid, large corrections risk central pontine myelinolysis.
- Where possible, perform frequent plasma sodium checks rather than using equations to calculate excess water.
- If the patient has LVF consider giving furosemide (20 mg IV PRN) and replacing urinary sodium with hypertonic saline aliquots.
- Hyponatraemia can occur with a normal osmolality if abnormal solutes (e.g. ethanol, ethylene glycol) have been ingested.
- Diuretics will affect urine osmolality and electrolytes; these should be stopped for >24 hours before urine osmolality and electrolyte measurement if a cause other than diuretics is considered likely.

Further reading
Adrogue HJ, et al. Hyponatraemia. *N Engl J Med* 2000; **342**(21): 1581–9.

☠ Hyperkalaemia

- Mild: 5.5–6.0 mmol/L.
- Moderate: 6.1–7.0 mmol/L.
- Severe: >7.0 mmol/L.

Causes

- Acute or chronic, oliguric renal failure.
- Metabolic acidosis.
- Addison's disease, aldosterone deficiency.
- Cell injury or ↑metabolism (e.g. rhabdomyolysis, crush injury, tumour lysis, haemolysis, or burns, malignant hyperthermia).
- Massive blood transfusion.
- Suxamethonium given to patients with the following conditions:
  - Major burns, spinal trauma, prolonged immobility, pre-existing ↑K⁺
- Excess intake of potassium (e.g. via infusions, medications, or diet).
- Drugs (e.g. spironolactone or amiloride, ACE inhibitors, ARAs, NSAIDs, pentamidine, β-blockers, digoxin overdose).

Presentation and assessment

Hyperkalaemia is often an incidental laboratory finding. Patients with chronically elevated levels may be asymptomatic; rapidly rising K⁺ levels influence the symptoms observed. Signs and symptoms may include:
- Neuromuscular: muscle cramps, fatigue, weakness, paraesthesia, paralysis (this may even present as failure to wean).
- ECG changes: tall tented T waves, slurring of ST segments into T waves, small P waves, prolonged PR interval, widened QRS, complete heart block, asystole or VF.
- GI: nausea, vomiting or diarrhoea.
- General effects: hyperkalaemia may potentiate the effects of 'lows'— low calcium, low sodium, low pH and low temperature.

Hyperkalaemia should be suspected in patients who have:
- Pre-existing renal failure, especially if dialysis has been missed.
- Dehydration and acidaemia (e.g. DKA).

Investigations

The patient's medications should be reviewed as a possible cause. Other investigations should be directed at confirming the diagnosis and cause:
- ABGs, or venous blood gases (acidaemia).
- U&Es (confirmation of serum K⁺ concentration, ↑urea/creatinine).
- Serum calcium (↓ in massive transfusion/renal failure; hypocalcaemia can exacerbate cardiac rhythm disturbances).
- CK (↑ in rhabdomyolysis, crush injury or burns).
- ECG (it is not essential to perform an ECG prior to treatment)
- Serum digoxin levels (if digoxin poisoning suspected).

Differential diagnoses

- Sampling error (tight tourniquet leading to crushed RBCs/haemolysis on sample arm, sample taken from near potassium-containing IV infusion).
- Severe leucocytosis, thrombocytosis (cells leak K⁺ in clotted sample).
- Blood sample left to rest a long time before testing.

Immediate management

- Give O_2 and support airway, breathing, and circulation as required.
- If the patient is mechanically ventilated consider temporarily increasing the ventilation rate to 'buy time' by decreasing acidosis/ inducing alkalosis and so lowering K^+ levels (K^+ moves into cells).
- Commence continuous ECG monitoring and obtain IV access.
- If hyperkalaemia is moderate or severe, or if the patient is symptomatic (or has ECG changes), and digoxin toxicity is not suspected:
  - Give calcium gluconate 10ml 10% over 2 minutes (or calcium chloride 3–5 ml of 10% solution IV over 3 minutes); has a cardioprotective effect only, will not lower potassium
  - The cardioprotective effect of calcium lasts ~1 hour; if ECG changes are present then these often resolve after calcium
  - Calcium may need to be repeated if hyperkalaemia persists
- If digoxin toxicity is suspected give calcium gluconate 10 ml 10% in 100 ml 5% glucose over 20 minutes.
- Give soluble insulin 15–20 units in 50 ml 50% dextrose IV over 15–30 minutes (glucose is not required if serum glucose>15 mmol/L).
- Salbutamol 5 mg nebulized (or other β agonists) may be added
  - Consider IV salbutamol 250 mcg in 50ml 0.9% saline over 15–30 minutes
- Sodium bicarbonate 8.4% 25–50 ml IV may be given if there is accompanying profound acidosis (mechanical ventilation may need to be ↑ if bicarbonate is given).

Further management

- Re-check K^+ level regularly to guide therapy; ABG analysers which allow K^+ analysis may be faster than sending formal laboratory samples.
- Consider polystyrene sulphonate resin (Calcium Resonium®) 15 g PO 8-hourly, or as 30 g enema (this requires colonic irrigation after 9 hours to remove K^+ from colon).
- Treat the cause (e.g. steroids for Addison's, FAB fragments for digoxin toxicity).
- Avoid suxamethonium.
- If hyperkalaemia does not respond to treatment proceed to dialysis.

Pitfalls/difficult situations

- It is important to note that insulin and salbutamol only move K^+ into cells; excess K^+ must eventually be removed from the body either in urine or via the bowels.
- If the patient is anuric, haemofiltration, or dialysis, is usually required.
- Hyperkalaemia can prolong neuromuscular blockade.
- If a rapid sequence intubation is required then consider using a modified technique without suxamethonium (e.g. with rocuronium).
- The rate of rise of K^+ governs arrhythmia potential, some patients with chronic renal failure and marked hyperkalaemia are quite stable.

Further reading

American Heart Association. Life-threatening electrolyte abnormalities. *Circulation* 2005; **112**: IV-121–5.
Evans KJ, et al. Hyperkalaemia: a review. *J Intensive Care Med* 2005; **20**(5):272–90.
Kuvin JT. Electrocardiographic changes of hyperkalaemia. *N Engl J Med* 1998; **338**: 662.

☼ Hypokalaemia

- Mild: 2.5–3.0 mmol/L.
- Severe: <2.5 mmol/L.

Causes

- ↓intake: malnutrition, omission from IV fluid, PN.
- Endocrine: SIADH, Cushing's syndrome, Conn's syndrome (Conn's should be suspected where there is a hypertensive, hypokalaemic alkalosis in a patient not taking diuretics).
- GI losses: diarrhoea, enemas or laxative abuse, vomiting or copious NG losses, intestinal fistula, rectal villous adenoma, pyloric stenosis, refeeding syndrome.
- Renal losses: magnesium depletion, haemofiltration losses, RTA, leukaemia (unknown mechanism).
- Drugs/toxins: diuretics (especially metolazone in the elderly), β agonists, steroids, thiopental infusions, theophylline, and aminoglycosides; liquorice abuse (pseudohyperaldosteronism, and less commonly glucocorticoid agonist effects); alcoholism.
- Transcellular shifts: insulin usage, alkalaemia, hypothermia, familial periodic paralysis.
- Rare syndromes: Gitelman syndrome, Liddle's syndrome, Bartter's syndrome, and Fanconi syndrome.

Presentation and assessment

Hypokalaemia may be an incidental laboratory finding. Signs and symptoms, when present, may include:

- Neurological: psychosis, delirium, hallucinations.
- Neuromuscular: muscle weakness, ↓tendon reflexes, paralysis, paraesthesia, cramps, hypotonia (this may present as respiratory failure, or difficulty weaning from ventilator).
- Cardiovascular: palpitations; ECG changes such as prolonged PR interval, ST depression, small/inverted T waves, visible U wave (after T), arrhythmias (SVT, VT, torsade de pointes).
- GI: abdominal cramps, constipation, nausea and vomiting.
- Renal: polyuria, nocturia, polydypsia.

Investigations

The patient's medications should be reviewed as a possible cause:

- ABGs, or venous blood gases (alkalaemia).
- U&Es (confirmation of serum K^+ concentration, AKI).
- Serum magnesium (coincident hypomagnesaemia is common).
- Serum calcium and phosphate (coexistent electrolyte disturbance).
- Digoxin level (if on digoxin; hypokalaemia can potentate arrhythmias).
- ECG (it is not essential to perform an ECG prior to treatment).

Differential diagnoses

- Sampling error: sample taken from near potassium-free IV infusion.
- Cushing's disease/syndrome; Conn's syndrome.
- Hypomagnesaemia; hypocalcaemia.

Immediate management

- Give O_2 and support airway, breathing, and circulation as required.
- Commence continuous ECG monitoring and obtain IV access.
- Where possible stop causative drugs.
- If symptoms or arrhythmias are life-threatening:
  - Give KCL replacement neat at 20 mmol/30 minutes *via central line only* (do not give replacement any more concentrated than 40 mmol/L via a peripheral line)
- If symptoms are moderate:
  - Give 40 mmol KCl in 1 L of fluid, this may be infused peripherally over 4–6 hours
  - Alternatively 40 mmol KCl in 100 ml of fluid may be infused via a central line over 4–6 hours
- If symptoms are mild and without arrhythmias use oral/NG therapy (e.g. using Sando-K®, 2–4 tablets TDS/QDS).
- Correct hypomagnesaemia which will antagonize attempts at potassium correction (magnesium sulphate 20 mmol, 5 g, in 100 ml 5% glucose over 1–2 hours).

Further management

- Monitor K^+ level hourly via ABG initially and treat underlying causes:
  - Discontinue laxatives and add in H_2 receptor antagonists and/or motility agents to decrease NG losses
- If diuretics are essential consider switching to potassium-sparing drugs (e.g. spironolactone or amiloride).

Pitfalls/difficult situations

- Potassium replacement in AKI or CKD may cause hyperkalaemia.
- Chronic hypokalaemia is better tolerated than acute hypokalaemia.
- Where patients have an associated acidaemia consider correcting hypokalaemia before or alongside acidaemia correction in order to avoid alkali-induced shift of potassium into cells.
- If bicarbonate is high then any hypokalaemia is likely to have been long-standing and may take up to 2 days to replace adequately.
- Take care to avoid hypokalaemia when treating DKA.
- Oral K^+ replacement may be limited by patient tolerance, some patients develop nausea or even GI ulceration.
- Surgery or interventional radiology may be required (e.g. renal artery stenosis, adrenal adenoma, intestinal obstruction, villous adenoma).
- Hypokalaemia increases the risk of digoxin toxicity.
- Maintaining K^+ levels of 3.5–4.5 mmol/L following myocardial injury or infarction may decrease the incidence of arrhythmias.
- Rebound hyperkalaemia may occur after thiopental infusion discontinuation (where the infusion has resulted in hypokalaemia correction).

Further reading

Gennari FJ. Current concepts: hypokalemia. *N Engl J Med* 1998; **339**:451–8.

Goyal A, et al. Serum potassium levels and mortality in acute myocardial infarction. *JAMA* 2012; **307**(2):195–6.

① Hypercalcaemia

- Normal: 2.2–2.5 mmol/L (ionized 0.9–1.1 mmol/L).
- Mild: 2.6–3.0 mmol/L.
- Moderate: 3.0–3.4 mmol/L.
- Severe: >3.4 mmol/L.
  Corrected calcium [mmol/L] = measured calcium + 0.02 × (40 − plasma albumin [g/L])

Causes

- Commonly 2° to malignancy, especially squamous-cell lung cancer, myeloma, breast cancer, or any cancer with bone metastases.
- Hyperthyroidism, phaeochromocytoma (MEN II), Addison's disease.
- 1° or tertiary hyperparathyroidism.
- Granulomatous disease (e.g. sarcoidosis, TB).
- Immobilization, Paget's disease, AIDS, advanced chronic liver disease.
- Renal failure (2° hyperparathyroidism).
- Familial benign hypocalciuric hypercalcaemia.
- Vitamin D intoxication, milk alkali syndrome, excess antacid ingestion, aluminium intoxication.
- Drugs: thiazide diuretics, lithium, theophylline.
- Hypophosphataemia (<1.4 mmol/L).

Presentation and assessment

Often identified as a result of blood tests, rather than clinically. Urgent treatment is required for calcium >3mmol/L. Symptoms are classically described as 'bones, stones, abdominal groans and psychic moans'.

- General: polyuria, polydipsia, dehydration, corneal calcification.
- Cardiovascular: raised BP, bradycardia, arrhythmias, cardiac arrest:
  - ECG changes: shortened QT, widened T wave
- Neurological: confusion, lethargy, depression, coma, hyper-reflexia, tongue fasciculations.
- GI: abdominal pain, anorexia, weight loss, peptic ulceration, nausea, vomiting, constipation, pancreatitis.
- Renal: kidney stones, renal failure.

Investigations

Underlying malignancy must be excluded.

- FBC (in various cancers: anaemia, leucocytosis, thrombocytopaenia).
- U&Es, (AKI, CKD), LFTs (liver disease).
- Serum calcium (to confirm the diagnosis).
- Serum phosphate (↓with thiazide use, ↑with immobilization/vitamin D intoxication).
- PTH levels (↑ 1° or tertiary hyperparathyroidism).
- ECG, CXR (malignancy, lytic bone lesions, hilar lymphadenopathy).
Further investigations may include:
- Urinary calcium, creatinine and sodium; serum ACE.
- 24-hour urinary calcium, urinary cAMP.
- Imaging investigations as indicated (e.g. skeletal survey for metastases, Paget's; CT/MRI /radionuclide imaging of parathyroids).

Differential diagnoses
- Falsely elevated levels: elevated serum protein levels, high paracetamol level, alcohol or hydralazine, and with haemolysis.

Immediate management
- Give O_2 and support airway, breathing, and circulation as required.
- Aggressively rehydrate with IV fluids (normally 0.9% saline).
- Give a loop diuretic e.g. furosemide (40 mg IV repeated as necessary).

Do not use a thiazide diuretics
- Consider dialysis if renal failure is present (use low-calcium dialysate).
- If calcium >3.4 mmol/L, give disodium pamidronate 30–90 mg in 1 L 0.9% saline IV over 4 hours (or given in divided doses over several days to a total of 90 mg).

Further management
- Aim to decrease serum calcium by 0.5 mmol/L over 1–2 days.
- Corticosteroids (e.g. prednisolone 120 mg/day) are commonly used in sarcoid, vitamin D toxicity, or haematological malignancy.
- Maintenance bisphosphonate treatments include: sodium clodronate PO 1.6 g/day, or disodium etidronate PO 7.5 mg/kg/day.
- Endocrinology or oncology referral may be required.
- Chemotherapy may decrease calcium in malignancy.
- Parathyroidectomy may be indicated.

Pitfalls/difficult situations
- It is ionized calcium which is physiologically active, therefore use corrected calcium level which eliminates the influence of serum albumin.
- Severe elevations in calcium levels may cause coma.
- Elderly patients may manifest symptoms from moderate elevations.
- Symptoms of malignancy may mask symptoms of hypercalcaemia.
- Hypercalcaemia associated with renal calculi, joint complaints, and ulcer disease is more likely to be due to hyperparathyroidism.
- Always consider malignancy, particularly if cachexia or bone pain are present; always consider hypercalcaemia in patients with multiple non-specific complaints and an associated lung mass.
- In moderate to severe hypercalcaemia anaesthetic agents may potentiate the risk of serious arrhythmias.
- Sodium calcitonin (8 units/kg/8 hours), an osteoclast inhibitor, is occasionally used (serum calcium fall is minimal and tachyphylaxis develops); rebound hypercalcaemia can occur after stopping therapy.
- Cinacalcet may be used for all forms of hyperparathyroidism; paricalcitol may be used for 2° hyperparathyroidism.

Further reading
Bilezikian JP. Management of acute hypercalcaemia *N Engl J Med* 1992; **326**: 1196–203.
Pecherstorfer M, et al. Current management strategies for hypercalcaemia. *Treat Endocrinol* 2003; **2**(4): 273–92.

☼ Hypocalcaemia

- Hypocalcaemia: <2.2 mmol/L (ionized <0.9 mmol/L)
  Corrected calcium [mmol/L] = measured calcium + 0.02 × (40 − plasma albumin [g/L])

Causes

- Sepsis (especially toxic shock syndrome), burns, or critical illness causing low albumin.
- Acute pancreatitis causing saponification of calcium by free fatty acids in peritoneum.
- Hypovitaminosis D: dietary deficiency, chronic renal failure.
- Transfusion of large quantities of citrated blood products.
- Malignancy: osteoblastic metastases and tumour lysis syndrome.
- Following surgery (small bowel syndrome, parathyroidectomy).
- Osteomalacia.
- Alkalosis or hyperventilation, causing reduction of ionized calcium fraction.
- Hypomagnesaemia, exacerbates hypocalcaemia and causes end-organ resistance to PTH.
- Hyperphosphataemia (binds calcium): chronic renal failure, rhabdomyolysis, parathyroidectomy.
- Drug administration: protamine, glucagon, heparin:
  - Bisphosphonates may cause rebound hypocalcaemia after being used to treat hypercalcaemia
  - Ethylene glycol poisoning
  - Citrate anticoagulation of renal replacement therapy with inadequate calcium replacement
- Over-hydration.

Presentation and assessment

Symptomatic patients with classical symptoms and signs require urgent evaluation and resuscitation.
- Neurological/neuromuscular symptoms:
  - Carpopedal spasm, cramp, tetany, convulsions, confusion
  - Chvostek's sign (tapping over the facial nerve, anterior to tragus of ear. stimulates facial twitching; positive in 10% of normocalcaemic individuals)
  - Trousseau's sign (inflating a BP cuff above systolic pressure causes local ulnar and median nerve ischaemia resulting in carpal spasm)
- Respiratory: wheeze, stridor, crepitations.
- Cardiovascular: arrhythmias, reduced cardiac output, hypotension, heart failure, angina:
  - ECG changes: prolonged PR interval, prolonged QT interval
- GI: dysphagia, diarrhoea, colic.

Investigations

- ABGs (some analysers are able to check ionized calcium, metabolic alkalosis, hypocapnia with hyperventilation).
- FBC, clotting profile (in massive transfusion or liver dysfunction).

- U&Es (raised urea/creatinine in renal failure).
- Serum calcium (to confirm the diagnosis).
- Serum phosphate (hyperphosphataemia suggests hypoparathyroidism or pseudohypoparathyroidism).
- Serum magnesium (hypomagnesaemia commonly coexists).
- LFTs, including albumin (to detect abnormal liver function; albumin concentration required to calculate 'corrected calcium').
- CK and urine myoglobin (trauma, burns, pancreatitis).
- Amylase, lipase (↑ in pancreatitis).
- Serum urate (raised in tumour lysis syndrome).
- Plasma PTH level.
- 12-lead ECG.

Differential diagnoses

- Sampling error: sample taken from near calcium-free IV infusion.
- Falsely depressed levels seen with iron dextran, heparin, oxalate, citrate, or hyperbilirubinaemia.

Immediate management

- Give O_2 and support airway, breathing, and circulation as required.
- Inotropic support may be required.
- Calcium supplementation:
  - Central administration is preferable as vasoconstriction and ischaemia can occur around tissues at the injection site
  - Give 10 ml 10% calcium chloride IV (2.25 mmol) over 10 minutes
  - Alternatively 10 ml 10% calcium gluconate IV over 10 minutes (slower onset)
- Calcium infusion may be needed (100 ml calcium gluconate 10% in 1 L 0.9% saline infused at an initial rate of 50 ml/hour).
- If hypocalcaemia is mild use oral/NG therapy (e.g. using Sandocal®, 1–2 tablets TDS/QDS).

Further management

- If respiratory alkalosis is present consider adjusting ventilator settings.
- Where spontaneous over-breathing is present in intubated patients consider deepening sedation to inhibit it.
- Correct any coexisting hypokalaemia and hypomagnesaemia.
- Consider enteral supplementation of calcium or vitamin D analogues.

Pitfalls/difficult situations

- Cardiac output or BP may rise during calcium administration.
- Do not administer in the same infusion line as sodium bicarbonate.

Further reading

Cooper MS, et al. Diagnosis and management of hypocalcaemia. Br Med J 2008; 336: 1298–302.
Marx SJ. Hyperparathyroid nnd hypoparathyroid disorders. N Engl J Med 2000; 343: 1863–75.

① **Hyperphosphataemia**

- Normal: 0.8–1.4 mmol/L
- Moderate: 1.5–2.0 mmol/L
- Severe: 2.1–4.0 mmol/L

Causes

- Renal failure (acute or chronic).
- Malignant disease (e.g. leukaemia, lymphoma, multiple myeloma).
- Tumour lysis syndrome.
- Trauma or burns (white phosphorus in particular).
- Excessive release from muscle stores (malignant hyperpyrexia, excessive exercise, rhabdomyolysis).
- Any cause of acidaemia.
- Ischaemic bowel.
- Hypothermia
- Haemolysis, out-of-date blood transfusion.
- Prolonged immobilization.
- Excessive intake or potassium phosphate treatment.
- Hypoparathyroidism, acromegaly, thyrotoxicosis, glucocorticoid withdrawal.
- Bisphosphonate therapy.
- Vitamin D intoxication and milk-alkali syndrome.
- Syndrome of familial intermittent hyperphosphataemia.

Presentation and assessment

Most patients are asymptomatic. If signs and symptoms occur, they are either 2° to the underlying cause, or 2° to the hypocalcaemia (see 📖 p.218), which occurs alongside hyperphosphataemia:

- General: cataracts, muscle cramps, Chvostek's sign, Trousseau's sign, perioral paraesthesia.
- Neurological: altered sensorium, delirium, ↓consciousness, seizures, coma.
- Cardiovascular: hypotension, cardiac failure.
  - ECG changes: prolonged PR interval, prolonged QT interval

Investigations

- ABGs (acidaemia).
- FBC (anaemia in haemolysis. ↓↑WCC in sepsis, leukaemia, lymphoma).
- U&Es (↑urea/creatinine and/or hyperkalaemia in AKI).
- Serum phosphate (to confirm the diagnosis).
- Serum calcium (usually ↑, may be ↓ in vitamin D intoxication and milk-alkali syndrome).
- Serum magnesium (often ↓), serum glucose.
- LFTs.
- Serum PTH level (↓ in vitamin D intoxication and milk-alkali syndrome).
- Serum CK and urinary myoglobin (↑ in trauma/burns).
- ECG.

Differential diagnoses
- Hypermagnesaemia.
- Hypercalcaemia or hypocalcaemia.

Immediate management
- Give O_2 and support airway, breathing, and circulation as required. Treatment of the hypocalcaemia, which occurs as symptoms arise, takes precedence (📖 p.218):
- Administration of insulin can hasten intracellular passage of phosphate as a temporizing measure.
- Oral phosphate binders may be given (some can cause hypercalcaemia), avoid aluminium containing binders as these may exacerbate renal failure.
- Where toxic ingestion has occurred, gastric lavage and oral phosphate binders may be appropriate.
- Consider using saline 0.9% with acetazolamide to increase urinary excretion.
- Renal replacement therapy may be needed for severe refractory cases or those with established renal failure.

Further management
- Continue to treat the underlying cause.

Further reading
Hartmut HH, et al. Management of hyperphosphataemia of chronic kidney disease: lessons from the past and future directions. *Nephrol Dial Transplant* 2002; **17**: 1170–5.

Thette L, et al. Review of the literature: severe hyperphosphatemia. *Am J Med Sci* 1995; **310**(4): 167–74.

☼ Hypophosphataemia

- Normal: 0.8–1.3 mmol/L
- Moderate: 0.3–0.7 mmol/L
- Severe: <0.3 mmol/L

Causes

- Critical illness, sepsis.
- Severe burns (transdermal fluid loss).
- Refeeding syndrome (after starvation, malabsorption or during hyperalimentation).
- Inadequate dietary intake (2° to vitamin D deficiency and phosphate deficiency).
- Chronic liver disease or alcoholism.
- Pancreatitis.
- Hyperparathyroidism, hypothyroidism, hyperaldosteronism.
- Lymphoma or leukaemia.
- Metabolic acidosis, or acute respiratory alkalosis.
- Neuroleptic malignant syndrome.
- Dialysis.
- Diuretic therapy (especially loop diuretics).
- Steroid therapy.
- After high-dose glucose and insulin therapy.
- Ingestion of phosphate binding antacids.
- Fanconi syndrome.

Presentation and assessment

Hypophosphataemia is most commonly found as an incidental finding in ICU. Where signs and symptoms are present they may include:
- General: metabolic acidosis, myopathy, rhabdomyolysis.
- Cardiovascular: cardiomyopathy, ↓cardiac output, ventricular ectopic beats.
- Respiratory: failure to wean, respiratory failure, left shift of the oxygen dissociation curve caused by ↓ 2,3 DPG levels.
- Neurological: encephalopathy, irritability, paraesthesia, seizures, coma.
- Haematological: leucocyte and erythrocyte dysfunction, reduced platelet half-life, haemolytic anaemia.

Investigations

- ABGs (acidaemia or alkalaemia).
- FBC (↓↑WCC in sepsis, leukaemia, lymphoma).
- U&Es (hypokalaemia in DKA treatment or alcoholism).
- Serum phosphate (to confirm/quantify the diagnosis).
- Serum calcium (↑ in 1° hyperparathyroidism, ↓ in vitamin D deficiency or malabsorption).
- Serum magnesium (↓levels suggest poor nutrition).
- Serum glucose (↓ in liver disease, raised in DKA, steroid use).
- LFTs (liver disease).
- Serum ammonia (hepatic encephalopathy).

- Serum lactate (may be ↑ in sepsis).
- Serum PTH level (raised in 1° / 2° hyperparathyroidism).
- Urinary fractional phosphate (>15% suggests hyperparathyroidism or 1° renal phosphate wasting; associated glycosuria and proteinuria suggests Fanconi syndrome).

Differential diagnoses

- Sampling error: sample taken from near phosphate-free IV infusion.
- Alcoholic ketoacidosis (ketoacidosis with normal glucose).
- Guillain–Barré syndrome (typical history, absence of electrolyte disorder).
- Uraemic encephalopathy.
- Rhabdomyolysis (myoglobinuria, renal failure).

Immediate management

- Give O_2 and support airway, breathing, and circulation as required.
- Treatment is normally reserved for those with severe or sustained hypophosphataemia:
  - IV therapy (usually reserved for phosphate <0.6 mmol/L): potassium acid phosphate 30 mmol over 4–6 hours, in 100 ml saline if given centrally, or in 1000 ml saline if given peripherally
  - Where patients are hyperkalaemic, sodium acid phosphate infusions may be used
  - Oral therapy is also available: Phosphate-Sandoz® 2 tablets TDS

Further management

- Continue to treat the underlying cause.

Pitfalls/difficult situations

- Replacing phosphate too rapidly may cause hypocalcaemia and metastatic calcification.

Further reading

Assadi F. Hypophosphatemia: an evidence-based problem-solving approach to clinical cases. *Iran J Kidney Dis* 2010; **4**(3): 195–201.

Bugg NC, et al. Hypophosphataemia. Pathophysiology, effects and management on the intensive care unit. *Anaesthesia* 1998; **53**(9): 895–902.

:⚙: Hypermagnesaemia

- Normal: 0.7–1.0 mmol/L.
- High: >2.5 mmol/L.

Causes

- Commonest cause is excessive intake or administration, most often due to:
  - Inadvertent IV magnesium overdose (e.g. when treating pre-eclampsia, asthma, or arrhythmias)
  - Magnesium-containing antacids, vitamins, or cathartics in patients with renal failure
  - Purgative abuse in anorexia nervosa
- Renal failure.
- Intestinal hypomotility: ↓elimination and ↑absorption.
- Tumour lysis syndrome and rhabdomyolysis.
- Adrenal insufficiency.
- Hypothyroidism, hypoparathyroidism.
- Extracellular volume contraction in DKA or severe dehydration.

Presentation and assessment

- General symptoms: skin flushing, light-headedness.
- Neurological: sedation, stupor, coma.
- Neuromuscular: weakness, disappearance of tendon reflexes:
  - Prolongation of neuromuscular blockade if muscle relaxants used
- Cardiovascular: hypotension, vasodilatation, bradycardia, arrhythmias (asystole, AF, intraventricular conduction delay), cardiac arrest:
  - ECG changes: prolonged PR interval, broad QRS complexes, heart block
- Respiratory: bronchodilatation, respiratory depression, failure to wean.
- Gastrointestinal: diarrhoea, nausea, vomiting.
- Haematological: impaired coagulation due to platelet clumping and delayed thrombin formation.

Signs of hypermagnesaemia	
Visible sign	*Magnesium level (mmol/L)*
• Abolition of knee jerk	3.0–5.5
• Risk of respiratory arrest	5.0–7.5
• All deep tendon reflexes abolished	>10
• Cardiac arrest	>15

Investigations

- ABGs.
- U&Es (↑urea/creatinine and/or hyperkalaemia in AKI).
- Serum magnesium (to confirm/quantify the diagnosis).

- Serum calcium (concurrent hypercalcaemia).
- Blood glucose.
- TFTs (hypothyroidism).
- PTH level (↓ in hypoparathyroidism).
- Serum CK, urinary myoglobin (rhabdomyolysis).
- ECG.

Differential diagnoses

- Hypercalcaemia, hyperkalaemia.
- Hypothyroidism and myxoedema coma.
- Rhabdomyolysis.
- Lithium toxicity.

Immediate management

- Give O_2 and support airway, breathing, and circulation as required.
- If severe or symptomatic;
  - Give 10 ml 10% calcium gluconate IV over 10 minutes, repeat dose if necessary
  - Give 50 ml 50% glucose and 10 units soluble insulin over 1 hour
  - Infuse saline 0.9%, at 1 L per hour initially, inducing a diuresis using furosemide 20–40 mg IV, this may be repeated as necessary
  - Dialysis with magnesium-free dialysate may be indicated in life-threatening situations

Further management

- Treat any precipitating cause (stop magnesium-containing infusions).

Pitfalls/difficult situations

- Except in iatrogenic overdose, hypermagnesaemia does not normally occur in isolation.
- Magnesium potentiates the effects of muscle relaxants.
- Avoid magnesium in patients with muscular dystrophies or myasthenia gravis.

Target plasma magnesium levels for therapies
Treatment description Target level (mmol/L)
- General therapeutic level   1.25–2.5
- Severe asthma   >1
- Pregnancy-induced hypertension   2–4
             1 g magnesium = 4 mmol magnesium.

Further reading

Noronha JL, et al. Magnesium in critical illness: metabolism, assessment and treatment. *Intensive Care Med* 2002; **28**(6): 667–79.

① Hypomagnesaemia

- Normal: 0.7–1.0 mmol/L
- Low: <0.7 mmol/L

Hypomagnesaemia complicates >20% of critical care episodes. Serum ionized magnesium concentration poorly reflects total body stores.

Causes

- Malabsorption/malnourishment (e.g. colitis, radiation injury, short bowel syndrome, elderly, chronic alcohol abuse).
- Refeeding syndrome.
- Diarrhoea, prolonged NG suction or drainage, bowel fistulae.
- Inadequate magnesium replacement with IV fluid therapy or PN.
- Metabolic acidosis, especially DKA with insulin administration.
- Pancreatitis.
- Renal losses (e.g. diuretic phase of AKI, interstitial nephritis, osmotic diuretics, hyperaldosteronism).
- Drugs (e.g. diuretics, digoxin, gentamicin, amphotericin, ciclosporin).
- Massive blood transfusion or volume overload.
- 'Hungry bone syndrome' following surgery for hyperparathyroidism.

Presentation and assessment

Hypomagnesaemia is a common incidental finding. When symptomatic it is associated with hypokalaemia, hypocalcaemia, and metabolic acidosis. Signs and symptoms may include:

- General: anxiety, confusion, depression, psychosis.
- Neurological/neuromuscular: coma, seizures, ataxia, vertigo, nystagmus, dysarthria, dysphagia, myoclonus, Trousseau's sign, Chvostek's sign, hyper-reflexia, weakness, muscle cramps.
- Cardiovascular: palpitations, hypertension, angina, arrhythmias (most commonly SVT or AF, less commonly VT/VF or torsade de pointes):
  - There is an ↑ risk of digoxin toxicity
  - ECG changes: prolonged PR and QT intervals, broadened QRS, inverted or peaked T waves, ST depression, U waves
- Respiratory: stridor 2° to laryngospasm.
- Life-threatening complications include: ventricular arrhythmias, laryngeal spasm and coronary vasospasm.

Investigations

- ABGs, U&Es (concurrent hypokalaemia).
- Serum magnesium (to confirm/quantify the diagnosis).
- Serum calcium, serum phosphate (both may be ↓).
- Serum glucose (rule out hypoglycaemia).
- LFTs and albumin (abnormal with cirrhosis, hypoalbuminaemia may lead to spurious hypomagnesaemia).
- ECG.

Differential diagnoses

- Sampling error: sample taken from near magnesium-free IV infusion.
- Hypocalcaemia, hypokalaemia, hypoalbuminaemia.

Immediate management

- Give O_2 and support airway, breathing, and circulation as required.
- Life-threatening complications such as stridor (📖 p.18), coma (📖 p.152), seizures (📖 p.160), and tachycardia (📖 p.138) should be treated alongside magnesium replacement.

Magnesium replacement/treatment regimens

- Asymptomatic, or minor symptoms:
  - Replacement infusion: 5 g (20 mmol $MgSO_4$)[1] over 1–2 hours; may need to be repeated, aim for symptom control with a plasma concentration >0.8 mmol/L
- Pre-eclampsia/eclampsia:
  - Magnesium sulphate IV 4 g (16 mmol $MgSO_4$)[1] over 5–10 minutes, followed by an infusion of 1 g/hour (4 mmol/hour) for at least 24 hours
  - A further dose of magnesium sulphate 2 g (8 mmol $MgSO_4$)[1] over 15–20 minutes can be given if further seizures occur; or the infusion rate may be ↑ to 2 g/hour
- Acute severe asthma:
  - Magnesium sulphate 2.5 g IV (10 mmol $MgSO_4$)[1] over 5–10 minutes
  - Followed by 12–25 g (50–100 mmol) over the next 24 hours
- AF or atrial flutter: consider a bolus of magnesium sulphate 2.5 g IV (10 mmol $MgSO_4$)[1] over 5–30 minutes, depending upon severity; followed by a replacement infusion if required, aiming for plasma concentration of 1.4–1.8 mmol/L.
- Torsade de pointes: give as per the severe asthma protocol.

[1] $MgSO_4$ infusions can be made up in ≥100 ml 0.9% saline or 5% glucose, and may be given via peripheral IV access, but at concentrations ≥20mmol/100 ml should be given via a CVC.

Further management

- Continue to treat precipitants; maintain magnesium level >0.8 mmol/L.
- Supplementation may be required in patients at risk of hypomagnesaemia, or symptomatic patients, even in the absence of low levels.

Pitfalls/difficult situations

- Magnesium is slow to equilibrate between plasma and intracellular spaces; serum magnesium may appear artificially elevated if measured too soon after a magnesium dose is administered.
- Profound magnesium depletion normally requires sustained/repeated correction of the hypomagnesaemia; hypomagnesaemia may cause hypocalcaemia, which does not resolve until magnesium is corrected.
- Hypomagnesaemia may potentiate hypokalaemia and hypocalcaemia.
- Rapid magnesium administration can cause flushing, muscle weakness, or hypotension; simultaneous volume resuscitation may be advisable.
- Alcohol withdrawal can be exacerbated by hypomagnesaemia.
- Acute MI: routine magnesium treatment is no longer recommended.

Further reading

Martin KJ, et al. Clinical consequences and management of hypomagnesemia. J Am Soc Nephrol 2009 ; 20(11): 2291–5.
Tong GM, et al. Magnesium deficiency in critical illness. J Intensive Care Med 2005; 20(1): 13–17.

:O: Diabetic ketoacidosis

DKA occurs almost exclusively in type 1 diabetes and is a state of absolute or relative insulin deficiency with hyperglycaemia, dehydration, ketonaemia and acidosis.

Causes

The causes of DKA have been described as 'the five I's':
- Infection, 30% of cases (commonly UTI, pneumonia, URTI, or skin).
- Incidental (new) diabetes, 25% of cases.
- Insufficient (or missed) insulin, 20% of cases.
- Infarction (e.g. MI, CVA, ischaemic bowel, peripheral vasculature).
- Intercurrent illness (e.g. diarrhoea and/or vomiting; almost any underlying condition can precipitate DKA).

Patients at high risk of complications include:
- The elderly.
- Pregnant women.
- Young people (18–25 years).
- Patients with pre-existing heart or kidney failure.
- Patients with other serious illness (e.g. severe sepsis).

Presentation and assessment

The diagnosis of DKA requires:
- Known diabetes mellitus or blood glucose >11 mmol/L.
- Ketonaemia ≥3.0 mmol/L, or urinary ketones ++ or more on dipstick testing.
- Venous pH <7.30 and/or venous bicarbonate <15 mmol/L.

Presenting signs and symptoms may include:
- General: 2–3-day history of gradual deterioration and ensuing dehydration, associated with polydipsia, polyuria:
  - Ill appearance, dry skin, or mucous membranes, reduced skin turgor
  - Hypothermia or fever if infection or infarction present
- Neurological/neuromuscular: ↓reflexes, drowsiness, coma (resulting from the fall in pH).
- Cardiovascular: tachycardia, hypotension.
- Respiratory: hyperventilation or breathlessness; characteristic Kussmaul's respiration with subjective dyspnoea:
  - Smell of acetone on the breath (described as similar to pear drops or nail varnish remover)
- GI: abdominal pain, nausea, and vomiting.

Investigations

- ABGs (metabolic acidosis with/without respiratory compensation):
  - Venous blood gases may be used as an alternative
- FBC (WCC often elevated).
- U&Es (AKI may be present with raised potassium, urea/creatinine).
- Serum glucose (>11 mmol/L, although acidosis can still exist at lower levels if insulin has only recently been used).
- Capillary ketones (using finger-prick ketone meter):

- Alternatively urinalysis for ketones (captopril can give a false positive test for urinary acetone; urinalysis may also suggest UTI)
- CRP (↑ if infection is a precipitant).
- LFTs, serum phosphate, magnesium, and calcium.
- Cardiac enzymes/troponins (↑ if MI is a precipitant).
- Blood, sputum, and urine cultures (if infection suspected).
- CXR (if pneumonia suspected).
- ECG (if MI suspected).

Differential diagnoses
- Sepsis.
- Renal failure.
- Salicylate overdose.
- Inborn errors of metabolism.
- Alcoholic ketoacidosis.
- Hyperosmolar hyperglycaemic syndrome.

Immediate management
- Give O_2 and support airway, breathing, and circulation as required.

The priority is to correct hypovolaemia
- Site large-bore IV cannula, central access may be needed in patients with major cardiac disease, autonomic nephropathy or the elderly.
- If hypotensive (systolic BP <90 mmHg) give 500 ml saline 0.9% IV[1] over 10–15 minutes; this should be repeated if BP remains low:
    - Ongoing hypotension should prompt investigation for an additional cause and appropriate additional resuscitation
- If systolic is >90 mmHg give 1000 ml 0.9% saline IV[1] over 1 hour.
- Ongoing fluids should be 1000 ml 0.9% saline IV[1] over 2 hours, *then*
    - 1000 ml 0.9% saline IV[1] over 2 hours, *then*
    - 1000 ml 0.9% saline IV[1] over 4 hours, *then*
    - Further fluid boluses over 4 and then 6 hours may be required
    - This regimen should be followed with caution in the elderly or those with cardiac disease and carefully titrated against CVP and clinical status, aiming to restore hydration status within 12–24 hours
- Potassium replacement according to protocol (see 📖 p.230); likely to be needed from the 2nd bag onwards.
- In unstable or severely acidotic patients insert arterial line to monitor replacement adequacy via ABGs.
- Catheterize if patient is oliguric or has a high serum creatinine.

Commence glycaemic correction with fluid resuscitation
- Give insulin infusion at 0.1 unit/kg/hour (of 50 units soluble insulin in 50 ml 0.9% saline).
- Continue long-acting insulins if normally used (e.g. Lantus®, Levemir®).
- Monitor capillary blood glucose and ketones (if available) hourly.
- Monitor venous bicarbonate and potassium after 1 hour and then 2-hourly.

[1] See 📖 Pitfalls/difficult situations.

Potassium replacement during resuscitation of DKA

Serum K+   *K+ replacement of infusion fluid*
- >5.5 mmol/L   Nil
- 3.5–5.5 mmol/L   40mmol/L
- <3.5 mmol/L   Senior review; additional potassium required

Aims of insulin therapy in treatment of DKA

- 0.5 mmol/L/hour reduction in capillary ketones, *or*
- 3 mmol/L/hour increase in bicarbonate and 3 mmol/L/hour decrease in glucose.
- Avoidance of hypoglycaemia and maintenance of normokalaemia.
Add 10% glucose 125 ml/hour if blood glucose falls below 14 mmol/L.

If the reductions in ketones, bicarbonate, or glucose are not achieved, increase 0.1 unit/kg/hour fixed rate insulin infusion in 1unit/hour increments until targets achieved (ensure infusion equipment is working correctly first).
  Continue fixed-rate insulin until capillary ketones <0.3 mmol/L, and venous pH>7.3 (and/or venous bicarbonate >18 mmol/L).

Potential indications for critical care admission

- Young people aged 18–25 years or elderly patients.
- Pregnant women.
- Patients with heart or kidney failure or other serious comorbidities.
- Severe DKA by following criteria:
  - Blood ketones above 6 mmol/L
  - Venous bicarbonate below 5 mmol/L
  - Venous pH <7.1
  - Hypokalaemia on admission (<3.5 mmol/L)
  - GCS <12
  - Oxygen saturations <92% on air (ABG required)
  - Systolic BP <90 mmHg
  - Pulse rate >100 or <60 beats/minute
  - Anion gap >16 [anion gap = $(Na^+ + K^+) - (Cl^- + HCO_3^-)$]

Further management

- Check electrolytes 4-hourly.
- Watch for arrhythmias due to fluxes in K^+ level (use ECG monitoring if potassium level is abnormal or there is cardiovascular instability).
- Gastroparesis is a common, consider placing an NGT (especially if marked vomiting is present).
- Investigate the cause of the disturbance that initiated the episode.
- Give thromboprophylaxis with LMWH.
- Monitor fluid balance, aiming for UOP >0.5 ml/kg/hour:

- Urinary catheterization is required if the patient has been anuric for 60 minutes
- Monitor for fluid overload, pulmonary oedema, or cerebral oedema.
- Refer to a diabetes team.
- Once ketonaemia and acidosis has resolved:
  - Convert to standard insulin sliding scale (see 📖 p.14) alongside maintenance IV fluids if the patient is *unable to eat and drink*, or
  - SC insulin if the patient is *able to eat and drink*

Pitfalls/difficult situations

- Plasma glucose is not always high, especially if there has been vomiting.
- High WCC may be seen, even in the absence of infection.
- Ketonaemia may result in falsely high creatinine levels.
- Hyponatraemia or hypernatraemia are common.
- Ketonuria does not mean ketoacidosis, alcohol may be the cause if glucose is normal.
- Amylase is often raised (by up to 10 ×) along with non-specific abdominal pain, even in the absence of pancreatitis; if pancreatitis is suspected consider US or CT imaging.
- If the patient requires mechanical ventilation, hyperventilate aggressively to maintain physiological compensation for acidosis and monitor ABGs.
- Avoid bicarbonate, even if the acidosis is severe (Ph <7); it can cause severe sodium overload, intracellular acidosis or cerebral oedema (relative CSF alkalosis will depress respiration which compromises respiratory compensation):
  - Bicarbonate therapy may occasionally be indicated in those with ketoacidosis and a normal anion gap as they have fewer ketones available to regenerate bicarbonate during insulin administration
- Hyperchloraemic acidosis caused by aggressive fluid resuscitation may complicate the recovery stage 12–24 hours later, clinical indices of recovery are usually reassuring by this stage:
  - Measuring serum chloride will assist in diagnosis
  - The choice of saline 0.9% is controversial; Hartmann's solution may avoid hyperchloraemic acidosis, and is used by some centres, but is not currently recommended in UK national guidelines as it is more complex to add potassium supplementation
- Repeated arterial blood sampling is painful and some diabetic patients become reluctant to present to hospital as a result; in most cases ABGs are not required, or venous gases may be used instead.
- Hypomagnesaemia commonly occurs with DKA fluid and insulin resuscitation; it is rarely severe and may not need replacement if the patient rapidly recovers and becomes able to eat and drink.

Further reading

Kitabchi AE, et al. Hyperglycemic crises in adult patients with diabetes: a consensus statement from the American Diabetes Association. *Diabetes Care* 2009; **32**: 1335–43.
Savage MW, et al. Joint British Diabetes Societies guideline for the management of diabetic ketoacidosis D. *Diabet Med* 2011; 28: 508–15.

:☼: Hyperosmolar hyperglycaemic state

Hyperosmolar hyperglycaemic non ketotic syndrome (HHS; also known as hyperosmolar non-ketotic crisis, HONK)) typically occurs in elderly type 2 diabetic patients. Compared with DKA the blood sugar is often very high, >35 mmol/L, and severe dehydration with no acidosis is present

Causes

- Any illness that results in dehydration or that leads to a decrease in insulin activity can precipitate HHS.
- Acute febrile illnesses account for the largest proportion of HHS cases.

Presentation and assessment

- Respiration is usually normal.
- Neurological symptoms predominate:
  - Confusion, agitation, or drowsiness are common
  - Coma is more frequent and mortality is much higher than in DKA
  - Presentation occasionally includes focal neurology, CVA, seizures
- Thrombotic events may occur (e.g. DVT, PE, MI).
- Biochemistry:
  - Acidosis is not usually present as there is sufficient insulin to prevent lipolysis and ketogenesis
  - Serum osmolality >340 mOsmol/kg

Investigations

(See also 📖 p.228.)
The same investigations as those required in DKA are suggested. The following differences may be apparent:
- ABGs (typically there is no acidaemia, pH >7.3; coexistent lactic acidosis considerably worsens the prognosis).
- Serum glucose (usually >35 mmol/L).
- Serum osmolality (>350 mOsmol/L).
- U&Es (severe dehydration causes a greater rise in urea than creatinine, and significant hypernatraemia may be hidden by the high glucose).
- Serum lactate.
- Plasma/urine ketones (no or mild ketosis only should be present).
- CRP (may be ↑ if infection a precipitant).
- Blood, urine, sputum cultures (if infection suspected).
- LP (if meningitis is suspected, and raised ICP has been ruled out).
- Cardiac enzymes/troponins (MI may be a precipitant).
- ECG (to exclude MI).
- CXR (looking specifically for any infective foci).
- CT head (if intracranial pathology is suspected).

Differential diagnoses

The differential diagnosis includes any cause of altered mental status:
- CNS infection or any other cause of sepsis.
- Electrolyte abnormalities (e.g. hypoglycaemia, hyponatraemia, uraemia, hyperammonaemia).

- Severe dehydration.
- Drug overdose.

Immediate management
- Give O_2 and support airway, breathing, and circulation as required.

Hypovolaemia correction
- Site large-bore IV cannula, central access may be needed in patients.
- If hypotensive (systolic <90 mmHg) give 500 ml saline 0.9% IV over 15–60minutes; this can be repeated if BP remains low.
- Ongoing hypotension should prompt investigation for an additional cause; inotropic support may be required.
- Replace fluids at a maximum of half the rate of DKA regime over 48 hours, as there is a risk of cerebral oedema:
  - There is no consensus on the rate of ongoing fluid replacement; one suggested rate is 100–200 ml/hour (rates of 250–500 ml/hour have also been used)
  - Replacement fluid should be 0.45% saline if plasma Na >150 mmol/L
- Potassium replacement according to protocol (see ☐ p.230); likely to be needed from the 2nd bag onwards.

Glycaemic correction
- Wait 1 hour before giving insulin as it may not be needed.
- Patients are often hypersensitive to insulin.
- Give insulin infusion at 0.1 unit/kg/hour (of 50 units soluble insulin in 50 ml 0.9% saline).
- Monitor capillary blood glucose hourly, and reduce insulin by 1 ml/hour as required, aiming for a blood glucose of 11–16 mmol/L.

Further management
- Check electrolytes and serum osmolality 4-hourly.
- Watch for arrhythmias due to fluxes in K^+ level (use ECG monitoring if potassium level is abnormal or there is cardiovascular instability).
- Correct serum phosphate and magnesium which often fall rapidly.
- Investigate the cause of the disturbance that initiated the episode.
- Monitor fluid balance, aiming for UOP >0.5 ml/kg/hour:
  - Urinary catheterization is likely to be required
- Monitor for fluid overload, pulmonary oedema, or cerebral oedema.
- Give thromboprophylaxis with LMWH; in severe cases full anticoagulation may be required.

Pitfalls/difficult situations
- HHS has also been reported in patients with type 1 DM.
- A combination of HHS and DKA may occur in the same individual.

Further reading
Kitabchi AE, et al. Hyperglycemic crises in diabetes. *Diabetes Care* 2009; **32**(7): 1335–43.

☼ Hypoglycaemia

- Normal glucose (fasting): 3.5–7.0 mmol/L.
- Hypoglycaemia: <2.8 mmol/L.

Hypoglycaemia commonly occurs in insulin-dependent diabetic patients, but can also occur in other conditions. Rapid recognition and correction is essential to avoid seizures/complications. Prolonged hypoglycaemia can cause brain damage. Symptoms can occur at normal blood sugar levels in diabetic patients, particularly where blood sugar control is poor.

For diabetic patients it is recommended that 4.0mmol/L is the lowest acceptable blood glucose level.

Causes

- Accidental/deliberate insulin/oral hypoglycaemic medication overdose.
- Inappropriate insulin/oral hypoglycaemics (e.g. given when NBM).
- Insulinoma.
- Other drugs, especially in combination with insulin/hypoglycaemic agents (e.g. NSAIDs, aspirin, β-blockers, quinine, co-trimoxazole, pentamidine, SSRIs, warfarin, MAO inhibitors, somatostatin analogues).
- Endocrine: Addison's, hypopituitarism, hypothyroidism.
- Other causes: hepatic failure, alcohol, starvation, severe sepsis.

In sedated patients signs and symptoms may be missed. Regular blood sugar monitoring is essential, especially in those at high risk:

- Long-term diabetic patients, or those with a history of hypoglycaemia.
- Patients on tight glycaemic control regimens.
- Severe hepatic dysfunction, impaired renal function, or dialysis therapy.
- IV insulin infusion without glucose infusion or enteral feed (malabsorption or cessation); or incorrect insulin administration.
- Patients on quinine therapy for malaria.
- Acute discontinuation of long-term steroid therapy.
- Prolonged hypothermia.

Presentation and assessment

- General: malaise, headache, nausea and vomiting.
- Autonomic symptoms: hunger, pallor, sweating, palpitations, tremor:
  - Tachycardia and tachypnoea
- Neuroglycopaenic symptoms:
  - Confusion, agitation, aggression
  - Focal neurological signs, blurred vision, dysphasia, ataxia
  - Drowsiness, seizures, coma.

Investigations

- Bedside blood sugar monitoring is adequate in most cases:
  - If this is low confirm with formal blood glucose readings.

Other investigations may be indicated:

- FBC (↑/↓ WCC in sepsis).
- Coagulation screen (deranged in hepatic failure or sepsis).
- U&Es, LFTs (deranged in hepatic failure).
- TFTs (deranged in hypothyroidism), serum cortisol (Addison's).
- Blood alcohol level, paracetamol, and salicylate levels.

- C-peptide (if an endogenous source of insulin is suspected).
- Blood, sputum, and urine cultures (if infection suspected).
- CXR (to exclude pneumonia).
- CT head, LP (if intracranial pathology/infection suspected).

Differential diagnoses
- Neurological disorder: stroke (e.g. stroke, epilepsy, meningitis).
- Psychosis.

Immediate management
- Give O_2 and support airway, breathing, and circulation as required.
- Treat any seizures (p.160) and simultaneously correct glucose.

Glucose correction
- If conscious and able to swallow, give oral sugary fluids or snacks
- If unconscious, having seizures, or aggressive:
  - Glucagon 1 mg IM (may take up to 15 minutes to take effect)
  - 20% glucose, 75–100 ml IV over 10–15 minutes, or
  - 10% glucose, 150–200 ml IV over 10–15 minutes
- Regularly monitor blood sugar:
  - Every 10 minutes until BM >4.0 mmol/L
- If patient is NBM consider ongoing 10% glucose IV 100 ml/hour.
- A continuous infusion of high-dose glucose (i.e. 50% glucose at 10–50 ml/hour, ideally given via CVC) may be required in resistant cases.

Further management
- Monitor potassium levels: replacement will be required for some patients who have been given large amounts of glucose.
- Adjust any insulin sliding scales to avoid further episodes.
- If no cause for hypoglycaemia is found, consider giving hydrocortisone 200 mg IV to exclude Addison's.
- Octreotide may help in cases of insulinoma.
- Give thiamine if alcoholism or malnutrition is suspected.

Pitfalls/difficult situations
- Check blood sugar in patients when confronted with seizures or coma.
- Hypoglycaemia occurring with long-acting sulphonylureas such as chlorpropamide or glibenclamide may be prolonged.
- Deliberate insulin overdose can cause intractable hypoglycaemia, which may recur; prolonged blood sugar monitoring will be required.
- Surgical excision of the insulin injection site has been attempted for large overdoses of long-acting insulin.
- In the elderly the effects of hypoglycaemia can mimic a stroke.

Further reading
Joint British Diabetes Societies Inpatient Care Group. *The hospital management of hypoglycaemia in adults with diabetes mellitus*, 2010. Available at: <http://www.diabetes.nhs.uk/our_publications/>.
Krinsley JS, et al. Severe hypoglycemia in critically ill patients: risk factors and outcomes. *Crit Care Med* 2007; 35(10); 2262–72.

☺ Addison's disease

Addison's disease (also called adrenal insufficiency or hypocortisolism) is an endocrine disorder caused by failure of the adrenal glands to produce enough cortisol and, in some cases, aldosterone.

An adrenal crisis can manifest with vomiting, abdominal pain, and cardio-vascular shock, usually 2° to a precipitating cause.

Causes

- Autoimmune adrenalitis (80%).
- Tuberculosis or malignant secondaries of the adrenal glands.
- Adrenal haemorrhage (Waterhouse–Friderichsen syndrome).
- Hypopituitarism.
- Drugs (e.g. metyrapone, aminoglutethimide, ketoconazole, etomidate infusions, rifampicin, phenytoin, phenobarbital.
- Physiological stressors (e.g. infection, trauma, surgery, sepsis, burns); these can also be crisis precipitants.
- Cessation of steroid therapy.

Presentation and assessment

- Weight loss, fatigue, weakness, myalgia, anorexia, dehydration.
- Precipitant symptoms: fever, night sweats (infection); flank pain (infarction).
- Hyperpigmentation may occur in chronic disease.
- Cardiovascular:
  - Postural hypotension
  - Shock, tachycardia, peripheral vasoconstriction, oliguria
  - Life-threatening arrhythmias
- GI:
  - Nausea and vomiting
  - Diarrhoea and abdominal pain (present in 20% of cases)
- Psychiatric features: asthenia, depression, apathy, and confusion.

Investigations

- ABGs (metabolic acidosis, respiratory failure).
- FBC (anaemia with normal MCV; moderate neutropaenia, relative eosinophilia/lymphocytosis).
- U&Es (likely to reveal hyponatraemia and hyperkalaemia with Na:K ratio <21:1; ↑urea/creatinine).
- Serum glucose (may show hypoglycaemia).
- Serum calcium (may be high but corrected calcium usually normal).
- Serum cortisol/ACTH, prior to hydrocortisone administration (baseline cortisol <400 nmol/L, and should be >1000 nmol/L in sick patients).
- 'Short Synacthen®' (250 ACTH given, cortisol measured at 0 and 30 minutes; if the 2nd cortisol is >500 nmol/L and >200 nmol/L greater than baseline, then Addison's is excluded).
- Blood, urine and sputum cultures.
- ECG (to exclude MI, PR/QTc prolongation).
- CXR (previous TB or bronchial carcinoma).
- AXR (adrenal calcification).

Differential diagnoses
- Acute abdomen.
- Septic shock.

Immediate management
- Give O_2 and support airway, breathing, and circulation as required.
  Do not delay treatment whilst awaiting urgent lab tests
- Take blood for cortisol (10 ml clotted sample) and ACTH (10 ml EDTA sample).
- Give hydrocortisone 200 mg IV stat followed by 100 mg QDS.
- Resuscitate with IV colloid or saline 0.9%.
- Inotropes/vasopressors may be required, but are likely to be ineffective unless cortisol replaced.
- Monitor blood glucose as there is a danger of hypoglycaemia.
- If hypoglycaemic give 75 ml 20% glucose IV.

Further management
- Diagnose and treat 1° /underlying cause.
- Guide fluid therapy using more invasive monitoring if necessary, so as to avoid extreme fluid overload.
- If response is poor, suspect other autoimmune diseases: check TFTs and coeliac serology.
- Consider fludrocortisone PO 50 mcg every other day, up to 0.15 mg daily.
- Hypoadrenalism related to sepsis can be treated with hydrocortisone 50 mg IV QDS for 7 days, a reducing dose is then given over 7 days.
- Dexamethasone can be used for steroid replacement for 48 hours before the Synacthen® test as it does not interfere with cortisol assays.

Pitfalls/difficult situations
- Unexplained abdominal symptoms could herald the disease.
- Perform a Synacthen® test if at all suspicious.

Equivalent doses of glucocorticoids	
• Dexamethasone:	0.75 mg
• Methylprednisolone:	4 mg
• Triamcinolone:	4 mg
• Prednisolone:	5 mg
• Hydrocortisone:	20 mg
• Cortisone acetate:	25 mg

Further reading

Albert SG, et al. The effect of etomidate on adrenal function in critical illness: a systematic review. *Intensive Care Med* 2011; **37**(6): 901–10.

Cooper MS, et al. Corticosteroid insufficiency in acutely ill patients. *N Engl J Med* 2003; **348**: 727–34.

Marik PE, et al. Adrenal insufficiency in the critically ill. *Chest* 2002; **122**(5): 1784–96.

:O: Thyroid storm

Thyroid storm (or hyperthyroid crisis) is a clinical syndrome marked by exaggerated manifestations of thyrotoxicosis. It represents the most serious complication of hyperthyroidism and carries a high mortality.

Causes

- Grave's disease.
- Hyperfunctioning thyroid multinodular goitre.
- TSH-secreting tumour.
- Radioiodine therapy.
- Excess thyroxine intake.
- Excess handling of thyroid gland intraoperatively.

Various conditions/treatments may trigger thyroid storm in susceptible individuals:

- Surgery or trauma.
- DKA.
- PE or MI.
- Sepsis.
- Labour.
- Drugs (e.g. ephedrine, atropine, contrast media).

Presentation and assessment

General signs/symptoms associated with hyperthyroidism may be present (e.g. goitre or ocular signs), as well as:

- Fever (>38.5°C) and often hyperpyrexia (>40°C):
  - Sweating, fatigue
- Cardiovascular: hypertension followed by hypotension:
  - Sinus tachycardia >140 beats/minute (often disproportionate to degree of fever)
  - AF, multifocal ventricular ectopics
  - Angina
  - Cardiac failure (30% of cases); typically high-output cardiac failure
- Respiratory: tachypnoea, dyspnoea:
  - If already ventilated: failure to wean, 'fighting' the ventilator
- Neurological: agitation, delirium, aggression, seizures, coma:
  - Hyporeflexia and myopathy are occasionally present
- GI: anorexia, weight loss:
  - Abdominal pain
  - Nausea, vomiting, diarrhoea
  - Hepatic failure, jaundice
- Renal failure (2° to rhabdomyolysis).

Investigations

Diagnosis is clinically based; no laboratory tests are diagnostic; a scoring system is available which may assist in making the diagnosis (Table 6.2). Do not delay treatment whilst awaiting lab results:

- TFTs: T3, free T4 and TSH (elevated T4/T3, suppressed TSH).
- ABGs (respiratory failure, metabolic acidosis).
- FBC (raised WCC).

- U&Es (hyperkalaemia).
- LFTs (raised transaminases and bilirubin).
- Serum calcium (hypercalcaemia).
- Serum magnesium (hypomagnesaemia).
- Serum CK (rhabdomyolysis may occur).
- Serum glucose (may be ↓).
- Blood, sputum and urine cultures (if infection suspected).
- Urinary myoglobin, urinary catecholamines (to exclude differential diagnoses).
- ECG (myocardial ischaemia/MI, arrhythmias, LV hypertrophy).
- CXR (if pulmonary oedema or pneumonia suspected).
- CT head (if intracranial pathology/infection needs to be excluded).

Differential diagnoses
- Malignant hyperpyrexia.
- Phaeochromocytoma.
- Serotonergic syndrome.
- Infection/sepsis.
- Anticholinergic or adrenergic drug intoxication.
- LVF/CCF.
- Hyperthyroidism, without thyroid storm.
- Essential hypertension.

Immediate management
- Give O₂ and support airway, breathing, and circulation as required.
  Symptom control is the priority, rather than correcting thyroid status:
- Do not await lab test confirmation of suspected diagnosis.
- Protect and support airway and breathing as required; relative hyperventilation is required to compensate for hypermetabolic state.
- Circulatory support with IV saline 0.9% may be required in view of large insensible losses from hyperpyrexia, diarrhoea, and vomiting:
  - ECG monitoring is required
- Replace glucose as required.
- Hyperpyrexia (see also 📖 pp.246 and 248) employ cooling measures:
  - Tepid sponging, axillae/femoral ice packs, cooling blankets
  - Peritoneal or NG lavage with ice cold fluid may be used
  - Haemofiltration or endovascular temperature-therapy catheter
  - Antipyretics: IV paracetamol 1g 6-hourly—*do not use NSAIDs or other drugs which displace thyroid hormone from binding sites*
  - Consider dantrolene as T4 causes calcium release similar to malignant hyperpyrexia (see 📖 p.246)
- Hyperadrenergic state:
  - Propranolol 1–5 mg IV up to 10 mg (can precipitate CCF); aim for pulse rate <100 beat/minute
  - As an alternative consider esmolol 250–500 mcg/kg loading then 50–100 mcg/kg/minute (but see later comments)
  - Reserpine 2.5–5 mg 6-hourly may be given.

- If already intubated/ventilated, sedation may be ↑ to obtund any exaggerated sympathetic responses
- Give IV hydrocortisone 200 mg 6-hourly or dexamethasone 2 mg IV 6-hourly (there is a relative deficiency of endogenous steroids)
- Excess T4/T3 treatment:
  - Propranolol and steroid (as earlier) in combination, reduces organification of iodine, inhibits iodide transport, and reduces peripheral conversion of T4 to T3 and reduces T4 release (*only propranolol has this effect*)

Further management
- Endocrinology referral will be required.
- Following IV loading, commence oral propranolol 20–40 mg 6-hourly.
- Start oral propylthiouracil PO 1 g loading dose, then 200–300 mg 6-hourly.

It is important to give propylthiouracil first, as iodine can cause ↑release of thyroid hormone:

- Monitor for signs of hepatic damage 2° to propylthiouracil.
- Following propylthiouracil, give oral Lugol's iodine 5–10 drops 6-hourly:
  - Alternatively: sodium iodide 500 mg IV 8-hourly, or
  - Potassium iodide 200–600 mg IV over 2 hours, then 2 g/day PO
- Consider carbimazole 60–120 mg/day PO (may cause agranulocytosis).
- Treat the precipitating cause.
- Correct electrolyte abnormalities.
- Plasmapheresis has been reportedly used as a life-saving measure.
- Correct any electrolyte derangement.
- If infection is suspected empirical antibiotic therapy will be required.

Pitfalls/difficult situations
- Identification of thyroid storm in patients may be easily mistaken for the physiological or pathophysiological response to the underlying trigger (e.g. trauma, sepsis).
- Insertion of an NG tube will be needed in some patients to facilitate the administration of essential medications.
- Cardioversion of arrhythmias is unlikely to be successful until the patient is biochemically euthyroid.
- β-blockade with propranolol may still be the drug of choice even in where cardiac failure is present.
- Thyroid hormone has a half-life of 3–6 days, amelioration of symptoms cannot occur until this vascular pool has been depleted; peritoneal dialysis or plasmapheresis may speed up vascular depletion.
- Oral colestyramine resin PO may bind thyroid hormone entering the gut, resulting in resin-hormone complex excretion.
- Drugs which increase thyroid hormone include NSAIDs, furosemide, phenytoin, heparin.
- 'Apathetic' hyperthyroid crisis occurs in some patients, and is associated with extreme weakness, fatigue, and hyporeflexia.

Table 6.2 Scale for the diagnosis of thyroid storm. Total >45 suggestive of thyroid storm

Temperature (°C)	Score
37.0–37.7	5
37.8–38.2	10
38.3–38.7	15
38.9–39.3	20
39.4–40.0	25
>40.0	30
CNS effects	
Absent	0
Agitation	10
Delirium, psychosis, extreme lethargy	20
Seizure, coma	30
GI or hepatic symptoms	
Absent	0
Diarrhoea, abdominal pain, nausea and vomiting	10
Jaundice	20
Tachycardia (beats/minute)	
90–109	5
110–119	10
120–129	15
130–139	20
≥140	25
Atrial fibrillation	
Absent	0
Present	10
Heart failure	
Absent	0
Mild (pedal oedema)	5
Moderate (bibasal crepitation)	10
Severe (pulmonary oedema)	20
Precipitant history	
Absent	0
Present	10

Further reading

Migneco A. et al. Management of thyrotoxic crisis. *Eur Rev Med Pharmacol Sci* 2005; **9**(1): 69–74.

Nayak B, et al. Thyrotoxicosis and thyroid storm. *Endocrinol Metab Clin North Am* 2006; **35**: 663–86.

Petry J, et al. Plasmapheresis as effective treatment for thyrotoxic storm after sleeve pneumonectomy. *Ann Thorac Surg* 2004; **77**: 1839–41.

:☼: Phaeochromocytoma and carcinoid syndrome

Phaeochromocytomas are catecholamine-producing tumours, which may present acutely, or coincidentally with another condition.

Carcinoid syndrome is a collection of features caused by a carcinoid tumour secreting serotonin, 5-hydroxytryptophan, and other mediators.

Causes

Phaeochromocytomas may present in isolation (10% malignant, 10% bilateral, 10% familial, 10% extra-adrenal) or as part of a syndrome: MEN 2a/b, von Recklinghausen's disease and von Hippel–Lindau disease.

Carcinoid tumours are found in stomach, bowel, pancreas, or bronchus. Factors that provoke release of mediators include tumour manipulation, catecholamine use, or the presence of liver metastases.

Presentation and assessment

Phaeochromocytoma

Signs/symptoms are more likely to manifest after painful procedures such as: endotracheal intubation or direct tumour manipulation; they are due to excessive sympathetic activity.
- General: anxiety, tremor, weakness, faintness, paraesthesia, cold extremities, pallor, drenching perspiration.
- Cardiovascular: hypertension (sustained or paroxysmal):
  - Myocardial ischaemia, palpitations, tachycardia, AF or VF
- Metabolic: unexplained lactic acidosis.

Carcinoid syndrome

Features vary in severity and depend upon the tumour location and subtype. Pre-existing features may include: cardiac valve abnormalities (TR), pulmonary stenosis and right heart failure. Features related to secretion of vasoactive substances include:
- General: flushing, nausea/vomiting, abdominal pain, diarrhoea, hyperglycaemia.
- CVS/RS: vasodilatation, hypotension, SVT, bronchoconstriction:
  - Haemoptysis and airway obstruction (in bronchial carcinoid)

Investigations

- ABGs (metabolic acidosis).
- U&Es (hypokalaemia, ↑urea in phaeochromocytoma).
- Glucose (hyperglycaemia).
- ECG (arrhythmias, LVH in phaeochromocytoma, RVH in carcinoid).
- CXR (pulmonary metastases in carcinoid).
- CT scan/US abdomen (to locate tumours/liver metastases).
- Phaeochromocytoma: 24-hour urine collection for VMA, catecholamines and metanephrine levels, and/or plasma catecholamines (if available):
  - Pentolinium suppression test (suppression will occur)
- Carcinoid: serum levels for of serotonin and/or 5 hydroxytryptophan:
  - Urine for 5 hydroxyindoleacetic (5HIAA) acid levels

Differential diagnoses
- Essential hypertension; inadequate sedation, analgesia, or anaesthesia.
- Hypertensive diseases: pre-eclampsia, thyroid storm.
- Inadvertent vasopressor bolus; or administration of indirect acting vasopressors (e.g. ephedrine) to patients taking MAOIs.
- Bronchospasm (e.g. anaphylaxis, asthma).

Immediate management
- Give O_2 and support airway, breathing, and circulation as required.
- Stop any avoidable stimulus, deepen any anaesthesia/sedation.
- Invasive monitoring if cardiovascularly unstable (arterial line, CVC).

Suspected phaeochromocytoma (adrenergic control)
- *Sole β-blockade may precipitate a hypertensive crisis due to unopposed alpha receptor stimulation.*
- Give phentolamine (non-selective α-blocker) 2–5 mg IV bolus and repeat as necessary to control hypertension:
  - Alternatively doxazosin PO 2–4 mg/day
- If further hypertensive control is required consider:
  - Magnesium sulphate 5 g (20 mmol) IV then 2 g/hour (8 mmol)
  - Sodium nitroprusside IV 0.5–1.5 mcg/kg/minute
- After alpha blockade established if HR >100 beats/minute, or there are frequent VEs, consider:
  - Labetalol 5–10 mg IV increments, or esmolol 1.5 mg/kg bolus IV

Suspected carcinoid
- Give nebulized ipratropium bromide 500 mcg and IV/inhalational steroids for bronchospasm (avoid β agonists).
- Commence fluid resuscitation for hypotension.
- Use phenylephrine 50–100 mcg boluses/IVI (can be given via a peripheral vein) for refractory hypotension.
- Give octreotide 50–100 mcg IV (this drug prevents the release, and block the peripheral actions of serotonin and other mediators).

Further management
- Phaeochromocytoma: stabilize on antihypertensive regimen:
  - The definitive treatment is excision of the 1° tumour
- Carcinoid: correct any electrolyte abnormalities:
  - Avoid hypoxia or hypercapnia which can increase mediator release.

Pitfalls/difficult situations
- The diagnosis is frequently not straightforward.
- The presence of RVF may complicate management of carcinoid.
- Phaeochromocytoma causes hypovolaemia masked by hypertension.
- Other endocrine abnormalities (e.g. Cushing's syndrome) may coexist.

Further reading
Kulke MH, et al. Carcinoid tumors. *N Engl J Med* 1999; **340**: 858–68.
Nguyen-Martin MA, et al. Phaeochromocytoma: an update on risk groups, diagnosis and management. *Hosp Physician* 2006; Feb: 17–24.

☠ Malignant hyperpyrexia and neurolept malignant syndrome

Malignant hyperpyrexia (MH) is an inherited disorder, which in susceptible individuals exposed to triggering agents causes intense muscle activity and a hypermetabolic state. Triggering agents are mostly used during anaesthesia, but critical care is required for on-going management.

Neurolept malignant syndrome (NMS) is a potentially fatal, idiosyncratic response to neuroleptic drugs and tranquillizers.

Causes
- MH:
  - Suxamethonium or volatile anaesthetic agents (e.g. isoflurane)
- NMS:
  - Caused by: phenothiazines, butyrophenones, thioxanthenes, lithium
  - May be triggered by exercise, exhaustion, or dehydration

Presentation and assessment
(See Boxes 6.1 and 6.2.)
- Muscle rigidity (or masseter spasm) and akinesia; metabolic acidosis.
- Rapid rise in core body temperature; sweating.
- Tachycardia, arrhythmias, autonomic impairment (labile BP).
- Complications of hyperpyrexia (see 🕮 p.248).

Investigations
(See also 🕮 p.248.)
- ABGs (acidosis, hypercapnia, low bicarbonate, hypoxia).
- FBC (↑WCC/platelets in NMS; thrombocytopaenia in DIC).
- Coagulation screen (↑PT/APTT, ↓fibrinogen in DIC).
- U&Es (hyperkalaemia, raised urea/creatinine).
- CK (raised in rhabdomyolysis); LFTs (may be deranged).
- Serum phosphate (may be raised), serum calcium (may be low).
- TFTs (to exclude the differential of hyperthyroidism).
- Blood, urine and sputum cultures (if infection suspected).
- Urine (for toxicology and/or myoglobinuria).
- ECG (if ischaemia is suspected), CXR (if infection suspected).
- Consider CT scan or lumbar puncture (if focal infection suspected).

Differential diagnoses
- Diseases associated with hyperthermia (e.g. sepsis, heat stroke).
- Diseases associated with rigidity (e.g. tetanus, Parkinson's disease).

Box 6.1 Management of a malignant hyperthermia crisis
Know where dantrolene is stored.

Recognition
- Unexplained increase in $ETCO_2$ *and* unexplained tachycardia *and* unexplained increase in O_2 requirement.
- Temperature changes are a late sign.

Immediate management
1. Stop all trigger agents, *call for help.*
2. Allocate specific tasks (use an action plan if available).
3. Use a new breathing circuit/system and *hyperventilate* 100% O_2.

4. Maintain anaesthesia with an intravenous agent.
5. *Abandon/finish* surgery as soon as possible.
6. Any muscle relaxation should be with a non-depolarizing neuromuscular blocking drug (e.g. atracurium).
7. Give dantrolene and initiate active cooling (avoid vasoconstriction).

Monitoring and treatment
- *Dantrolene*: 2.5 mg/kg IV bolus; repeat 1-mg/kg boluses as required to 10 mg/kg maximum (for a 70-kg adult: *initial bolus of 9 dantrolene vials*, each 20-mg vial mixed with 60 ml H_2O; further boluses of 4 vials dantrolene repeated up to 7 times).
- Hyperkalaemia: calcium chloride, glucose/insulin, $NaHCO_3$
- Arrhythmias: magnesium/amiodarone/metoprolol.
  - *Avoid* calcium channel blockers (interacts with dantrolene)
- Metabolic acidosis: hyperventilate, $NaHCO_3$
- Myoglobinaemia: urinary alkalinization, may require RRT later.
- DIC: FFP, cryoprecipitate, platelets.
- Check serum CK as soon as possible.
- Continuous monitoring: core and peripheral temperature, SpO_2, $ETCO_2$, invasive BP, ECG, CVP.
- Repeated blood tests: ABGs, U&Es (potassium), FBC (haematocrit/platelets), coagulation studies.

Follow-up
- Continue monitoring on ICU, repeat dantrolene as necessary.
- Monitor for acute kidney injury and compartment syndrome.
- Repeat CK.
- Consider alternative diagnoses (sepsis, phaeochromocytoma, thyroid storm, myopathy).
- Counsel patient and family members; refer to an MH unit[1].

[1] The UK MH Investigation Unit, Academic Unit of Anaesthesia, Clinical Sciences Building, Leeds Teaching Hospitals NHS Trust, Leeds LS9 7TF. Direct line: 0113 206 5270. Fax: 0113 206 4140, Emergency Hotline: 07947 609601.

Reproduced with the kind permission of the Association of Anaesthestists of Great Britain and Ireland.

Box 6.2 Management of neurolept malignant syndrome
- *Stop causative agents.*
- Supportive management/cooling as in hyperthermia (see 📖 p.248).
- Consider the following drug therapy: dantrolene (use MH guidelines), diazepam, levodopa (orally), bromocriptine, amantadine.

Further management
- Repeat drug therapy if required.
- Continue monitoring and support therapy for at least 72 hours.
- Otherwise follow management plan for hyperpyrexia (see 📖 p.249).

Further reading
Adnet P, et al. Neuroleptic malignant syndrome. Br J Anaesth 2000; 85(1): 129–35.

Glahn KPE, et al. Recognizing and managing a malignant hyperthermia crisis: guidelines from the European Malignant Hyperthermia Group. Br J Anaesthesia 2010; 105(4): 417–20.

AAGBI/British MH Association. Malignant hyperthermia crisis. London: AAGBI, 2011.

⚙ Hyperthermia and heat injury

- Hyperthermia is defined as a *core body temperature* >38°C.
- Severe hyperthermia is >40.5°C sustained for >1 hour.

At >42°C cellular enzymes cease to function, proteins are denatured, and there is extensive damage to endothelium, nervous tissue and the liver.

Causes

Factors that increase body heat production, or ↓dissipation:
- Environmental exposure (heat exhaustion).
- Infection, sepsis.
- Burns (probably due to resetting of central thermostat).
- Acute hepatic failure.
- Mismatched blood transfusion (release of pyrogens).
- Endocrine disorders (e.g. hyperthyroidism, phaeochromocytoma).
- CNS disorders (e.g. head injury, SAH, meningitis, encephalitis, seizures).
- Toxicity (e.g. amphetamines, including ecstasy, salicylates, cocaine, phencyclidine, lysergic acid diethylamide/LSD).

A number of factors can predispose to developing hyperthermia:
- Dehydration, hyperactivity/overexertion.
- Illnesses: Parkinsonism, delirium tremens, psychosis, cardiovascular disease, autonomic dysfunction, endocrine dysfunction.
- Anticholinergics and phenothiazines (↓sweating).
- Salicylates (uncoupled oxidative phosphorylation).
- Diuretics (dehydration).
- Tricyclics/MAOI's (muscle rigidity, ↓sweating).
- α/β-blockers (↓heat loss).
- Sympathomimetics (↑ heat production, vasoconstriction).
- Hallucinogenics (↓sweating, ↑ metabolism).

Presentation and assessment

- Apathy, malaise, headache, dizziness, confusion, muscle rigidity/dystonia, ataxia, focal neurological signs, syncope, seizures, coma.
- Nausea and vomiting.
- Tachycardia, arrhythmias, wide pulse pressure, hypotension.
- Hyperventilation, exhaustion, hypercapnia, metabolic acidosis.

Prolonged, untreated hyperthermia can lead to:
- Cardiovascular failure, and/or ARDS.
- Muscle damage/rhabdomyolysis; lactic acidosis; liver dysfunction.
- DIC (denatured clotting factors; endothelial damage).
- Renal failure (due to dehydration, hypotension, rhabdomyolysis).
- Hypernatraemia, hypo/hyperkalaemia, hypocalcaemia.

Investigations

- ABGs (metabolic acidosis, hypercapnia).
- FBC (↑WCC/platelets in NMS, ↓platelets in DIC).
- Coagulation screen (↑PT/APTT, ↓fibrinogen in DIC).
- U&Es (hyperkalaemia, raised urea/creatinine), LFTs (may be deranged).
- Serum phosphate (↑), serum calcium (↓).

6

- CK (↑ in rhabdomyolysis), TFTs (exclude hyperthyroidism).
- Blood, urine and sputum cultures.
- Urine analysis (for toxicology and myoglobinuria).
- ECG (arrhythmias, if ACS suspected).
- CXR, CT scan or LP (if infection suspected).

Differential diagnoses
- Specific syndromes causing hyperpyrexia (e.g. toxic epidermal necrolysis, NMS, MH, thyroid storm).

Immediate management
- Give O_2 and support airway, breathing, and circulation as required.
- Give IV fluids, ideally guided by CVP and other invasive haemodynamic monitoring in cardiovascularly unstable patients.
- Start cooling as soon as possible; options include:
  - Antipyretics (paracetamol and/or NSAIDs)
  - Peripheral cooling using exposure, tepid sponging, and fans
  - Cooling blankets and mattresses
  - Cold IV fluid infusions
  - Cold irrigation of: stomach, bladder, peritoneum, pleural spaces
  - Use of intravascular cooling systems (i.e. CoolGard™)
  - Haemofiltration using cold fluids
- Sedation and ventilation along with neuromuscular block may be required to reduce heat production:
  - Hyperventilate to compensate for ↑ CO_2 production

Further management
- Active cooling should continue until core temperature reaches <38°C.
- Continue to monitor for DIC, metabolic acidosis, and electrolyte imbalance during and after cooling; correct electrolytes if required.
- Treat arrhythmias if these cause haemodynamic compromise.
- Consider supportive measures for rhabdomyolysis (📖 p.268).
- Treatment of seizures may be required (see 📖 p.160).
- Ventilatory and inotropic/vasopressor support may be required.
- Drug therapy with paracetamol or NSAIDS may be effective in patients with hyperthermia due to proven infection/SIRS.
- Alpha antagonists have been used to vasodilate to improve heat.

Pitfalls/difficult situations
- Peripheral cooling causes vasoconstriction and may prevent heat loss.
- Peripheral temperature in a vasoconstricted patient will not reflect central temperature.
- Be prepared to treat severe arrhythmias.

Further reading
Laupland KB. Fever in the critically ill medical patient. *Crit Care Med* 2009; **3**(S): S273–S278.
Trujillo MH, et al. Multiple organ failure following near-fatal exertional heat stroke. *J Intensive Care Med* 2009; **24**(1): 72–8.

☼ Hypothermia

- Mild hypothermia: 32–35°C.
- Moderate hypothermia: 28–32°C.
- Severe hypothermia: <28°C.

Hypothermia is defined as a *core temperature* of <35°C.

Temperature measured at peripheral sites (skin) may be up to 2°C lower than that measured at central sites (close to the core). In states of poor circulation, this difference may increase.

Temperature measured in the rectum, oesophagus, nasopharynx, and tympanic membrane approximates core temperature.

Causes

The common causes of hypothermia in critical care are:
- Environmental injury.
- Postoperative patient after prolonged/extensive surgery.
- Postoperative patient after cardiac surgery (cardiopulmonary bypass).
- Massive blood/fluid transfusion.
- Exposed body surfaces (especially burns).
- Extracorporeal procedures: haemodialysis/haemofiltration, ECMO.
- Irrigation of body cavities: peritoneal, bladder.
- Hypometabolic states: hypothyroidism, hypoglycaemia, hypopituitarism, adrenal insufficiency.
- Toxicity: alcohol, barbiturates, central depressants, antidepressants.

A number of factors can predispose to developing hypothermia:
- Immobility, or major trauma/immersion injuries.
- Impaired consciousness.
- Extremes of age.
- Autonomic neuropathy.
- Malnutrition.
- Renal failure.

Presentation and assessment

Mild hypothermia (32–35°C):
- General: shivering, with resultant ↑ oxygen demand.
- Respiratory: dyspnoea, ↑rate/depth of breathing.
- Cardiovascular: vasoconstriction, tachycardia, ↑cardiac output.
- Neurological: confusion/lethargy, dizziness, ataxia, dysarthria.
- Renal: ↑renal blood flow with resultant diuresis.
- Other: platelet and clotting factor function is progressively impaired.

Moderate/severe hypothermia (28–32°C):
- Progressive depression of organ function occurs.
- General: shivering stops at very low temperature (i.e. <32°C).
- Respiratory: reduced respiratory rate/depth, depression of cough reflex, apnoea (<24°C).
- Cardiovascular: bradycardia, progressive cardiovascular depression:
  - ECG changes include: bradycardia, prolonged PR and QT intervals, 'J' wave (<33°C), AF, VF (<28°C)
- Neurological: hyporeflexia/areflexia, coma, dilated pupils.

- Renal: oliguria and associated AKI.
- Haematology: neutropaenia, thrombocytopaenia (splenic sequestration).
- Other: hyperglycaemia (reduced insulin secretion and peripheral insulin resistance); hypoglycaemia may occur with prolonged hypothermia:
  - Mixed respiratory and metabolic acidosis.

In a sedated patient/postoperative patient, the following may be present:
- At mild/moderate hypothermia:
  - Inappropriately excessive sedation; slow postoperative recovery
  - Bradycardia or arrhythmias
  - Loss of reflexes
  - Metabolic acidosis

Prolonged untreated hypothermia can lead to:
- Infections (e.g. pneumonia, surgical site infection).
- ARDS.
- Renal failure.
- Bowel ischaemia.
- Pancreatitis.
- Rhabdomyolysis.
- DIC.

Investigations

- ABGs (mixed metabolic and respiratory acidosis:
  - Allow for temperature correction of PaO_2; partial pressure of oxygen may appear artificially high when measured during hypothermia; approximate correction factor for oxygen is 7% per °C
- FBC (WCC may be raised if infection present).
- U&Es (hyperkalaemia, raised urea/creatinine).
- Serum glucose (hypoglycaemia/hyperglycaemia may be present).
- Serum magnesium, phosphate, and calcium (Mg^{2+}/PO_4^- may be ↓).
- CK (↑ with rhabdomyolysis).
- Amylase (↑ with pancreatitis).
- TFTs (to exclude hypothyroidism).
- Serum cortisol (to exclude adrenal insufficiency).
- Blood, urine and sputum cultures (if infection suspected).
- Urine analysis (for toxicology, proteinuria, and myoglobinuria).
- ECG.
- CXR (to exclude infection, identify ARDS).

Differential diagnoses

Although most severe cases of hypothermia are associated with environmental injury, it can coexist with, or be the result of, medical illnesses, especially:
- Hypometabolic states: hypothyroidism, hypoglycaemia, hypopituitarism, adrenal insufficiency.
- Toxicity: alcohol, barbiturates, central depressants, antidepressants.
- Stroke.

Immediate management
- Give 100% O_2 (shivering increases O_2 demand by 200–500%).
- Support airway, breathing, and circulation as required.
- Confirm hypothermia using a suitable low-reading thermometer (oesophageal, rectal, or bladder).

Cardiac arrests
(See also 📖 p.98.)
- If resuscitation is required, the ALS protocol should be adjusted for hypothermia:
  - At <30°C, resuscitative drugs will not be effective, and should be withheld until temperature is corrected to >30°C
  - At <30°C, 3 DC shocks can be tried, if unsuccessful no further shocks should be given until the temperature is >30°C
  - Start active re-warming and continue CPR and ventilation
  - At 30°C the lowest recommended dose of the drugs can be given at twice the recommended interval in the ALS protocol
- CVC access is extremely important due to sluggish peripheral circulation.
- Invasive haemodynamic monitoring is mandatory.

Rewarming and general resuscitation
Mild hypothermia (32–35°C):
- Rewarm gradually using passive means:
  - Remove any wet clothing, and replace with dry garments
  - Keep in a warm environment
  - Apply blankets (consider using foil or 'space' blankets)
Moderate hypothermia (<32°C):
- Rewarm more aggressively
  - Warmed, humidified O_2
  - Warmed IV fluids (avoiding fluids containing lactate may be advisable; liver capacity to metabolize lactate may be reduced)
  - Heat lamps
  - Heated forced-air air blankets
  - Warmed fluid mattresses
- Careful cardiovascular monitoring for arrhythmias and hypotension.
- Aim for up to a 1 °C increase in core temperature per hour.
Severe hypothermia (<28°C), in addition to that already listed:
- Consider rewarming using gastric, bladder, colonic or peritoneal lavage with warmed fluids in patients with stable cardiac rhythms.
- If significant cardiac arrhythmias are present consider:
  - Intravascular warming systems (i.e. CoolGard™)
  - Pleural/thoracic lavage with warm saline
  - Extracorporeal warming using a modified bypass technique, a 'level one' fluid warmer, haemodialysis/haemofiltration with a warmed circuit
  - Formal cardiac bypass (spontaneous cardiac output is not required)
- Rewarming at rates >2°C/hour have been shown to reduce mortality in cases of severe hypothermia.

- Volume expansion will be required during rewarming, use CVP as a guide.
- Avoid rapid changes in pH; severe metabolic acidosis (pH <7.1) may be corrected using a bicarbonate infusion.
- Monitor blood glucose levels (early moderate hyperglycaemia should be tolerated later as hypoglycaemia can occur with rewarming).
- Active resuscitation should continue until core temperature ≥35°C.

Further management
- When not associated with immersion, hypothermia is commonly associated with sepsis; empirical antibiotics may be required.
- Monitor for DIC, metabolic acidosis, and electrolyte imbalance during and after rewarming; correct any electrolyte changes.
- Avoid hyperventilation.
- Treat arrhythmias if these cause haemodynamic compromise.
- Give thiamine 250 mg IV if there is history of ↑ alcohol intake.
- If temperature is slow to correct suspect hypothyroid or Addisonian crisis; consider treatment with liothyronine 20 mcg IV and hydrocortisone 200 mg IV, repeated as necessary.
- Infection commonly occurs with hypothermia, antibiotic treatment may be indicated.
- Treat any frostbite/gangrene.

Pitfalls/difficult situations
- Profound bradycardia or bradypnoea may be present in hypothermic patients, allow as much as 1 minute to confirm their presence/absence.
- Rough handling/inappropriate CPR may precipitate arrhythmias.
- The possibility of hypothermia 2° to an underlying disease should be considered, and causes looked for.
- Many drugs are ineffective at hypothermic temperatures and may cause rebound/unwanted side effects as the patient is rewarmed.
- Core temperature may drop during rewarming (this 'after-drop' is probably due to temperature equilibration between core and periphery rather than return of cold blood from the peripheries).
- In endocrine disorders and sepsis the cause of hypothermia may be initially difficult to diagnose.
- Be prepared to treat severe arrhythmias during hypothermia and rewarming.
- Death cannot be easily diagnosed in a hypothermic patient, CPR along with rewarming and active management should continue until core temperature is >35°C.
- Assessment of neurological status is also impaired during hypothermia
- MOF is common after profound and prolonged hypothermia.

Further reading
American Heart Association guidelines for cardiopulmonary resuscitation and emergency cardio-vascular care. Hypothermia. *Circulation* 2005; **112**:IV136–IV138.
Davis PR, et al. Accidental hypothermia. *J R Army Med Corps* 2006; **152**: 223–33.
Epstein E, et al. Accidental hypothermia *Br Med J* 2006; **332**: 706–9.
Vassal T, et al. Severe accidental hypothermia treated in an ICU: prognosis and outcome. *Chest* 2001; **120**(6): 1998–2003.

Renal

① /:☼: **Fluid balance disorders**

Fluid balance disorders include hypovolaemia (oligaemia), dehydration/acute fluid depletion, and hypervolaemia/fluid overload. Careful attention to fluid balance is essential in ICU. Patients are likely to require 'maintenance' fluids in addition to any fluid resuscitation.

Causes

Hypovolaemia (see also Shock, ☐ p.104) occurs when there is a decrease in the volume of circulating blood. It can be accompanied by a decrease in total body water (dehydration/acute fluid depletion); but can also occur where there is an overall increase in total body water, due to fluid leaking out of the intravascular space (e.g. in sepsis). Causes include:

- Haemorrhage (see ☐ p.112), or burns (transdermal fluid loss).
- 'Third-space' losses (e.g. fluid leaking into the interstitial compartment, or oedema caused by diseases such as sepsis or pancreatitis):
  - This may occur rapidly, especially where surgical/radiological drainage of large amounts of ascites or pleural fluid (especially transudate) promotes rapid reaccumulation of fluid
- Severe dehydration.
- Aggressive negative balance with RRT.

Dehydration/acute fluid depletion

- Inadequate intake or inadequate fluid resuscitation.
- ↑Increased fluid losses:
  - GI: diarrhoea, vomiting
  - Renal: polyuria/diuresis (diuretic therapy, DKA, DI)
  - Other: severe burn injury, hyperpyrexia/heatstroke
  - Aggressive negative balance with RRT.

Hypervolaemia/fluid overload

- Iatrogenic.
- Renal failure (acute kidney injury or chronic kidney disease).
- Polydipsia.
- Chronic heart failure.
- Cirrhosis.
- Nephrotic syndrome.

Presentation and assessment

Fluid balance/volume status assessment will include:

- The patient's fluid charts (and anaesthetic charts).
- Any history of diarrhoea, vomiting, diuresis.

Hypovolaemia may present as shock (see Shock, ☐ p.104, and Haemorrhage, ☐ p.114). Signs and symptoms of fluid depletion may include:

- General: thirst, skin turgor, dry mucous membranes, sunken eyes:
  - Pyrexia may be present if it is associated with the cause of fluid loss
- Neurological: altered mental state, ↓consciousness, syncope.
- Cardiovascular: tachycardia, normotension or hypotension:
  - ↑ capillary refill time
  - Cold peripheries, mottling
  - ↓ JVP/CVP

- ↑cardiac output or CVP (if monitored) in response to straight leg raising (45° for 4 minutes) or a fluid bolus
- Renal: anuria/oliguria, raised urea and creatinine:
  - Polyuria may be present if it is associated with the cause (i.e. DKA)
  - Metabolic acidosis
- GI: vomiting or diarrhoea may be present.
- Haematology: raised Hct and Hb (haemoconcentration).
- Other: hypernatraemia, raised serum osmolality, raised serum lactate.

Acute fluid overload signs and symptoms may include:
- General: peripheral/dependent oedema, or enlarged and tender liver, ascites may be present *if* there is acute-on-chronic overload.
- Respiratory: pulmonary oedema may occur.
- Cardiovascular: tachycardia, raised JVP (>4 cm from sternal angle), CVP (>15 cmH$_2$O), or PAOP (>18 mmHg):
  - Gallop rhythm, S3 may be present
  - Hypotension may be present if cardiogenic shock is present
- Renal: pre-existing renal failure or oliguria may be present, polyuria may also be present.
- Haematology: lowered Hct and Hb (haemodilution).
- Other: hyponatraemia, ↓serum osmolality (↑ serum chloride and or sodium may be present in iatrogenic hypervolaemia).

Investigations
- ABGs (hypoxia, acidaemia).
- FBC, coagulation screen.
- U&Es, LFTs (including serum albumin).
- Serum lactate.
- Serum magnesium, calcium, and phosphate.
- Serum glucose (to exclude hyperglycaemic states), capillary ketones.
- Serum osmolality.
- TFTs, serum cortisol (if hypoadrenalism or hypothyroidism suspected).
- Serum CRP.
- Septic screen (blood, urine, sputum cultures, if infection is suspected).
- Stool culture and CDT testing, if diarrhoea present.
- Cardiac enzymes (if a myocardial infarct is suspected).
- 12-lead ECG and echocardiography (if cardiogenic shock suspected).
- CXR (if pulmonary oedema or infection suspected).
- CVP or cardiac output measurement, or echocardiography may help define intravascular fluid balance status.
- Urinalysis (both dipstick and urinary U&Es/osmolality).

Differential diagnoses
Dehydration/acute fluid depletion
- Hyperosmolar hyperglycaemic state.
- Meningitis.
- Adrenal insufficiency or hypothyroidism.

Acute fluid overload
- Cardiac failure.
- TUR syndrome.

Immediate management

- Give O_2 as required, support airway, breathing, and circulation.
- Manage shock/hypotension as required (🕮 p.104).
- Manage major haemorrhage if required (🕮 p.112).

Dehydration/acute fluid depletion

- Assess patient fully, including age, weight, working diagnosis, co-morbidities, and volume status (CRT, HR, BP, C/JVP, UOP):
  - Urinary catheterization is likely to be required
- Prescribe appropriate fluid challenge:
  - 250–500 ml IV gelatin colloid (e.g. Gelofusine®) over 15–60 minutes
  - In patients who are very small, elderly with IHD, or known to have poor LV function consider reducing fluid challenge to 200 ml over 30–60 minutes
  - In fit healthy severely dehydrated patients (e.g. patients with severe DKA) consider speeding initial fluid challenges up to 1000 ml over 15–30 minutes
- Review patient following fluid challenge noting changes in haemodynamic and urinary variables.
- Prescribe further fluid challenges as appropriate, and review again.
- Prescribe maintenance fluids (usually crystalloids) and resuscitation fluids (crystalloids or colloids) separately.

Acute fluid overload

- Treat pulmonary oedema if present (🕮 p.86).
- Consider monitoring degree of overload using CVP measurement.
- Potential therapies include:
  - Diuresis: furosemide IV 20–40 mg (requires functioning kidneys)
  - Vasodilatation using GTN IV infusion if patient is normo- or hypertensive (1 mg/ml at 0–15 ml/hour) and/or morphine IV 2–10 mg (repeated doses may accumulate in renal failure)
  - Fluid removal using renal replacement therapy
  - If in extremis consider venesecting 200–400 ml of blood whilst preparing other treatments

Further management

Electrolyte abnormalities associated with acute fluid balance problems:

- Hyponatraemia/hypernatraemia; hypokalaemia/hyperkalaemia.
- Calcium (hypocalcaemia in massive blood transfusion, pancreatitis).
- Phosphate (hypophosphataemia; hyperphosphataemia in acute renal failure 2° to tubular obstruction, e.g. tumour lysis syndrome).
- Magnesium (hypomagnesaemia 2° to marked diuresis).
- Acid–base problems associated with fluid balance problems include:
  - Hyperchloraemic metabolic acidosis 2° to excessive replacement with 0.9% sodium chloride
  - Hypochloraemic hypokalaemic metabolic alkalosis 2° to HCl loss with persistent vomiting, or excess NG aspirates
  - Metabolic acidosis 2° to diabetic ketoacidosis
  - Metabolic acidosis 2° to excess bicarbonate loss from small bowel fistula, or ureteroenterostomy.

Pitfalls/difficult situations

- The optimal degree of fluid resuscitation in acute hypovolaemia, and the point at which to initiate inotropes/vasopressors is unclear.
- Glucose containing fluids such as 5% glucose spread into interstitial and intracellular fluid spaces, whilst the oncotic pressure generated by colloids keeps fluid within the intravascular space for longer; as an approximation regarding intravascular fluid replacement 1 L of colloid is equivalent to 2–3 L of saline 0.9% is equivalent to 8–9 L of 5% glucose:
  - There is very little evidence to advocate the use of colloids (including human albumin solution) over crystalloids, or vice-versa
  - 'Balanced' solutions may avoid hyperchloraemic acidosis
- Hypotonic fluids may exacerbate cerebral oedema and increase ICP in head-injured patients; human albumin solution is not recommended in cases of TBI.
- Salt loading should be avoided in hepatic failure.
- Fluid accumulation during critical care management may be associated with ↑ length of time weaning from mechanical ventilation.

Prescribing maintenance fluids

(See also Tables 7.1 and 7.2.)

- Daily fluid requirements: ~40 ml/kg/day or 1.5 ml/kg/hour:
  - Increase if there are large losses from urine, diarrhoea, vomiting, or skin (e.g. burns losses)
- Daily electrolyte requirements: sodium 1–2 mmol/kg/day,[1] potassium ~0.5–1 mmol/kg/day.[2]

In practice, U&Es should be regularly checked and potassium supplementation given as required. Maintenance fluids may be adjusted according to plasma sodium, for example:

- Na+ <135 mmol/L: 0.9% saline.
- Na+ 135–145 mmol/L: Hartmann's or glucose 4%/saline 0.18%.
- Na+ >145 mmol/L: 5% glucose.

Maintenance fluids may also be provided in the form of enteral feed or PN.

[1] Larger daily amounts of sodium are regularly given to critically ill patients, especially during acute resuscitation. Hyponatraemic/hypo-osmolar fluids should be avoided in head injuries; sodium-containing fluids should be avoided if possible in liver failure.
[2] Potassium requirements may be ↑ by certain diseases or medications, or ↓ by renal failure or tissue destruction.

Further reading

Antonelli M, et al. Hemodynamic monitoring in shock and implications for management. *Intensive Care Med* 2007; **33**: 575–90.

National Heart, Lung, and Blood Institute ARDS Clinical Trials Network, et al. Comparison of two fluid-management strategies in acute lung injury. *N Engl J Med* 2006; **354**: 2564–75.

Powel-Tuck J, et al. *British consensus guidelines on intravenous fluid therapy for adult surgical patients. (GIFTASUP).* London: NHS National Library of Health, 2008.

Perel P, et al. Colloids versus crystalloids for fluid resuscitation in critically ill patients. *Cochrane Database Syst Rev* 2011; **3**: CD000567. DOI: 10.1002/14651858.CD000567.pub4.

SAFE study Investigators. A comparison of albumin and saline for fluid resuscitation in the intensive care unit. *N Engl J Med* 2004; **350**: 2247–56.

SAFE study Investigators. Saline or albumin for fluid resuscitation in patients with traumatic brain injury. *N Engl J Med* 2007; **357**: 874–84.

Table 7.1 Commonly available IV fluids

Fluid	Other names/similar solutions	Na⁺	K⁺	Cl⁻	Other	pH
Saline 0.9%	Saline; 'normal' saline	154	0	154		5
Glucose 4%/0.18% saline	5% Glucose saline; 4% and a fifth	30	0	30		4
'Balanced' crystalloids	Compound sodium lactate; Ringer's lactate; Hartmann's	131	~5	~110	Ca²⁺ 2; Lactate ~30	6.5
5% glucose		0	0	0	Glucose 50 (g/L)	4
Sodium bicarbonate 8.4%		1000				8
'Standard' colloids	Gelofusine®, Haemaccel®, starch solutions; human albumin solution 4.5% (HAS)	~150	Haemaccel® ~5	Haemaccel® 125–145	Haemaccel® Ca²⁺ ~6	~7.4
'Balanced' colloids	Volulyte®; Tetraspan®, Isoplex®, Geloplasma®	137–150	4–5	100–118	Mg²⁺ 0.9–1.5; Ca²⁺ 0–2.5; lactate or acetate ~24–34	4.5–7.4

Table 7.2 Commonly available IV colloids

Fluid	General information	Indications	Complications
Albumin	Available as 4.5% and 20% preparations Molecular weight ~68 kDa	Unclear: shown to be as safe as crystalloids for acute resuscitation Provides plasma expansion for ~4 hours	Theoretical risk of transmission of nvCJD; prepared from pooled donors
Blood (packed red cells)	Expands intravascular compartment only Increases oxygen carriage.	Haemorrhage, anaemia	Immune reaction, infection, immunosuppression
Dextrans	Polysaccharide products of sucrose Classified by their molecular weights Dextran 70: molecular weight 70,000 kDa	Provides volume expansion for ~12 hours	Alters platelet function; incidence of allergic reactions; rouleaux formation affects crossmatching
Gelatins	Widely variable molecular size (typically 30,000 kDa) Excreted by unchanged kidney Long shelf life	Provides plasma expansion for ~4 hours	Anaphylaxis
Starches	Hetastarch®: 450,000 kDa Haes-steril®: 200,000 kDa Voluven®/Volulyte®/Tetraspan®: 130,000 kDa Most as 6% or 10% solutions	Provides volume expansion for ~24 hours	May impair coagulation: factors VII & vWF; may accumulate in RES if large volumes given (>33ml/kg/24hour); may cause pruritus; some formulations associated with AKI

⊙ Acute kidney injury

Acute kidney injury (AKI; previously called acute renal failure, ARF) is defined as kidney injury occurring within 48 hours, involving an absolute increase in serum creatinine of ≥26.4 μmol/L, or an increase in serum creatinine to 1.5 × baseline value, or oliguria of <0.5 ml/kg/hour for 6 hours (in the absence of, for example, acute catheter obstruction).

Causes

Pre-renal causes

• Dehydration, caused by inadequate intake or:
  • GI losses (e.g. diarrhoea, vomiting)
  • Renal losses (e.g. polyuria/diuresis caused by diuretics, DKA, DI)
  • Other losses (e.g. burn injury, hyperpyrexia, heat exhaustion)
• Hypotension (e.g. septic, cardiogenic, or haemorrhagic shock).

Intra-renal causes

• Drug toxicity (e.g. NSAIDs and ACE inhibitors, particularly in combination with pre-renal failure; radiocontrast agents).
• Rhabdomyolysis.
• Renal artery obstruction (e.g. stenosis, emboli, or aortic surgery).
• Venous obstruction (e.g. intra-abdominal compartment syndrome).
• Vasculitis (e.g. SLE, PAN).
• Thrombotic disease (e.g. HUS/TTP, DIC).
• Infections (particularly streptococcal and TB).
• Primary glomerulonephritis.
• Carcinoma (e.g. myeloma).

Post-renal causes

• Ureteric obstruction (e.g. calculi, carcinoma, retroperitoneal fibrosis, or disruption following surgery such as emergency hysterectomy).
• Prolonged bladder outflow obstruction (e.g. clot, tumour, neurogenic bladder, catheter obstruction).

AKI is more likely to develop in patients with chronic kidney disease (CKD). Severe renal impairment (grades 4–5) affects 0.4% of the population. Individuals at risk include patients with:
• Vasculitis, diabetes, or hypertension.
• Cardiac failure.
• Previous renal or aortic surgery.

Classification of chronic kidney disease

• Stage 1: kidney damage with normal or ↑ GFR[1] (≥90).
• Stage 2: kidney damage and mildly ↓ GFR[1] (60–89).
• Stage 3: moderately ↓ GFR[1] (30–59).
• Stage 4: severely reduced GFR[1] (15–29).
• Stage 5: kidney failure (established renal failure), GFR[1] <15.

[1] GFR is measured in ml/minute/1.73m²

Adapted from Concise UK CKD guidelines, ⚲ www.renal.org and from American Journal of Kidney Diseases, 'KDOQI Guideline on stratification and classification of CKD', 39, 2, pp. S46–S75, Copyright 2002, with permission from Elsevier and the National Kidney Foundation.

Presentation and assessment

Features of AKI include:
- Anuria or oliguria (<0.5ml/kg/hour), the commonest presenting feature.
- Features of fluid overload (e.g. pulmonary oedema) may occur.
- Metabolic acidosis and/or hyperkalaemia may develop.
- Serum creatinine (and urea) will increase over time.

Other signs and symptoms may include:
- General: thirst and/or skin turgor if fluid depletion is present:
  - Pyrexia may be present if there is associated infection
- Neurological: altered mental state, ↓ consciousness.
- Respiratory signs and symptoms: tachypnoea, dyspnoea, gasping or sighing breathing (Kussmaul's breathing):
  - $PaCO_2$ is often <3.5 kPa due to compensatory hyperventilation
- Cardiovascular :
  - In shock: tachycardia, hypotension, ↑ capillary refill time and ↓ JVP/CVP
  - In fluid overload: tachycardia, raised JVP (>4 cm from sternal angle), CVP (>15 cmH$_2$O), or PAOP (>18 mmHg)
  - ECG changes associated with hyperkalaemia: tall tented T waves, slurring of ST segments into T waves, small P waves, prolonged PR interval, widened QRS, complete heart block, asystole or VF
- GI: nausea and vomiting; diarrhoea may be present.
  - IAP may be raised
- Other: evidence of trauma or compartment syndrome may be present.

Investigations

- ABGs (metabolic acidosis with/without respiratory compensation).
- FBC, coagulation studies.
- U&Es (serial measurements to monitor potassium and creatinine).
- LFTs (if hepatorenal syndrome suspected).
- Serum CK (raised in rhabdomyolysis), serum CRP.
- Serum magnesium, calcium, and phosphate.
- Serum glucose, serum osmolality.
- Septic screen (blood, urine, sputum cultures if infection suspected).
- Stool culture (if diarrhoea present).
- 12-lead ECG (if hyperkalaemia or cardiogenic shock suspected).
- Consider renal US (or abdominal CT), or rarely IVU.
- Urinalysis (urine dipstick).
- Urine U&Es, osmolality (±microscopy for cells, casts, crystals).
- Urine for myoglobin or Bence-Jones protein (if rhabdomyolysis or myeloma suspected).
- Consider autoantibody screen, complement concentrations, serum immunoglobulins and electrophoresis.
- Renal biopsy may be required for certain conditions.

Differential diagnoses

- Traumatic renal rupture (urine collecting in abdomen).
- LVF/pulmonary oedema.
- Catheter obstruction.

Immediate management

• Give O_2 as required; support airway, breathing, and circulation.

Treatment of complications

• Treat pulmonary oedema as per protocol (📖 p.86).
• Hyperkalaemia may need rapid correction (see 📖 p.212):
  • If signs of potassium toxicity are present give calcium chloride IV 3–5 ml of 10% solution over 3 minutes for cardioprotecton (unless digoxin toxicity suspected)
  • IV soluble insulin 10–15 units soluble insulin in 50 ml 50% glucose over 30–60 minutes may be required
• Severe acidosis (Ph <7.1) may be transiently controlled with boluses of sodium bicarbonate 8.4% IV 25–50 ml.

Renal support

• Stop any nephrotoxins (e.g. NSAIDs).
• Insert a urinary catheter and monitor urine output and fluid balance.
• Exclude outflow obstruction:
  • Washout the bladder to ensure the urinary catheter is patent
  • Consider renal tract imaging (renal US or CT abdomen) if ureteric obstruction/hydronephrosis is a possibility
  • If ureteric of bladder obstruction is present obtain urological advice (a suprapubic catheter or nephrostomy may be required)
• Optimize renal perfusion:
  • Give fluid challenges as required; CVP measurement may help
  • Avoid hypotension, using vasopressors/inotropes if required, aiming for a MAP %70 mmg (or as close to normal values as possible). Monitor and treat raised IAP (📖 p.284).

Renal replacement therapy

• Indications for RRT can be found on 📖 p.266.
• Within ICU/HDU this is usually continuous veno-venous haemofiltration (CVVH, CVVHF), HD or a combination (e.g. CVVHDF); HF and HD are considered equivalent.
• Insert a dialysis line for RRT (📖 p.536), correct clotting abnormalities prior to insertion, confirm catheter position with a CXR (if within SVC territory) prior to use.
• Anticoagulation will be required in most patients requiring RRT:
  • Avoid anticoagulation in patients with coagulopathy
• CVVH fluid balance should be prescribed, there are 3 possibilities:
  • Net balance to the patient is negative (useful in fluid overload where an hourly negative balance of 50–100 ml is usually sufficient; higher rates may be used, but the patient should be monitored for cardiovascular decompensation)
  • Net balance to the patient is even (the CVVH machine will have to be adjusted regularly to ensure that any fluid boluses, e.g. from drugs, are removed)
  • Balance to the *machine* is even (net balance to the *patient* will be positive as any fluid boluses will accumulate).

Complications of renal replacement therapy

Cardiac arrest

If cardiac arrest occurs, clamp the vascular access catheter lumens and stop CVVH, *unless* the cause is hyperkalaemia (keep the filter running) or hypovolaemia (wash the filter blood back into the patient).

Hypotension/cardiovascular collapse

Hypotension commonly occurs on commencement of CVVH (especially where extracorporeal circuits are chemically, rather than steam, sterilized). Hypotension normally resolves rapidly, but may require colloid boluses (250 ml IV) and/or low dose inotrope boluses (metaraminol IV 0.5–1 mg). Where patients are shocked or cardiovascularly unstable inotrope infusions may be commenced before starting CVVH. Exclude bleeding (from the circuit, or as a result of anticoagulation).

Metabolic derangement

CVVH will usually correct hyperkalaemia within a few hours and control metabolic acidosis within a day. If they persist consider whether potassium-releasing, or acidosis-causing, processes are still at work.

Potassium supplements are commonly added to the replacement fluid after the first day to prevent the development of hypokalaemia. Persistent lactataemia may be improved by using lactate-free replacement fluid.

Pressure alarms

CVVH machines vary in design, but pressure alarms may include:
* Transmembrane pressure (TMP) or filter pressure (FP): increasing pressures indicate filter clotting, check clotting and consider a further fluid bolus; or change filter.
* Arterial and venous pressures: high pressures indicate a problem with arterial and venous access; consider rotating, flushing or changing the line. High blood flow is desirable (≥200 ml/minute) as this will deliver high ultrafiltration rates, this relies on good vascular access.
* Blood leak or air-in-the-circuit alarms: the circuit should be fully inspected and problems corrected.

Filter clotting

Unless anticoagulation is contraindicated (coagulopathy, thrombocytopaenia, imminent or recent surgery) an IV heparin infusion (~500–1000 units/hour) should be used to minimize filter clotting. INR and APTT should be checked first. A loading dose of 500–2000 units may be given. The lowest dose possible to maintain filter patency should be given. Target APTTR is 1.5–2.5; target ACT is 150–180 seconds.

Over-anticoagulation

If over-anticoagulation occurs, heparin should be stopped until APTT returns to normal. If it is associated with major haemorrhage consider giving protamine IV (5 mg slowly, then review). Epoprostenol IV 5.2 ng/kg/minute is an alternative, but can cause hypotension. Citrate anticoagulation is supported by some machines.

Further management

- The underlying cause of the AKI should be actively sought and treated.
- Many drug doses will require adjustment where AKI or CKD is present, discuss with pharmacy and/or nephrology specialists.
- Monitor U&Es, including magnesium and phosphate.
- Monitor the patient's temperature.
- RRT may be discontinued intermittently in stable patients to look for evidence of renal recovery:
  - Return of urine output
  - Maintenance of acid–base, electrolyte, and fluid balance
  - 'Plateau' development of elevated creatinine and urea, and their eventual decrease

---

Indications for renal replacement therapy

- Significant fluid volume overload (e.g. causing, or likely to cause, pulmonary oedema).
- Hyperkalaemia (symptomatic, >7.0 mmol/L, or rapidly increasing)
- Significant metabolic acidosis –pH | 7.15).
- Symptomatic uraemia (usually >40 mmol/L).
- Haemodialysis may be indicated in some forms of poisoning (ethanol, methanol, ethylene glycol, salicylates, theophylline, lithium).

Patients who are known to be dialysis-dependent prior to ICU/HDU admission should be treated with RRT before the listed indications develop.

Pitfalls/difficult situations

- Low-dose dopamine or furosemide boluses/infusions have not been shown to prevent the onset of AKI.
- Consultation with nephrologists may be required in situations, especially if chronic renal supportive therapy is likely to be required.
- Complications of RRT may be found on 📖 p.265.
- AKI with deranged urea and creatinine commonly persists for 2–3 weeks, and in some cases renal function never recovers.
- In patients not receiving RRT furosemide infusions may be used to improve urine output; this will not alter outcome, but may improve fluid balance management.
- Polyuria is common in the recovery phase of AKI; care must be taken to avoid hypovolaemia.
- IV contrast (i.e. when used during angiography or CT scanning) is known to cause contrast-induced nephropathy (CIN):
  - Ensuring adequate hydration prior to administration will help
  - IV N-acetylcysteine 150 mg/kg prior to contrast *may* help
  - CVVH may also be required after IV contrast exposure
- Hypothermia may occur in patients undergoing CVVH and aggressive rewarming is required:
  - Pyrexia may be masked by CVVH induced hypothermia
- High-volume haemofiltration has also been used as a treatment for severe sepsis/septic shock, but it is unlikely to alter outcome.

Modes of renal replacement therapy

- Continuous ambulatory peritoneal dialysis (CAPD)[1]
- Haemodialysis (HD)[2,3]
- Haemofiltration (HF):
  - Continuous arterio-venous haemofiltration (CAVH, CAVHF)[4]
  - Continuous veno-venous haemofiltration (CVVH, CVVHF)
  - Continuous veno-venous haemo-diafiltration (CVVHD, CVVHDF)

[1] CAPD is less effective in critically ill patients, is rarely possible where abdominal conditions exist, and may complicate other therapies (e.g. by splinting the diaphragm); it is only occasionally used in ICU/HDU.

[2] HD may precipitate haemodynamic instability in critically ill patients compared with CVVH.

[3] Electrolyte imbalance, acidosis, and volume overload may be corrected more rapidly with HD.

[4] CAVH is only rarely used, unlike CVVH it does not require an extracorporeal pump and relies on systolic BP to drive blood, and is less efficient where shock is present (the risks associated with arterial cannulation are also present).

Classification/staging system for AKI

Stage 1
- Increase in serum creatinine of ≥ 26.4 μmol/L or increase to 1.5–2 × baseline value; or
- Urine output of <0.5 ml/kg/hour for "6 hours.

Stage 2
- Increase in serum creatinine to 2–3 × baseline value; or
- Urine output of <0.5ml/kg/hour for "12 hours.

Stage 3
- Increase in serum creatinine to more than 3 × baseline value; or serum creatinine of ≥ 354 μmol/L with an acute increase of at least 44 μmol/L; or
- Urine output of <0.3ml/kg/hour for 24 hours, or anuria for 12 hours.

Reproduced with permission from the Acute Kidney Injury Network (AKIN) guidelines, 2007, adapted from the RIFLE Criteria (Risk, Injury, Failure, Loss, End-stage), 2004 also copyright of the Acute Kidney Injury Network.

Further reading

Barrett BJ, et al. Preventing nephropathy induced by contrast medium. N Engl J Med 2006; 354: 379–86.

John S, et al. Renal replacement strategies in the ICU. Chest 2007; 132: 1379–88.

Marik PE. Low-dose dopamine: a systematic review. Intensive Care Med 2002; 28: 877–83.

Mehta RL, et al. Acute Kidney Injury Network: report of an initiative to improve outcomes in acute kidney injury. Crit Care 2007; 11: R31.

Pannu N, et al. Renal replacement therapy in patients with acute renal failure: a systematic review. JAMA 2008; 299(7): 793–805.

Pavelsky PM. Indications and timing of renal replacement therapy in acute kidney injury. Crit Care Med 2008; 36(s): S224–S228.

Stewart J, et al. Adding insult to injury: a review of the care of patients who died in hospital with a primary diagnosis of acute kidney injury (acute renal failure). London: National Confidential Enquiry into Patient Outcome and Death, 2009.

Van Wert R, et al. High-dose renal replacement therapy for acute kidney injury: systematic review and meta-analysis. Crit Care Med 2010; 38: 1360–9.

:O: Rhabdomyolysis/crush syndrome

Rhabdomyolysis occurs when widespread muscle breakdown causes the release of intracellular products, (e.g. potassium, phosphate, myoglobin).

Causes

- Trauma/environmental injury: crush injury, compartment syndrome (typically lower limb), burns, electrocution, heatstroke.
- Ischaemia/vascular occlusion: following surgery (e.g. vascular surgery), prolonged immobility (e.g. collapse or overdose), sickle cell disease.
- Muscle overactivity: seizures, dystonia, malignant hyperpyrexia, status asthmaticus, alcohol withdrawal.
- Immune-mediated: dermatomyositis, polymyositis, paraneoplastic.
- Toxins/drugs, including: ecstasy, cocaine, alcohol, methadone, envenomation, statins, amphetamines, barbiturates, hemlock, drugs causing malignant hyperpyrexia (e.g. suxamethonium, anaesthetic volatile agents); the list of drugs associated with rhabdomyolysis is extensive.
- Congenital disorders of metabolism (e.g. McArdle's disease).

Patients at greater risk of developing AKI include those with more severe muscle injury, or hypotension/dehydration; or pre-existing CKD.

Presentation and assessment

Features of rhabdomyolysis include:
- General: lethargy and malaise, or pyrexia may be present:
  - Other trauma, or skin erythema/blistering may indicate crush injury
- Neuromuscular: muscular pain, tenderness and stiffness:
  - Tense, swollen compartments with paraesthesia may be present
- Cardiovascular: pale and pulseless peripheries may be present:
  - Tachycardia and hypertension; hypotension occurs with reperfusion
  - ECG changes associated with hyperkalaemia (e.g. tall tented T waves, ST segments slurred into T waves, small P waves, prolonged PR interval, widened QRS, complete heart block, asystole, VF)
- Respiratory: tachypnoea/dyspnoea, due to pain or metabolic acidosis:
  - $PaCO_2$ may be <3.5 kPa due to compensatory hyperventilation
- Renal: characteristic dark brown urine:
  - Oliguria (<0.5 ml/kg/hour), or anuria; metabolic acidosis
- GI: nausea and vomiting may be present.
- Neurological: altered mental state, ↓ consciousness.
- Other: hyperkalaemia, hypercalcaemia and hyperphosphataemia.

Investigations

- ABGs (metabolic acidosis with/without respiratory compensation).
- FBC, coagulation studies (DIC may be present).
- Serum CK (usually >200 iu/L in rhabdomyolysis, values >20,000 iu/L are not uncommon, CKMB should remain low).
- U&Es (high creatinine to urea ratio suggests rhabdomyolysis, >10 μmol/L:1 mmol/L; serial monitoring of potassium levels).
- LFTs, serum magnesium, calcium, and phosphate.
- 12-lead ECG (if hyperkalaemia suspected).
- Urine dipstick (myoglobin will show as positive for blood).

- Laboratory urinalysis for myoglobin.
- Compartment manometry (>30 mmHg confirms the diagnosis).

Differential diagnoses
- Other causes of AKI (see 📖 p.262).

Immediate management
- Give O_2 as required, and support airway, breathing, and circulation.
- In the case of trauma, crush injury, or unconsciousness, complete a basic ABC 1° survey:
  - Use spinal precautions (spinal board, hard collar, sand bags and strapping); if intubation is required use in-line manual stabilization
  - Obtain an 'AMPLE' history (📖 p.2)
  - Assess neurological state and treat accordingly (📖 p.152)
- Involve orthopaedic specialists in trauma or compartment syndrome:
  - Fasciotomy is indicated if diastolic BP minus compartment pressure is <30 mmHg
- Hyperkalaemia may be temporarily controlled by IV soluble insulin 15–20 units in 50 ml 50% glucose over 30–60 minutes (this may not be sufficient if muscle damage is profound):
  - Boluses of sodium bicarbonate 8.4% IV 25–50 ml may help to control hyperkalaemia and acidosis as a temporizing measure
  - RRT may be required to treat hyperkalaemia, acidosis or fluid overload (myoglobin is not removed by CVVH/HD).

Methods aimed at avoiding AKI
- Aggressive fluid loading is required aiming for a UOP >2 ml/kg/hour:
  - Invasive monitoring will be required
  - Urinary alkalinization with sodium bicarbonate 1.24% (IV 500 ml) aiming for a urine pH >6 may improve myoglobin excretion

Further management
- In severe cases of crush injury causing severe hyperkalaemia and acidosis, limb amputation may be required.
- Regularly monitor U&Es, including magnesium and phosphate.
- Perform 2° and tertiary surveys as soon as appropriate.

Pitfalls/difficult situations
- Aggressive fluid resuscitation with AKI may lead to pulmonary oedema.
- Recognition of compartment syndromes in burn victims is often difficult due to overlying soft tissue injury.
- Open fractures may still cause a compartment syndrome.
- Consider the possibility of rhabdomyolysis in all obtunded patients.

Further reading
Gonzalez D. Crush syndrome. *Crit Care Med* 2005; **33**(1): S34–S41.
Hunter JD, et al. Rhabdomyolysis. *Cont Educ Anaesth Crit Care Pain* 2006; **6**(4): 141–3.
Shapiro ML, et al. Rhabdomyolysis in the intensive care unit. *J Intensive Care Med* 2011; DOI 10.1177/0885066611402150.
Tiwari, A, et al. Acute compartment syndromes. *Br J Surg* 2002; **89**(4): 397–412.

Gastrointestinal and hepatic

☠ Gastrointestinal haemorrhage

Haemorrhage may occur in the upper (oesophagus, stomach, or duodenum) or lower GI tract (small bowel or colon). Severity can vary greatly from trivial to immediately life-threatening. It may be the cause of critical care admission, or occur as a complication of ICU care.

Causes

Upper GI
- Pre-existing peptic ulcer disease (with/without *Helicobacter pylori* infection).
- 'Stress' ulceration which is associated with critical illness and shock, renal failure, or burns.
- Drugs:
  - NSAIDs (including aspirin)
  - SSRIs
  - Steroids or anticoagulants (in combination with NSAIDs/SSRIs)
- Oesophageal (or gastric) varices.
- Malignancy.
- Mallory–Weiss tear.

Lower GI
- Infection or inflammation (e.g. diverticulitis, Crohn's disease).
- Malignancy (including polyps).
- Trauma.
- Angiodysplasia/vascular malformations.
- Ischaemic colitis.
- Radiation colitis/enteropathy.
- Haemorrhoids.

Minor lesions (e.g. gastric erosions or haemorrhoids) may cause major GI bleeds where patients are coagulopathic (e.g. anticoagulated, or thrombocytopaenic).

Presentation and assessment

GI signs and symptoms may be relatively non-specific:
- Abdominal pain (occasionally epigastric in nature).
- Nausea, vomiting, or diarrhoea.
- Evidence of chronic liver disease (e.g. jaundice, ascites, spider naevi, asterixis, encephalopathy).

Evidence of bleeding:
- Haematemesis or blood aspirated from an NG tube (may be fresh blood or 'coffee-ground').
- Small/occult GI bleeds may be a cause of unexplained anaemia.
- Fresh PR blood (if source is below the duodenum/ ligament of Treitz).
- Melaena may occur with upper or lower GI bleeding, typically within 24–48 hours of a bleeding event.

Major bleeds may cause features associated with haemorrhage (see 📖 p.112), including:
- General: pallor and anaemia.
- Cardiovascular: tachycardia, hypotension, ↑capillary refill time.

- Respiratory: tachypnoea/dyspnoea.
- Renal: oliguria (<0.5 ml/kg/hour), metabolic acidosis.
- Neurological: syncope, ↓ consciousness.

Investigations

- Crossmatch blood.
- ABGs (acidaemia).
- FBC (anaemia, thrombocytopaenia).
- Coagulation screen, including fibrinogen (to identify new coagulopathy, or quantify the effects of anticoagulants):
  - Thromboelastography may help in rapid correction of coagulation
- U&Es (urea will be raised with enteric absorption of blood, raised urea/creatinine with AKI).
- LFTs (liver failure/dysfunction may be present).
- ECG (if cardiac ischaemia suspected).
- CXR (subdiaphragmatic air will occur with perforation).
- GI endoscopy (upper or lower GI endoscopy is the definitive way of diagnosing GI bleeds, although the presence of large volumes of blood may obscure the actual bleeding point).
- Angiography, or radiolabelled bleeding scan.

Differential diagnoses

- Haemoptysis.
- Epistaxis/pharyngeal bleeding (swallowed blood may be regurgitated).
- Occult haemorrhage from any cause; shock from any cause.

Immediate management

- Give O$_2$ as required, support airway, breathing, and circulation.
- Endotracheal intubation may be required to protect the airway in certain situations:
  - Where there is ↓ consciousness
  - Where there is torrential bleeding and/or oesophageal manipulation (e.g. endoscopy or insertion of a Sengstaken tube)
  - Induction of anaesthesia may provoke cardiovascular instability
- Obtain large-bore venous access (ideally 2 × 14g cannulae).
- Ensure blood is crossmatched, aggressively correct coagulopathies.
- Circulatory resuscitation will be required:
  - Start fluid resuscitation as clinically appropriate, initially with crystalloid/colloid followed by blood/blood products as required
  - Reverse anticoagulation if required
  - In major GI haemorrhage consider giving vitamin K IV 10 mg, and tranexamic acid IV 1 g (there is mixed evidence that tranexamic acid is beneficial)
  - Urinary catheterization and fluid balance monitoring is required
  - Invasive CVP monitoring may be required
  - Inotropic/vasopressor support for circulation as necessary

Lower GI bleeding

- Colonoscopy (or sigmoidoscopy for distal sources) is the investigation of choice.

- Alternatively consider CT/angiography in lower GI bleeding if the patient is stable.
- Surgery or angiographic embolization may be required in severe cases.

Upper GI bleeding
- Upper GI endoscopy is the investigation of choice in major GI haemorrhage:
  - Endoscopic therapies may be applied to bleeding lesions, visible vessels, or ulcers with an adherent blood clot
  - Adrenaline injections may be combined with thermal or mechanical treatments
- Where endoscopic treatments are only partially successful (e.g. because of large volumes of blood), or if a rebleed would most likely be fatal, they should be repeated within 24 hours.
- Where endoscopic treatments fail proceed to:
  - Interventional radiology (selective arterial embolization), *or*
  - Surgery
- After endoscopy high-dose proton pump inhibition should be commenced using omeprazole IV 80 mg bolus followed by an infusion of 8 mg/hour for 72 hours (alternatively pantoprazole may be used).

Variceal upper GI bleeding
- Terlipressin IV 2g 6-hourly should be administered before endoscopy.
- Upper GI endoscopy should be undertaken with oesophageal variceal band ligation or gastric variceal sclerotherapy.
- Uncontrollable variceal bleeding may require temporary insertion of a Sengstaken Blakemore (SSB) tube (or equivalent, e.g. Minnesota, or Linton Nachlas tubes).
  - Sedation (and almost certainly intubation/ventilation) is likely to be required in order to tolerate Sengstaken tubes
- After endoscopic treatment terlipressin should be continued for 48 hours:
  - Alternatively octreotide SC 100–200 mcg 6-hourly, or IV 20–50 mcg/hour, may be used

Further management
- Careful cardiovascular monitoring and serial FBC measurement should be undertaken.
- Avoid steroids, SSRIs, and NSAIDs where possible.
- An NGT may be sited at endoscopy (depending upon the lesion); it should be left to drain.
- In patients with chronic liver disease and upper GI variceal bleeding, antibiotic therapy should be commenced (e.g. ciprofloxacin IV 1 g daily for 7 days).
- Further variceal bleeding may be prevented by commencing β-blocker or nitrate therapy.

- Transjugular intrahepatic porto-systemic shunting (TIPSS) may be considered for patients with oesophageal varices.
- H .pylori identification/eradication may be required in the long term.

Pitfalls/difficult situations

- Patients should ideally be stabilized before endoscopy but this is not always possible with ongoing bleeding.
  - Endoscopy may need to be performed on ICU or in theatres; a surgical team may need to be 'standing by' in the end of a failure to endoscopically gain control of the bleeding
- Rise in urea and drop in haemoglobin may be the only initial sign that a bleed is present in the intubated patient.
- In some cases the source of bleeding may not be found, angiography or labelled scans should be considered.
- Aortoenteric fistulas may present with relatively small GI bleeds prior to a catastrophic haemorrhage.
- Prophylaxis against stress ulceration should include enteral feeding:
  - Consider giving ranitidine IV (50 mg 8-hourly) or PO/NG (150 mg 12-hourly); or omeprazole IV 40 mg daily; or sucralfate NG (2 g 8-hourly)

Further reading

Barkun A, et al. International consensus recommendations for managing patients with nonvariceal upper gastrointestinal bleeding. Ann Internal Med 2010; 152(2): 101–13.

Jalan R, et al. UK Guidelines on the management of variceal haemorrhage in cirrhotic patients. BSG guidelines in gastroenterology. Gut. 2000; 46(S III): iii1–iii15.

Scottish Intercollegiate Guidelines Network. Management of acute upper and lower gastrointestinal bleeding. Edinburgh: Scottish Intercollegiate Guidelines Network, 2008.

ⓘ **Acute severe pancreatitis**

Acute inflammation of the pancreas may cause local tissue destruction and a generalized inflammatory response causing distal organ failure.

Causes

- Post-procedure (e.g. after ERCP or biliary surgery).
- Alcohol (up to 40% of cases).
- Neoplasms (pancreatic).
- Cystic fibrosis, or Cold (hypothermia).
- Rheology (e.g. vasculitis/SLE, hypoperfusion, ischaemia).
- Endocrine (hypercalcaemia).
- Anatomical/functions abnormalities.
- Triglycerides/hyperlipidaemia.
- Idiopathic.
- Trauma (especially blunt abdominal trauma).
- Infections (especially mumps, rubella, EBV, HIV, CMV).
- Stones/gall stones (up to 35% of cases).
- Toxins (e.g. steroids, azathioprine, didanosine, pentamidine, envenomation).

Presentation and assessment

- General: pyrexia, marked 'third-space' loss (i.e. oedema, ascites, pleural effusions).
- Abdominal/GI: abdominal pain (often radiating to the back):
  - Nausea and vomiting, diarrhoea may also occur
  - Cullen's sign (umbilical bruising)
  - Grey Turner's sign (flank bruising)
- Cardiovascular: tachycardia, hypotension.
- Respiratory: tachypnoea/dyspnoea due to pain or metabolic acidosis.
  - Respiratory distress and/or hypoxia may occur due to abdominal splinting or pleural effusion
- Renal: oliguria (<0.5 ml/kg/hour), AKI, metabolic acidosis.
- Other:
  - Super-added infection/sepsis (typically respiratory or abdominal)
  - Hypocalcaemia
  - Hyperglycaemia
  - Multiple organ failure

Investigations

- ABGs (metabolic acidosis is common; hypoxia).
- FBC (raised WCC; thrombocytopaenia in DIC).
- Coagulation screen (↑ PT/APTT, ↓ fibrinogen in DIC).
- U&Es, (raised urea/creatinine if AKI develops).
- LFTs (jaundice or liver dysfunction, especially with gall stone disease or malignancy).
- Serum amylase and lipase (raised in pancreatitis, but moderate rises may be non-specific).
- Serum glucose (hyperglycaemia is common).
- Serum calcium (hypocalcaemia is common).

- Serum magnesium and phosphate, and serum CRP.
- Blood, urine and sputum culture (if infection is suspected).
- CXR, AXR (raised hemidiaphragm, pleural effusions, basal atelectasis, or pulmonary infiltrates may be present).
- US abdomen (to evaluate the biliary tract or identify gall stones).
- CT abdomen, contrast-enhanced (to confirm the diagnosis and assess severity); indications for CT include:
  - Hyperamylasaemia, clinically severe disease, temperature >39°C
  - Ranson score >3, APACHE II score >8
  - Failure to improve after 72 hours of conservative treatment
  - Acute deterioration
- CT abdomen should be repeated after 48–72 hours to identify and delineate any complications/necrosis which may have developed.

Differential diagnoses
- Bowel obstruction/perforation, or bowel ischaemia.
- Cholecystitis/cholangitis.
- Renal colic.
- MI.
- Pneumonia.
- DKA.

Immediate management
- Give O_2 as required, support airway, breathing, and circulation.
- In severe cases respiratory support may be required using NIV or mechanical ventilation:
  - Drainage of massive pleural effusions may improve lung function
  - Drainage of severe ascites to improve ventilation has been described
- Aggressive fluid resuscitation is likely to be necessary, with inotropic/ vasopressor support as required:
  - Urinary catheterization and fluid balance monitoring is required
  - Invasive monitoring of CVP may be required
  - CO monitoring may be helpful if CVS instability is present
- Analgesia (e.g. morphine PCA or infusion) and antiemetics should be prescribed.
- Correct coagulopathy/electrolyte disturbance:
  - Hypocalcaemia may be corrected with calcium chloride 10% IV (10 ml)
  - Hyperglycaemia is likely to require an IV insulin sliding scale
- The severity of the pancreatitis should be assessed using a scoring system (📖 p.279).

Further management
- Regular reassessment of oxygenation/fluid balance is required.
- Maintain glycaemic control (serum glucose 6–10 mmol/L).
- Intra-abdominal pressure monitoring should be commenced in patients with severe abdominal distension and/or oliguria unresponsive to blood pressure and fluid status correction.

- Renal replacement therapy may become necessary.
- NGT enteral feeding is possible in most patients (80%) but an NJ tube may be needed:
  - PN may be used in patients in whom a 7-day trial of enteral feeding has failed
- If gallstone obstruction is suspected ERCP should be performed (ideally within 24–72 hours of onset):
  - Early cholecystectomy may be indicated
- Be vigilant for complications, including:
  - Pancreatic necrosis, abscess or pseudocyst formation
  - Diabetes mellitus; hypocalcaemia
  - Pancreatic encephalopathy
  - Sepsis
- Early sepsis is likely to be extra-pancreatic in origin (e.g. pneumonia).
- Pancreatic necrosis may result in super-added pancreatic infection:
  - Routine antimicrobial prophylaxis is not generally recommended (although the evidence is inconclusive, and some centres still use prophylaxis)
  - Where infection is suspected (e.g. by the presence of gas on radiological imaging) radiologically-guided fine-needle aspiration should be attempted
  - Where infection or abscess is confirmed, antibiotics (e.g. meropenem 1 g IV 8-hourly) and radiologically guided drainage should be undertaken
  - In severe cases surgical pancreatic necrosectomy may become necessary, but it should be noted that delayed surgery is associated with better survival than surgery undertaken early
- Indications for surgical referral include infected pancreatic necrosis or pancreatic abscess, persistent biliary peritonitis.

Pitfalls/difficult situations

- An APACHE II score >8 is associated with a severe attack; identifying severe cases early enables rapid aggressive intervention.
- CT scanning within 48 hours may underestimate necrosis but initial scan may help with differential diagnosis.
- Timing of surgical intervention can be difficult, early intervention is associated with higher mortality.
- Pseudocyst formation is common (10% of cases), but rarely needs urgent treatment.
- There is little evidence at present that drug therapy such as octreotide is of any benefit.
- Pancreatitis complicated by *Candida* infections is associated with worse outcomes, and empiric antifungal cover may be needed in severe infections (e.g. using an echinocandin such as caspofungin).
- Other factors associated with severity/worse outcome include:
  - Pleural effusion present on admission
  - CRP >150 mg/L within first 48 hours of symptoms
  - Obesity (BMI >30)
  - Proven necrosis >30%
  - Persistent organ failure

Pancreatitis severity scoring

Ranson criteria (score 1 for each of the following):[1]

- At presentation:
  - Age >55
  - Blood glucose > 11 mmol/L
  - White cell count >16 × 10⁹/L
  - Lactate dehydrogenase (LDH) >400 iu/L
  - AST >250 iu/L
- Within 48 hours after presentation:
  - Haematocrit fall by >10%
  - Serum calcium <2 mmol/L
  - Base deficit >4 mmol/L
  - Blood urea rise >1 mmol/L
  - Fluid sequestration >6 L
  - PaO_2 <8 kPa.

Score 0–2 < 1% mortality Score 3–4 15% mortality
Score 5–6 40% mortality Score >6 ~100% mortality

Modified Glasgow scale (≥3 in 48 hours predicts severe disease)[2]

- Age >55.
- PaO_2 <8 kPa.
- WCC >15 × 10⁹/L.
- Serum calcium <2 mmol/L.
- ALT >100iu/L.
- Lactate dehydrogenase (LDH) >600 iu/L.
- Blood glucose >10 mmol/L.
- Serum albumin <32 g/L.
- Blood urea >16 mmol/L.

Computed tomography grading

A radiological grading system is also used ranging from A (normal) to D (the most severe grade, associated severe inflammation, necrosis or infection).

[1] Reprinted with permission from the Journal of the American College of Surgeons, formerly Surgery Gynaecology & Obstetrics. 'Prognostic signs and the role of operative management in acute pancreatitis'. Randon JHC, Rifkind KM, Roses DF, et al., *Surg Gynecol Obstet* 1974;139:69–81.

[2] Reproduced from *Gut*, S.L. Blamey et al., 'Prognostic factors in acute pancreatitis', 25, 12, pp.1340–1346, copyright 1984, with permission from BMJ Publishing Group Ltd.

Further reading

Balthazar et al. Acute pancreatitis: assessment of severity with clinical and CT evaluation. *Radiology* 2002; **223**(3): 603–13.

Mier J, et al. Early versus late necrosectomy in severe necrotizing pancreatitis. *Am J Surg* 1997; **173**: 71–5.

Skipworth JRA, et al. Acute pancreatitis. *Br J Intenisve Care* 2010; **20**(4): 105–15.

UK Working Party on Acute Pancreatitis. UK guidelines for the management of acute pancreatitis. *Gut* 2005; **54**(SIII): iii1–iii9.

van Santvoort, et al. A step-up approach or open necrosectomy for necrotizing pancreatitis. *N Engl J Med* 2010; **362**: 1491–502.

Villatoro E, et al. Antibiotic therapy for prophylaxis against infection of pancreatic necrosis in acute pancreatitis. *Cochrane Database Syst Rev* 2010; **5**: CD002941. DOI: 10.1002/14651858. CD002941.pub3.

Whitcomb, D. Acute pancreatitis. *N Engl J Med* 2006; **354**: 2142–50.

① The acute abdomen

An acute abdomen (critical illness associated with marked abdominal signs, chiefly tenderness and rigidity) may be the cause of admission to ICU, or may occur whilst in critical care.

Causes

- Generalized peritonitis due to perforated viscus (large bowel, small bowel, gastroduodenal ulcer):
  - Anastomotic breakdown should be suspected after surgery, especially if there was contamination and a 1° anastomosis
  - Traumatic perforation should be suspected where there is penetrating injury, or where there is blunt trauma causing major bruising or fractures of the spine, rib or pelvis
- Infection from a bowel perforation or leak, or from another cause (e.g. spontaneous bacterial peritonitis, or in patients receiving CAPD).
- Generalized peritonitis due to peritoneal irritation:
  - Haemorrhage (e.g. traumatic splenic rupture, ectopic pregnancy, a ruptured AAA, or surgical bleeding)
  - Bile leak (following biliary injury or after surgery)
  - Urine leak (following bladder trauma, or associated with surgery)
- Localized peritonitis: diverticulitis, cholecystitis, appendicitis, abscesses.

Presentation and assessment

Features associated with an acute abdomen include:
- General: pyrexia; marked 'third-space' losses (e.g. oedema, ascites), with associated hypovolaemia; shoulder-tip pain.
- Abdominal/GI:
  - Abdominal pain causing rigidity and prostration, with rebound and guarding (bowel obstruction may also cause colic)
  - Abdominal distension; absent, or altered, bowel sounds
  - Anorexia or lack of NG absorption, or large NG aspirates
  - Nausea and vomiting, diarrhoea, or bowel obstruction
  - An abdominal mass, or incarcerated hernias, may be present
  - If there has been recent surgery fluid may be present in wound drains (e.g. blood, faecal contents, urine)
- Cardiovascular: hypotension, tachycardia (or occasionally a relative bradycardia); haemorrhage will result in associated signs (📖 p.112).
- Respiratory: tachypnoea/dyspnoea due to pain or metabolic acidosis.
  - Respiratory distress may occur due to abdominal splinting
- Renal: oliguria (<0.5 ml/kg/hour), AKI, metabolic acidosis, lactataemia.
- Other: sepsis, multiple organ failure, raised WCC.

Investigations

- Crossmatch blood.
- ABGs (hypoxia, metabolic acidosis).
- FBC (raised WCC; thrombocytopaenia if DIC develops).
- Coagulation screen (↑ PT/APTT, ↓ fibrinogen in DIC).
- U&Es (raised urea/creatinine if AKI develops).
- LFTs (jaundice or liver dysfunction, especially with gall stone disease).

- Serum amylase and lipase (to exclude pancreatitis).
- Serum glucose, magnesium, phosphate, calcium.
- β-HCG (to exclude pregnancy).
- ECG and cardiac enzymes (to exclude cardiac ischaemia).
- Blood, sputum, urine, and surgical samples (wound, tissue or drain fluid) for culture.
- CXR (air under the diaphragm, basal atelectasis may be present).
- AXR (check for enlarged bowel or sentinel loops).
- US (may rapidly reveal presence of blood), or CT abdomen.

Differential diagnoses
- Thoracic diseases (e.g. MI, pneumonia).
- Intraluminal disease (e.g. gastroenteritis, colitis).
- Other diseases (e.g. DKA, sickle cell crises, drug withdrawal).

Immediate management
- Give O₂ as required, support airway, breathing, and circulation.
- In severe cases endotracheal intubation and ventilation will be required to stabilize the patient prior to surgery.
- Give analgesia; keep patient NBM and insert a NGT.
- Commence aggressive fluid resuscitation:
  - Urinary catheterization and fluid balance monitoring is required
  - Inotropic/vasopressor support for circulation as necessary
  - Invasive monitoring may be required
- Obtain surgical advice:
  - Where the patient is cardiovascularly unstable and probably actively bleeding, treat as for haemorrhage (☐ p.112) and consider rapid surgical intervention
  - Where infection is suspected the patient may proceed to laparotomy/laparoscopy once they have been optimized
- Empirical antibiotics for suspected bowel perforation: piptazobactam IV 4.5 g 8–hourly and gentamicin IV 5 mg/kg daily.

Further management
- If infection is present treat as for sepsis (☐ p.322 and ☐ p.346).
- Measure IAP and monitor for IAH (☐ p.284).
- Enteral feeding may be possible after large bowel surgery; PN may be required after small bowel surgery, but can be safely delayed.

Pitfalls/difficult situations
- AXRs and erect CXRs are difficult to obtain on ventilated patients, CT abdomen may more appropriate despite the risks of transfer.
- Patients are often less stable immediately following surgery.
- Abdominal signs may be absent in sedated (or paralysed) patients.

Further reading

Crandall M, et al. Evaluation of the abdomen in the critically ill patient: opening the black box. Curr Opin Crit Care 2006; 12(4): 333–9.
Manterola C, et al. Analgesia in patients with acute abdominal pain. Cochrane Database Syst Rev 2007; 3: CD005660. DOI: 10.1002/14651858.CD005660.pub2.

⚙ Acute bowel ischaemia

Acute bowel ischaemia may present with subtle symptoms and is associated with a high mortality (up to 50–100%).

Causes

- Superior mesenteric artery emboli (associated with AF, cardiac hypokinesia, cholesterol emboli, or valvular lesions).
- Arterial occlusion as a result of atherosclerosis, vasculitis, trauma, or dissecting aortic aneurysm.
- Non-occlusive mesenteric ischaemia (e.g. caused by cardiac failure or septic shock; after cardiopulmonary bypass).
- Venous occlusion:
  - Procoagulant disorders (e.g. antiphospholipid syndrome)
  - Secondary venous occlusion (e.g. pancreatitis, malignancy, paraneoplastic syndrome, trauma, inflammatory bowel disease)
- Extravascular obstruction (e.g. volvulus, band adhesions, incarcerated hernias, intussusception).

Presentation and assessment

Most abdominal signs (i.e. rigidity and distension) occur late, by which time hypotension and severe acidaemia are commonly present.

- General: mildly raised WCC, pyrexia (occurs late).
- Abdominal/GI:
  - Abdominal pain, initially without significant tenderness
  - Sudden vomiting or diarrhoea (sometimes bloody) may occur
  - Nausea and abdominal distension may develop
  - Absent, or altered, bowel sounds
  - Anorexia or lack of NG absorption, or large NG aspirates
  - Ischaemic bowel may perforate
  - Incarcerated femoral or inguinal hernias may be present
- Cardiovascular: tachycardia (hypotension is a late finding):
  - AF may be present
  - May coexist with MI or recent cardiac surgery
- Respiratory: tachypnoea/dyspnoea due to pain or metabolic acidosis.
- Renal: oliguria (<0.5 ml/kg/hour) and developing AKI are common:
  - Metabolic acidosis and lactataemia develop very rapidly
- Other: sepsis, multiple organ failure.

Suspect further ischaemic bowel in any patient who has had a recent small bowel resection for ischaemia.

Investigations

- Crossmatch blood.
- ABGs (hypoxia, metabolic acidosis).
- FBC, coagulation studies.
- U&Es (hyperkalaemia, raised urea/creatinine if AKI develops).
- LFTs (LDH and ALP commonly raised).
- Serum glucose (hyperglycaemia may occur).
- Serum CK (often raised).
- Serum amylase (often mildly raised, high levels suggest pancreatitis).
- Serum magnesium, calcium, phosphate (hyperphosphataemia).

- Blood, sputum, urine culture.
- Stool sample (for CDT and culture if diarrhoea present).
- Consider checking stool for FOB.
- ECG and cardiac enzymes (AF, cardiac ischaemia).
- CXR (air under the diaphragm if perforation present, basal atelectasis).
- AXR ('thumb printing', distended bowel, or sentinel loops).
- Doppler US (may identify proximal occlusive disease).
- CT abdomen (thickened bowel wall, pneumatosis intestinalis, mesenteric oedema).

Differential diagnoses

- Pancreatitis.
- AAA.
- Renal colic.
- Bowel obstruction, or perforation; or infective colitis.

Immediate management

- Give O_2 as required, support airway, breathing, and circulation.
- Commence aggressive fluid resuscitation:
  - Urinary catheterization and fluid balance monitoring is required
  - Inotropic/vasopressor support for circulation as necessary
  - Invasive monitoring may be required
- Give analgesia, keep patient NBM and insert NGT.
- If there is strong clinical suspicion obtain a CT abdomen with angiography, followed by surgical advice:
  - Laparotomy and bowel resection is often required
  - Where there are no peritoneal signs, but angiography reveals thrombus, anticoagulation (for venous thrombosis) may be possible; or thrombolysis (for arterial thrombosis in high-risk patients)

Further management

- Avoid hypotension.
- AKI/ metabolic acidosis often develops after surgery, requiring RRT.
- Sepsis is common, antibiotics are likely to be required.
- Measure IAP and monitor for IAH (📖 p.284).
- Enteral feeding is occasionally possible after large bowel surgery; PN may be required after small bowel resection.

Pitfalls/difficult situations

- Patients often become cardiovascularly unstable as the bowel is handled.
- Incarcerated hernias are easy to miss.
- Vasopressors may exacerbate ischaemia.
- Non-occlusive mesenteric ischaemia has been treated with papaverine vasodilatation.

Further reading

AGA Technical review on intestinal ischemia. *Gastroenterology* 2000; **118**: 954–68.

Sreenarasimhaiah J. Diagnosis and management of intestinal ischaemic disorders. *Br Med J* 2003; **326**: 1372–6.

⊙ Intra-abdominal hypertension

Rises in intra-abdominal pressure (IAP) can lead to abdominal compartment syndrome (ACS) where blood flow to retro-peritoneal/intra-peritoneal contents (especially kidneys) becomes compromised.

Grades of intra-abdominal hypertension (IAH)

IAH grades	Intra-abdominal pressure
• Normal (non-ventilated)	0 (5–7 mmHg in ICU patients)
• Grade I (mild)	12–15 mmHg (16–20 cmH$_2$O)[1]
• Grade II (moderate)	16–20 mmHg (21–28 cmH$_2$O)
• Grade III (severe)	21–25 mmHg (29–35 cmH$_2$O)
• Grade IV (extreme)	>25 mmHg (>35 cmH$_2$O)

ACS exists if IAP remains >20mmHg and new organ dysfunction occurs.

[1] May be seen during mechanical ventilation, after surgery and in the obese.

Reproduced with permission from the World Society of the Abdominal Compartment Syndrome.

Causes

The risk factors for IAH include:
• Trauma (especially blunt abdominal trauma, ACS develops in up to 15% of patients); pelvic fractures; massive transfusion.
• Severe burns (especially with abdominal wall eschar formation).
• Ascites or visceral oedema: infection, liver failure, pancreatitis, massive fluid resuscitation (>5 L in 24 hours); peritoneal dialysis.
• Peritonitis, intra-abdominal abscesses.
• Pneumoperitoneum, haemoperitoneum, haematoma.
• Abdominal surgery (especially with 1° closure, 'damage control' laparotomy, incisional hernia repair, or retained surgical packs).
• Bowel obstruction, ileus, volvulus.
• Mechanical ventilation (especially with high levels of PEEP or prone positioning).
• Obesity (BMI >30).
• Tumour (abdominal or retroperitoneal).
• Pneumonia, or sepsis from other causes.
• Acidaemia (pH <7.2); hypothermia (<33°C); coagulopathy.

Presentation and assessment

IAH may be only be diagnosed by measuring IAP. A high index of suspicion is required to initiate measurement (Fig. 8.1). Features of IAH may include:
• General: sepsis may develop (related to bacterial translocation).
• Abdominal/GI: tense abdomen:
   • Abdominal wounds may dehisce; fasciitis may occur
   • Hepatic function may become deranged
   • Anastomotic breakdown or bowel ischaemia may occur
• Cardiovascular: tachycardia, hypotension, ↓ CO (due to IVC obstruction and ↑ afterload, all worse in hypovolaemia):

- CVP and PAOP may remain high due to transmitted IAP
- Respiratory: respiratory distress may occur due to abdominal splinting:
  - Reduced lung/chest wall compliance leads to ↑ airway pressures in ventilated patients:
  - Hypercapnia (due to ↑ deadspace) and hypoxia
- Renal: oliguria and metabolic acidosis, despite adequate BP:
  - AKI with raised urea and creatinine may develop
- Other: lactataemia may develop.

Investigations

- ABGs (hypoxia, hypercapnia, metabolic acidosis).
- FBC, coagulation studies.
- U&Es (raised urea/creatinine if AKI develops).
- LFTs, serum glucose.
- Serum amylase (exclude pancreatitis).
- CXR (air under the diaphragm if perforation present, basal atelectasis).
- CT abdomen (slit-like IVC compression, tense retroperitoneal infiltration and ↑ AP to transverse diameter ratio may be present; there may be evidence of intra-abdominal pathology).

Immediate management (see also Fig. 8.2)

- Give O_2 as required, support airway, breathing, and circulation.
- Respiratory support (NIV or mechanical ventilation) may be needed.
- IAP should be measured (see 🕮 p.550):
  - Grade I: maintain normovolaemia
  - Grade II: hypervolaemic resuscitation
  - Grade III: consider surgical decompression
  - Grade IV: decompression and re-exploration
- Aggressive fluid resuscitation is likely to be required:
  - Ensure urinary catheterization and fluid balance monitoring
  - Inotropic/vasopressor support for circulation as necessary
- Abdominal perfusion pressure (APP) should be calculated (MAP − IAP); APP should be maintained at ≥60 mmHg.
- Sedation, supine body position and neuromuscular blockade should be considered (to improve abdominal wall compliance).
- An NGT should be inserted to decompress intraluminal contents; prokinetics and enemas may also be required.
- Abdominal eschars present on burns victims may be divided
- Consider paracentesis of abdominal fluid, or percutaneous drainage of haematomas or abscesses.
- Surgical decompression is the treatment of choice for ongoing ACS causing severe organ failure; the abdomen may need to be left open.

Further management

- Venous stasis is common, thromboprophylaxis should be used.
- Regular repeated measurement of IAP should continue.

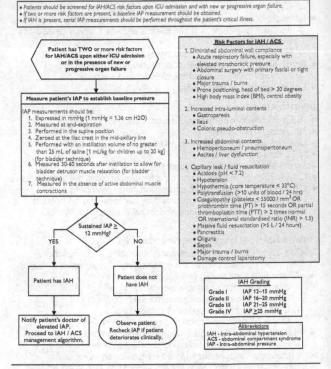

- Patients should be screened for IAH/ACS risk factors upon ICU admission and with new or progressive organ failure.
- If two or more risk factors are present, a baseline IAP measurement should be obtained.
- If IAH is present, serial IAP measurements should be performed throughout the patient's critical illness.

Patient has TWO or more risk factors for IAH/ACS upon either ICU admission or in the presence of new or progressive organ failure

Measure patient's IAP to establish baseline pressure

IAP measurements should be:
1. Expressed in mmHg (1 mmHg = 1.36 cm H2O)
2. Measured at end-expiration
3. Performed in the supine position
4. Zeroed at the iliac crest in the mid-axillary line
5. Performed with an instillation volume of no greater than 25 mL of saline [1 mL/kg for children up to 20 kg] (for bladder technique)
6. Measured 30–60 seconds after instillation to allow for bladder detrusor muscle relaxation (for bladder technique)
7. Measured in the absence of active abdominal muscle contractions

Sustained IAP ≥ 12 mmHg?

YES → Patient has IAH → Notify patient's doctor of elevated IAP. Proceed to IAH / ACS management algorithm.

NO → Patient does not have IAH → Observe patient. Recheck IAP if patient deteriorates clinically.

Risk Factors for IAH / ACS

1. Diminished abdominal wall compliance
   - Acute respiratory failure, especially with elevated intrathoracic pressure
   - Abdominal surgery with primary fascial or tight closure
   - Major trauma / burns
   - Prone positioning, head of bed > 30 degrees
   - High body mass index (BMI), central obesity

2. Increased intra-luminal contents
   - Gastroparesis
   - Ileus
   - Colonic pseudo-obstruction

3. Increased abdominal contents
   - Hemoperitoneum / pneumoperitoneum
   - Ascites / liver dysfunction

4. Capillary leak / fluid resuscitation
   - Acidosis (pH < 7.2)
   - Hypotension
   - Hypothermia (core temperature < 33°C)
   - Polytransfusion (>10 units of blood / 24 hrs)
   - Coagulopathy (platelets < 55000 / mm³ OR prothrombin time (PT) > 15 seconds OR partial thromboplastin time (PTT) > 2 times normal OR international standardised ratio (INR) > 1.5)
   - Massive fluid resuscitation (>5 L / 24 hours)
   - Pancreatitis
   - Oliguria
   - Sepsis
   - Major trauma / burns
   - Damage control laparotomy

IAH Grading	
Grade I	IAP 12–15 mmHg
Grade II	IAP 16–20 mmHg
Grade III	IAP 21–25 mmHg
Grade IV	IAP ≥25 mmHg

Abbreviations

IAH - intra-abdominal hypertension
ACS - abdominal compartment syndrome
IAP - intra-abdominal pressure

Fig. 8.1 Algorithm for assessment of intra-abdominal hypertension. Reproduced with permission from the World Society of the Abdominal Compartment Syndrome, 2006.

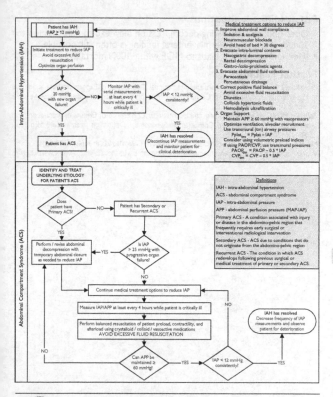

Fig. 8.2 Algorithm for the management of intra-abdominal hypertension.
Reproduced with permission from the World Society of the Abdominal
Compartment Syndrome, 2006.

Pitfalls/difficult situations

- Open abdomen following decompression may lead to fluid loss (up to 20 L/day) and hypothermia; enteral feeding is often still possible.
- If left untreated ACS leads to MOF with ~100% mortality.

Further reading

Cheatham ML, et al. . Results from the International Conference of Experts on Intra-abdominal Hypertension and Abdominal Compartment Syndrome. II. Recommendations. *Intensive Care Med* 2007; **33**: 951–62.

Malbrain MLNG, et al. Results from the International Conference of Experts on Intra-abdominal Hypertension and Abdominal Compartment Syndrome. I. Definitions. *Intensive Care Med* 2006; **32**(11): 1722–32.

Maerz L, et al. Abdominal compartment syndrome. *Crit Care Med* 2008; **36**(4s): s212–s215.

World Society of the Abdominal Compartment Syndrome website: ℘ <http://www.wsacs.org/>

:O: Hepatic failure, hepatic encephalopathy, and hepatorenal syndrome

Fulminant liver failure is defined as severe impairment of hepatic function or severe hepatocyte necrosis after liver injury in the absence of pre-existing liver disease.

Hyper-acute liver failure exists if encephalopathy appears within 7 days of jaundice; acute liver failure if it appears within 8–28 days; and subacute if it appears between 29 days and 12 weeks. It is a syndrome rather than a disease, and so has a number of triggering aetiologies.

Hepatorenal syndrome (HRS) is the development of renal failure in patients with severe liver disease in the absence of any other identifiable cause of renal pathology.

Causes

- Drugs/toxins (e.g. paracetamol, the most common cause, sulphonamides, phenytoin, isoniazid, MAOIs, ecstasy, tetracycline, yellow phosphorus, *Bacillus cereus* toxin):
  - Idiosyncratic drug reactions (e.g. halothane, NSAIDs, rifampicin, valproic acid, disulfiram)
- Infection (e.g. HAV, HBV, HCV, CMV, EBV, HSV, adenovirus, haemorrhagic fever viruses).
- Toxins (e.g. *Amanita phalloides* mushrooms, carbon tetrachloride).
- Alcohol.
- Autoimmune hepatitis.
- Malignancy (e.g. lymphoma, metastases).
- Pregnancy related (e.g. acute fatty liver of pregnancy, HELLP syndrome).
- Metabolic (e.g. Wilson's disease, Reye's syndrome, galactosaemia, hereditary fructose intolerance, tyrosinaemia).
- Vascular (e.g. right heart failure, Budd–Chiari syndrome, veno-occlusive disease, ischaemic hepatitis).
- Other (e.g. neurolept malignant syndrome, heat stroke, sepsis).

Hepatorenal syndrome may:
- Occur spontaneously in the setting of progressive liver failure.
- Be associated with spontaneous bacterial peritonitis (SBP), sepsis, and large paracentesis without albumin replacement.
- Arise from compensatory renal vasoconstriction secondary to systemic vasodilatation.

Two types of hepatorenal syndrome exist:
- Type 1; acute form: rapidly progressive renal failure occurs spontaneously in patients with severe liver disease (may be associated with SBP).
- Type 2; chronic form: deterioration occurs over months, typically in patients with diuretic resistant ascites.

Presentation and assessment

Hepatic failure may be associated with a history of viral illness, drug (paracetamol), or alcohol intake.

Signs of chronic liver failure are not commonly present unless the present illness is 'acute-on-chronic':
- General: jaundice.
- Cardiovascular: vasodilatation, hyperdynamic circulation, lowered BP (predominantly diastolic) and tachycardia
  - ↑ cardiac output and ↓ SVR
  - Spikes of hypertension may indicate cerebral oedema
- Respiratory: hypoxia due to ↑ shunt fraction
  - Pulmonary aspiration, atelectasis, or chest infection
  - ARDS (up to 10% of patients)
- Abdominal/GI: abdominal pain and retching (particularly with paracetamol poisoning)
  - Splenomegaly is typically absent in most cases, its presence may indicate Wilson's disease or lymphoma
- Renal: HRS may occur.

Hepatic encephalopathy can be caused by acute fulminant hepatic failure, chronic liver failure decompensation, GI bleed, or trauma.
- Grade 1: mild drowsiness, impaired cognition.
- Grade 2: increasing drowsiness, confusion but conversant.
- Grade 3: obeys simple commands but marked confusion.
- Grade 4: responds only to painful stimuli, or not responsive.
- Cerebral oedema is common with grade 3/4 hepatic encephalopathy.
- Systemic hypertension, pupillary abnormalities, decerebrate posturing, hyperventilation, seizures and loss of brainstem reflexes may occur.

Features associated with a worse prognosis in hepatic failure include:
- Bleeding complications: GI bleeding is common; subconjuctival haemorrhage (in paracetamol poisoning); prolonged PT and low-grade DIC.
- Metabolic complications: hypoglycaemia, hyponatraemia, hypokalaemia, hypophosphataemia, lactic acidosis.
- Infections: pneumonia, UTI or sepsis.

Investigations
- Group and save.
- ABGs (metabolic acidosis).
- FBC (raised WCC in infection, thrombocytopaenia in chronic disease).
- Coagulation screen (deranged clotting).
- U&Es.
- LFTs (albumin may be normal initially, AST and ALT may be >40 × normal initially but will fall with progression of damage).
- Serum glucose (hypoglycaemia occurs, monitor hourly).
- Serum magnesium, calcium, phosphate (hypophosphataemia and hypomagnesaemia are common); serum ammonia level.
- Drug screen (paracetamol).
- Viral serology (HAV-IgM, HbsAg; HBcore-IgM; EBV, CMV, HSV).

- Blood, urine, sputum cultures (infections are common precipitants and are more common in patients with liver failure); ascitic fluid culture.
- Urinary osmolality and electrolytes.
- ECG (multiple VEs, heart block, bradycardia common).
- CXR.
- CT head (to exclude other causes of encephalopathy).
- Abdominal US (metastases, lymphoma, venous patency, ascites).
- Liver biopsy (rarely required).
- Consider EEG (slow voltage waveforms in encephalopathy).

Hepatorenal syndrome

The diagnosis of HRS requires the exclusion of other causes of renal failure in patients with liver disease. General signs and symptoms may include fatigue/malaise, systemic vasodilatation, hypotension, high cardiac output and evidence of liver failure/ ascites. The diagnostic criteria for HRS include:
- Chronic or acute liver disease with advanced hepatic failure and portal hypertension.
- Low GFR, as indicated by serum creatinine >225 µmol/L or creatinine clearance <40 ml/minute.
- Absence of shock, ongoing bacterial infection, or recent treatment with nephrotoxic drugs; absence of excessive fluid losses (including gastrointestinal bleeding).
- No sustained improvement in renal function following expansion with 1.5 L of isotonic saline.
- Proteinuria <0.5 g/day, and no ultrasonographic evidence of renal tract disease.

Additional criteria *not* required for diagnosis but commonly present:
- Urine volume <500 ml/day.
- Serum sodium <130 mmol/L; urine sodium <10 mmol/L; urine osmolality >plasma osmolality.
- Urine RBC <50 per high field.

Differential diagnoses
- Sepsis.
- Poisoning.
- Causes of encephalopathy (📖 pp.152 and 192):
  - Meningitis/encephalitis, stroke, intracranial haematoma
  - Hypoxia or hypercapnia
  - Endocrine abnormality: hypopituitarism, myxoedema, Addison's
  - Hypo/hyperthermia
  - Electrolyte disturbance: hyponatraemia, hypoglycaemia, hyper- and hypo-osmolar states.

The differential diagnoses of hepatorenal syndrome include:
- Hypovolaemia.
- GI bleed.
- Sepsis.
- Paracetamol overdose.
- Acute tubular necrosis.
- Glomerulonephritis.

Immediate management

- Give O_2 as required, support airway, breathing, and circulation.
- Endotracheal intubation and mechanical ventilation is likely to be required in grade 3 or 4 encephalopathy if the GCS <9 or the patient is not protecting their airway.
- Insert large peripheral venous cannulae for volume expansion:
  - Start volume expansion with crystalloids or colloids
  - Urinary catheterization and fluid balance monitoring is required
  - Inotropic/vasopressor support for circulation as necessary
  - Invasive monitoring will be required, FFP cover may be required for central line insertion
- Check blood sugar (aim for >3.5 mmol/L):
  - Correct hypoglycaemia with a glucose bolus if required (e.g. 25%, 25 ml solution IV)
  - A continuous infusion of high-dose glucose (i.e. 50% glucose at 10–50 ml/hour, ideally given via a central line) may be required
- Monitor and correct any electrolyte imbalance.

Hepatic encephalopathy

- Insert an NGT and drain any blood in stomach.
- Give lactulose to achieve 2–3 bowel motions per day.
- Correct electrolyte imbalance.
- Correct coagulopathy before invasive procedures.
- Consider metronidazole PO 500 mg 8-hourly.
- Consider early ICP monitoring in grade 3 and 4 encephalopathy, maintain CPP >50 mmHg:
  - Nurse with 30° head-up tilt
- Aggressively treat any seizures according to protocol (📖 p.160).

Hepatorenal failure

- Consider volume expansion with up to 1.5 L salt-poor albumin.
- Invasive CVP and BP monitoring will be required.
- Consider cardiac output monitoring.
- Inotropic/vasopressor support for circulation as necessary.
- Give terlipressin IV 2 mg 12-hourly.
- Exclude reversible causes/precipitating factors.
- If required commence a non-nephrotoxic broad-spectrum antibiotic.

Further management

- Discuss all acute cases with a liver transplant unit, transfer to a regional unit may be indicated, liver transplant may be indicated.
- MARS may be used as a bridge-to-transplant.
- Give N-acetylcysteine IV (see 📖 p.460) in paracetamol poisoning.
- Penicillamine and vitamin E may be required in Wilson's disease.
- Aggressively treat any infection; antibiotics and antifungals may be recommended as prophylaxis if there is no evidence of infection.
- Monitor for glucose, DIC, metabolic acidosis, and electrolyte imbalance and correct abnormalities.
- Correct coagulopathies with vitamin K IV (10 mg once only); FFP and platelets if required.

- Enteral feeding should be commenced, TPN should be used in the presence of ileus.
- Maintain adequate nutrition (protein restriction is not recommended).
- Treat raised ICP with mannitol (100 ml 20%) unless renal failure present in which case use haemofiltration.
- Avoid sedation if possible (it may be required for ICP control).
- Thiopental infusion may be required to reduce cerebral metabolic rate if there is persistent seizure activity.
- Discuss cases of renal failure with a nephrology specialist:
  - Avoid/stop any nephrotoxic drugs
  - Consider paracentesis (giving 10 g albumin replacement for every litre of ascites drained)
  - Diuretics, octreotide and N-acetylcysteine have all been used, there is little evidence that they improve outcome
  - Renal replacement therapy can be used to support the patient until the liver recovers

---

Transplant criteria for patients with acute liver failure

Paracetamol overdose
- pH <7.30 (irrespective of grade of encephalopathy), *or*
- PT >100s (INR >6.5) and serum creatinine >300 μmol/L (3.4 mg/dl) with grade III or IV encephalopathy

Non-paracetamol
- PT >100s (INR >6.5), irrespective of encephalopathy grade *or 3 of*:
  - PT >50s (INR >3.5)
  - Unfavourable aetiology (non-paracetamol, not Hep A or B)
  - Jaundice to encephalopathy >7 days
  - Age <10 years or >40 years
  - Bilirubin >300 μmol/L (>17.6 mg/dl).

With kind permisssion from Springer Science+Business Media, *Current Treatment Options in Gastroenterology*, 'Fulminant Hepatic Failure', 6, 6, 2003, pp.473–479, Albert J. Chang.

Pitfalls/difficult situations

- Early referral to specialist centre is important.
- Volume status can be difficult to assess.
- The presence of ARDS, renal failure, and grade 4 encephalopathy are associated with worse prognosis.
- The cause of the hepatic failure may not be clear, or hepatic failure may be due to 'acute on chronic' disease.
- Distribution and metabolism of the drugs will be altered, consult hepatologists and pharmacists on dose adjustments.
- Severe fluctuations in blood glucose are common; hypoglycaemia is a consequence of ↑ circulating insulin, impaired gluconeogenesis and an inability to mobilize liver glycogen.
- Respiratory alkalosis due to hyperventilation may occur; may be exacerbated by metabolic alkalosis due to hypokalaemia, or continuous gastric aspiration.

- In patients with fulminant hepatic failure or decompensated chronic liver disease, the presence of a metabolic acidosis that does not respond to volume loading is associated with a very poor outlook.
- Encephalopathy may be very difficult to in intubated patients; acute confusional state may have been obvious pre-intubation (stage 1), but deep coma despite cessation of sedation may indicate stage 4.
- Cerebral oedema requires high index of suspicion to detect (irreversible brain injury is associated with ICP >30 mmHg, or CPP <40 mmHg):
  - ICP monitoring is the only reliable way to detect raised intracranial pressure, but this may not be possible unless an ICP bolt can be placed (specialist neurosurgical centre)
- Clotting factors, as well as platelets, may be required prior to any invasive procedure; response to replacement therapy may only be temporary.
- Scrupulous attention to asepsis is paramount; 80% of patients will develop superadded urinary or respiratory tract infections, often with atypical organisms.
- Patients with advanced liver disease are at risk of hepatic hydrothorax, portopulmonary hypertension, and hepatopulmonary syndrome (pathological pulmonary vasodilatation).

Further reading

Arroyo V, et al. Definition and diagnostic criteria of refractory ascites and hepatorenal syndrome in cirrhosis. *Hepatology* 1996; **23**(1): 164–76.

Dagher L, et al. The hepatorenal syndrome. *Gut* 2001; **49**; 729–37.

Devlin J, et al. Indications for referral and assessment in adult liver transplantation: a clinical guideline. British Society of Gastroenterology. *Gut* 1999; **45**(S6): VI1–VI22.

Findlay JY, et al. Critical care of the end-stage liver disease patient awaiting liver transplantation. *Liver Transplant* 2011; **17**: 496–510.

Hemprich U, et al. Respiratory failure and hypoxemia in the cirrhotic patient including hepatopulmonary syndrome. *Curr Opinion Anaesthesiol* 2010; **23**: 133–8.

Kunze K. Metabolic encephalopathies. *J Neurol* 2003; **245**: 1150–1159.

Lai WK, et al. Management of acute liver failure. *BJA CEPD* 2004; 4(2):40–43.

Ortega R, et al. Terlipressin therapy with and without albumin for patients with hepatorenal syndrome: results of a prospective, nonrandomized study. *Hepatology* 2002; **36**: 941–948.

Riaz Q, et al. Acute liver failure. *Gastroenterology* 2001; **33**(3): 191–198.

Sizer E, et al. Acute liver failure in the ICU. In: *Yearbook of intensive care and emergency medicine*, pp. 847–57. Berlin: Springer-Verlag, 2003.

Stravitz RT, et al. Intensive care of patients with acute liver failure: recommendations of the U.S. Acute Liver Failure Study Group. *Crit Care Med* 2007; **35**(11): 2498–508.

Haematology and oncology

⚙ **Blood product transfusion and transfusion reactions**

Blood product transfusion is common in critically ill patients. The risks and expense associated with transfusion require that practitioners use products appropriately and can manage complications.

Indications
- Packed red cells:
  - Major haemorrhage (see major haemorrhage protocol, 📖 p.115)
  - Correction of symptomatic or severe anaemia
  - Sickle cell crises (see 📖 p.310)
- FFP, cryoprecipitate, platelets:
  - Major haemorrhage (see major haemorrhage protocol, 📖 p.115)
  - Clotting derangement (see 📖 p.302)
- Human albumin solution:
  - Fluid resuscitation (except in cases of TBI)
  - Plasma exchange
  - Paracentesis of ascites, spontaneous bacterial peritonitis, hepatorenal syndrome

Compatibility
Compatibility predominantly applies to packed red cells and FFP, and should obey the following rules:
- Packed red cells:
  - Blood group O patients can only receive group O blood
  - Group A patients can receive group O or A blood
  - Group B patients can receive group O or B blood
  - Group AB patients can receive O, A, B, or AB blood
  - Female patients of child-bearing age must only receive Rhesus D negative blood
  - Patients with Rhesus D negative blood should preferentially receive Rhesus D negative units, but can receive positive units if necessary
  - Other red blood cell antigen/antibody reactions should be ruled out by a crossmatch wherever possible
- FFP:
  - Patients should preferentially receive units of the same group as their own blood
  - All patients can receive A, B, or AB, but it may need checking to ensure it does not contain a high titre of anti-A or anti-B activity
  - Only group O patients can receive group O FFP.

Blood conservation strategies
Where major haemorrhage (>1000 ml or >20% estimated blood volume) is predicted in a critically ill patient (e.g. a patient with critical illness who has to undergo a major surgical procedure) consider:
- Administering antifibrinolytics: tranexamic acid IV (loading dose 1g); protamine is no longer recommended.
- Perioperative cell salvage.

Haemoglobin transfusion triggers

A conservative blood transfusion policy should be used within critical care. The transfusion trigger should be

- Ongoing bleeding/early septic shock: 8–10 g/dl
- Known ischaemic heart disease: 10 g/dl
- Symptomatic anaemia (e.g. dyspnoeic): 9–10 g/dl
- All other cases: 7–9 g/dl
- It is also suggested that patients with burns, cerebrovascular disease or head injury should share a transfusion trigger of 8–10 g/dl

Safety requirements

Transfusion of blood products requires a 'zero-tolerance' approach to sampling, prescribing, and administration (Fig. 9.1), and should include:

- Crossmatch samples should be taken from one patient at a time:
  - Patients should be identified by full name, date of birth and hospital/NHS number (by wrist band and verbally if possible)
  - Sample tubes should be hand-written at the bedside
- All products should be prescribed using a record which contains full patient identification as just described.
- Administration of blood products should only occur after a 2-person check of blood products, prescription and patient identification:
  - Any errors should prompt the administration to be abandoned
  - Details of the transfusion, including start/finish times and serial numbers should be recorded

There is a legal requirement to keep a traceable record of all blood products transfused in Europe.

Special measures

This refers to the need for irradiated or CMV negative blood products. In the following cases transfusion should be discussed with a haematologist in case special measures are required:

- Patients who have had, or who may require, haematopoietic stem cell transplants ('bone marrow transplants').
- Patients with Hodgkin's disease, ALL, or aplastic anaemia.
- After purine analogues (e.g. fludarabine), or pentostatin.
- Patients with CLL treated with Campath 1H (alemtuzumab).

Patient refusal

Adult patients, in particular Jehovah's Witness patients, have an absolute right to refuse blood product transfusions. This may differ from patient to patient and some techniques, such as cell salvage, may be acceptable to some. This should be discussed in detail with them.

Complications

- Acute transfusion reaction:
  - Hypotension, fever, or allergic reactions occurring within 24 hours of a transfusion

- Error in transfusion requirements or administration; inappropriate/unnecessary transfusion:
  - Failure to adhere to 'cold chain', or excessive administration time (>3.5 hours)
  - Use of expired red cells
  - Failure to administer anti-D
  - Failure to apply special measures (irradiated/CMV negative products)
  - Over-transfusion as a result of blood sample laboratory errors or over-enthusiastic transfusion prescribing
- Haemolytic transfusion reaction:
  - Most commonly occurs if ABO incompatible blood transfused, but can involve uncommon antibodies, or bacterial overgrowth
  - Associated with fever/rigors, chest, back or abdominal pain, sweating, tachycardia and hypotension, tachypnoea and cyanosis, oliguria, haemoglobinuria, DIC
  - Can be acute or delayed in onset
  - More common in patients with sickle cell disease
- Transfusion associated circulatory overload (TACO):
  - Within 6 hours of a transfusion, any 4 of: tachypnoea/dyspnoea, tachycardia, hypertension, pulmonary oedema, peripheral oedema
- Transfusion-related acute lung injury (TRALI):
  - Occurs within 6 hours of plasma administration (FFP and platelets), resulting in hypoxia, hypotension, fever, and CXR findings consistent with pulmonary oedema (with a normal/low CVP)
- Transfusion associated dyspnoea (TAD):
  - New respiratory distress within 24 hours of transfusion which is not TACO or TRALI
- Transfusion-associated graft-versus-host disease:
  - Fever, rash, liver dysfunction, diarrhoea, pancytopaenia and marrow hypoplasia <30 days after transfusion
- Transfusion transmitted infection:
  - Fever, sepsis or infection associated with the transmission of infections such as: bacteria, malaria, HIV, hepatitis viruses, or new-variant Creutzfeldt–Jakob disease
- Post-transfusion purpura:
  - Thrombocytopaenia 5–12 days after red cell transfusion

Further reading

Association of Anaesthetists of Great Britain and Ireland. *Management of anaesthesia for Jehovah's Witnesses*. London: AAGBI, 1999.

Hebert PC, e al. A multicenter, randomized, controlled clinical trial of transfusion requirements in critical care (TRICC). *N Engl J Med* 1999; **340**: 409–17.

McClelland DBL, et al. *Handbook of transfusion medicine*, 4th edn. London: United Kingdom Blood Services, 2007.

SAFE study Investigators. A comparison of albumin and saline for fluid resuscitation in the intensive care unit. *N Engl J Med* 2004; **350**: 2247–56.

SAFE study Investigators. Saline or albumin for fluid resuscitation in patients with traumatic brain injury. *N Engl J Med* 2007; **357**: 874–84.

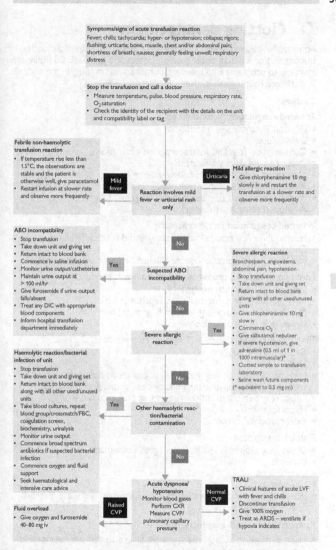

Fig. 9.1 Management of acute transfusion reactions. Reproduced from the *Handbook of transfusion medicine*, 4th edn, United Kingdom Blood Services, 2007.

:⚙: Clotting derangement

Abnormally delayed blood clotting may occur due to deficiencies in amount and/or function of coagulation factors and platelets. Clinically, this may lead to problems with bleeding, purpura, and bruising. In the critically ill, deranged haemostasis is often multifactorial.

Causes

Acquired coagulation factor deficiency
- Dilution 2° to massive transfusion.
- Liver failure.
- Consumption (e.g. DIC, extracorporeal circulation).
- Drugs (e.g. heparin, warfarin).
- Nutritional deficiency, particularly vitamin K.
- Autoantibodies (e.g. lupus anticoagulant, anti-Factor VIII antibody).
- Primary fibrinolysis (e.g. burns, neurosurgery, malignancy).
- Amyloid (Factor X deficiency).

Inherited coagulation factor deficiency
- Haemophilia A (Factor VIII deficiency) and B (Factor IX deficiency, Christmas disease).
- von Willebrand's disease (Factor VIII deficiency/platelet dysfunction).

Thrombocytopaenia, caused by reduced platelet production
- Marrow infiltration by malignancy.
- Marrow failure (e.g. critical illness, sepsis, viruses).
- Nutritional deficiency (e.g. vitamin B_{12}, folate).
- Drugs (e.g. cytotoxics, alcohol).

Thrombocytopaenia, caused by ↑ platelet consumption
- DIC (see 📖 p.306).
- HUS/TTP.
- Immune destruction (e.g. heparin-induced thrombocytopaenia (HIT, see 📖 p.305), idiopathic thrombocytopaenic purpura, HIV, SLE).
- Drugs (e.g. penicillins, anticonvulsants, antituberculous drugs).
- Hypersplenism.
- Extracorporeal circuits.

Platelet dysfunction
- Drugs (e.g. aspirin, NSAIDs, clopidogrel, abciximab).
- Uraemia.
- Liver failure.
- Leukaemias.
- Inherited platelet disorders (rare), e.g. Glanzmann's disease, Bernard–Soulier syndrome.

Presentation and assessment

- Haemorrhage, including intraoperative failure to achieve haemostasis.
- Oozing from wounds and drain sites.
- Spontaneous bleeding, bruising, or purpura (atypical sites such as muscles and joints may be involved).
- Incidental finding on haematological investigation.

Investigations

Basic investigations should include:
- G&S.
- FBC (includes platelets).
- Coagulation screen (PT, APTT and TT) and fibrinogen.
- U&Es, LFTs.

Involvement of a haematologist is required in many cases as more specialized haematological tests may be indicated, for example:
- Blood marrow film and/or bone marrow aspirate.
- Antiplatelet antibody tests/autoantibody screen.
- Platelet function tests.
- Specific coagulation factor levels.
- FDPs, D-dimers.

Differential diagnoses

- Meningococcal, streptococcal septicaemia; infective embolic rashes.
- Ongoing bleeding.
- Over anticoagulation.
- Lab error, or sample contamination (i.e. from IV drip arm).

Immediate management

Give O_2 as required, support airway, breathing, and circulation.
- If the patient is clinically shocked, begin fluid resuscitation, following a major haemorrhage protocol if appropriate (see 📖 p.115)
- Maintain a high index of suspicion for 'surgical' or other bleeding and stop local bleeding where possible:
  - In postoperative patients or following trauma
  - Following invasive procedures and line insertion
  - In patients at risk of GI bleeding
- Send urgent blood for crossmatch, FBC and coagulation screen
- Avoid hypothermia and acidosis (both impair coagulation)
- Avoid/stop NSAIDS, anticoagulants; avoid IM injections
- In cases of major trauma or major haemorrhage 1 g IV tranexamic acid may decrease the amount of blood loss due to fibrinolysis.

Coagulopathy

- 10–15 ml/kg[1] FFP, will rapidly reverse of clotting factor deficiency: aim for an INR <1.5 in the bleeding patient
- If fibrinogen is low (<1.0 g/L), often associated with massive transfusion and DIC, give cryoprecipitate
- Warfarin overdose (only needs rapid correction if there is bleeding/ risk of bleeding):
  - Can be rapidly corrected with IV prothrombin complex concentrate (concentrated factors II, VII, IX, and X) and/or more slowly with vitamin K IV 10 mg (takes ~4–12 hours to be effective)
- Heparin overdose (often rapidly excreted if renal function normal), if the heparin infusion is stopped APTT should normalize in 2–4 hours
  - Can be corrected with IV protamine (slowly over 10 minutes): 1 mg/100 units of heparin

Thrombocytopaenia
- In cases of haemorrhage, DIC, massive transfusion, or where surgical Intervention is required aim for a platelet count >50 × 10⁹/L
- In cases of major trauma or requiring CNS surgery aim for a platelet count >100 × 10⁹/L
- In chronic thrombocytopaenia without bleeding aim for a platelet count >10 × 10⁹/L
- 1 adult dose[2] will raise the platelet count by ~10 × 10⁹/L
- 'Antiplatelet' drugs should be stopped; irreversible drugs such as clopidogrel or aspirin mean that transfusion may be necessary despite apparently normal platelet numbers

[1] 1 bag of FFP is ~300 ml.

[2] 1 adult dose of platelets = 5 units.

Further management
- Ongoing transfusion necessitates regular coagulation studies and platelet counts, as does critical illness.
- Ongoing bleeding in the face of normal coagulation studies and platelet numbers should prompt a thorough search for a *surgical* cause.
- Avoid hypothermia, acidosis, and correct hypocalcaemia (calcium is an important cofactor in the coagulation cascade).
- Thrombocytopaenia/platelet dysfunction:
  - Involvement of a haematologist is indicated if no cause is apparent as bone marrow biopsy or specialist tests to diagnose and quantify abnormal platelet function may be required
  - Immune thrombocytopaenia (ITP) is treated with IV immunoglobulin and steroids; platelets are rarely indicated
  - Thrombotic thrombocytopaenic purpura/haemolytic uraemic syndrome (HUS/TTP) requires specialist haematology/renal input; platelet transfusions may result in further thromboses
  - Dialysis and desmopressin can be used in the setting of platelet dysfunction 2° to uraemia

Pitfalls/difficult situations
- Irreversible 'antiplatelet' drugs, particularly aspirin and clopidogrel, should be stopped 5–10 days before surgery and invasive procedures.
- FFP and cryoprecipitate take up to 30 minutes to thaw.
- Platelets are held centrally and may time to reach peripheral hospitals.
- Be careful with NGT or urinary catheter insertion in the coagulopathic.
- In coagulopathic patients minor trauma can cause catastrophic bleeds.

Further reading
Balikai G, et al. Haemotological problems in intensivse care. *Anaesthes Intensive Care Med* 2009; **10**(4): 176–8.

DeLoughery TG. Thrombocytopaenia in critical care patients. *J Intensive Care Med* 2002; **17**(6): 267–82.

George JN. Evaluation and management of pateints with thrombotic thrombocytopenic purpura. *J Intens Care Med* 2007; **22**(82): 82–91.

Keeling D et al. The management of heparin induced thrombocytopaenia. *Br J Haematol* 2006; **133**: 259–69.

Clotting function tests
- Prothrombin time (PT; normal 12–14 seconds):
  - Assesses factor VII activity (extrinsic coagulation pathway)
  - Prolonged in liver disease, warfarin, vitamin K deficiency
- Activated partial thromboplastin time (APTT; normal 25–35 seconds):
  - Assesses factors VIII, IX, XI, XII (intrinsic coagulation pathway)
  - Normal PT and prolonged APTT suggests heparin use, or inherited defect (von Willebrand's disease, antiphospholipid syndrome, haemophilia)
  - Prolonged APTT and PT: liver disease, DIC, warfarin
- Thrombin time (TT; normal 10–12 seconds):
  - Assesses thrombin and fibrinogen (common clotting pathway)
  - Prolonged with heparin, fibrinogen defect, FDPs
  - Prolonged APTT, PT, and TT: heparin, defective fibrinogen
- Platelet count (thrombocytopaenia is a count <150 × 10⁹/L):
  - Does not assess platelet function
- Fibrinogen (normal 2–4g/L):
  - Reduced in DIC and severe liver disease
- Fibrin degradation products (FDPs, normal 10mg/L) and D-dimers:
  - ↑ in DIC

Heparin-induced thrombocytopaenia (HIT)
Thrombocytopaenia in patients exposed to heparins may be caused by HIT, an antibody-mediated disease that reduces platelet survival and can trigger thromboses. Scoring systems help assess the probability:
- Thrombocytopaenia:
  - 2 points: fall in platelet count of >50%, or nadir 20–100 × 10⁹/L
  - 1 point: fall in platelet count of 30–50%, or nadir 10–19 × 10⁹/L
  - 0 points: fall in platelet count of <30%, or nadir <10 × 10⁹/L
- Timing (heparin exposure = day 0):
  - 2 points: onset day 5–10 (or day 0 if heparin within past 100 days)
  - 1 point: onset >day 10, or dates unclear
  - 0 points: onset day 1–4
- Thrombotic events or skin lesions:
  - 2 points: new thrombus or skin necrosis
  - 1 point: progressive/recurrent or suspected thrombus
  - 0 points: no events
- Other potential causes:
  - 2 points: no other cause
  - 1 point: other possible causes
  - 0 points: other definite cause
Score 0–3: low risk; 4–5 intermediate risk; 6–8 high risk. If HIT is likely:
- Stop all heparin/LMWH.
- Perform ELISA antigen assays (or serotonin release assay).
- Anticoagulate with danaparoid or lepirudin (avoid warfarin).
- Platelet transfusions are rarely necessary.

☼ Disseminated intravascular coagulation

DIC is a 'consumptive' coagulopathy characterized by abnormal, widespread intravascular coagulation and fibrinolysis leading to loss of coagulation factors and platelets. Bleeding and microvascular thrombosis causing organ damage can occur.

Causes

There are many causes of DIC, including:
- Sepsis (60% of cases).
- Trauma (especially crush injury and tissue necrosis), and burns.
- Obstetric emergencies: severe pre-eclampsia, abruption, amniotic fluid embolism/anaphylactoid syndrome of pregnancy, IUFD.
- Anaphylaxis.
- Transfusion reactions and haemolysis.
- Malignancy: e.g. mucinous adenocarcinomas, promyelocytic leukaemia.
- Pancreatitis and/or liver failure.
- Heat stroke.
- DKA.
- Autoimmune disease.
- Toxins: snake bites, recreational drugs.

Presentation and assessment

Widespread bleeding, deranged coagulation, low fibrinogen and a low platelet count suggest a diagnosis of DIC. Assay of fibrin degradation products (FDPs) may also be helpful.

Acute DIC
- Bleeding may predominate:
  - Petechiae and ecchymoses (purpura fulminans)
  - Oozing at puncture sites and mucous membranes
  - Haemorrhage, typically GU, GI, pulmonary or intracranial
- Microvascular thrombi affecting any organ may predominate, typically skin (ischaemia), kidneys (AKI, oliguria), lungs (hypoxia, dyspnoea, cyanosis), brain (delirium, coma), GIT, liver, heart and pancreas.

Chronic DIC
- Bleeding may be milder, embolic events may still occur.
- Chronic DIC may be clinically silent, disturbing laboratory values only.

Investigations

- FBC (↓ platelets).[1]
- Blood film/smear may show schistocytes (90% of chronic DIC and 50% of acute DIC), leucocytosis with a left shift, and thrombocytopaenia.
- Coagulation studies (prolonged PT, APTT, and TT).[1]
- Fibrinogen (↓).[1]
- FDPs, D-dimers (both ↑).

1 A chronic, compensated form can exist with 'supranormal' values of PT and APTT; normal or mildly elevated fibrinogen; normal or slightly low platelets.

DISSEMINATED INTRAVASCULAR COAGULATION **307**

DIC scoring system

- Platelet count—2 points: $<50 \times 10^9/L$; 1 point: $50–100 \times 10^9/L$; 0 points: $>100 \times 10^9/L$
- Elevated D-dimer or fibrin degradation products—2 points: strong increase; 1 point: moderate increase; 0 points: no increase
- Prolonged PT—2 points: >6 seconds; 1 point: 3–6 seconds; 0 points: <3 seconds
- Fibrinogen level—1 point: <1 g/L; 0 points: >1 g/L

A score ≥5 is compatible with overt DIC, repeat daily.
A score <5 may be suggestive of non-overt DIC, repeat every 1–2 days.

Reproduced from Taylor FB, Toh CH, Hoots WK, et al. Towards Definition, Clinical and Laboratory Criteria, and a Scoring System for Disseminated Intravascular Coagulation. *Thromb Haemost* 2001; 86: 1327–30, with permission.

Differential diagnoses
- HUS/TTP.
- HELLP.
- HIT.
- Bone marrow failure from any cause.

Immediate management
- Give O_2 as required, support airway, breathing, and circulation.
- Maintain adequate oxygenation and intravascular volume (minimize the effects of any thromboses).
- The cornerstone of management is aimed at correcting the underlying cause (e.g. IV antibiotics, surgical drainage, delivery of placenta).
- Manage haemorrhage appropriately (p.112).
- Correct coagulopathy if bleeding, or before invasive procedures:
  - Aim to maintain platelets $>50 \times 10^9/L$

Further management
- Involvement of a haematology specialist is essential.
- Once the trigger for DIC is removed FDP levels should fall, and fibrinogen levels should rise in 3–6 hours if liver function is adequate.

Pitfalls/difficult situations
- If venous/arterial thrombosis or vascular skin infarction is present commence an IV heparin infusion (aim for an APTT ratio of 1.5–2.5).
- The use of activated protein C is no longer advocated.
- In critically ill patients with DIC who are not bleeding, prophylactic dose LMWH is recommended.
- Antifibrinolytics (e.g. tranexamic acid) are generally not recommended (except in a hyperfibrinolytic states such as promyelocytic leukaemias).

Further reading
Levi M, et al. Guidelines for the diagnosis and management of disseminated intravascular coagulation. *Br J Haematol* 2009; **145**: 24–33.
Senno SL, et al. Disseminated intravascular coagulopathy (DIC): pathophysiology, laboratory diagnosis, and management. *J Intensive Care Med* 2000; **15**(3): 144–58.

① Neutropaenia

Neutropaenia with a neutrophil count $<1 \times 10^9$/L is associated with ↑ risk of infection. Absolute neutrophil counts, rate of fall, and duration of suppression correlate with severity of infection.

Neutropaenic sepsis is often defined as a pyrexia ≥38°C for 2 hours with a neutrophil count $<1.0 \times 10^9$/L.

Causes

A low index of suspicion for neutropaenia should be maintained in any patient with severe infection or trauma, having radio- or chemotherapy, having antithyroid drugs, or with autoimmune disease.

Acquired

- Cytotoxic drug therapy.
- Marrow infiltration by malignancy or fibrosis.
- Idiopathic aplasia and myelodysplasia.
- Infection, especially viral (e.g. EBV, CMV, HIV), TB, and brucellosis
- Radiotherapy.
- Drugs: antithyroid drugs (e.g. carbimazole), sulphonamides, cephalosporins, and penicillins.
- Hypersplenism.
- Autoimmune destruction (e.g. SLE, rheumatoid arthritis, Goodpasture's syndrome).
- Felty's syndrome (rheumatoid arthritis, splenomegaly, neutropaenia).
- Severe trauma.
- Nutritional deficiency, particularly vitamin B_{12} and folate.

Inherited

- Congenital agranulocytosis (Kostmann syndrome): presents in infancy.
- Cyclic neutropaenia (cyclic variations in cell counts over a several week period).

Presentation and assessment

Neutropaenia is commonly asymptomatic and may be an incidental finding. Infections may be superficial affecting the oral mucosa, skin, sinusitis/pharyngitis, or systemic with life-threatening septicaemia. The classical signs of infection (📖 p.322) are often lacking.

Investigations

Unexplained neutropaenia requires urgent investigation. A thorough history (including drugs and over-the-counter medications) and clinical examination is vital. Haematological guidance is necessary as further testing may include blood films and bone marrow biopsy. Other tests include:

- FBC and blood film.
- Antinuclear antibodies, rheumatoid factor.
- Vitamin B_{12} and folate.

Differential diagnoses

- Sampling error/lab error.

Immediate management

- Give O_2 as required, support airway, breathing, and circulation.
- Drugs which may be implicated should be stopped.

Treat infection/sepsis urgently:

- Investigate the infection source, taking samples/cultures as required:
  - Blood cultures (peripheral and venous/arterial catheter samples)
  - Urine culture (and screening for legionella/pneumococcal antigen)
  - Sputum/BAL culture (and immunofluorescence/PCR; AFB/fungal culture)
  - Throat viral swabs
  - Skin swabs
  - Stool samples (including C. difficile toxin screening)
  - Viral serology (e.g. EBV, CMV, hepatitis, HSV, VZV, HIV)
  - CXR
  - CSF
- Parenteral antimicrobial therapy is crucial and microbiological advice must be sought in the context of the neutropaenic patient.
- Empirical antibiotic therapy might include piptazobactam IV 4.5g 8-hourly +/– gentamicin up to 5 mg/kg daily.
- Obtain microbiological reassessment if no improvement by 72 hours.
- Surgical drainage of collections, or indwelling line removal may be required.

Further management

- Measures should be instigated to protect the neutropaenic patient from infective complications:
  - Patient isolation, particularly if the neutrophil count <1 × 10^9/L, with strict infection control procedures ('reverse-barrier' nursing)
  - Minimize invasive procedures; use sterile techniques
  - Fastidious patient hygiene
  - Use NIV to avoid/ minimize duration of invasive ventilation
  - Routine antifungal/antiviral prophylaxis, if appropriate
  - Avoiding foods at risk of microbial contamination (e.g. salads)
  - Monitor for signs of infection, with regular bacteriological screening
- Recombinant human granulocyte-colony stimulating factor (rhG-CSF) may be used to improve neutrophil production in certain conditions.

Pitfalls/difficult situations

- Neutropaenia 2° to severe infection places the patient in a poorer prognostic group.
- Neutropaenia as a side effect of radio- or chemotherapy often has to be tolerated using measures to avoid infective complications.
- Atypical infections are more common in this population; empirical blind, broad-spectrum antibiotics may be required initially.

Further reading

Marti Marti F et al. Management of febrile neutropaenia: ESMO clinical recommendations. *Ann Oncol* 2009; **20**(s4): iv166–iv169.

Penack O, et al. Management of sepsis in neutropenic patients: guidelines of the infectious diseases: guidelines from the infectious diseases working party of the German Society of Hematology and Oncology. *Ann Oncol* 2011; **22**(5): 1019–29.

:☼: Severe haemolysis

Severe haemolysis causes premature destruction of RBCs compromising organ function. It may be intravascular or extravascular. In critically ill patients anaemia may be severe as compensation for ongoing haemolysis may be compromised by bone marrow suppression.

Causes

Acquired immune
- Autoimmune: warm or cold antibody mediated; may be idiopathic or 2° (e.g. lymphoma, SLE).
- Isoimmune (e.g. transfusion reaction).
- Drug induced (e.g. high-dose penicillin, methyldopa, quinine).

Acquired non-immune
- Direct chemical toxicity (e.g. lead poisoning).
- Infection related (e.g. sepsis, malaria).
- Traumatic (e.g. prosthetic valves).
- Haemolytic uraemic syndrome (HUS)/TTP.
- HELLP syndrome (see ⬚ p.436).
- DIC (see ⬚ p.306).

Inherited
- Haemoglobinopathies (e.g. sickle cell disease, thalassaemia).
- Membrane disorders (e.g. hereditary spherocytosis).
- Enzyme defects (rare), (e.g. G6PD: decompensation with haemolysis and anaemia may occur after sulfonamide administration).

Microangiopathic haemolytic anaemia (MAHA) describes haemolysis resulting from red cells becoming damaged by turbulent flow (i.e. prosthetic valves) or fibrin-rich small vessels (i.e. HUS/TTP, DIC).

Presentation and assessment

- Transfusion-related haemolysis may cause: chest pain, SOB, headache, rash, jaundice, rigors, cardiovascular collapse, multi-organ failure.
- Sickle cell crises are characterized by pain (ischaemia), classically in long bones and soft tissues, but any site may be involved:
    - Chest symptoms, neurological involvement, renal impairment, GI sequelae, thrombocytopaenia and liver failure may supervene
- HUS/TTP: fever, neurological signs, AKI and thrombocytopaenia.
- Other causes of haemolysis may present with: cardiovascular collapse; severe anaemia; coagulopathy or DIC; jaundice; acute renal failure.
- Splenomegaly suggests reticuloendothelial (extravascular) haemolysis, CLL, SLE, or hereditary spherocytosis.

Investigations

- Crossmatch.
- ABGs (may reveal a metabolic acidosis).
- FBC (anaemia; thrombocytopaenia e.g.; in HUS/TTP, DIC, SLE, CLL).
- Blood film (fragmented cells; sickle cells; immature RBC forms, (e.g. reticulocytes, suggesting an increase in marrow production)).
- Coagulation screen, fibrinogen, FDPs; haptoglobins (reduced).
- U&Es, LFTs (elevated unconjugated bilirubin), LDH (↑).

- Urine dipstick, urinalysis (urinary urobilinogen).
- Plasma and urine assays of free Hb (raised in intravascular haemolysis).
- Direct Coombs testing (indicating an immune aetiology).
- Hb electrophoresis (to diagnose haemoglobinopathies).
- Glucose-6-dehydrogenase screen.
- Blood/sputum/urine cultures and/or viral serology.
- CXR (segmental infiltrate in sickle chest disease; pneumonic changes).

Differential diagnoses
- Liver failure.
- Sepsis.
- Haemorrhage.

Immediate management
- Give O_2 as required, support airway, breathing, and circulation
- Aggressive fluid resuscitation may be required.
- Obtain a full history and examination, e.g. sickle cell disease, recent transfusion (of ABO incompatible blood), or drugs.
- If transfusion-related haemolysis is suspected, follow the guidelines on 🕮 p.301.
- Obtain haematological advice and:
  - Stop any potentially implicated drugs or transfusions
  - Transfuse blood if Hb <7 g/dl, or if anaemic with CVS compromise/IHD
- Corticosteroids or IVIG may be required for autoimmune haemolysis.

If sickle cell disease is suspected:
- Management centres around oxygenation, maintaining circulating volume, peripheral perfusion, normothermia, and correcting acidosis.
- Adequate analgesia is essential and opioids are commonly required
- Transfusion is likely to be indicated if Hb <6 g/dl.
- Chest crises may require mechanical ventilatory support (e.g. NIV).
- Antibiotics may be required if an infective cause is suspected.
- Obtain haematological advice which may include:
  - Exchange transfusion in cases with: chest crisis, cerebral infarct, severe painful crisis, splenic sequestration, priapism, severe sepsis
  - The temporary suspension of hydroxycarbamide treatment (associated with myelosuppression)
  - Continuation of asplenism prophylaxis (penicillin V)
- Anticoagulation is not routinely required.

Further management
- Supportive measures may be required (e.g. haemofiltration).
- Folate replacement may be necessary.
- Patients with sickle cell disease should have/have had prophylactic vaccines for influenzae, pneumococcus, meningococcus, and HiB.

Further reading
George JN. Evaluation and management of patients with thrombotic thrombocytopenic purpura. *J IntensiveCare Med* 2007; **22**: 82–91.
Montalambert M. Management of sickle cell disease. *Br Med J* 2008; **337**: 626–30.

① Vasculitic crises

Vasculitis may be 1° or 2° and causes destructive, inflammatory changes to the blood vessel walls. It may result in wall thickening, stenosis, and occlusion, with subsequent organ ischaemia.

Clinical presentation varies according to histological type of inflammation, and the distribution/calibre of involved blood vessels. Expert guidance from rheumatology/renal/respiratory/haematology physicians will be suggested by the pattern of involvement.

Causes

Causes of vasculitic crises (i.e. involving organ impairment), include:
- 1°:
  - Wegener's granulomatosis
  - Goodpasture's syndrome/anti-GBM disease
  - Giant cell arteritis (large arteries)
  - Microscopic polyarteritis (small and medium arteries)
  - Henoch–Schönlein purpura (small vessels)
- 2°:
  - SLE
  - Infective endocarditis
  - Malignancy (e.g. leukaemia/ lymphoma)
  - Rheumatoid arthritis
  - Drug reactions
  - Type 2 cryoglobulinaemia (commonly associated with HCV)
  - Infections (e.g. syphilis, leptospirosis, hepatitis, EBV, CMV, TB)

Presentation and assessment

Infection may precipitate a vasculitic crisis in predisposed individuals. 2° vasculitis may present alongside the symptoms and signs of the 1° illness. Presenting features may include:
- General: pyrexia, weight loss and malaise, myalgia, arthralgia/arthritis:
  - Rashes and nodules, splinter haemorrhages, purpura, rash
  - Epistaxis and nasal discharge, sinusitis
- Respiratory: cough, dyspnoea, haemoptysis.
- Renal: AKI, haematuria, proteinuria.
- Neurological: confusion, fits, focal neurological impairment, peripheral polyneuropathy, CVA, encephalopathy.
- Gut: abdominal pain, nausea, vomiting, hepatomegaly, splenomegaly.
- Vascular: hypertension, extremity claudication, BP difference between limbs, bruits.

Vasculitis should be suspected in any patient with unexplained deterioration in the presence of coexisting chronic rheumatological disease, HCV, malignancy, or new drug therapy.

Investigations

- ABGs.
- FBC, coagulation screen (DIC may supervene).
- U&Es, LFTs.
- Serum CK (elevated with muscle involvement).

- Serum ESR and CRP.
- Blood/sputum/urine cultures and/or viral serology.
- Autoimmune screen: ANCA (classically cANCA in Wegener's and microscopic polyarteritis, pANCA in Churg Strauss); ANA/dsDNA (positive in SLE); anti-GBM.
- Urine dipstick (proteinuria, haematuria, casts).
- ECG (and ECHO if infective endocarditis suspected).
- CXR and/or CT chest (pneumonic changes; ground glass appearance, septal thickening, nodules).
- Consider renal/skin biopsy.

Differential diagnoses
- Sepsis.

Immediate management
- Give O_2 as required, support airway, breathing, and circulation
- Stop any potentially implicated drugs
- Airway or pulmonary disease/haemorrhage (📖 p.84) may require ventilatory support
- Pulmonary oedema may occur requiring treatment (📖 p.86)
- Cardiac monitoring will allow early identification of arrhythmias
- Invasive haemodynamic monitoring should be considered and careful fluid balance measurement undertaken
- Seizures should be treated appropriately (📖 p.160)
- Infection and sepsis should be sought and treated aggressively according to local microbiological guidelines

Further management
- 1° vasculitis treatment requires immunosuppression with high dose steroid and/or cyclophosphamide/methotrexate therapy.
- Plasma exchange may be of benefit in renal disease; expert involvement is obligatory.
- IVIG is first-line therapy in Kawasaki disease.
- Management of 2° vasculitis will involve treatment of the underlying pathology.
- RRT may be required for acute renal failure (see 📖 p.266).
- Consider IV heparin therapy in large vessel vasculitis.
- Angioplasty with stent insertion or graft implantation may be required.

Pitfalls/difficult situations
- In certain conditions blindness and/or deafness may occur.
- Tracheal involvement may lead to development of subglottic stenosis and airway compromise.

Further reading
Semple D, et al. Clinical review: Vasculitis on the intensive care unit – part 1: diagnosis. *Crit Care* 2005; **9**(1): 92–7.
Semple D, et al. Clinical review: Vasculitis on the intensive care unit – part 1: treatment and prognosis. *Crit Care* 2005; **9**(2): 193–7.

① Tumour lysis syndrome

Tumour lysis syndrome (TLS) is potentially fatal and occurs when rapid tumour cell destruction, typically 1–5 days after cancer treatment, releases intracellular ions and metabolic by-products into the circulation.

The main principles of management include starting prophylactic treatment in high-risk patients, early recognition of complications and prompt instigation of supportive therapy.

Causes

Common causes include chemotherapy, monoclonal antibodies, steroids, radiotherapy, and radiofrequency ablation of susceptible tumours:
- Bulky, aggressive, treatment-sensitive tumours.
- Non-Hodgkin's lymphoma.
- Acute leukaemias with high blast cell counts.
- It may occur spontaneously with Burkitt's lymphoma and some leukaemias.

It is more likely in cases where there is:
- Elevated pre-treatment uric acid.
- Elevated pre-treatment LDH (>2 × normal).
- Poor renal function.

Presentation and assessment

The biochemical changes associated with tumour lysis syndrome include:
- Hyperphosphataemia.
- Hypocalcaemia.
- Hyperkalaemia.
- Hyperuricaemia.

Signs and symptoms (commonly seen in first 48–72 hours post cancer therapy) may include:
- General: malaise, nausea, vomiting, anorexia, lethargy.
- Cardiovascular:
  - Arrhythmias of hyperkalaemia (see 🕮 p.212)
  - ECG changes: tall tented T waves, slurring of ST segments into T waves, small P waves, prolonged PR interval, widened QRS, complete heart block, asystole or VF
  - Fluid overload, pulmonary oedema
- Neuromuscular: muscle cramps, tetany.
- Neurological: seizures or syncope, muscle cramps, tetany, paraesthesia.
- Renal: oliguria, AKI.

Investigations

- ABGs (metabolic acidosis with high anion gap).
- FBC.
- U&Es, LFTs (hyperkalaemia, renal impairment).
- Serum calcium, phosphate, magnesium ($\downarrow Ca^{2+}$, $\downarrow Mg^{2+}$, $\uparrow PO_4^{4-}$).
- Serum urate (hyperuricaemia).
- ECG (evidence of hyperkalaemia).
- LDH (may be elevated).

Differential diagnoses
- Sampling error.
- Trauma, burns.
- Tissue ischaemia (ischaemic bowel).
- Haemolysis.
- Pancreatitis.
- Rhabdomyolysis.
- AKI.
- Malignant hyperthermia.
- Heat stroke.

Immediate management
Emergency treatment
- Give O_2 as required, support airway, breathing, and circulation
- Commence ECG and fluid balance monitoring
- Aggressive fluid resuscitation is likely to be required
- Treat hyperkalaemia/hyperphosphataemia (📖 pp.212 and 220):
  - If ECG changes are present give calcium chloride 3–5 ml of 10% solution IV over 3 minutes (has a cardioprotective effect only, will not lower potassium)
- Treat hyperuricaemia with IV rasburicase (IV 200 mcg/kg daily)
- Haemodialysis may be required for severe hyperkalaemia, hyperphosphataemia or AKI, indications include:
  - Intractable hyperkalaemia
  - Fluid overload
  - Profound metabolic acidosis
  - Anuria/oliguria
- Occasionally it may be necessary to aid serum uric acid excretion using sodium bicarbonate to alkalinize urine (see 📖 pp.269 and 456)

Preventative measures (which should be started before cancer therapy)
- IV hydration from 24–48 hours pre-chemotherapy to 72 hours post-chemotherapy, aiming for a urine output of 3 L/day
- Closely monitor U&Es, uric acid, calcium, phosphate, LDH, ABGs for 72 hours after treatment is commenced
- Allopurinol prophylaxis (600 mg/day PO) may be started 24–48 hours pre-chemotherapy
- Consider oral phosphate binders
- Consider leucopheresis in the case of high blast cell counts

Further management
- Renal and oncological advice should be obtained early.

Pitfalls/difficult situations
- Exclude ureteric obstructive nephropathy with renal US.

Further reading
Howard SC, et al. The tumour lysis syndrome. Review article. *N Engl J Med* 2011; **364**: 1844–54.

① Superior vena cava obstruction

A characteristic clinical picture arises when the venous drainage of the superior vena cava (SVC) territory is obstructed resulting in venous congestion (if occurring acutely), or the development of a collateral circulation into the azygous, intercostal, epigastric, femoral and vertebral veins (if occurring chronically).

Causes

Malignant (80%)
- Small cell lung cancer.
- Non-small cell lung cancer.
- Mediastinal/thoracic lymphoma (non-Hodgkins).
- Germ cell tumours.
- Breast cancer.

Non-malignant (20%)
- Indwelling central venous lines; venous strictures/thrombosis.
- Retrosternal thyroid goitre or thymoma.
- Sarcoid.
- Infection (e.g. TB, syphilis).
- Cystic hygroma.

Presentation and assessment

When SVC obstruction develops slowly the collateral circulation has time to develop and signs/symptoms may be mild. Acute SVC obstruction can present as an emergency with the following:
- Tachypnoea, dyspnoea, and cough.
- Hoarse voice, stridor.
- Headache, nasal stuffiness, stupor, coma.
- Upper body plethora:
  - Facial 'fullness' and collar tightness; loss of venous neck pulsation
  - Oedema of face and arms
  - Distended neck and arm veins (which remains if arms are raised)
  - Dusky/cyanosed skin discolouration of upper chest, arms and face
- Symptoms improved by sitting upright and leaning forwards:
  - Symptoms worsen on bending over/ lying flat

Investigations

- FBC, coagulation screen.
- U&Es, LFTs, Ca^{2+}.
- CXR (widened mediastinum, right-sided chest mass).
- CT/MRI or (to identify external compression or thrombosis).
- Invasive contrast venography (to identify obstruction).
- Doppler US neck vessels.

Differential diagnoses

- Acute airway obstruction.
- Cardiac tamponade or tension pneumothorax.
- Angio-oedema.
- Axillary thrombosis.

Immediate management

- Give O_2 as required, support airway, breathing, and circulation.
- Elevate the head of the bed.
- Secure the airway and ensure breathing/ventilation is adequate; endotracheal intubation may be required.
- Ensure adequate IV access; lower limb IV access is preferable, especially when inducing anaesthesia, as severe SVC obstruction leads to a very slow arm-brain time.
- Consider corticosteroids and diuretics if cerebral/laryngeal oedema is present (although efficacy questionable).
- If due to thrombosis: consider thrombolysis, anticoagulation, removal of CVC line.

Further management

- Where an oncological cause is suspected, obtain oncology advice:
  - Attempts may be required to obtain a histological diagnosis (i.e. from biopsies of accessible lymph nodes)
  - Urgent chemotherapy or radiotherapy may be advised, especially if SVC obstruction is the first presenting symptom of malignancy
- SVC stenting or SVC bypass may be appropriate in some cases.

Pitfalls/difficult situations

- Survival depends on the course of the underlying disease.
- If untreated, life expectancy is approximately 30 days.
- An equivalent pathology of the inferior vena cava exists though lower-body swelling is often initially attributed to other causes.
- Patients may be so agitated that induction of anaesthesia is required.
- The relaxation associated with anaesthesia may precipitate lower airway obstruction in patients with mediastinal masses.

Further reading

National Institute for Health and Clinical Excellence. *Stent placement for vena caval obstruction.* London: NICE, 2004.

Wilson LD, et al. Superior vena cava syndrome with malignant causes. *N Engl J Med* 2007; **356**: 1862–9.

⊙ Cord compression

Cord compression affects up to 5% of patients with cancer and is an important source of morbidity such as pain, vertebral collapse, and disability. Management depends on the close collaboration between oncologists, spinal surgeons and radiologists. Management decisions are based on the patient's degree of neurodisability, speed of onset, duration and site of compression; as well as the type of 1° tumour, presence of metastases, and likely prognosis.

Causes

Metastatic spread from:
• Breast (29%).
• Lung cancer (14%).
• Prostate (14%).
• Lymphoma (5%).
• Myeloma/renal (4%).

Presentation and assessment

General

• Back pain (severe, unremitting pain, preventing sleep; exacerbated by straining/coughing).
• Local bony tenderness.
• Radicular nerve pain.
• Muscle weakness.
• Sensory loss.
• Bladder/bowel dysfunction.
• Autonomic dysfunction (occurs late; carries poor prognosis).
• Respiratory distress if high C-spine involvement.

Spinal cord compression

• Symmetrical and profound weakness.
• ↑or absent knee/ankle reflexes.
• ↑plantar reflexes.
• Symmetrical level of sensory loss.
• Late loss of sphincter control or painless urinary retention.
• Rapid progression.

Cauda equina (lesion below L1)

• Asymmetrical flaccid paraparesis.
• Sensory loss: saddle to L1.
• Spared sphincters.
• Variable progression.

Conus medullaris (sacral segments):

• Symmetrical weakness.
• ↑ knee reflexes; ↓ ankle reflexes.
• ↑ plantar reflexes.
• Saddle distribution sensory loss.
• Early loss of sphincter control.
• Variable progression.

Investigations

- ABGs and spirometry assessment if respiratory compromise suspected.
- AP/lateral spinal X-rays (may show vertebral collapse).
- MRI (to confirm diagnosis within 24 hours of pain/neurology onset).
- CT (may be required to assess stability or plan surgical approach).

Differential diagnoses

- Epidural haematoma or abscess.
- Paraneoplastic neuropathy.
- Cord damage may also be caused by trauma or infection.

Immediate management

- Give O_2 as required, support airway, breathing, and circulation
- Nurse patient flat in neutral alignment with log-rolling
- Appropriate analgesia
- Seek spinal surgical/neurosurgical and/or oncology opinion as the following may be required:
  - High IV dose steroids (e.g. loading dose of 16 mg IV dexamethasone followed by 16 mg/daily for 5–7 days)
  - Bisphosphonates may be appropriate for myeloma, or breast/prostate metastases
  - Vertebroplasty/kyphoplasty/surgical decompression and/or internal fixation
  - Surgical decompression to prevent permanent disability from acute compression or to reduce pain resistant to analgesics
  - Local radiotherapy if unsuitable for surgery (e.g. complete quadra/paraplegia lasting >24 hours)

Further management

- Multidisciplinary approach is required, especially for rehabilitation.
- Monitor haemodynamics as autonomic instability may develop.
- Chest physiotherapy, thromboprophylaxis, bladder and bowel continence management, and good pressure area care are vital.

Pitfalls/difficult situations

- If ventilation is compromised (e.g. VC <15 ml/kg, or VC <1 L) ventilatory support is likely to be necessary.
- Prolonged nerve damage (i.e. >24 hours) is unlikely to be salvageable.
- High-dose steroids may trigger tumour lysis syndrome if lymphoma is present (see 📖 p.314).
- Pre-treatment function is the main guide to post-treatment mobility.
- Good prognostic indicators include: minimal neuropathology pre-treatment, ability to walk pre-treatment, lack of previous radiotherapy, 1° breast cancer, solitary/minimal spinal metastases, absence of visceral metastases.

Further reading

National Institute for Health and Clinical Excellence. *Metastatic spinal cord compression: diagnosis and management of patients at risk of or with metastatic spinal cord compression.* London: NICE 2008.

Infections

☼ Sepsis

(See also septic shock, 🕮 p.118.)
Systemic inflammation has a loose, clinical definition, the systemic inflammatory response syndrome (SIRS), which can be caused by many diseases that result in admission to critical care. When the cause is infection sepsis may develop 25–30% of ICU admissions are initially associated with sepsis. Severe sepsis has a mortality of 40–50%.

Diagnostic criteria

Sepsis

Proven or suspected infection and 1 or more of:
- Temperature >38°C or <36°C.[1]
- Heart rate >90/minute.[1]
- Respiratory rate >20/minute or $PaCO_2$ <4.3 kPa.[1]
- WCC >12 × 10^9/L, <4 × 10^9/L, or >10% immature (band) forms.[1]
- Altered mental status.
- Hyperglycaemia (>7.7 mmol/L) in the absence of diabetes.
- Significant oedema or positive fluid balance (>20 ml/kg in 24 hours).
- Raised CRP or procalcitonin (>2 standard deviations).
- Arterial hypotension (MAP <70 mmHg, systolic <90 mmHg, or a decrease in systolic >40 mmHg).
- Arterial hypoxia (PaO_2/FiO_2 ratio <40 kPa).
- Urine output <0.5 ml/kg/hour despite fluid resuscitation.
- Raised creatinine (↑ by >44.2 µmol/L).
- INR >1.5 or APTT >60 seconds or platelet count <100 × 10^9/L.
- Ileus (absent bowel sounds).
- Serum bilirubin >70 µmol/L.
- Lactate >1.6 mmol/L.
- Mottling or ↑ capillary refill time.

Septic shock

Sepsis with associated hypotension, or hypoperfusion (e.g. oliguria) after adequate fluid resuscitation.

Severe sepsis

- Sepsis with evidence of organ dysfunction:
  - ALI with PaO_2/FiO_2 ratio <33 kPa without pneumonia
  - ALI with PaO_2/FiO_2 ratio <27 kPa with pneumonia
  - Urine output <0.5 ml/kg/hour despite fluid resuscitation
  - Lactate >1.6 mmol/L
- Platelet count <100 × 10^9/L, or INR >1.5.
- Creatinine >177 µmol/L.
- Serum bilirubin >34 µmol/L.

[1] SIRS is the response to a variety of clinical insults resulting in with ≥2 of the first 4 signs.

Causes

Causes of SIRS include: infection, trauma or burns, pancreatitis, infarction: myocardial, intracerebral, bowel, pulmonary embolism, drug and alcohol withdrawal, massive blood transfusion.

Infections causing sepsis may be community or hospital/health-care acquired (ICU acquired is a subset). Common sites of infection include:
- Respiratory (~38%).
- Device related (~5%).
- Wound/soft tissue (~9%).
- Genitourinary (~9%).
- Abdominal (~9%).
- Endocarditis (~1.5%).
- CNS (~1.5%).

The natural defences against infection may be disrupted by:
- Trauma, burns, or major surgery (especially GI, GU surgery, or debridement of localized infections).
- Intestinal obstruction/distension; gut ischaemia or perforation.
- Endotracheal intubation or tracheostomy.
- Indwelling intravascular catheters, urinary catheters and wound drains.
- Intravenous infusions of fluids, drugs and nutrition.

In immunocompromised patients unusual, multiple or opportunistic infections (e.g. fungal) may be seen. Common causes of immunocompromise include:
- Drug treatment: chemotherapy, steroids.
- Haematopoietic stem cell transplants.
- Radiation injury.
- AIDS.
- Malnutrition, alcohol/drug abuse, or prolonged systemic disorders (including renal failure, hepatic failure, malignancy, multiple infections).
- Multiple trauma, major surgery, multiple blood transfusions.

Presentation and assessment
Presentation of infections, SIRS and sepsis varies according to infection site/type, and comorbidities. Non-localizing signs/symptoms include:
- General: pyrexia (or hypothermia, particularly in the elderly or immunocompromised), sweats, rigors.
- Respiratory: tachypnoea and hypoxia.
- Cardiovascular: tachycardia (bradycardia may be a pre-terminal sign):
  - Peripheral vasodilatation (warm peripheries); or peripheral shut-down (cold peripheries) usually as late manifestation
  - ↑cardiac output if monitored, (though it may decrease in severe sepsis) and ↓ systemic vascular resistance
  - Poor perfusion (metabolic acidosis, raised lactate)
  - Hypertension or hypotension/shock
  - ↓ JVP, CVP, or PAOP
  - Arrhythmias, particularly AF, atrial flutter or VT
  - Angina, or evidence of cardiac ischaemia
  - Peripheral/dependent oedema
- Neurological: agitation, confusion, diminished consciousness, syncope.
- Renal: oliguria, raised urea and creatinine.
- GI: anorexia, nausea and vomiting.
- Haematology: raised or lowered WCC; DIC.
- Other: raised inflammatory markers (CRP, ESR, PCT).
- Multiorgan dysfunction syndrome, or failure (MODS or MOF).

Investigations

- ABGs (metabolic acidosis, hypoxia).
- FBC (raised/lowered WCC, thrombocytopaenia/thrombocytosis).
- Coagulation screen, including D-dimers and fibrinogen (DIC, D-dimers may also be raised in response to inflammation).
- U&Es, LFTs (renal/hepatic dysfunction, hyponatraemia).
- Serum calcium, magnesium, phosphate.
- Serum glucose (hypo/hyperglycaemia).
- ECG.

Some investigations may also confirm the likelihood of sepsis, or identify the source or type of organisms involved:
- CRP (and to a lesser extent ESR; CRP is raised in inflammation, particularly so with infection).
- Serum procalcitonin (PCT; used in some centres to help differentiate inflammation from infection).
- Serum (and urine) antigen or antibody tests may be available for some organisms, including:
  - *Legionella* and *Pneumococcal* antigens are routinely tested in urine
  - *Mycoplasma*
  - Many viruses (HIV, HTLV, hepatitis A/B/C/D/E, EBV, CMV)
  - Protozoal or helminthic infections
- Bacteriology, 1 or more of the following samples:
  - Septic screen: blood,[1] urine, and sputum cultures
  - Wound swabs; drain fluid (wound, chest, or other drains)
  - Nose and throat swabs (for culture and/or viral PCR)
  - Stool (for culture or for toxin detection, e.g. *C. difficile* toxin)
  - CSF (LP may also reveal other findings, 🕮 p.574)
  - If any invasive lines are removed, line-tips may be sent for culture
  - Some institutions take brush samples from CVCs
  - BAL samples (samples may be sent for bacterial, fungal, specialist culture or tests, e.g. AFBs for TB; viral PCR; immunofluorescence, galactomannan)
  - Samples of 'tapped' fluid (e.g. ascites, pleural fluid)
  - Speculum exam and vaginal swabs
- Gram stains may be useful where rapid identification of any organism is significant (e.g. in CSF), or where unusual organisms are significant (e.g. gut organisms in pleural fluid); in other situations they do not aid diagnosis (e.g. Gram stain of BAL samples).
- CXR (pneumonia, mediastinitis, perforated viscus).
- US and/or CT scan of chest, abdomen (including renal and hepatic), head, or pelvis for evidence of a collection.
- Echocardiography (TTE or TOE) for suspected endocarditis or to assess any LV dysfunction.

Differential diagnoses

- Any non-infectious disease which causes an inflammatory response.
- Infection from another site.

1 Blood cultures should be taken from every invasive line, as well as 1–2 percutaneous venous samples; percutaneous venous stabs should be taken from different sites to minimize the risk of skin contamination.

Immediate management
- Give O_2, titrate to SaO_2 of 94–98%.

Airway: endotracheal intubation may be required.
- Where infection or threatens airway patency.
- Where there is ↓consciousness (GCS ≤8).
- To facilitate mechanical ventilation.

Breathing: ensure breathing/ventilation is adequate.
- Fatigue may lead to respiratory failure; CPAP and/or non-invasive BIPAP may be indicated.
- Mechanical ventilation may optimize oxygenation in severe shock.
- Respiratory infections may compromise breathing and require mechanical ventilation.

Circulation: support should be commenced in patients with hypotension or elevated serum lactate.
- Large peripheral venous cannulae are required.
- Arterial and/or central venous cannulation should be undertaken as soon as feasible, checking coagulation studies and platelets first.
- Resuscitate with crystalloids/colloids, (in first 6 hours), aiming for:
  - MAP ≥65 mmHg
  - CVP 8–12 mmHg (12–15 mmHg if mechanically ventilated)
  - Urine output ≥0.5 ml/kg/hour
  - CVC oxygen saturations ≥70% (or mixed venous >65%)
- If venous SaO_2 not achieved consider:
  - Further fluid resuscitation or dobutamine up to 20 mcg/kg/minute
  - Packed red cells transfusion if Hb < 7g/dl, (10g/dl if there is cardiac ischaemia or ongoing haemorrhage); or to achieve a haematocrit of ≥30% if venous oxygen saturation <70% despite a CVP of 8–12 mmHg (this latter target is disputed by some authorities)
- Measurement of CO (e.g. oesophageal Doppler, pulse contour analysis) and SVR estimation will allow assessment of the effects of fluids and the need for vasopressors.
- Vasopressor therapy with noradrenaline 0.05–3 mcg/kg/minute or dopamine 0.5–10 mcg/kg/minute (via a central catheter) is indicated when fluid challenge fails to restore BP/organ perfusion.

Infection identification and control
- Treat any identifiable underlying cause, make a full survey for likely sources of infection, take a focused clinical history, and review notes and charts where possible.
- Take all appropriate cultures; ensure 1–2 percutaneous blood culture samples, also sample blood from each intravascular catheter
- Commence appropriate antibiotics ideally within 1st hour of treatment: respiratory (📖 p.334), abdominal (📖 p.346), wound/soft tissue (📖 p.342), GU (📖 p.344), endocarditis (📖 p.338), CNS (📖 p.340).
- Remove intravascular access devices that are a potential infection source after establishing other vascular access.
- Arrange surgery, if required, to remove focus of infection.

Further management

- Admit the patient into suitable critical care facility.
- Continue invasive monitoring of respiratory and circulatory status.
- Monitor and treat complications, including ARDS, DIC, metabolic acidosis, and electrolyte imbalance.

Infection

- Use infection control procedures where resistant or highly infectious agents are suspected (📖 p.382).
- Report any notifiable diseases (📖 p.380).
- Reassess antimicrobial regimen within 72 hours and adjust according to culture results; following advice from microbiology, aim to de-escalate antimicrobial therapy from broad spectrum to targeted therapies:
  - Monitor for superadded or ICU-acquired infections (e.g. VAP)
  - If there is no improvement repeat all cultures and consider adding therapy for unusual organisms (e.g. antifungals)
  - If there is a suspicion of 2° infections consider changing indwelling catheters or vascular access lines

Adjunctive therapies

- Activated protein C is no longer recommended.
- Low-dose steroids:(hydrocortisone 50–75 mg IV 6 hourly for 7 days, with or without fludrocortisone 50 mcg PO daily) may be of benefit in patients requiring vasopressors (mixed evidence).
- 'Care bundles' should be used to minimize the risk of 2° infections (see 📖 p.383).

Treat or prevent complications

- Vasopressor resistant septic shock (VRSS) may occur, where hypotension and tissue hypoperfusion cannot be corrected with standard vasopressor/inotropic therapy; the following have been tried but have little evidence to support their routine usage:
  - Vasopressin infusion 0.01–0.04 units/minute IV infusion
  - Alternatively consider terlipressin 1 mg IV 8hourly
  - Methylene blue IV may improve haemodynamic status
- Respiratory:
  - ARDS: use a lung protective ventilation strategy (📖 p.53)
  - Use a weaning protocol where appropriate
- Renal:
  - Do not use 'renal dose' dopamine
  - Correct severe metabolic acidosis; use continuous veno-venous haemofiltration (CVVH) or intermittent haemodialysis if necessary
  - Avoid bicarbonate therapy for lactic acidosis if pH ≥7.15
- Haematology:
  - Do not use erythropoietin to treat sepsis-related anaemia
  - Use FFP/fibrinogen to correct clotting abnormalities if there is bleeding, or invasive procedures are planned
  - Minimize the use of blood products by following a restrictive transfusion policy for blood and for platelets (see 📖 pp.299 and 304)
  - Do not use antithrombin therapy
- Other measures (see also 📖 p.10):

- Provide stress ulcer prophylaxis (e.g. ranitidine 50 mg IV TDS) if appropriate; unless contraindicated use DVT prophylaxis; maintain serum glucose <10 mmol/L (avoiding hypoglycaemia); use a sedation protocol and scoring system
- Consider antipyretics and/or peripheral cooling for pyrexia; avoid hyperpyrexia (temperature >40°C)
- Enteral nutrition may maintain integrity of gut mucosal barrier; PN may be required in some situations (e.g. small bowel damage)

Pitfalls/difficult situations

- Cause/source of infection may not be clear, consider non-obvious locations (retro-peritoneal space, vertebrae).
- The diagnosis of sepsis requires proven or *suspected* infection.
- Examples of proven infection include: positive cultures, Gram stain or PCR; evidence of infection (e.g. pus) in an otherwise sterile area, such as peritoneum or CSF; CXR changes of pneumonia; evidence of bowel perforation; stigmata of meningococcal septicaemia.
- Fungal infections are often overlooked, suspect it in cases of 2° infections, and in immunocompromised patients.
- DIC may be difficult to treat, seek expert haematology advice.
- Patients with impaired renal function (or on CVVH/IHD) may require alterations to medication doses, discuss with pharmacy.
- Adapt antimicrobial regimens for patients with penicillin allergy.
- Mixed pictures of shock often occur with sepsis coexisting with other causes such as cardiac failure.
- Have a low threshold for suspecting vascular access catheters as a source for bacteraemia.
- Organisms are often not found in culture (in up to 40% of cases).
- Factors associated with a poor prognosis include: age >70 years, ARDS, leucopaenia, hypothermia, DIC, multiple-organ (>2) failure.

Further reading

Albert M, et al. Utility of Gram stain in the clinical management of suspected ventilator-associated pneumonia. Secondary analysis of a multicenter randomized trial. *J Crit Care* 2008; **23**: 74–81.

Dellinger RP, et al. Surviving Sepsis Campaign: international guidelines for management of severe sepsis and septic shock. *Intensive Care Med* 2008; **34**: 17–61.

Harrison DA, et al. The epidemiology of severe sepsis in England, Wales and Northern Ireland, 1996 to 2004: secondary analysis of a high quality clinical database, the ICNARC Case Mix Programme Database. *Crit Care* 2006; **10**:R42 (doi:10.1186/cc4854).

Kumar A, et al. Duration of hypotension before initiation of effective antimicrobial therapy is the critical determinant of survival in human septic shock. *Crit Care Med* 2006; **34**(6): 1589–96.

Kwok ESH, et al. Use of methylene blue in sepsis: a systematic review. *J Intensive Care Med* 2006; **21**:359–63.

Otero RM, et al. Early goal-directed therapy in severe sepsis and septic shock revisited: concepts, controversies, and contemporary findings. *Chest* 2006; **130**: 1579–95.

Rivers E, et al. Early goal directed therapy in the treatment of severe sepsis and septic shock. *N Engl J Med* 2001; **345**:1368–77.

Russell JA, et al. Vasopressin versus norepinephrine in patients with septic shock. *N Engl J Med* 2008; **358**(9): 877–87.

Sprung CL, et al. Hydrocortisone therapy for patients with septic shock (CORTICUS). *N Engl J Med* 2008; **358**: 111–24.

⚠ Fever

Within intensive care a core body temperature ≥38.3°C is considered a significant fever.

Causes

Within ICU the commonest cause of pyrexia is infection:
- Intravascular devices and implants.
- Pneumonia, VAP.
- Intra-abdominal collections.
- Colitis (especially *C. difficile*).
- UTI, urinary catheter related sepsis.
- Sinusitis (especially if using nasogastric or naso-endotracheal tubes).
- Surgical site infections.
- 'Occult', unusual, or difficult to culture infections (e.g. infective endocarditis (IE), CNS infections, viruses (including CMV, fungal, TB).

Non-infectious causes:
- Postoperative fever.
- Drug fever (e.g. β-lactam related), or drug withdrawal (e.g. alcohol).
- Malignancy: lymphoma, leukaemia, solid cell tumours (especially renal), tumour lysis syndrome.
- Connective tissue diseases: SLE, RA, PMR, sarcoid, vasculitis.
- Infarction: myocardial, intracerebral, bowel, PE, fat emboli, stroke.
- Venous thrombosis.
- Inflammation: SIRS, ARDS, cytokine storm, hepatitis, pancreatitis, burns, gout, Dressler syndrome, immune reconstitution syndrome, Jarisch–Herxheimer reaction, transplant rejection.
- Endocrine/metabolic: adrenal insufficiency, thyroid storm, malignant hyperpyrexia, NMS.
- Blood product transfusion.

Presentation and assessment

Pyrexia may be associated with other evidence of infection, including:
- Tachypnoea, tachycardia, rigors, sweats.
- Complications of sepsis (see 📖 p.322).
- Raised WCC and/or inflammatory markers.

Other signs and symptoms may help identify the cause of the infection:[1]
- Altered mentation: meningitis (TB, cryptococcal, carcinomatous, sarcoid), brucellosis, typhoid fever.
- Arthritis/arthralgia: SLE, infective endocarditis, Lyme disease, lymphogranuloma venereum, Whipple's disease, brucellosis, inflammatory bowel disease.
- Animal contact: brucellosis, toxoplasmosis, cat scratch disease, psittacosis, leptospirosis, Q fever, rat bite fever.
- Cough: tuberculosis, Q fever, typhoid fever, sarcoidosis, *Legionella*.
- Epistaxis: Wegener's granulomatosis, relapsing fever, psittacosis.
- Epididymo-orchitis: TB, lymphoma, polyarteritis nodosa, brucellosis, leptospirosis, infectious mononucleosis.

- Hepatomegaly: lymphoma, disseminated TB, metastatic carcinoma of liver, alcoholic liver disease, hepatoma, relapsing fever, granulomatous hepatitis, Q fever, typhoid fever, malaria, visceral leishmaniasis.
- Lymphadenopathy: lymphoma, cat scratch disease, TB, lymphomogranuloma venereum, infectious mononucleosis, CMV infection, toxoplasmosis, HIV, brucellosis, Whipple's disease, Kikuchi's disease.
- Renal angle tenderness: perinephric abscess, chronic pyelonephritis.
- Splenomegaly: leukaemia, lymphoma, TB, brucellosis, subacute bacterial endocarditis, cytomegalovirus infection, EBV mononucleosis, rheumatoid arthritis, sarcoidosis, psittacosis, relapsing fever, alcoholic liver disease, typhoid fever, Kikuchi's disease.
- Splenic abscess: subacute bacterial endocarditis, brucellosis, enteric fever, melioidosis.
- Conjunctival suffusion: leptospirosis, relapsing fever, Rocky Mountain spotted fever.
- Subconjunctival haemorrhage: infective endocarditis, trichinosis, leptospirosis.
- Uveitis: TB, sarcoidosis, adult Still's disease, systemic lupus erythematosus, Behçet's disease.

Investigations

- FBC and differential (check for eosinophils).
- CRP, ESR.
- U&Es, LFTs, serum amylase, TFTs.
- Blood culture from all lines, and a peripheral 'stab'.
- Samples for culture with/without microscopy, Gram stain, fungal culture, AFBs:
  - Samples from all drains and any effusions that can be tapped
  - Sputum; ideally BAL or protected specimen if intubated (for culture, immunofluorescence, PCR)
  - Swabs from nose, throat, naso-pharynx and perineum (for culture and/or viral PCR)
  - Urine (also do a dipstick test)
  - Serum for HIV (and possibly also toxoplasmosis, brucellosis, coxiellosis, EBV, CMV)
  - If diarrhoea is present stool culture and *C. difficile* toxin testing
  - If neurological symptoms present CT and/or LP
  - Blood smear if malaria a possibility
- ECG.
- CXR.
- Consider TTE or TOE if endocarditis is suspected.
- Other imaging: US of abdomen, CT of any suspect area (especially after major surgery), sinus X-rays, white cell scans.
- Consider autoantibody screens (ANA, ANCA, RF); GI endoscopy; BM biopsy and culture, lymph node biopsy (if lymphadenopathy present); temporal artery biopsy.

Differential diagnoses

- Exclude measurement errors (check core temperature if possible).

Immediate management

- Give O_2 as required, support airway, breathing, and circulation
- Review the patient's history including, including drug history, sexual history, travel, occupation and exposure to animals.
- Look for any obvious site of infection including;
  - Eyes, ears, mouth, PR/PV (exclude the presence of tampons)
  - Cannulae, epidural and catheter entry sites for redness/pus
  - Skin especially the back of the patient and buttocks
  - Check for enlarged lymph nodes
- Review all previous investigations, looking for changes in inflammatory markers, WCC, ↑ insulin requirements, alteration in oxygen requirements, ↑ lactate, reduced absorption of feed
- If the patient is unwell start empirical treatment with different broad spectrum antibiotics to those used previously, covering for HAIs (e.g. meropenem IV 500 mg 8-hourly and vancomycin IV 500 mg 6-hourly)

Further management

- Remove as many non-essential invasive devices as possible, especially if blood drawn from a line produces a positive blood culture.
- If blood cultures remain negative but the patient is still clinically unwell, continue broad-spectrum antibiotics for 48 hours and review.
- Consider introducing antifungal medications if the patient condition is deteriorating and the fever remains high.
- Treat with antipyrexial agents with/without surface cooling if there is limited cardiovascular reserve, brain injury, or pyrexia is >39.5°C.

Pitfalls/difficult situations

- Pyrexia precedes other signs for ≥3 days in some infections, including viral hepatitis, EBV, measles, leptospirosis, typhoid.
- TTE is often technically difficult on mechanically ventilated patients.
- Hypothermia may also be associated with infection.
- If temperature persists despite 5–7 days of adequate antibiotic cover stop antibiotics for 12 hours, re-culture, and start different antibiotics.
- CVVH often causes low temperatures and can mask signs of fever.
- Patients may become colonized, but not infected with, organisms.
- Consider the possibility of rare/tropical infections; or biological agents.
- Immunocompromised patients may be at risk from unusual infections which are difficult to identify/culture (see HIV, 📖 p.376, and neutropaenia, 📖 p.308); in neutropaenia micro-organisms may include:[2]
  - Lung: *Pseudomonas aeruginosa, Pneumococci,* Alpha-haemolytic streptococci, *Acinetobacter* species, *Klebsiella, Aspergilllus*
  - Abdomen: *E. coli, Pseudomonas aeruginosa, Clostridium* spp., *Enterococcus* spp., *Klebsiella* spp.
  - Urogenital: *E. coli, Klebsiella* spp., *Pseudomonas aeruginosa,*
  - Soft tissue: *S. aureus,* Alpha-haemolytic streptococci
  - Intravascular catheters: coagulase negative staphylococci, *Corynebacteriae, Propionibacterium* species, *Candida* spp.
  - Unknown: coagulase negative staphylococci, *E. coli, Enterococcus* spp.

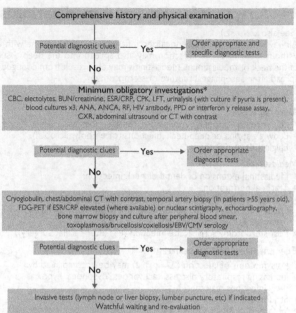

*Peripheral blood smear should be done at this stage if patient has recently travelled to malaria
endemic areas or if CBC suggests bone marrow involvement. CBC=complete blood count;
BUN=blood urea nitrogen; ESR=erythrocyte sedimentation rate; CRP=C-reactive protein;
CPK=creatine phosphokinase; LFT=liver function test; ANA=antinuclear antibody;
ANCA=antineutrophilic cytoplasmic antibody; RF=rheumatoid factor;
PPD=purified protein dervative; CXR=chest radiograph; CT=computed tomography;
FDG-PET=fluoro-2-deoxy-D-glucose-positron emission tomography;
EBV=Epstein-Barr virus, CMV=cytomegalovirus.

Fig. 10.1 Algorithm for the evaluation of fever of unknown origin. Reproduced
from *British Medical Journal*, Varghese GM, et al. Investigating and managing pyrexia
of unknown origin in adults, **341**: 878–81. Copyright 2010, with permission from
BMJ Publishing Group Ltd.

References

1. Varghese GM, et al. Investigating and managing pyrexia of unknown origin in adults. *Br Med J*
2010; **341**: 878–81.
2. Penack O, et al. Management of sepsis in neutropenic patients: guidelines of the infectious
diseases: guidelines of the infectious diseases working party of the German Society of
Hematology and Oncology. *Ann Oncol* 2011; **22**(5): 1019–29.

Further reading

Laupland KB. Fever in the critically ill medical patient. *Crit Care Med* 2009; **3**(S): S273–S278.
Marik PE. Fever in ICU. *Chest* 2000; **117**: 855–69.
O'Grady NP, et al. Guidelines for evaluation of new fever in critically ill adult patients: 2008 update
from the American College of Critical Care Medicine and the Infectious Diseases Society of
America. *Crit Care Med* 2008; **36**: 1330–49.

:⊙: **Airway infections and mediastinitis**

(See also 📖 p.32.)
Airway infections can cause localized inflammation and oedema with or
without systemic sepsis. Infection may also spread into the deep tissues
of the neck or mediastinum. Mediastinitis may also result from contiguous
spread after oesophageal rupture or sternotomy.

Causes

Airway infections
- Pharyngeal, retropharyngeal, or peri-tonsillar abscess.
- Ludwig's angina or deep-neck infections (often polymicrobial).
- Epiglottitis or diphtheria.

Mediastinitis
- Mediastinal extension of dental or neck infection.
- Tracheal perforation.
- Oesophageal perforation (traumatic, post-surgical anastomotic
  breakdown, spontaneous/Boerhaave syndrome); associated with
  malignancy or infection (e.g. TB).
- Post-sternotomy surgical site infection (e.g. after cardiac surgery).

Presentation and assessment

Signs/symptoms of infection (📖 p.322) may be accompanied by:
- Increasing respiratory distress, tachypnoea, dyspnoea, hypoxia.
Airway infections may cause:
- Stridor.
- 'Hunched' posture; sitting forward, mouth open, tongue protruding.
- 'Muffled' or hoarse voice, sore throat, painful swallowing, drooling .
- Neck swelling, or trismus.
Mediastinitis may be associated with:
- A history of coughing, choking, or vomiting (Boerhaave syndrome).
- Recent oesophageal surgery or endoscopy.
- Signs associated with pneumothorax, or hydrothorax (i.e. percussion
  note and auscultation changes); most commonly left sided.

Investigations

(See 📖 p.324.)
Other investigations will depend on the presentation, but may include:
- Throat swabs.[1]
- Lateral soft tissue neck X-ray may demonstrate swelling and loss of
  airway cross-section ('thumb print' and 'vallecula' signs).
- Laryngoscopy (indirect or fibreoptic).[1]
- CT or MRI of head and neck; or CT scan of chest.
- CXR (pneumomediastinum, pneumothorax or hydrothorax).
- Oesophagoscopy.
- Water soluble contrast swallow (or barium swallow).

1 Airway interventions in a patient with a partially obstructed airway can provoke complete airway
obstruction.

Differential diagnoses

• Airway foreign body or tumour; traumatic pneumo- or haemothorax

Immediate management

• Give O_2 as required, support airway, breathing, and circulation.
Airway infections
• Airway intubation or tracheostomy is required in severe cases; anaesthetic and ENT input will be required (see 📖 p.33)
• Obtain IV access and consider steroids (dexamethasone 8 mg IV)
Oesophageal perforation
• Keep patient NBM
• Insert intercostal chest drain(s) as indicated by X-ray findings
Suggested empirical antimicrobials
• Epiglottitis: cefotaxime 1–2 g IV 12-hourly
• Deep-seated neck infections: clindamycin 600 mg IV 6-hourly, benzyl penicillin 600 mg IV 6-hourly, and metronidazole 500 mg IV 8-hourly
• Diphtheria: clarithromycin 500 mg IV 12-hourly, and possibly anti-toxin (if strain is toxin producing)
• Oesophageal perforation: piptazobactam IV 4.5 g 8-hourly and gentamicin IV 5 mg/kg daily and fluconazole IV 400 mg daily

Further management

• Airway or dental abscesses should be assessed by ENT specialists in case surgical drainage or dental extraction is required.
• Thoracic surgical advice should be sought where mediastinal collections or oesophageal perforation are suspected; early presentation of an oesophageal perforation may be amenable to repair.
• Oesophageal perforation will require feeding to be post-pyloric (nasojejunal, or jejunostomy) or parenteral.
• In cases of airway infection assess for airway swelling (laryngoscopy/cuff-leak test) prior to extubation.

Pitfalls/difficult situations

• In cases of airway infection, delaying intubation may make a difficult intubation impossible.
• Spontaneous oesophageal rupture may present very late with gross contamination of the pleura and a large hydropneumothorax; small-bore chest drains are often insufficient.

Further reading

Ames WA, et al. Adult epiglottitis: an under-recognized, life-threatening condition *Br J Anaesth* 2000; **85**: 795–7.

Ridder GJ, et al. Descending necrotizing mediastinitis: contemporary trends in etiology, diagnosis, management, and outcome. *Ann Surg* 2010; **251**(3): 528–34.

Kaman L, et al. Management of esophageal perforation in adults. *Gastroenterol Res* 2010; **3**(6): 235–44.

Khan AZ, et al. Boerhaave's syndrome: diagnosis and surgical management. *Surgeon* 2007; **5**(1): 39–44.

⚙ Pneumonia and empyema

(See also 📖 p.62.)
Pneumonia can occur as a result of infection acquired in the community or in hospital/health-care settings. In hospitalized patients, oropharyngeal overgrowth of enteric organisms, *Pseudomonas*, or *Candida* amongst the flora increases the risk of pneumonia after aspiration/micro-aspiration; pneumonia caused by drug-resistant organisms is also more common.

Abscesses may occur within the lung, or infection may spread from the lung to a parapneumonic effusion, resulting in an empyema. The mortality from lung abscess or empyema is 10–20%.

Causes

Pneumonia-causing organisms vary according to where it is acquired:
- Community acquired pneumonia (CAP).
- Hospital acquired pneumonia (HAP) or health-care associated pneumonia (HCAP).
- Aspiration pneumonia or ventilator-acquired pneumonia (VAP).

Infection may be caused by:
- 'Typical' organisms (*S. pneumoniae, H. influenzae*).
- 'Atypical' organisms (i.e. insensitive to penicillins: *Legionella, Mycoplasma, Chlamydophila* species, *Coxiella burnetti*).
- Viruses (e.g. influenza A and B).
- Uncommon organisms, often associated with chronic illness and hospitalization (*S. aureus, M. catarrhalis, K. pneumonia, Pseudomonas, E. coli, Enterobacter, Acinetobacter*).

Where there is no response to treatment or the patient is immunocompromised consider less common causes:
- 'Unusual' organisms: TB, *Pneumocystis jiroveci, Stenotrophomonas, Cryptococcus neoformans*.
- Resistant species: MRSA, resistant *Pseudomonas*.
- Viral: varicella, CMV.
- Fungal: *Candida* spp., Aspergillus.

Empyema:
- Community-acquired empyema is most commonly associated with streptococcal infections (50%), as well as *Staphylococci*, anaerobes and Gram-negative organisms.
- Hospital-acquired empyema is often caused by *S. aureus* (including MRSA), as well as *Pseudomonas, E. coli,* and *Enterobacter*.

Lung abscess:
- Organisms include aerobic organisms (*S. aureus, H. influenzae, Klebsiella* species, *S. milleri, S. pyogenes*) and anaerobes (*Prevotella, Bacteroides, Fusobacterium* spp.); often polymicrobial.
- Associated with *S. aureus, K. pneumonia,* and *Pseudomonas*.
- Associated with bronchial carcinoma, aspiration, prolonged pneumonia, liver disease, dental disease, and IV drug use (septic embolization).

See Table 10.1 for incidence of pneumonia-causing organisms.

Presentation and assessment

Signs and symptoms of infection (📖 p.322) may be accompanied by:
- Increasing respiratory distress, tachypnoea, dyspnoea.
- Cough, purulent sputum, haemoptysis, or pleuritic chest pain.
- Features of coexisting disease (e.g. COPD or bronchiectasis).
- CXR changes of collapse, consolidation or parapneumonic effusion.

Atypical pathogens should be suspected where the following are present:
- Dry cough and/or multisystem involvement (e.g. headache, abnormal LFTs, elevated serum creatine kinase, hyponatraemia).
- A history of travel, pets, high-risk occupations, comorbid disease.
- Immunosuppressive disease or therapy.

HAP, HCAP, VAP, or aspiration should be suspected in patients where:
- Symptoms occur ≥48 hours after hospital admission.
- The patient is readmitted ≤10 days after discharge from hospital.
- Residence in a nursing home or extended care facility where there is recent or prolonged antibiotic use (e.g. leg ulcer treatment).
- Receiving care for a chronic condition.
- Patients with a neurological injury or ↓ consciousness level.
- Difficulty swallowing (e.g. stroke, Parkinson's disease), or NG feeding.
- In patients mechanically ventilated for >48 hours by means of an ETT or tracheostomy, where there is:
  - Worsening oxygenation or ↑ sputum production
  - Indices of infection (pyrexia, WCC, CRP, culture results)
  - CXR changes on routine films

Empyema: pleural effusion is a common ICU finding, suspect infection if:
- Sepsis or inflammatory markers do not resolve.
- Imaging suggests fibrin stranding or loculation.
- Pleural tap reveals fluid that is turbid or has decreased pH.

Multiple drug resistance (MDR) may be present if:
- HAP/HCAP/VAP are suspected.
- The patient has been on prolonged antibiotic therapy, or there is a failure to respond to appropriate antibiotics.
- Immunosuppressive disease or therapy is present.
- The patient is receiving care for a chronic condition (e.g. dialysis).
- The patient, their relatives, or the place where they are treated, are known to be associated with multidrug-resistant pathogens.

Investigations

(See 📖 pp.63 and 324.)
Also consider:
- ABGs (hypoxia, acidosis, or respiratory alkalosis).
- FBC (WCC may be high, >12, or low <4 × 10⁹/L; neutrophilia).
- U&Es (↓Na; ↑urea/creatinine).
- LFTs (non-specific abnormalities); coagulation screen (↑INR, DIC).
- CRP (↑); CK (occasionally ↑: Legionella, H1N1).
- CXR (infiltrates, consolidation, effusion, or cavitation).
- Culture of blood and sputum (possibly including AFB for TB).
- Urine for Pneumococcal antigen and Legionella antigen.
- Viral throat swab PCR.

- Bronchoscopy or non-directed BAL (if safe to do so) testing for:
  - Culture and sensitivity (including AFBs, fungus, *Legionella*)
  - Immunofluorescence (e.g. influenza, *Pneumocystis, Mycoplasma*)
  - Other: viral PCR; galactomannan (*Aspergillus*)
- Pleural fluid (if present) for microscopy, culture (±AFBs) and pneumococcal antigen:
  - Also assess for pH (pH testing is unnecessary if pleural fluid is cloudy or turbid), protein, LDH, cytology, glucose, and amylase
- Imaging: US and/or CT chest.

Differential diagnoses

- Pneumonia: acute MI/pulmonary oedema; PE, pneumothorax, pneumonitis, vasculitis, sarcoidosis, or malignancy.
- Empyema:
  - Transudative effusions: LVF, liver cirrhosis, hypoalbuminaemia, hypothyroidism, PE, nephrotic syndrome
  - Exudative effusions: malignancy, autoimmune disease, pancreatitis, rheumatoid arthritis, drug-related (e.g. amiodarone, phenytoin).

Immediate management

Follow guidelines on 🕮 pp.62 and 325.
- 100% O_2 initially, then titrate to SpO_2 or blood gas results
- Support airway, breathing, and circulation.

Suggested empirical antimicrobials

- CAP: co-amoxiclav 1.2 g IV 8-hourly and clarithromycin 500 mg 12-hourly:
  - If associated with influenza add flucloxacillin IV 2 g 6-hourly
- Aspiration pneumonia: co-amoxiclav IV 1.2 g 8-hourly:
  - For severe, in-hospital aspiration add gentamicin IV 5 mg/kg daily
- Atypical pathogens suspected: co-amoxiclav IV 1.2 g 8-hourly and clarithromycin IV 500 mg or levofloxacin IV 500 mg 12-hourly
- HAP/HCAP/VAP: piptazobactam 4.5 g IV 8-hourly ± linezolid 600 mg IV 12-hourly (avoid using previously used antibiotics)
- In immunocompromised patients, or where any of the following are suspected treat accordingly:
  - *Pneumocystis jiroveci*: co-trimoxazole IV 120 mg/kg/day for 3 days, followed by 90 mg/kg/day for a further 18 days (and steroids)
  - Fungal infections: liposomal amphotericin B IV (dose depends upon formulation)
  - Viral infections: influenza, oseltamivir PO/NG 75 mg 12-hourly; herpes, aciclovir IV 10 mg/kg 8-hourly; CMV, ganciclovir IV 5 mg/kg 12-hourly
  - TB: seek advice from respiratory or infectious diseases specialists
- MDR organisms suspected add:
  - MRSA: linezolid IV 600 mg 12-hourly, or vancomycin IV 500 mg 6-hourly
  - Resistant *Acinetobacter*: amikacin IV 7.5mg/kg 12-hourly

Further management

(See also 📖 pp.65 and 326.)
- Report notifiable diseases such as *Legionella* (see 📖 p.380).
- Pleural fluid drainage is indicated if:
  - The fluid is cloudy or turbid
  - The pH is <7.2 and infection is suspected
  - Infection is identified on Gram stain or culture
  - The effusion is loculated
  - Clinical condition deteriorates and infection is suspected
- Complications such as empyema or abscess may require surgical treatment.

Pitfalls/difficult situations

- Malignancies or foreign bodies may give rise to pneumonia, empyema, or lung abscesses.
- Pneumonia, and especially lung abscesses, may be polymicrobial.
- Consider *Legionella* where there is evidence of other organ failure (especially renal) and/or a community outbreak.
- If necrotizing pneumonia caused by a PVL-producing strain of *S. aureus* is suspected see 📖 p.356.

Table 10.1 Incidence of pneumonia-causing organisms

	Within hospital	Within ICU setting
S. pneumoniae	39.2%	21.6%
H. influenzae	5.2%	3.8%
Legionella	3.6%	17.8%
S. aureus	1.9%	8.7%
M. catarrhalis	1.9%	
Gram-negative bacilli	1%	1.6%
Mycoplasma	10.8%	2.7%
Chlamydophila	13.1%	

Further reading

American Thoracic Society. Guidelines for the management of adults with hospital-acquired, ventilator-associated, and healthcare-associated pneumonia. *Am J Respir Crit Care Med* 2005; **171**: 388–416.

Lim WS, et al. British Thoracic Society Guidelines for the management of community acquired pneumonia in adults: update 2009. *Thorax* 2009; **64**(sIII): iii1–iii55.

Maskell NA, et al. BTS guidelines for the investigation of a unilateral pleural effusion in adults. *Thorax* 2003; **58**(S2): ii8–ii17.

Masterton RG, et al. Guidelines for the management of hospital-acquired pneumonia in the UK: Report of the Working Party on Hospital-Acquired Pneumonia of the British Society for Antimicrobial Chemotherapy. *J Antimicrob Chemother* 2008; **62**: 5–34.

Walters J, et al. Pus in the thorax: management of empyema and lung abscess. *CEACCP* 2011; **11**(6): 229–33.

① Infective endocarditis

Infective endocarditis (IE) is sometimes also referred to as bacterial endo-carditis, or subacute bacterial endocarditis (SBE). It can be caused by bac-teria or fungi, which initially cause heart valve vegetation, followed by later valve destruction and abscess formation.

Causes

- Underlying aortic or mitral valve disease; or rheumatic disease.
- Prosthetic heart valves, or other intracardiac devices (e.g. pacemakers or defibrillators).
- IV drug use or chronic vascular access (e.g. haemodialysis).

Infective organisms include:

- Viridans *Streptococci* (e.g. *S. mutans*, *S. mitis*, *S. sanguis*, *S. salivarius*, *Gemella morbillum*); associated with oral/dental infections.
- *S. milleri*, *S. anginosus* (associated with abscess formation).
- *S. aureus* (including MRSA); coagulase negative staphylococci.
- Enterococci (e.g. *E. faecalis*, *E. faecium*, *E. durans*).
- Gram-negative 'HACEK' group bacilli (e.g. *Haemophilus* species, *Actinobacillus actinomycetemcomitans*, *Cardiobacterium hominis*, *Eikenella corrodens*, *Kingella* spp.).
- *Coxiella burnetii*, *Bartonella*, *Chlamydophila*/*Chlamydia* (associated with negative blood cultures).
- Fungi (e.g. *Candida* spp.).

Presentation and assessment

Fever is the most common sign; other signs/symptoms of infection (📖 p.322) may be accompanied by:

- Heart murmurs (especially regurgitant).
- New heart failure or conduction abnormalities.
- Left-sided (mitral or aortic) phenomenon:
  - Osler's nodes; Janeway lesions; splinter haemorrhages; purpuric lesions; Roth spots
  - Metastatic abscesses or infarcts (lung, heart, brain)
  - Splenomegaly
  - Glomerulonephritis; microscopic haematuria
- Right-sided (tricuspid or pulmonary) phenomenon:
  - Pulmonary embolism or abscess.

Infection may be more likely if:

- Suspicious organisms are cultured.
- Dental infections are present.
- There is evidence of IV drug abuse (i.e. 'track' marks).
- Intracardiac devices or prosthetic valves are present.
- Known cardiac valve defects or a previous history of endocarditis.

Investigations

(See 📖 p.324.)
Also consider:

- Serial blood cultures (from multiple sites, repeated every 24–48 hours).
- Serial CRP measurements.

- Serology (especially for *Coxiella burnetti*, *Bartonella*, *Chlamydia*, *Candida*, *Aspergillus*).
- Urine dipstick (microscopic haematuria).
- ECG (conduction abnormalities).
- Transthoracic/transoesophageal echocardiography (vegetations, abscesses, valve aneurysms/pseudoaneurysms, valve perforation, prosthetic valve dehiscence).
- Cardiac CT or MRI.
- Tissue sample culture (following surgery).

Differential diagnoses

- MI, PE.
- Systemic infections causing multiple abscesses.

Immediate management

Follow guidelines on 📖 p.325.
- Give O₂ as required, support airway, breathing, and circulation.
- Treat heart failure (📖 p.122) and arrhythmias (📖 pp.132 and 138).

Suggested empirical antimicrobials

- Flucloxacillin IV 2 g 6-hourly and gentamicin IV 1 mg/kg 8-hourly.
- Prosthetic valves or severe infection/complications: vancomycin IV 500 mg 6-hourly, gentamicin IV 1 mg/kg 8-hourly, and rifampicin IV 600 mg 12-hourly.
- If immunocompromised add IV liposomal amphotericin B (dose depends upon formulation).
- Antibiotics should be tailored to cultured organisms, as resistant streptococci, enterococci, and HACEK organisms may respond better to other antimicrobial combinations.
- Culture-negative endocarditis may require the addition of doxycycline or fluoroquinolones.

Further management

- Surgery may need to be considered where there is:
  - Gross valve regurgitation causing haemodynamic compromise
  - Prosthetic valve endocarditis
  - Perivalvular abscesses or very large vegetations
  - Resistant organisms (e.g. MRSA)

Pitfalls/difficult situations

- Endocarditis treatment may require prolonged antimicrobial therapy.

Further reading

Baddour LM, et al. Infective endocarditis: diagnosis, antimicrobial therapy, and management of complications. *Circulation* 2005; **111**: e394–e433.

Beynon RP, et al. Infective endocarditis. *Br Med J* 2006; **333**: 334–9.

Elliott TSJ, et al. Guidelines for the antibiotic treatment of endocarditis in adults: report of the Working Party of the British Society for Antimicrobial Chemotherapy. *J Antimicrob Chemother* 2004; **54**: 971–81.

Habib G, et al. Guidelines on the prevention, diagnosis, and treatment of infective endocarditis. *Eur Heart J* 2009; **30**: 2369–413.

⚙ **Neurological infections**

(See also 📖 p.188.)
Meningitis is the inflammation of the meninges surrounding the brain and spinal cord. Encephalitis refers to inflammation of the brain parenchyma. Intracranial abscesses may also occur.

Causes

- Meningitis/encephalitis is commonly caused by:
  - *S. pneumoniae* and *N. meningitides*
  - Nosocomial infections including *E. coli*, *Pseudomonas* spp., *Klebsiella*, and *Acinetobacter*
  - *Listeria*, TB, *Toxoplasma* and fungal infections (e.g. *Cryptococcus* and *Histoplasma*) are more common in the immunocompromised
  - *S. aureus* and *S. epidermis* are more common following surgery
  - Viral infections include herpes simplex, coxsackie enteroviruses, measles, mumps and rubella (if not vaccinated)
  - *H. influenzae B* is less common due to mass HiB inoculation
- Intracranial abscesses can occur as:
  - Haematogenous spread (including endocarditis and dental sepsis)
  - Contiguous spread (including progression of meningitis; or chronic sinusitis or otitis media)
  - Following neurosurgery, penetrating injury
  - They are also more common in immunocompromised patients

Presentation and assessment

(See also 📖 p.188.)
Signs and symptoms of infection (📖 p.322) may be accompanied by:
- Meningism: headache, neck-stiffness, vomiting, photophobia, lethargy.
- Neurological signs: focal neurological signs, seizures, altered mental state, ↓ consciousness, papilloedema (often absent or late).
- In the immunosuppressed and elderly classical signs may be absent; behavioural changes and low-grade fever may be the only signs.
- Chronic sinus pain, postnasal drip or otitis media (occasionally accompanied by cholesteatoma) are associated with subdural abscesses.

Investigations

(See 📖 pp.189 and 324.)
- Blood cultures, drain fluid culture.
- Serum PCR (or antigen tests) for *N. meningitidis*.
- Throat/nasopharyngeal swabs (both for culture and PCR).
- Rash scrapings or skin pustule aspirates (for culture/PCR).
- CT head and/or MRI.
- LP (see 📖 p.574; opening pressure, CSF for urgent Gram stain and microscopy, PCR, protein, glucose with paired serum sample)—depending on CT/MRI results LP may be contraindicated.
- If *Cryptococcus* or *Toxoplasmosis* are present consider HIV testing.

Differential diagnoses

- Subarachnoid haemorrhage.
- Malignancy, malignant infiltration.
- Autoimmune/vasculitic process.

Immediate management
- Give O_2 as required, support airway, breathing, and circulation.
- Treat the systemic effects of sepsis and meningococcal sepsis as appropriate (📖 pp.325 and 348).
- Treat ↓ consciousness and seizures (📖 pp.152 and 160).

If you suspect bacterial meningitis do not delay treatment. Even if the GP/admitting physician has already given benzyl penicillin.

Suggested empirical antimicrobials
- Ceftriaxone 2 g IV 12-hourly.
- If abscess is suspected add metronidazole IV 500 mg 8-hourly.
- If viral meningitis is suspected add aciclovir IV 10 mg/kg 8-hourly.
- If following neurosurgery add flucloxacillin IV 2 g 6-hourly (vancomycin IV 500 mg 6-hourly if MRSA).
- In elderly or immunocompromised patients consider adding amoxicillin IV 1 g 6-hourly.
- In the immunocompromised add gentamicin IV 5 mg/kg daily and liposomal amphotericin B IV (dose depends upon formulation) and aciclovir IV 10 mg/kg 8-hourly.
- For suspected bacterial meningitis or abscesses with mass effect give dexamethasone 10 mg IV 6-hourly with first dose of antibiotic.
- If an LP Gram stain becomes available, adjust antimicrobials.

Further management
- Report notifiable diseases (📖 p.380).
- Manage patients in an HDU/ICU setting.
- Intracranial abscesses or hydrocephalus require neurosurgical referral.
- Raised ICP may occur (see 📖 p.186).
- Consider re-culturing the CSF if there is slow clinical improvement.
- New focal neurology will require a repeat CT head.

Pitfalls/difficult situations
- LP is contraindicated if raised ICP (📖 p.186) or abscess is suspected, if there is any doubt await the results of a CT head first.
- Herpes simplex meningoencephalitis may present with personality and behavioural changes; if there is any suspicion start acyclovir.
- CSF pleocytosis has a number of causes including: partially treated bacterial meningitis, TB, Lyme disease, sarcoidosis, Behçet's disease.
- In very rare cases of meningococcal meningitis prophylaxis for staff may be required (e.g. if they had performed mouth-to-mouth resuscitation).

Further reading
Chadwick DR. Viral meningitis. *Br Med Bull* 2006; **75&76**: 1–14.
Meningitis Research Foundation website: ⅍ <http://www.meningitis.org/>
Rappaport ZH, et al. Intracranial abscess: current concepts in management. *Neurosurg Quart* 2002; **12**(3): 238–50.
Stephens DS, et al. Epidemic meningitis, meningococcaemia and *Neisseria meningitides*. *Lancet* 2007; **369**: 2196–210.
Van de Beek D, et al. Community-acquired bacterial meningitis in adults. *N Engl J Med* 2006; **354**: 44–53.

① Skin and orthopaedic infections

Skin, soft-tissue, bone and joint infections can occur after a loss of tissue integrity (e.g. compound fractures, burns, bites and stings), or after haematogenous spread.

Causes

Skin infections
- Cellulitis, abscess formation or wound infection.
- Necrotizing infections (e.g. necrotizing fasciitis, Fournier's gangrene).

Joint infections
- Septic arthritis, of healthy, prosthetic or damaged joints (e.g. by RA).
- Osteomyelitis.

Common organisms include:
- Soft tissue infections are often polymicrobial involving 1 or more of Gram-positive (*Staphylococci*, *Streptococci*), Gram-negative (*Enterococci*), and anaerobes (*Bacteroides*, *Peptostreptococcus*).
- Soft tissue infections causing fasciitis may be toxin producing (e.g. PVL-SA, or β-*haemolytic streptococci*).
- Soft-tissue infections causing myonecrosis may be clostridial (e.g. *C. perfringens* or *C. septicum*).
- Rare soft-tissue infections include *Vibrio vulnificus* (a water-borne infection) and fungal infections (e.g. *Rhizopus* and *Mucor*).
- Septic arthritis is most commonly caused by *S. aureus* (including MRSA) and *Streptococci*; but may involve *H. influenzae*, *N. gonorrhoea*, *E. coli*, *Salmonella*, TB, *P. aeruginosa*.

Presentation and assessment

Signs/symptoms of infection (📖 p.322) may be accompanied by:
- A medical history of immunocompromise, chronic disease (e.g. diabetes, alcoholism or renal failure); or IV drug use.
- Recent skin trauma (sometimes very minor) or chronic ulceration; recent joint replacement; recent intra-articular steroid injection.
- Obvious abscesses, frank pus in wounds, wound drains or in urine.
- Skin, or joint, erythema, swelling, and pain.
- Crepitus, vesicles or blistering (or black eschars in fungal infections).
- Lymph node enlargement.

Necrotizing skin infection spreads along the superficial or deep fascial planes, or causes muscle necrosis. It most commonly occurs on the legs, abdomen, perineum or groin (Fournier's gangrene affects men involving scrotum, perineum or penis) causing:
- Rapidly progressive cellulitis (over hours).
- Skin may become grey and necrotic in appearance.
- Severe pain, though affected skin is often anaesthetized.
- Systemic disturbance (septic shock, DIC, AKI, metabolic acidosis).

Investigations

(See 📖 p.324.)
Also consider:
- Serum CK, CRP and ESR.

- Synovial fluid microscopy, Gram stain and culture (for septic arthritis).
- Blood cultures; pus or debrided skin samples for cultures.
- Joint/soft-tissue X-rays CT scan (joint destruction, tissue necrosis, emphysema).
- US imaging of hips (may be useful) in hip septic arthritis.
- MRI (may detect osteomyelitis, particularly of the spine).

Differential diagnoses

- Any cause of rash, erythema or skin discolouration (e.g. TEN, toxic shock, drug-rash, meningococcal septicaemia).
- Any cause of myalgia or joint pain (e.g. arthritis, influenza, gout).

Immediate management

Follow guidelines on 🔲 p.325.

- Give O_2 as required, support airway, breathing, and circulation.
- Analgesia will be required.
- Surgery may be required:
  - Surgical debridement will be required for necrotizing fasciitis
  - CT imaging for suspected necrotizing fasciitis should not delay surgical exploration
  - Arthroscopy/joint washout may be required for septic arthritis

Suggested empirical antimicrobials

- Septic arthritis: vancomycin IV 500 mg 6-hourly and ceftriaxone IV 2 g 12-hourly.
- Necrotizing infections: piptazobactam IV 4.5 g 8-hourly, clindamycin IV 900 mg to 1.2 g 6-8 hourly, and linezolid IV 600 mg 12-hourly (add antifungals if fungal infection suspected; doxycycline if Vibrio suspected).
- Severe surgical wound infection: vancomycin IV 500 mg 6-hourly and gentamicin IV 5 mg/kg daily and metronidazole IV 500 mg 8-hourly.

Further management

- Repeated surgery/surgical debridement may be required.
- Tetanus immunoglobulin with/without vaccine may be required.

Pitfalls/difficult situations

- There is a high mortality associated with necrotizing fasciitis and surgical debridement is often radical.
- Osteomyelitis may complicate trauma or joint/infection.
- Compartment syndrome may complicate necrotizing fasciitis.
- STDs are associated with septic arthritis.
- A high index of suspicion for contaminated wounds is required (e.g. rabies, botulism, tetanus).

Further reading

Coakley G, et al. BSR & BHPR, BOA, RCGP and BSAC guidelines for management of the hot swollen joint in adults. *Rheumatology* 2006; **45**: 1039–41.

Mathews CJ, et al. Bacterial septic arthritis in adults. *Lancet* 2010; **375**: 846–55.

Moran E, et al. The diagnosis and management of prosthetic joint infections. *J Antimicrob Chemother* 2010; **65**(S3): iii45–iii54.

Ustin JS, et al. Necrotizing soft-tissue infections. *Crit Care Med* 2011; **39**(9): 2156–62.

① Urological infections

Urinary tract infection (UTI) may be upper (pyelonephritis) or lower (cystitis). Infection typically ascends from the urethra, but occasionally occurs via haematogenous spread. Sepsis caused by UTIs is often referred to as urosepsis.

Bacteriuria alone does not necessarily indicate a UTI, particularly in older, female patients, or those with indwelling urinary catheters.

Causes

UTIs are classified as uncomplicated, or complicated (i.e. associated with a structural/functional GU tract abnormality; or with immunodeficiency).

Common infective organisms include:
- Enterobacteriaceae (e.g. *E. coli*, *Klebsiella* spp.).
- Gram-positive cocci (e.g. *Enterococci*, *S. saprophyticus*).
- *Proteus* species.
- *Pseudomonas*.
- TB, *Salmonella* and *S. aureus* can cause UTIs after haematogenous spread.
- *Candida* species occasionally cause UTIs in catheterized patients.

UTIs are associated with
- Sexual activity.
- Indwelling urinary catheters.
- Urinary tract malformations (e.g. polycystic kidney disease).
- Renal calculi.
- Urinary obstruction (including acute hydronephrosis, or chronic urinary retention caused by prostatic hypertrophy).
- Recent urological surgery.
- Neurogenic bladder.
- Diabetes mellitus.
- Immunosuppression.

Presentation and assessment

Signs/symptoms of infection (📖 p.322) may be accompanied by:
- Back pain or renal colic; suprapubic pain.
- Dysuria, urinary frequency.
- Haematuria, cloudy urine.
- In the elderly the only symptom may be altered mental state.

UTIs may be difficult to identify in catheterized patients with no localizing signs; and may be the source of occult infection in ICU patients.

Investigations

(See 📖 p.324.)
Also consider:
- U&Es (renal function may be deranged).
- Urine for culture (mid-stream urine, MSU, or catheter-specimen urine, CSU); catheterized patients will have evidence of colonization without infection (a positive culture typically has >10^5 organisms/ml).
- Urine dipstick (positive if nitrates or leukocyte esterases are present).

- Renal tract imaging to identify calculi or hydronephrosis:
  - US kidney and bladder
  - Pelvic X-ray (kidney ureter bladder, KUB)
  - Intravenous urogram (IVU)
  - CT abdomen (with/without urogram)

Differential diagnoses

- Renal infarct.
- Renal or GU tract tumour.
- Drug-induced haemorrhagic cystitis.

Immediate management

Follow guidelines on 📖 p.325.
- Give O_2 as required, support airway, breathing, and circulation
- Analgesia is likely to be required, especially if colic is present

Suggested empirical antimicrobials

- Community-acquired infection: co-amoxiclav IV 1.2 g 8-hourly
- Severe or hospital-acquired infection: piptazobactam IV 4.5 g
  8-hourly and gentamicin IV 5 mg/kg daily
- If penicillins have already been administered give meropenem 500 mg
  8-hourly
- Immunocompromised: consider adding fluconazole IV 400 mg daily

Further management

- Urological referral may be required:
  - If ureteric obstruction occurs for: nephrostomy, 'double-J' stent,
    suprapubic catheterization or difficult urethral catheterization
  - If emphysematous pyonephritis or cystitis, or renal tract abscesses
    are present
- Change catheters where chronic infection/colonization is suspected.

Pitfalls/difficult situations

- Occasionally consider TB (send early morning urines for AFBs),
  schistosomiasis, or fungal infections.
- Aggressively treat bacteriuria in the presence of pregnancy or a
  transplanted kidney.
- If neurogenic bladder is possible perform a full neurological
  assessment.
- If prostatitis is present consider using fluoroquinolone antibiotics.
- Urinary infection that rapidly recurs may indicate underlying
  obstruction or calculi.
- Resistant bacteria are common in UTIs.

Further reading

Grabe M, et al. *Guidelines on urological infections.* European Association of Urology, 2009. Available
at: 🖰 www.uroweb.org/gls/pdf/Urological Infections 2010.pdf.
Scottish Intercollegiate Guidelines Network. *Management of suspected bacterial urinary tract infection in adults.* Edinburgh: SIGN, 2006.

① **Abdominal infections**

Abdominal infections include peritonitis caused by upper or lower gut perforation, cholangitis/cholecystitis, and infective colitis. Peritonitis caused by bowel perforation has a high associated mortality.

Causes

- Large bowel perforation (caused by obstruction/tumour, or breakdown of anastomoses); diverticulitis; appendicitis.
- Gastroduodenal/small bowel perforation (associated with ulcers or trauma).
- Cholecystitis/cholangitis (often associated with gall stones).
- Tubo-ovarian abscess.
- Infected pancreatic necrosis.
- Peritonitis 2° to CAPD infection.
- Spontaneous bacterial peritonitis (SBP, associated with liver disease and/or ascites).
- Infected colitis (most commonly due to *C. difficile* infection).

Infection is often polymicrobial, involving Gram-negative organisms (e.g. *E. coli*, *Klebsiella* spp., *Proteus* and *Pseudomonas*), Gram-positive enterococci, and anaerobes (e.g. *Bacteroides*, *Clostridia*, *Peptostreptococci*).

- *S. aureus* and coagulase-negative streptococci may be involved, particularly after surgery or CAPD.
- Viridans streptococci may be involved in SBP.
- *Candida* is occasionally involved.
- Rarer infections include TB and actinomycosis.

Presentation and assessment

(See also 📖 pp.280 and 322.)
Signs/symptoms of infection may be accompanied by:
- Recent history of abdominal operation.
- Abdominal pain, rebound, guarding, which may localize.
- Abdominal distension; bowel obstruction, or diarrhoea.
- Nausea and vomiting; anorexia (or failure to absorb NG feed).
- Jaundice; frank ascites (distension, shifting dullness, fluid waves).

Investigations

(See 📖 p.324.)
Also consider:
- ABGs (metabolic acidosis, raised lactate).
- FBC (leucocytosis), CRP.
- Serum LFTs, calcium, amylase or lipase (to identify liver dysfunction or pancreatitis).
- Cultures of surgical/radiological aspirates, tissue samples, or drain fluid.
- Tap and culture ascites if SBP is suspected (also send for Gram staining, amylase, glucose, protein, LDH, triglycerides, and cytology).
- If diarrhoea is present send stool for *C. difficile* toxin; if toxin is negative consider culture (and microscopy if there is recent travel).
- CXR (sub-diaphragmatic air may be present).
- Imaging: CT abdomen; US abdomen.
- Lower GI endoscopy (if colitis suspected).

Differential diagnoses

- Any cause of abdominal pain (e.g. pseudo-obstruction, pancreatitis, porphyria, DKA, sickle crisis).
- Any cause of diarrhoea (e.g. NG feed intolerance, ischaemic colitis).

Immediate management

- Give O_2 as required, support airway, breathing, and circulation
- Analgesia may be required
- Abdominal catastrophe is likely to require aggressive fluid and/or vasopressor resuscitation
- Surgical referral is required for a patient with an acute abdomen:
  - Laparotomy may be required
  - US or CT guided percutaneous abscess drainage may be possible

Suggested empirical antimicrobials

- Perforation/peritonitis, biliary infection, or SBP: piptazobactam IV 4.5 g 8-hourly
  - Add gentamicin IV 5mg/kg daily in severe cases
  - Consider adding fluconazole IV 400 mg daily
  - If previous CAPD consider adding vancomycin IV 500 mg 6-hourly (dose will depend on dialysis regimen)
- Suspected *C. difficile*: metronidazole PO/NG 400 mg 8-hourly or vancomycin PO/NG 125 mg 6-hourly
- If there is no NG access then use metronidazole IV 500 mg 8-hourly (there may be some limited biliary excretion)

Further management

- The use of a stool management system for patients with diarrhoea may prevent cross-contamination.
- Percutaneous drainage/ERCP may be needed for obstructive jaundice.
- Stop proton pump inhibitors if possible in patients with *C. difficile*.

Pitfalls/difficult situations

- CT imaging may be negative, even in the presence of gross faecal or biliary contamination.
- *C. difficile* may be difficult to treat on ICU, requiring the continuation of prokinetics (despite diarrhoea) to enable oral treatment; and possibly even rectal antimicrobial instillation, or surgical resection.
- *C. difficile* diarrhoea may be difficult to spot in patients with stomas.
- Strict isolation and hand-washing (with soap *not* alcohol gel) is required if *C. difficile* is suspected.

Further reading

Mazuski JE, et al. The Surgical Infection Society guidelines on antimicrobial therapy for intra-abdominal infections: an executive summary. *Surg Infect* 2002; 3(3): 161–73.

Sartelli M. A focus on intra-abdominal infections. *World J Emerg Surg* 2010; 5:9.

Shannon-Lowe J, et al. Prevention and medical management of *Clostridium difficile* infection. *Br Med J* 2010; 340: 641–6.

Solomkin JS, et al. Diagnosis and management of complicated intra-abdominal infection in adults and children: guidelines by the Surgical Infection Society and the Infectious Diseases Society of America. *Clin Infect Dis* 2010; 50: 133–64.

:☺: Meningococcal sepsis

Neisseria meningitidis can cause meningitis/meningoencephalitis (see 📖 p.340) or fulminant sepsis that can be rapidly fatal. A combination of the two can also occur with meningitis signs/symptoms predominating.

Causes

Risk factors for meningococcal sepsis include:
- Communal living (e.g. university halls of residence or army barracks).
- Overcrowding and social deprivation.
- Smoking or recent URTI (↑ risk of nasopharyngeal carriage):
  - Passive smoking is a risk factor for invasive disease
- Complement deficiencies (↑ risk of re-infection).

Presentation and assessment

- General: rapidly deteriorating flu-like presentation with:
  - Pyrexia, myalgia
  - Rash: purpuric (or sometimes petechial) lesions on abdomen and/ or lower limbs, coalescing into ecchymoses
- Respiratory: tachypnoea and hypoxia; pulmonary oedema may develop, especially associated with aggressive fluid resuscitation:
  - ARDS may develop
- Cardiovascular: tachycardia and hypotension (often severe):
  - Cardiovascular compromise may rapidly develop
  - Pericarditis may develop
- Neurological: agitation, confusion, diminished consciousness.
  - Meningitis may also occur with or without septicaemia (📖 p.188).
- Renal: oliguria, raised urea and creatinine (AKI may develop):
  - Metabolic acidosis
- GI: anorexia, diarrhoea, nausea and vomiting.
- Haematology: DIC.
- Musculoskeletal: septic arthritis or reactive arthritis may occur.

Investigations

(See also 📖 p.324.)
- ABGs (compensated metabolic acidosis with elevated lactate levels).
- FBC (WCC may be high or low, Hb and platelets may be low).
- Coagulation studies, including fibrinogen (DIC may be present).
- Serum glucose (often low), U&Es, LFTs.
- Blood culture × 2 (*N. meningitidis* may be difficult to culture).
- Blood EDTA bottle for antigen detection and for PCR.
- Skin lesion scrapings or fluid aspiration (culture or PCR).
- Nasopharyngeal/throat swabs.
- CT brain (if reduced consciousness and focal neurological signs). LP is not indicated for patients with meningococcal sepsis.

Differential diagnoses

- Severe bacterial sepsis, especially *Streptococcus pneumoniae* or *Haemophilus influenza*; particularly where a rash or DIC is present.
- Toxic shock syndrome.
- Viral haemorrhagic fevers (if there is a history of travel).

Immediate management

- Give O_2 as required, support airway, breathing, and circulation
- Airway: endotracheal intubation may be required:
  - Where there is ↓consciousness (GCS ≤8)
  - To facilitate mechanical ventilation
- Ensure breathing/ventilation is adequate:
  - Mechanical ventilation may be needed to optimize oxygenation in severe shock or pulmonary oedema
- Circulatory support should be commenced:
  - Large peripheral venous cannulae are required
  - Repeated fluid boluses (20 ml/kg) will be required to treat hypotension (pulmonary oedema is common, particularly once ≥30 ml/kg of IV fluid boluses have been given)
  - Inotropic/vasopressor support is likely to be required
  - Use early goal directed treatment (CVP 8–12 mmHg; MAP ≥65 mmHg; UOP ≥0.5 ml/kg/hour; $ScvO_2$ or SvO_2 ≥70%)
  - Arterial and/or central venous cannulation should be undertaken as soon as feasible, checking coagulation studies and platelets first.

If meningococcal septicaemia is suspected, do not delay treatment. Commence antibiotic therapy immediately:
- Antimicrobial treatment: ceftriaxone 2g IV 12-hourly
- If benzyl penicillin is given by GP/admitting physician, a 3rd-generation cephalosporin (e.g. ceftriaxone) should still be administered

Further management

Same as for sepsis and septic shock (📖 pp.326 and 120).
- Transfer to HDU/ICU.
- Cardiac output monitoring is likely to be required as myocardial depression is often more severe than with other types of sepsis:
  - Calcium replacement may be improve myocardial function
- Renal replacement therapy is likely to be required.
- Modify antimicrobial treatment according to blood culture results and microbiological advice.
- Platelets often fall, but transfusion should be reserved for those with a high risk of bleeding.
- Check limbs regularly as DIC and purpura fulminans can cause occlusion of vessels and amputation may be required.

Pitfalls/difficult situations

- The speed of onset from innocuous symptoms to death can be in <2 hours and delay in antibiotic administration may be fatal.
- The rash may present as a 'simple' maculopapular rash; it may be difficult to see on pigmented skin; it may even be absent.

Further reading

Scottish Intercollegiate Guidelines Network. *Management of invasive meningococcal disease in children and young people. A national clinical guideline.* Edinburgh: SIGN, 2008.
Thompson MJ, et al. Clinical recognition of meningococcal disease in children and adolescents *Lancet* 2006; **367**: 397–403.

① Legionella pneumonia

(See also Pneumonia 🕮 pp.62 and 334.)
Pneumonia caused by *Legionella* spp. (90% *L. pneumophila*, 5–10% *L. micdadei*) accounts for 2–5% of CAPs. It is one of the 'atypical' pneumonias (i.e. not treatable with penicillins) and can cause multi-system derangement (with a mortality of 10–15%), which is sometimes termed Legionnaire's disease.

Causes

Legionella is spread by exposure to aerosolized infected water:
• Contaminated water storage tanks.
• Air conditioning units.
• Windscreen wiper water.
Legionnaire's disease is more common in:
• The middle aged or elderly.
• Smokers.
• Chronic alcoholics.
• Patients with chronic illness (e.g. diabetes, COPD or renal failure).
• Males are twice as likely to be affected as females.

Presentation and assessment

Legionella is often contracted through travel (abroad > domestic) and there is ↑prevalence in the summer and autumn. It can also be healthcare-acquired. The incubation period is 1–19 days (median 6 days).

Systemic complications are more common than in other pneumonias, and may be out of proportion to the degree of respiratory involvement. Signs and symptoms may include:
• General: flu-like presentation with fevers, sweats and rigors.
• Respiratory: tachypnoea and hypoxia:
  • Dry cough
  • Pleuritic chest pain is common
• Cardiovascular: tachycardia:
  • Cardiovascular compromise may develop (more common than in other pneumonias)
• Renal: oliguria, raised urea and creatinine (AKI may develop).
• GI: abdominal pain, vomiting and diarrhoea are common.
• Neurological: confusion, diminished consciousness, cerebellar signs.

Investigations

(See also 🕮 p.324.)
• ABGs (hypoxia, metabolic acidosis).
• FBC (a moderate increase in WCC with a lymphopaenia may occur).
• U&Es (marked hyponatraemia and raised urea/creatinine are common).
• LFTs (often deranged and with low albumin).
• Serum CK (occasionally raised).
• Serum CRP (raised).
• Blood cultures × 2 (organism is difficult to grow and must be specifically requested; can take 10 days to culture).

- Sputum, endotracheal aspirate, or BAL (culture, immunofluorescence or PCR); culture must be specifically requested:
  - Species identification aids source tracing
- Urinary antigen testing (highly specific, but may not detect all types).
- Serum for legionella antigen (IgG testing can take up to 10 days).
- ECG.
- CXR (rapidly progressing patchy shadowing).

Differential diagnoses
- Other organisms which cause CAP.
- Always consider TB as a cause of pneumonia in patients with multisystem involvement who fail to respond to conventional treatment.

Immediate management
- Give O_2 as required, support airway, breathing, and circulation:
  - Assess degree of pneumonia according to CURB-65 score (🕮 p.64)
  - Respiratory support/mechanical ventilation is commonly required
- Send appropriate investigations (see 🕮 Investigations).
- Treat as CAP, empirical antibiotics may include:
  - Co-amoxiclav IV 1.2g 8-hourly and clarithromycin IV 500 mg 12-hourly
  - When diagnosis is confirmed add ciprofloxacin IV 500 mg 12-hourly

Further management
- Transfer to HDU/ICU.
- Rifampicin may be an alternative to fluoroquinolones.
- Antibiotic duration depends upon disease severity.
- Public health should be informed.
- Sepsis care bundles should be implemented (see 🕮 p.10).

Pitfalls/difficult situations
- Patients are often disproportionately sicker than those with CAP.
- Hypoxia and confusion may make patients non-compliant with therapy.
- 20% of patients develop ARDS.
- Pericardial and myocardial involvement may occur.
- Systemic involvement, especially hyponatraemia, liver and neurological changes, makes the diagnosis more likely.

Further reading
Lim WS, et al. British Thoracic Society Guidelines for the management of community acquired pneumonia in adults: update 2009. *Thorax* 2009; **64**(sIII): iii1–iii55.

Masterton RG, et al. Guidelines for the management of hospital-acquired pneumonia in the UK: Report of the Working Party on Hospital-Acquired Pneumonia of the British Society for Antimicrobial Chemotherapy. *J Antimicrob Chemother* 2008; **62**: 5–34.

:☼: Tetanus

Tetanus is caused by a neurotoxin, tetanospasmin, released by *Clostridium tetani*, a Gram-positive anaerobic bacillus. The toxin is irreversible and prevents neurotransmitter release causing muscle rigidity/spasm and autonomic instability. Recovery occurs with nerve terminal regrowth.

Causes

Four forms of tetanus are described: local, cephalic, neonatal, and the most common form generalized. Risk factors include:
- Inadequate or absent vaccination history.
- Penetrating trauma (often trivial).
- Drug abusers, especially if SC or IM injectors (associated with infected batches of illegal drugs, and occurs in outbreaks).

Presentation and assessment

Symptom onset occurs 2–60 days after inoculation. Often the injury is trivial. Signs and symptoms may include:
- General: sore throat, hypersecretion (saliva, bronchial), hyperpyrexia.
- Neuromuscular:
  - Early symptoms include neck stiffness, dysphagia, and trismus
  - Muscle spasms develop in facial muscles, 'risus sardonicus' (facial muscles are often affected first due to shorter axonal pathways)
  - Later spasms become more widespread with neck and back rigidity with/without hyperextension
  - Spasms are often triggered by innocuous stimuli and are extremely painful, and can damage muscles, tendons, joints, and bones
- Respiratory: spasms can cause laryngospasm and/or ventilation may be impaired, causing respiratory arrest.
- Cardiovascular: autonomic instability develops a few days after spasms have commenced and can cause tachycardia and hypertension, bradycardia, asystole and profound hypotension.
- GI: ileus.
- Neurological: seizures may occur.

Investigations

(See also 📖 p.324.)
   Tetanus is a clinical diagnosis.
- ABGs (may show high lactate and metabolic acidosis).
- FBC, U&Es, LFTs, serum CK.
- Blood cultures/wound swabs (30% of wound cultures grow organism).
- X-rays of any suspected fracture sites.

Differential diagnoses

- Acute dystonic reactions.
- Epilepsy.
- Chorea.
- Meningitis/encephalitis or SAH.
- Strychnine poisoning.
- Rabies.
- Drug withdrawal states.

Immediate management

- Give O_2 as required, support airway, breathing, and circulation.
- Consider elective endotracheal intubation and mechanical ventilation; the commonest cause of death is from laryngospasm and respiratory muscle paralysis.
- Nurse in a darkened room with minimal stimulation
- Control muscle spasm and autonomic instability:
  - Heavy sedation with diazepam, or midazolam, and morphine is required (doses may be very high)
  - Refractory spasms may require neuromuscular blockade

Prevent further toxin damage and release:

- Give human tetanus antitoxin IM 5,000–10,000 iu.
  - One dose is required as the half-life is 23 days, it neutralizes circulatory toxin but not that bound intraneuronally
  - Side effects include fevers, shivers, and hypotension; the rate of infusion should be slowed if this occurs
- Reduce toxin load by debriding any infected tissue.
- Give metronidazole IV 500 mg 8-hourly for 7–10 days to eradicate any bacterium left.

Further management

- 2° agents which may be used for muscle spasms include baclofen, dantrolene, and chlorpromazine.
- Refractory autonomic instability may respond to:
  - Clonidine (centrally acting α-2 adrenergic agonist)
  - Magnesium sulphate infusion, 20 mmol/hour adjusted to achieve plasma concentrations of 2.5–4.0 mmol/L
- Prolonged mechanical ventilation may require a tracheostomy.
- Treatments aimed at reducing complications of neuromuscular weakness or paralysis include:
  - Respiratory infections: regular physiotherapy and tracheal toilet
  - NG or PEG feeding; bowel care may be needed
  - DVT/PE: compression stockings or LMWH
  - Skin damage, joint contractures: pressure area care, physiotherapy
- Watch for nosocomial infections, fractures, or rhabdomyolysis.
- Immunization is required in the convalescent period.
- Public health need to be informed as tetanus is a notifiable disease.

Pitfalls/difficult situations

- Clinical suspicion is important to institute early effective management.
- Sudden cardiac arrest is common and may be due to high catecholamine levels or a direct effect of the toxin on the myocardium.
- Recovery of function may take months.

Further reading

Cook TM, et al. Tetanus a review of the literature. Br J Anaesth 2001; 87(3): 477–87.
Taylor AM. Tetanus. Cont Educ Anaesth Crit Care Pain 2006; 6(3): 101–4.

☼ Botulism

The toxin of *Clostridium botulinum* causes botulism. The toxin blocks the pre-synaptic release of acetylcholine at neuromuscular junction, parasympathetic terminals and autonomic ganglia. The toxin has 6 subtypes (A–F), but A, B, and E cause the illness.

Causes

Clostridium botulinum may be:
- Food-borne (symptoms in <18 hours of contaminated food ingestion).
- Associated with IV, or SC/IM ('popping') drug abuse with 'black tar heroin' (this leads to SC wounds that promote growth of the organism)
- Associated with infected wounds (rare).
- Associated with intestinal overgrowth and toxin production (rare in infants, exceptionally rare in adults).
- There have also been case reports of inhaled botulinum, and of parenteral administration of unlicensed cosmetic preparations.

Presentation and assessment

Signs and symptoms include:
- Cranial nerve involvement occurs first, including:
  - Extraocular muscles (blurred vision, diplopia); ptosis
  - Dilated pupils, and an inability to accommodate
  - Dysphagia (and possibly regurgitation); dysarthria
  - Pharyngeal collapse and airway obstruction may occur
- Autonomic: dry mouth, postural hypotension, dizziness:
  - 'Normalization' of blood pressure normally occurs later
- Descending neurological/neuromuscular involvement with progressive muscular weakness leading to symmetrical paralysis:
  - Pharyngeal and then upper and lower limb muscles in severe cases
  - Deep tendon reflexes may be lost
  - Respiratory failure due to muscle weakness may occur, but potentially without obvious external signs of agitation
  - Sensation is normally preserved, although paraesthesia has been reported
- GI: nausea, vomiting, constipation and ileus are common.

The speed and degree of progression are variable. Poor prognosis is indicated by limb and respiratory weakness, age >20 years, and illness caused by type A toxin.

Investigations

(See also 📖 p.324.)
- ABGs (hypoxia, hypercapnia).
- Serum and stool assay for *Clostridium* toxin:
  - Vomitus may also be sent, as can debrided wound material
- LP will be normal (protein will be raised with Guillain–Barré).
- PFTs.
- ECG, CXR.
- Tensilon test to exclude myasthenia gravis.
- Nerve conduction studies to exclude Guillain–Barré.

- EMG studies will show abnormal patterns (neuromuscular junction block with normal axonal conduction).
- CT/MRI head (may reveal stroke).

Differential diagnoses

Of the differentials, only botulism will cause outbreaks.
- Guillain–Barré; poliomyelitis.
- Stroke; viral encephalitis.
- Spinal cord injury (especially epidural abscess or haematoma).
- Myasthenia gravis; Eaton–Lambert syndrome.
- Tick paralysis; shellfish poisoning.

Immediate management

- Give O_2 as required, support airway, breathing, and circulation
- Airway may become compromised; if the protective reflexes of the upper airway are diminished, early intubation must be considered
- Assess adequacy of ventilation using FVC and FEV_1:
  - If FVC <15 ml/kg, or FVC <predicted TV, or failure to expectorate secretions occurs than supportive ventilation is indicated
  - Repeat PFTs 4-hourly
  - Other indications for ventilation may include hypercapnia and/or CXR changes (pneumonia, atelectasis)

Prevent further toxin damage and release

- Give 10,000 units of trivalent anti-toxin immediately; contact the Health Protection Agency duty officer for out-of-hours supply, and information on further dosing:
  - Anticipate minor allergic reactions and keep antihistamines and steroids ready for administration
- Give benzylpenicillin IV 1.2 g 6-hourly, and metronidazole IV 500 mg 8-hourly
- In cases of wound infection debridement is indicated
- Consider gastric lavage to remove toxins (patients with bulbar weakness require endotracheal intubation before lavage)

Further management

- Transfer to HDU/ICU; recovery may be very protracted.
- Continue assessment and management of airway/breathing problems:
  - Treatment of pneumonia if present.

Pitfalls/difficult situations

- Dilated and non-reactive pupils in an alert patient is a distinguishing feature of botulism; pupils may, however, remain dilated but reactive.

Further reading

Sobel J. Botulism. Clin Infect Dis 2005; 41: 1167–73.
UK Health Protection Agency website: ℘ <http://www.hpa.org.uk>
Wenham T, et al. Botulism. Cont Educ Anaesth Crit Care Pain 2008; 8(1): 21–5.

:O: Toxic shock syndrome and Panton–Valentine leucocidin infections

Toxic shock syndrome (TSS) is caused by toxin-producing Gram-positive staphylococci or streptococci (streptococcal toxic shock is sometimes termed toxic shock-like syndrome; TSLS). The site of infection is often localized to skin/soft-tissue, vaginal tract or respiratory tract; but the toxins produce systemic manifestations.

Other *Staphylococcus aureus* strains (both MRSA and MSSA) may be able to produce PVL toxin (PVL-SA), causing necrosis and white blood cell destruction. PVL-SA involves skin and soft tissue, but septic arthritis, polymyositis and community-acquired necrotizing pneumonia can occur.

Causes
- Toxic shock syndrome is associated with:
  - Menstruation, tampons, or female barrier contraception
  - Any wound infection (including: postoperative wounds, insect bites, burn injury, herpes zoster infections)
- PVL-SA is associated with:
  - Close-contact community outbreaks (e.g. within households, sport-clubs, gyms, prisons, military training camps)

Presentation and assessment

TSS may present with signs and symptoms of localized or systemic infection/sepsis (📖 p.322), and may be accompanied by:
- General: fever, diffuse macular rash (may be similar to sunburn or a drug reaction); desquamation is often a late sign.
- Mucous membranes: vaginal, oropharyngeal, conjunctival oedema.
- Acute respiratory distress (ARDS).
- Cardiovascular: tachycardia and hypotension (systolic ≤90 mmHg).
- CNS: altered consciousness with no focal neurology.
- GI: diarrhoea or vomiting.
- Renal and hepatic dysfunction.
- Haematological: DIC/thrombocytopaenia.
- Muscular/soft-tissue: myalgia, myositis, skin necrosis.

PVL-SA may present with signs and symptoms of localized or systemic infection/sepsis (📖 p.322), and may be accompanied by:
- Abscesses, cellulitis, and tissue necrosis affecting children/young adults.
- Diarrhoea and vomiting.
- Marked leucopaenia.
- Pneumonia with CXR changes (infiltrates with effusions, and later cavitation) with/without haemoptysis.

Investigations
(See 📖 p.324.)
- ABGs.
- FBC (leucocytosis; leucopaenia in PVL-SA; ↓ platelets in TSS).
- Coagulation screen (for DIC).
- U&Es (↑ urea/creatinine, especially in TSS).

- LFTs († bilirubin and/or transaminases in up to 40% of TSS cases).
- Serum CK (often elevated) and CRP (likely to be very high).
- Cultures: blood cultures (rarely positive in TSS); vaginal swabs; throat swabs; urine culture; wound swabs; BAL if appropriate.
- CXR (multilobar infiltrates in PVL-SA pneumonia).

Differential diagnoses

- Any cause of sepsis, including meningococcal septicaemia.
- Necrotizing fasciitis/cellulitis; staphylococcal scalded skin syndrome.
- Measles, leptospirosis, Rocky Mountain spotted fever (for TSS).
- Community-acquired pneumonias, anthrax (for PVL-SA pneumonia).

Immediate management

(As for sepsis 📖 p.325.)
- Give O_2 as required, support airway, breathing, and circulation.
- Ensure breathing/ventilation is adequate:
  - Mechanical ventilation may be needed to optimize oxygenation
- Circulatory support should be commenced:
  - Large peripheral venous cannulae are required
  - Fluid boluses will be required to treat hypotension
  - Inotropic/vasopressor support is likely to be required
  - Use early goal directed treatment (CVP 8–12 mmHg; MAP ≥65 mmHg; UOP ≥0.5 ml/kg/hour; $ScvO_2$ or SO_2 ≥70%)

Treatment of infection

- Remove the source of infection: wound drainage (or removal of foreign body, including tampons) may have to be undertaken while the patient is still being resuscitated.
- Empirical cover for TSS, TSLS, or PVL-SA may include clindamycin IV 900 mg to 1.2g 6–8 hourly with linezolid IV 600 mg 12-hourly.

Further management

Same as for sepsis and septic shock (📖 pp.120 and 326).
- Apply infection control measures where pneumonia is present (surgical masks for endotracheal intubation and closed tracheal suctioning).
- In severe disease (e.g. multiple-organ failure or PVL-SA pneumonia) IVIG should be considered at a dose of 2 g/kg (or 1 g/kg/day for 2 days).
- Rifampicin may be used in PVL-SA if there is clindamycin resistance.

Pitfalls/difficult situations

- Immediate removal of source of infection is crucial.
- Rapid onset of syndrome requires rapid response for resuscitation.
- Electrolyte derangement and rhabdomyolysis may occur.
- Rash may be similar to acute drug reactions.
- Flucloxacillin is not recommended in PVL-SA pneumonia.

Further reading

Health Protection Agency. *Guidance on the diagnosis and management of PVL-associated Staphylo-coccus aureus infections (PVL-SA) in England*. London: HPA, 2008.
Lappin E, et al. Gram-positive toxic shock syndromes. *Lancet Infect Dis* 2009; **9**: 281–90.

:○: Anthrax

Bacillus anthracis, the bacterium responsible for anthrax, is carried by large herbivores, and can exist as spores within soil. It is a toxin-producing organism. It was previously known as 'wool-sorter's disease'.

Causes

There are 3 types of anthrax:
- Cutaneous anthrax: contracted from infected animals or untreated animal skins, bone, or blood, or from IV drug use with contaminated drugs (typically heroin).
- Injection anthrax: illicit drug use.
- Inhalational anthrax: from spore inhalation (e.g. during the processing of animal skins, after deliberate release, or after smoking heroin; inhalational anthrax is very rare).
- Intestinal anthrax: from the ingestion of infected meat (exceptionally rare).

Person-to-person transmission does not occur with inhalational anthrax, and is easily prevented in cutaneous anthrax by universal precautions (see 📖 p.382).

Presentation and assessment

The incubation period is usually 1-7 days, but may be up to 60 days.
- Cutaneous: pruritus initially, followed by a lump with marked surrounding oedema (typically on the head or forearms; often painless):
  - The swelling blisters and then ulcerates and develops a depressed necrotic centre; often painless
  - Focal lymphadenopathy may develop
  - Signs of IV drug use may be present (i.e. 'track marks')
- Inhalational symptoms: severe sweating, fever, myalgia, non-productive cough and chest pain:
  - Progresses to severe dyspnoea and ARDS
  - Haemorrhagic mediastinitis results in mediastinal widening on CXR
- Neurological: headache and meningism/meningitis may occur.
- GI: nausea/vomiting, abdominal pain, GI bleed, ascites (may be due to 1° intestinal anthrax, or spread from other sites):
  - Oropharyngeal anthrax can occur with associated dysphagia
- General symptoms of sepsis may develop in all cases: malaise, fever, rigors, shock, severe sepsis.

Investigations

(See also 📖 p.324.)
- Crossmatch.
- FBC, U&E, CRP, lactate (all may be only minimally changed).
- Coagulation screens.
- Blood cultures and EDTA blood sample for PCR testing:
  - Skin lesion tissue for Gram stain and culture
  - Serum sample for toxin/antibody testing
  - Pleural fluid aspirate (haemorrhagic)

- LP, if meningitic, for Gram stain and culture (haemorrhagic with neutrophils and Gram positive bacilli).
- CXR (parenchymal infiltrates, hilar lymphadenopathy, mediastinal widening, pleural effusions).
- CT chest and/or head.

Microbiological samples should be classified as 'high risk' and their handling discussed with microbiology departments.

Differential diagnoses

- Cutaneous: syphilis, cellulitis, tularaemia, mucormycosis.
- Inhalational: atypical pneumonia, mediastinitis, PE, MI.
- Intestinal: amoebic dysentery, *Shigella*, typhoid.

Immediate management
(See Fig. 10.2.)
- Give O_2 as required, support airway, breathing, and circulation.
- Coordinate treatment with microbiology, infectious diseases, surgical teams (if skin involvement is present), and the Health Protection Team.
- Necrotic tissue should excised (for sampling, and then debridement).

Suggested empirical antimicrobials
- Ciprofloxacin IV 400 mg 12-hourly, clindamycin IV 900 mg to 1.2 g 6–8 hourly, and benzylpenicillin IV 1.2 g 6-hourly:
  - Where there is cutaneous involvement add flucloxacillin IV 500 mg 6-hourly and metronidazole IV 500 mg 12-hourly
- Anthrax 'antitoxin' (anthrax immune globulin IV) may be of benefit; discuss with microbiology.

Further management
- Management on ICU/HDU will be required.
- Debridement may cause marked blood loss.
- Pleural/ascitic fluid contains toxin and will require drain insertion.

Pitfalls/difficult situations
- Although anthrax is very responsive to antibiotics, the mortality associated with systemic infection, haemorrhagic mediastinitis, or meningitis is very high.
- Compartment syndrome may occur with cutaneous anthrax.
- Thrombocytopaenia is thought to herald the onset of severe shock.

Further reading
Bushra M, et al. Fatal inhalational anthrax with unknown source of exposure in a 61-year-old woman in New York City. *JAMA* 2002; **287**(7): 858–62

Health Protection Scotland. *Interim clinical guidance for the management of suspected anthrax in drug users.* Edinburgh: Health Protection Scotland, 2010.

Shafazand S. Inhalational anthrax. *Chest* 1999; **116**(5): 1369–76

UK Health Protection Agency website: <http://www.hpa.org.uk>

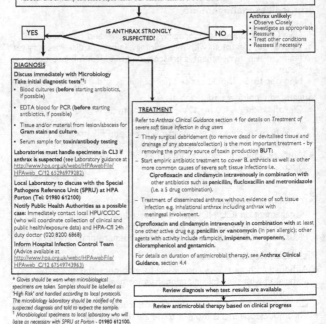

Anthrax infection suspected in a drug user

Any drug user who presents with:
- **Severe soft tissue infection**, including **possible necrotising fasciitis or cellulitis/abscess** particularly if associated with tissue oedema (often marked). This can present as a **compartment syndrome**
- **Signs of severe sepsis** even without evidence of soft tissue infection
- **Meningitis** (particularly haemorrhagic meningitis). Also be suspicious if drug users present/ have CT evidence suggestive of subarachnoid haemorrhage/intracranial bleed)
- Signs and symptoms of **inhalational anthrax**
  - Flu-like illness, progressing to severe respiratory difficulties and shock
  - Chest x-ray signs (pleural effusions, mediastinal widening, paratracheal fullness, hilar fullness, parenchymal infiltrates)
  - Progressively enlarging haemorrhagic pleural effusions are a consistent feature
- **Respiratory symptoms** may also be accompanied by signs and symptoms suggesting meningitis or intracranial bleeding in the rapidly advancing stages of the disease process due to haematogenous spread
- Cases of **disseminated anthrax** whether 'injectional' or inhalational may present with a variety of symptoms such as abdominal pain, nausea, vomiting, diarrhoea, gastrointestinal haemorrhage, ascites etc., suggestive of either GI involvement or actual gastrointestinal anthrax

NB A drug user may also present with the signs and symptoms of classical cutaneous anthrax (see algorithm: Clinical evaluation and management of persons with possible cutaneous anthrax). In the recent outbreak, the presentation has been one of mainly soft tissue sepsis rather than classical features of black eschar.

IS ANTHRAX STRONGLY SUSPECTED?

YES

NO → Anthrax unlikely:
- Observe Closely
- Investigate as appropriate
- Reassure
- Treat other conditions
- Reassess if necessary

DIAGNOSIS

Discuss immediately with Microbiology
Take initial diagnostic tests[1]:
- Blood cultures (**before starting antibiotics**, if possible)
- EDTA blood for PCR (**before starting antibiotics**, if possible)
- Tissue and/or material from lesion/abscess for Gram stain and culture
- Serum sample for toxin/antibody testing

Laboratories must handle specimens in CL3 if anthrax is suspected (see Laboratory guidance at http://www.hpa.org.uk/webc/HPAwebFile/HPAweb_C/12 65296979282)

Local Laboratory to discuss with the Special Pathogens Reference Unit (SPRU) at HPA Porton (Tel: 01980 612100)

Notify Public Health Authorities as a possible case: Immediately contact HPU/CCDC (who will coordinate collection of clinical and public health/exposure data) and HPA-Cfl 24h duty doctor (020 8200 6868)

Inform Hospital Infection Control Team
(Advice available at http://www.hpa.org.uk/webc/HPAwebFile/HPAweb_C/12 67549743963)

* Gloves should be worn when microbiological specimens are taken. Samples should be labelled as 'High Risk' and handled according to local protocols. The microbiology laboratory should be notified of the suspected diagnosis and told to expect the sample.
[1] Microbiological specimens to local laboratory who will liaise as necessary with SPRU at Porton - 01980 612100.

TREATMENT

Refer to *Anthrax Clinical Guidance* section 4 for details on *Treatment of severe soft tissue infection in drug users*

- Timely surgical debridement (to remove dead or devitalised tissue and drainage of any abscess/collection) is the most important treatment - by removing the primary source of toxin production **BUT:**
- Start empiric antibiotic treatment to cover B. anthracis as well as other more common causes of severe soft tissue infections i.e.
  Ciprofloxacin and clindamycin intravenously in combination with other antibiotics such as **penicillin, flucloxacillin and metronidazole** (i.e. a 5 drug combination).

- Treatment of disseminated anthrax without evidence of soft tissue infection e.g. Inhalational anthrax including anthrax with meningeal involvement.

Ciprofloxacin and clindamycin intravenously in combination with at least one other active drug e.g. **penicillin or vancomycin** (in pen allergic); other agents with activity include **rifampicin, imipenem, meropenem, chloramphenicol and gentamicin.**

For details on duration of antimicrobial therapy, see **Anthrax Clinical Guidance**, section 4.4

Review diagnosis when test results are available

Review antimicrobial therapy based on clinical progress

See also **Anthrax Clinical Guidance** at http://www.hps.scot.nhs.uk/anthrax/documents/clinical-guidance-for-use-of-anthrax-immune-globulin-v12-1-2001-03-19.pdf

Fig. 10.2 Evaluation and management of suspected anthrax in a drug user. Reproduced with permission from the Health Protection Agency.

⚠ **Enteric fever (typhoid)**

Enteric fever is caused by infection with *Salmonella enterica* with a serovar of Typhi or Paratyphi, causing typhoid and paratyphoid respectively. It is endemic in Africa, South America, and the Indian subcontinent.

Causes

- Spread is mostly faeco-oral, but can be food or water borne.
- May be more likely if gastric acidity is reduced.
- Chronic carrier state can be present in 1-3% of infected patients one year after treatment of acute illness.

Presentation and assessment

The incubation period is 7–21 days; occurrence is rare 1 month after return from an endemic area. General signs and symptoms of infection (📖 p.322) may be accompanied by:

- General: malaise, headache (a very common symptom), chills, sweats, myalgia, sore throat and cough:
  - Gradual rise of temperature in the 1st week
  - Epistaxis is common
  - Erythematous lesions, that blanch on pressure (rose spots) appear on upper abdomen in up to 30% of patients
  - Cervical lymphadenopathy
- Cardiovascular: a relative bradycardia is common (tachycardia is uncommon).
- Respiratory: pneumonia may occur.
- GI: anorexia, pain, nausea, vomiting, constipation, diarrhoea can all be seen (constipation occurs early, diarrhoea late):
  - Jaundice
  - GI bleeding
  - Acute abdomen due to bowel perforation may occur, typically in the 2nd or 3rd week of infection
  - Splenomegaly or hepatomegaly may be seen
- Neurological: agitation/delirium is common; coma, seizures, encephalopathy, and meningism occur in up to 5% of patients.
- Renal: UTIs may occur.

5–10% of patients present with toxic shock or multi-system dysfunction.

Investigations

(See also 📖 p.324.)
Also consider:

- FBC (initially, <7 days, a raised WCC may be seen; more commonly, and particularly >7 days, pancytopaenia occurs).
- U&Es; coagulation screen (DIC may be present).
- LFTs (commonly deranged in the first 7 days).
- Urinalysis (proteinuria, pyuria, casts).
- CXR (infiltrates may occur).
- AXR (subdiaphragmatic gas may be seen in bowel perforation).
- CT head will be required if neurological complications present.

- Cultures:
  - <7 days: blood cultures positive in up to 90% of patients
  - >7 days: blood cultures are generally negative, but urine and stool cultures are likely to be positive
  - Bone marrow cultures may be appropriate, but are more invasive
- Serology is no longer recommended.

Differential diagnoses
- Pneumonia.
- Febrile illnesses (e.g. malaria, TB, leptospirosis, viral infections).
- Meningitis/encephalitis.
- Diarrhoea-causing illnesses (e.g. *C. difficile* colitis, cholera, *Shigella*).

Immediate management
- Give O$_2$ as required, support airway, breathing, and circulation
- Aggressive fluid resuscitation is likely to be required
- Invasive monitoring and vasopressor support may be required in unstable patients
- In severe toxaemia give dexamethasone IV 3 mg/kg followed by 1 mg/kg 6-hourly

Suggested empirical antimicrobials
- Give cefotaxime IV 1 g 12-hourly

Further management
- Supportive measures will be required, as in sepsis (p.326).
- Careful management of electrolyte balance is required.
- Antipyretic therapy may be required.
- Typhoid is a notifiable disease, public health must be informed.
- Continuing assessment and management of complications is required:
  - Pneumonia
  - UTIs
  - Cholecystitis
  - Haemolytic anaemia
  - Meningitis
  - Peripheral neuropathy
  - Osteomyelitis
  - Intestinal perforation, abscess formation and/or intestinal haemorrhage: may require surgery

Pitfalls/difficult situations
- Chloramphenicol has previously been standard antibiotic therapy, but outbreaks of drug resistance have occurred; resistance to co-trimoxazole and ampicillin is also common.
- Ciprofloxacin may be used but there are increasing levels of resistance.

Further reading
Bhutta ZA. Current concepts in the diagnosis and treatment of typhoid fever. *Br Med J* 2006; **333**: 78–82.
Bhutta ZA. Typhoid fever: current concepts. *Infect Dis Clin Pract* 2006; **14**(5): 266–72.
Warr C. Tropical enteritides. *Curr Anaesth Crit Care* 2004; **15**: 157–64.

① Malaria

Malaria is caused by a bite from the infected female *Anopheles* mosquito. After a variable amount of time in the liver, injected sporozoites, invade RBCs destroying them and releasing merozoites. The destruction of RBCs and the immune response to foreign proteins causes a profound physiological disturbance and the clinical features of malaria.

Causes

Malaria is caused by *Plasmodium vivax*, *Plasmodium ovale*, *Plasmodium malariae*, or *Plasmodium falciparum* (potentially the most dangerous of the malaria causing organisms).

Risk factors for malaria include:
- Travel to (or through) endemic areas.
- Inadequate prophylactic measures (or the co-administration of enzyme inducing medications, decreasing the effect of prophylaxis).
- 'Airport malaria' can occur, typically amongst baggage handlers and ground-crew.

Severity is ↑ in:
- People from non-endemic areas (i.e. travellers).
- Children.
- Pregnant women.

Presentation and assessment

A full history of travel to or through endemic areas should be ascertained, including whether prophylaxis has been used. Incubation period is typically 7–10 days, but can be longer.

Signs and symptoms may include:
- General: fever (not always the classical tertian or quartan fever):
  - Rigors, chills and sweats
  - Muscular aches and pains
  - Jaundice or anaemia may be clinically apparent
- Respiratory: tachypnoea (hypoxia or pulmonary oedema may develop).
- Cardiovascular: tachycardia (cardiovascular compromise may develop).
- Renal: oliguria, raised urea and creatinine (AKI may develop):
  - Metabolic acidosis
- GI: abdominal pain, anorexia, nausea and vomiting:
  - Hepatosplenomegly may be found
- Neurological: confusion, behavioural changes, diminished consciousness, headache (cerebral malaria):
  - Upper motor neuron signs may occur

Severe malaria is defined as parasitaemia with 1 or more of:
- Impaired consciousness, or multiple seizures.
- Respiratory distress, or pulmonary oedema.
- Circulatory collapse.
- Severe anaemia, abnormal bleeding, haemoglobinuria, or jaundice.
- Hypoglycaemia.
- Metabolic acidosis.

Investigations

Chemoprophylaxis should be stopped on admission to hospital as it may interfere with parasite detection:

- ABGs (initially respiratory alkalaemia, later metabolic acidosis).
- FBC (thrombocytopaenia and/or anaemia may be seen).
- Blood film (thick and thin films) for parasite recognition and count:
  - Often 2–3 films are needed over a period of several hours to confirm diagnosis (thick film detects parasites; thin film allows species identification and staging of parasite differentiation as well as quantification of percentage of parasitized RBCs)
  - Regular films are needed throughout treatment to assess effectiveness of therapy
  - Parasite count: <2% mild; 2–5% moderate; >5% severe
- Malaria rapid diagnostic tests (MRDT antigen blood tests) or parasite DNA PCR from blood are available in some centres.
- Coagulation screen, including D-dimers and fibrinogen (DIC may occur).
- U&Es (raised urea and creatinine).
- LFTs (elevations in AST and bilirubin reflect haemolysis).
- Serum glucose (hypoglycaemia; needs rechecking hourly).
- Blood/sputum/urine culture (other infections may be present).
- β-HCG (pregnancy increases the risk of malaria becoming severe).
- Urinalysis (to exclude infections and check for haemaglobinuria).
- CT head may be required (may exclude other diagnosis; in cerebral malaria cerebral oedema may be seen, as may diffuse hypodensity with sparing of the basal ganglia).

World Health Organization (WHO) criteria for severe *P. falciparum* malaria

One or more of the following in a patient with *P. falciparum* malaria:

- Coma/impaired consciousness.
- Prostration/extreme weakness.
- Failure to feed.
- >2 seizures in 24 hours.
- Respiratory distress or pulmonary oedema on CXR.
- Systolic BP <70 mmHg or circulatory collapse.
- Clinical jaundice or other organ dysfunction.
- Haemoglobinuria.
- Spontaneous bleeding.
- Hypoglycaemia (<2.2 mmol/L).
- Severe normocytic anaemia (Hb <5 g/dl).
- Acidaemia/acidosis (pH <7.3, HCO_3 <15 mmol/L).
- Hyperlactataemia (>5 mmol/L).
- Acute kidney injury (serum creatinine >265 µmol/L).
- Hyperparasitaemia (>2%/100,000/µL in low intensity transmission areas, or >5% in areas of high/stable malaria transmission intensity).

Reproduced from Guidelines for the treatment of malaria, 2nd edition, WHO, 2010, with permission. ℘ http://whqlibdoc.who.int/publications/2010/9789241547925_eng.pdf

UK definition of severe/complicated P. falciparum malaria in adults

Any of the following in a patient with *P. falciparum* malaria:
- Coma/impaired consciousness, or seizures.
- Renal impairment (oliguria <0.4 ml/kg/hour or creatinine >265 μmol/L.
- Acidaemia (pH <7.3).
- Hypoglycaemia (<2.2mmol/L).
- Pulmonary oedema or ARDS.
- Hb <8 g/dl.
- Spontaneous bleeding/DIC.
- BP <90/60 mmHg.
- Haemoglobinuria (without G6PD deficiency).

Reprinted from *Journal of Infection*, 54, 2, David G. Lalloo *et al.*, 'UK malaria treatment guidelines', pp.11–111, Copyright 2007, with permission from Elsevier.

Differential diagnoses
- Influenza/SARS/Viral haemorrhagic fevers.
- Meningitis.
- Hepatitis.
- Leptospirosis.
- Typhoid.

Immediate management

(See also Fig. 10.3.)
- Give O_2 as required, support airway, breathing, and circulation.
- Obtain IV access and rehydrate as necessary:
  - Avoid over-hydration which may exacerbate cerebral or pulmonary oedema/ARDS (aim for CVP <10 cmH$_2$O)
- Check serum glucose, if hypoglycaemic give 20–50 ml of 50% dextrose

Treatment of parasitaemia

See also ◻ p.367 for treatment algorithm.
- IV treatment is indicated for:
  - Patients with severe or complicated malaria
  - Patients with >2% parasitaemia
  - Those unable to swallow
  - Pregnant women
- Quinine IV 20 mg/kg in 5% dextrose over 4 hours (maximum dose 1400 mg), then 10 mg/kg over 4 hours 8-hourly, for 48 hours or until patient can swallow (monitor ECG); if IV treatment is continued >48 hours reduce dose to 12-hourly:
  - Quinine can be given orally when the patient is able to absorb effectively (600 mg 8-hourly)
- Quinine should be accompanied by a second-line drug: doxycycline (200 mg daily), or clindamycin (450 mg 8-hourly) continued for 7 days.
- An alternative regimen of artesunate is possible IV 2.4 mg/kg at 0 hours, 12 hours, 24 hours and then daily (use if heart disease or very high parasitaemia are present, or if quinine resistance is suspected, i.e. travel in SE Asia); this should also be accompanied by doxycyline.
- Other regimens are on the Health Protection Agency website.

Further management

- Transfer to HDU/ICU.
- Monitor the effectiveness of therapy with 4-hourly blood films to show a reduction in parasite count; counts may rise initially, but should fall by ≥25% of admission value within 48 hours.
- Invasive monitoring is required in severe malaria.
- Exchange transfusion may be considered for patients with severe disease and very high parasite counts (indications include >30% parasitaemia or >10% with indicators of severe disease/organ failure).
- For fevers, consider using antipyretics with/without surface cooling.
- Complications include AKI, ARDS, DIC, hypoglycaemia, metabolic acidosis, and seizures:
  - Seizures should be treated aggressively (📖 p.160), check glucose and U&Es, once other causes have been excluded cerebral malaria is the most probable cause (which is a poor prognostic marker)
  - Haemofiltration may be indicated for renal failure/acidaemia/electrolyte imbalance
- Infections occur alongside malaria (Gram-negative sepsis is particularly common and often precipitates circulatory collapse):
  - If clinical suspicion exists consider commencing broad-spectrum antibiotics after blood cultures

Pitfalls/difficult situations

- 3 negative blood films in 72 hours are required to exclude malaria.
- Occasionally incubation period can be in excess of 6 months.
- Suspicion is essential in the prompt recognition of the disease, even in those who have taken prophylaxis.
- Deterioration can occur rapidly (within hours).
- Presentation with hypoglycaemia, convulsions, or acidosis is associated with a poorer outcome.
- Do not reduce the dose of drugs if renal failure is present.
- Complications can occur with even low levels of parasitaemia.
- Sometimes the parasite is difficult to find, treat on clinical suspicion and treat for the most severe form: *P. falciparum*.

Further reading

Lalloo DG, et al. UK malaria treatment guidelines. *J Infection* 2007; **54**: 111–21.
Pasvol G. The treatment of complicated and severe malaria. *Br Med Bull* 2005; **75–76**(1): 29–47.
Sarkar PK et al. Critical care aspects of malaria. *J Intensive Care Med* 2010; **25**: 93–103.
UK Health Protection Agency website: 🖰 <http://www.hpa.org.uk>.
Whitty CJM. Malaria: An update on the treatment of adults in non-endemic countries. *Br Med J* 2006; **333**: 241–5.
WHO. *Guidelines for the treatment of malaria*, 2nd edn. Geneva: WHO, 2010.

Important information
- Malaria occurs in the tropics and sub-tropics
- Adherence to chemoprophylaxis does not exclude malaria
- Patients with malaria may deteriorate rapidly
- All cases should be discussed with a specialist with current experience of managing malaria
- Notify all cases to the local health protection unit, send blood films to reference laboratories

Triage
All febrile or ill patients with a history of travel to a malaria area in the prior 6 months should be assessed urgently (Incubation for non-falciparum infection may occasionally be greater than 6 months)

For those within 3 weeks of return, discuss infection control requirements (eg viral haemorrhagic fever (VHF), avian influenza or SARS) with the duty microbiologist but do NOT delay blood film

Early diagnosis and assessment of severity is vital to avoid malaria deaths

Expert Advice
Local infectious disease unit or
Liverpool 0151 706 2000
London 0845 155 5000
Ask for duty tropical doctor

Useful information
British National Formulary
UK malaria treatment guidelines:
Lalloo DG et al. J Infect 2007;
54: 111-21
from www.hpa.org.uk or
www.britishinfectionsociety.org

Key points in history and examination – no symptoms or signs can accurately predict malaria
- Symptoms are non-specific, but may include: fever/sweats/chills, malaise, myalgia, headache, diarrhoea, cough, jaundice, confusion and seizures
- Consider country of travel, including stopovers, and date of returns; falciparum malaria is most likely to occur within 3 months of return, but this may be longer in those who have taken chemoprophylaxis or partial treatment. The incubation period for malaria is at least 6 days
- Consider what malaria prophylaxis was taken (ie drug, dose & adherence): Correct prophylaxis with full adherence does not exclude malaria
- Consider other travel-related infections: eg typhoid fever, hepatitis, dengue fever, avian influenza, SARS, HIV, meningitis/encephalitis and VHF
- Examination findings are non-specific

Urgent investigations – all patients should have:
- Thick & thin blood films and malaria rapid antigen test. Send to laboratory immediately and ask for a result within one hour
- Full blood count (FBC) for thrombocytopenia, urea & electrolytes (U&Es), liver function tests (LFTs) and blood glucose
- Blood culture(s) for typhoid and/or other bacteraemia
- Urine dipstick (for haemoglobinuria) and culture. If the patient has diarrhoea, send faeces for microscopy and culture
- Chest radiograph to exclude community-acquired pneumonia

If falciparum malaria is confirmed
- Ask the laboratory to estimate the parasite count – ie % of RBCs parasitised
- Clotting screen, arterial blood gases and 12-lead ECG are required in complicated infection (see below)
- Do a pregnancy test if there is a possibility of pregnancy: pregnant women are at higher risk of severe malaria

Blood tests show

Non-falciparum malaria
- Vivax — Outpatient therapy
- Ovale — usually appropriate
- Malariae — depending on clinical judgement

Falciparum malaria
- Falciparum
- Mixed infection
- Species not characterised

Admit all cases to hospital
Assess severity on admission

No evidence of malaria
A single negative film and/or antigen test does not exclude malaria

- Stop prophylaxis until malaria excluded
- Empirical therapy for malaria should be avoided unless the patient is severely ill. Seek expert advice before commencing this (see contact numbers above)

Blood films daily for 2 more days

- Malaria is unlikely with 3 negative blood films. Consider other travel and non-travel illness
- Finish chemoprophylaxis

Non-falciparum antimalarials
Chloroquine (base) 600mg followed by 300mg at 6, 24 and 48 hours. In vivax and ovale after treatment of acute infection use primaquine (30mg base/day for vivax, 15 mg/day for ovale) for 14 days to eradicate liver parasites; G6PD must be measured before primaquine is given – seek expert advice if low

Falciparum antimalarials
Uncomplicated:
a) Oral quinine 600mg/8h plus doxycycline 200mg daily (or clindamycin 450mg/8hr) for 7 days
OR
b) Malarone® 4 'standard' tablets daily for 3 days
OR
c) Riamet® (if weight >35kg, 4 tablets then 4 tablets at 8, 24, 36, 48 and 60 hours

Complicated malaria = one or more of:
- Impaired consciousness (measure GCS and MSQ) or seizures — check blood glucose urgently
- Hypoglycaemia
- Parasite count ≥2% (lower counts do not exclude severe malaria)
- Haemoglobin ≤8g/dl
- Spontaneous bleeding/disseminated intravascular coagulation
- Haemoglobinuria (without G6PD deficiency)
- Renal impairment or electrolyte/acid-base disturbance (pH <7.3)
- Pulmonary oedema or adult respiratory distress syndrome
- Shock (algid malaria), may be due to Gram negative bacteraemia

Essential features of general management
- Commence antimalarials immediately (see boxes)
Severe malaria
- Consider admission to high dependency/intensive care
- Seek early expert advice from an infection or tropical unit
- Oxygen therapy
- Careful fluid balance (observe JVP, lying/sitting BP and urine output). Avoid hypovolaemia. Over-hydration may induce pulmonary oedema: consider CVP monitoring
- Monitor blood glucose regularly (especially during IV quinine)
- ECG monitoring (especially during IV quinine)
- 4-hourly observations until stable: pulse, temperature, BP, RR, SaO₂, Urine output & GCS. Regular medical review until stable
- Repeat FBC, clotting, U&Es, LFTs and parasite count daily
- In shock, treat for Gram negative bacteraemia

Falciparum antimalarials
Complicated or if patient is vomiting:
EITHER Quinine 20mg/kg loading dose (no loading dose if patient taking quinine or mefloquine already) as IVI in 5% glucose over 4hr and then 10mg/kg as IVI over 4h every 8 hr plus oral doxycycline 200mg daily for 7 days (In pregnancy, use IV/oral clindamycin 450mg/8hr). Max dose quinine 1.4 g

OR If available, artesunate intravenously 2.4mg/kg at 0, 12, 24 hrs then daily to complete a course of seven days plus doxycycline or clindamycin as above

When patient is stable & able to swallow, switch to oral quinine 600mg/8hr plus doxycycline 200mg daily (or clindamycin 450mg/8hr) to complete 7 days

BRITISH INFECTION SOCIETY   Health Protection   February 2007

K210

Fig. 10.3 Malaria assessment algorithm. Reproduced with permission from the Health Protection Agency.

:⚙: Viral haemorrhagic fevers

Viral haemorrhagic fevers (VHFs) are a group of illnesses endemic in Africa, South America, and various regions of Asia; the main complicating feature is haemorrhage. Suspected cases occur within 21 days of leaving endemic area. All cases should be discussed with an Infectious diseases specialist and instruction followed regarding isolation, handling of blood, and pathological specimens.

Causes

- Argentine, Bolivian, Brazilian, and Venezuelan haemorrhagic fevers.
- Crimean-Congo haemorrhagic fever (CCHF).[1]
- Dengue fever.
- Ebola.[1]
- Hantaan
- Kyasanur Forest disease.
- Lassa fever.[1]
- Marburg fever.[1]
- Olmsk haemorrhagic fever.
- Rift valley fever.
- Yellow fever.

Presentation and assessment

See Tables 10.2 and 10.3.

[1] These are considered high-risk infections as person-to-person spread can occur.

Table 10.2 Signs and symptoms of VHFs

Infection	Signs and symptoms
Crimean Congo haemorrhagic fever	High-grade pyrexia; malaise; headache; pain in limbs and loins; anorexia, nausea, vomiting and abdominal pain; haemorrhagic complications; CNS involvement occurs in 15–20% of cases.
Dengue fever	The 1st exposure leads to systemic illness resembling viral fever; the 2nd exposure to a different serotype leads to haemorrhagic complications.
	High-grade pyrexia; headache; joint pains; maculopapular rash.
	2nd exposure: haemorrhagic shock (presentation will depend on the site of bleeding and amount of blood loss).
Ebola virus fever	High-grade pyrexia; sore throat; headache; joint pains; abdominal pain; vomiting; maculopapular rash; haemorrhagic complications.
Lassa fever	High-grade pyrexia; sore throat (pharyngitis); retrosternal pain; proteinuria; haemorrhagic complications (presentation will depend on the site of bleeding and amount of blood loss).
Marburg fever	Similar to Ebola.
Yellow fever	In first 3 days of onset: high-grade pyrexia; headache; muscle pains; vomiting.
	In the following days: haemorrhagic complications; jaundice; relative bradycardia; renal failure; DIC; multi-system dysfunction.

Table 10.3 Viral haemorrhagic fevers

	Spread	Incubation period	Common area of origin
Crimean-Congo haemorrhagic fever	Contact with infected livestock or ticks Human to human transmission	1–12 days	East and West Africa, but also Dubai, Iraq, Pakistan, India, Turkey, Greece, Albania, Afghanistan
Dengue fever	Mosquito to human transmission It can also spread as an epidemic	3–15 days	Asia and Africa
Ebola virus fever	It can also spread as an epidemic Human to human transmission	2–21 days	Zaire, Sudan, Côte D'Ivoire, Gabon
Lassa fever	Rodent to human, human to human transmission	3–21 days	West Africa
Marburg fever	Human to human transmission	3–16 days	Uganda
Yellow fever	Mosquito to human transmission	3–15 days	Equatorial regions of Africa and South America

Investigations

(See also 📖 pp.324 and 365.)

If VHFs other than Dengue and Yellow fever are considered likely **do not take blood samples until authorized to do so** by an infection diseases expert. Investigations may include:

- ABGs (hypoxia or metabolic acidosis).
- FBC and differential (leucocytosis or leucopaenia may be present).
- ESR and CRP.
- G&S; sickle cell screen; G6 phosphate dehydrogenase deficiency screen.
- Coagulation screen.
- U&Es (renal failure may occur); LFTs.
- Serum CK, amylase, calcium, and glucose.
- Blood films (thick films are not recommended) to identify malaria.
- Diagnostic PCR and serological tests (paired testing of acute and convalescent sera is recommended).
- EBV screen.
- CXR.

Any samples must be classed as high risk and treated according to local protocols; the laboratory should liaise with the Health Protection Agency:
- Wherever possible closed sampling systems should be used.
- No fingerprick tests should be undertaken where VHF is suspected.
- The point-of-testing of samples (including ABGs) should be discussed with an infectious diseases expert.

Differential diagnoses
- Malaria (the commonest alternative diagnosis).
- Enteric fevers, leptospirosis.
- Chikungunya, rickettsial infections.
- Other differentials include rheumatic fever and viral hepatitis.

Immediate management
- Give O_2 as required, support airway, breathing, and circulation
- A full and detailed history should be taken, documenting any travel, contact with animals, outdoor activities, or medical work (including postmortem work)
- Isolation and protection should be implemented as an initial precaution (see 📖 p.382):
  - VHF agents with person-to-person spread (CCHF, Ebola, Lassa, Marburg) all require high-security isolation
  - Protective measure should include a protective gown and a waterproof protective apron; latex gloves; a particulate filter face mask; eye protection; the exception to this would be individuals in a deliberate aerosol release exposure zone (📖 p.384)
  - Scrupulous hand-washing is required as normal
  - Decontamination
- In severe toxaemia treat as septic shock (see sepsis 📖 p.118):
  - Severe shock is common and will require aggressive fluid resuscitation with/without vasopressors
- Ribavirin has been used for the treatment of Lassa fever and CCHF

Further management
- Supportive measures for sepsis are required.
- Continue assessment and management of complications, obtain haematological advice on blood and blood product replacement.
- The involvement of an infectious diseases specialist is essential.
- VHF infection is considered a notifiable disease, public health must be informed.
- Wherever possible within the UK patients should be managed in a high-security infectious diseases unit:
  - Coppetts Wood Hospital, North London
  - Newcastle General Hospital

Pitfalls/difficult situations

- Malaria must be excluded, but concurrent viral infection may occur.
- Toxaemia and haemorrhagic complications carry high mortality.
- Late transmission of Marburg and Lassa fever may occur.
- The disposal of dead bodies should be treated as a biohazard risk.

Further reading

Advisory Committee on Dangerous Pathogens. *Management and control of viral haemorrhagic fevers.* London: HMSO, 1996.

CDC Special Pathogens website: ℳ <http://www.cdc.gov/ncidod/dvrd/spb/index.htm>.

Stollenwerk N, et al. Bench-to-bedside review: Rare and common viral infections in the intensive care unit – linking pathophysiology to clinical presentation. *Crit Care* 2008; **12**(4): 219.

UK Health Protection Agency website: ℳ <http://www.hpa.org.uk/infections>.

:☼: Pandemic influenza and SARS

Pandemics occur when an infectious disease spreads through a population over a large geographical area. Many respiratory viruses have the potential to mutate and spread rapidly through populations who have little or no immunity to the new mutation. The WHO monitors influenza pandemics and in recent years declared the H1N1 subtype ('swine flu') to be at stage 6, global pandemic.

Viral pandemics are marked by rapid spread and ↑illness severity, in particular pneumonia. Mortality is ↑ in 'at-risk' groups, but it is often ↑mortality in younger patients that is most striking.

Other recent viruses that may still have the potential to develop into pandemics include H5N1 influenza A subtype ('avian flu'), and SARS-CoV (severe acute respiratory syndrome associated coronavirus).

Presentation and assessment

- Symptoms are often non-specific: fever, cough, sore throat, rhinorrhoea, myalgia, conjunctivitis, diarrhoea, and respiratory distress.
- Symptoms may initially be quite benign but it is the speed of deterioration to unresponsive hypoxia that is the hallmark of these diseases.
- Where there is respiratory involvement pneumonia of any cause should be considered (see 📖 p.334).
- Pandemic influenza strains may displace seasonal flu and be associated with younger patients (often <65 years), fever (>38°C), WCC (<12 × 10⁹), bilateral CXR changes, and absence of confusion.
- H5N1 influenza and SARS should be considered where there is a history of recent (<10 days) travel to an area where SARS may re-emerge (e.g. Honk Kong, mainland China, Vietnam), combined with fever, cough or respiratory distress, and CXR infiltrates.
- Contact with a patient suspected to have H5N1 influenza or SARS should also prompt consideration of the diagnosis.
- Close contact (<1 m) with potentially infected birds is also associated with H5N1 influenza.

Investigations

- ABGs.
- FBC (lymphopaenia is common).
- Coagulation studies (thrombocytopaenia, APTT may be ↑ in SARS).
- U&Es, LFTs (commonly deranged).
- Serum CK, serum CRP, and serum LDH (all often ↑).
- CXR (often initially normal but bilateral infiltrates common).
- Blood and sputum cultures (to exclude other infections).
- Urine and/or serum for *Legionella* and *Strep. pneumoniae* antigen.
- Nasopharyngeal swabs for viral PCR testing.
- Endotracheal aspirate or BAL (if patient's trachea has been intubated).
- SARS: serum for antibody testing, or sputum/nasopharyngeal aspirates for PCR.
- Influenza viruses: nasopharyngeal aspirate, throat swab, endotracheal aspirate or BAL for PCR, immunofluorescence or viral culture.

Differential diagnoses
- Pneumonia (community or hospital acquired).
- Other pneumonitis (e.g. varicella, chemical).
- Acute pulmonary oedema.
- ARDS.

Immediate management
- Give O_2 as required, support airway, breathing, and circulation.
- Treatment is supportive.
- Isolate patient and use strict infection precautions (see 🕮 p.382).
- Treat as for pneumonia (🕮 p.334).
- Early intubation is likely to be essential not only for maximal oxygen delivery but to allow full respiratory therapy to be given without the risk of contamination to staff.
  - Non-invasive ventilation is thought to increase spread of infected respiratory particles
  - A lung protective strategy is essential
  - A restrictive fluid administration regimen is thought to help, even in the presence of inotrope dependence
- Where hypoxia is refractory high frequency oscillator ventilation and prone positioning may aid oxygenation in the short term:
  - Consideration for early referral to a regional ECMO centre may be needed
- For H1N1 and H5N1 infections prescribe oseltamivir PO/NG 75 mg 12-hourly for 5 days. If critically ill, increase to 150 mg 12-hourly for 10 days.
  - Zanamivir IV may be available on a named-patient basis (inhaled zanamivir may be used in patients who are not ventilated but has been reported to 'clog' ventilators)

Pitfalls/difficult situations
- Pregnancy is associated with a higher mortality, as are other 'at risk' conditions (e.g. immunosuppression, diabetes mellitus; chronic respiratory, heart, liver, renal disease, and neurological conditions).
- Desaturation is often associated with a pneumothorax, which tend to be more common in this group of patients.
- Absorption of oseltamivir is not consistent in the critically ill patient and can have significant GI side effects.
- Steroid use remains controversial.
- Where immunization is available it should be provided for staff.
- 'Surge' and triage plans should be in place in case of a rapid increase in casualties, and a potential decrease of available staff (see 🕮 p.498).

Further reading
Beigel J. Influenza. *Crit Care Med* 2008; 36(9): 2660–6.
Centers for Disease Control and Prevention website: 🕾 http://www.cdc.gov/
Kamming D, et al. Anaesthesia and SARS. *Br J Anaesth* 2003; **90**(6): 715–18.
UK Health Protection Agency website: 🕾 <http://www.hpa.org.uk>
Writing Committee of the Second World Health Organization Consultation on Clinical Aspects of Human Infection with Avian Influenza A (H5N1) Virus, et al. Update on avian influenza A (H5N1) virus infection in humans. *N Engl J Med* 2008; **358**: 261–73.

ⓘ HIV and critical illness

Human immunodeficiency virus causes a chronic, incurable destruction of the immune system with consequential opportunistic infections causing acquired immune deficiency syndrome (AIDS).

The outcome of HIV-positive patients admitted to ITU with non-HIV related illnesses is the same as those who are HIV negative.

Causes

The viruses HIV1 and HIV2 both cause HIV infection and can be transmitted by sexual contact, blood-to-blood contact, mucous membrane contact, or vertical transmission. The following is a list of behaviours associated with a higher risk of contracting HIV, but it should be noted that there is a small but increasing group of individuals who acquire HIV infection through heterosexual sex in the UK.

* Men who have sex with men.
* IV drug abusers.
* People who have had sex with individuals from areas of high prevalence (e.g. sub-Saharan Africa).
* Sex workers.
* Health workers who suffer needlestick injuries.
* People who received transfusions of infected blood products (no longer a significant risk factor in Western countries).

Presentation and assessment

* Early HIV infection (CD4 count >350 at time of diagnosis).
* Late HIV infection (CD4 count of 200–350 at time of diagnosis).
* Very late HIV infection (CD4 count <200 at time of diagnosis).

The term AIDS is now rarely used unless describing one of the AIDS defining conditions.

Patients with HIV infection are likely to require critical care involvement because of:

* Diseases affecting immunocompetent individuals (HIV infection is incidental).
* Severe pneumonia (especially pneumocystis pneumonia,[1] PCP).
* Neurological disease (toxoplasmosis, cryptococcus, 1° CNS lymphoma and progressive multifocal leucoencephalopathy).
* Drug reactions:
  * NRTI drugs have been associated with: hepatitis, lactic acidosis bone marrow suppression, and pancreatitis
  * NNRTI drugs are associated with TEN (see 📖 p.422)
  * PI drugs are associated with GIT upset and pancreatitis
* Liver failure (hepatitis B or C co-infection can accelerate morbidity associated with HIV and increase the likelihood of liver failure).

---

[1] Also known as *Pneumocystis jiroveci.*

AIDS-related illness
- Candidiasis of bronchi, trachea, or lungs; or of the oesophagus.
- Cervical cancer, invasive.
- Coccidioidomycosis, disseminated or extrapulmonary.
- Cryptococcosis, extrapulmonary.
- Cryptosporidiosis, chronic intestinal (>1 month's duration).
- Cytomegalovirus disease (other than liver, spleen, or nodes).
- Cytomegalovirus retinitis (with loss of vision).
- Encephalopathy, HIV-related.
- Herpes simplex: chronic ulcer(s) (>1 month's duration); or bronchitis, pneumonitis, or esophagitis.
- Histoplasmosis, disseminated or extrapulmonary.
- Isosporiasis, chronic intestinal (>1 month's duration).
- Kaposi's sarcoma.
- Lymphoma, Burkitt's (or equivalent term).
- Lymphoma, immunoblastic (or equivalent term).
- Lymphoma, 1°, of brain.
- *Mycobacterium avium* complex or *Mycobacterium kansasii*, disseminated or extrapulmonary.
- *Mycobacterium tuberculosis* (pulmonary or extrapulmonary).
- *Mycobacterium*, other species or unidentified species, disseminated or extrapulmonary.
- *Pneumocystis jiroveci (carinii)* pneumonia (PCP).
- Pneumonia, recurrent.
- Progressive multifocal leucoencephalopathy.
- *Salmonella* septicaemia, recurrent.
- Toxoplasmosis of brain.
- Wasting syndrome due to HIV.

Adapted from *1993 revised classification system for HIV infection and expanded surveillance case definition for aids among adolescents and adults.* National Center for Infectious Diseases Division of HIV/AIDS.

Investigations
Investigations will vary according to presenting disease, but pneumonia and sepsis are very common and the following may be required:
- ABGs.
- FBC, coagulation studies.
- U&Es, LFTs.
- Serum CRP.
- HIV testing (see 📖 Pitfalls/difficult situations), CD4+ count, and HIV viral load.
- BAL (bacterial culture, immunofluorescence, atypical and fungal culture, TB, viral and PCP PCR).
- Consider serology for CMV, *Toxoplasma* and *Cryptococcus*.
- CXR (classically PCP has diffuse alveolar infiltrates; not always seen).
- CT or MRI head if there is a neurological presentation.
- LP (if ICP is not raised), send sample for protein, glucose, culture, Gram staining, Indian ink for *Cryptococcus*, TB, viral panel (e.g. HSV, EBV, VZV, J-C virus) cytology. Opening pressure measurement (important in the treatment of cryptococcal meningitis).

Immediate management

- Give O_2 as required, support airway, breathing, and circulation
- The treatment for all HIV related conditions is supportive.

PCP

- Suggested by dry cough, gradual onset of breathlessness, desaturation on exercise, and diffuse shadowing on CXR.
- NIV or mechanical ventilation may be required depending on the condition of the patient
- Pneumothoraces are common.
- If hypoxia (PaO_2<9.3 kPa or SpO_2 <92%) is present give:
  - Cotrimoxazole IV 120 mg/kg/day for 3 days, followed by 90 mg/kg/day for a further 18 days
  - Prednisolone PO (40 mg 12-hourly for 5 days, followed by 40 mg daily for 5 days, followed by 20mg daily for 11 days), or
  - If unable to take oral medications, methylprednisolone IV at 75% of this dose (i.e. 70mg daily for the first dose)[1]
  - Steroids are ineffective unless administered within 72 hours of commencing anti-PCP therapy
- Antibiotic therapy should also be provided which will cover common pneumonia-causing organisms as well, e.g. piptazobactam IV 4.5 g 8-hourly and clarithromycin IV 500 mg 12-hourly.
- Antifungal therapy may also be required.

Neurological disease

- Treatment and management is as for meningitis/encephalitis (📖 pp.188 and 340).
- Suggested empirical antimicrobials include ceftriaxone 2 g IV 12 hourly and amoxicillin IV 1 g 6-hourly and liposomal amphotericin B IV (dose depends upon formulation) and aciclovir IV 10 mg/kg 8-hourly.
- Where toxoplasmosis is suspected the treatment of choice is sulfadiazine PO (15 mg/kg 6-hourly) combined with pyrimethamine PO (200 mg loading dose then 50 mg/day) and folinic acid supplementation PO (10–15 mg/day).
- Where CMV encephalitis is suspected the treatment of choice is ganciclovir IV (5 mg/kg 12-hourly).

[1] There is significant variation within recent journal articles regarding the dose of methylprednisolone used for this indication, with some using up to 240 mg/day.

Further management

- Involve the HIV team early to help with diagnosis and management.
- Highly active anti-retroviral therapy (HAART) is occasionally given in the acute setting, and may prescribed by the HIV team:
  - Immune reconstitution inflammatory syndrome (IRIS) may occur in severely ill patients
  - Many medications are difficult to give (usually administered PO)
  - HAART drugs have multiple drug interactions
- PCP treatment may take up to 5–7 days to work. Second-line agents include clindamycin, primaquine, atovoquone, dapsone and pentamidine.

Pitfalls/difficult situations

- Infections may be unusual, multiple, or have atypical presentations.
- Consent is required for HIV testing. Where patients are unable to consent, but knowledge of the patient's HIV status is in the patient's immediate clinical interests (i.e. it is likely to affect differential diagnosis and treatment decisions) then testing may be undertaken.
- Disclosure of the HIV test results to close contacts at risk of the infection is allowed but should ideally wait until the patient is able to give consent; where the patient is unlikely to survive disclosure is also allowed—follow the advice of the local HIV team.
- Disclosure of HIV test results to relatives who are not at risk is not allowed, even after the death of the patient.
- Needlestick injuries—postexposure prophylaxis should not be delayed awaiting consent for HIV testing.
- TB is common in HIV patients and is more infectious.

Potential HIV exposure management

Potential HIV exposure can occur as a result of percutaneous injury (e.g. needlestick injury) or exposure of broken skin or mucous membranes to another body fluid. Non-blood stained saliva, urine, vomit, and faeces are *all considered safe*.

- Stop the procedure
- For skin injuries: encourage bleeding (do not suck wounds), wash wound with soap and water, and cover with a waterproof dressing
- For eye and mouth splash incidents: irrigate with plenty of water
- Complete an incident form
- Check the patient: are they considered to be at high risk of carrying HIV? For example, someone who is known to have:
  - HIV (or is ill with suspected HIV infection)
  - Had sexual contact with someone HIV+
  - Refused an HIV test
  - Used drugs
  - Had male homosexual sex
  - Worked in the sex industry
  - Lived in, or travelled to, Africa
- Contact Occupational Health or Infectious Diseases department, according to local guidelines. Their instructions may include:
  - Consenting patient for blood tests
  - Attend for blood testing yourself
  - Taking prophylactic retroviral therapy

Further reading

Corona A, et al. Caring for HIV-infected patients in the ICU in the highly active antiretroviral era. *Curr HIV Res* 2009; **7**(6): 569–79.

Dockrell DH, et al. Pulmonary opportunistic infections. *HIV Med* 2011; **12**(S2):25–42.

Nelson M, et al. Central nervous system opportunistic infections. *HIV Med* 2011; **12**(S2): 8–24.

⑦ **Notifiable diseases**

Registered medical practitioners who attend patients known, or suspected to have a notifiable disease have a statutory duty to notify a 'Proper Officer' of the Local Authority. Within hospitals, Microbiology, or Infectious Diseases, departments often do this. Notification should be sent to the Proper Officer within 3 days, or verbally within 24 hours if the case is considered urgent. Clinical *suspicion* of a notifiable infection is all that is required; do not wait for laboratory confirmation before notification.

List of notifiable diseases
- Acute encephalitis.
- Acute meningitis.
- Acute poliomyelitis.
- Acute infectious hepatitis.
- Anthrax.
- Botulism.
- Brucellosis.
- Cholera.
- Diphtheria.
- Enteric fever (typhoid or paratyphoid fever).
- Food poisoning.
- Haemolytic uraemic syndrome (HUS).
- Infectious bloody diarrhoea.
- Invasive group A streptococcal disease and scarlet fever.
- Legionnaires Disease.
- Leprosy.
- Malaria.
- Measles.
- Meningococcal septicaemia.
- Mumps.
- Plague.
- Rabies.
- Rubella.
- Severe acute respiratory syndrome (SARS).
- Smallpox.
- Tetanus.
- Tuberculosis.
- Typhus fever.
- Viral haemorrhagic fever.
- Whooping cough.
- Yellow fever.

List of causative agents

Bacillus anthracis; *Bacillus cereus* (only if associated with food poisoning); *Bordetella pertussis*; *Borrelia* spp.; *Brucella* spp; *Burkholderia mallei*; *Burkholderia pseudomallei*; *Campylobacter* spp.; Chikungunya virus; *Chlamydophila psittaci*; *Clostridium botulinum*; *Clostridium perfringens* (only if associated with food poisoning); *Clostridium tetani*; *Corynebacterium diphtheria*; *Corynebacterium ulcerans*; *Coxiella burnetii*; Crimean-Congo haemorrhagic fever virus; *Cryptosporidium* spp; Dengue virus; Ebola virus; *Entamoeba histolytica*; *Francisella tularensis*; *Giardia lamblia*; Guanarito virus; *Haemophilus influenzae* (invasive); Hanta virus; Hepatitis A, B, C, delta, and E viruses; Influenza virus; Junin virus; Kyasanur Forest disease virus; Lassa virus; *Legionella* spp.; *Leptospira interrogans*; *Listeria monocytogenes*; Machupo virus; Marburg virus; measles virus; mumps virus; *Mycobacterium tuberculosis* complex; *Neisseria meningitides*; Omsk haemorrhagic fever virus; *Plasmodium falciparum, vivax, ovale, malariae, knowlesi*; Polio virus (wild or vaccine types); Rabies virus (classical rabies and rabies-related lyssaviruses); *Rickettsia* spp.; Rift Valley fever virus; Rubella virus; Sabia virus; *Salmonella* spp.; SARS coronavirus; *Shigella* spp.; *Streptococcus pneumoniae* (invasive); *Streptococcus pyogenes* (invasive); Varicella zoster virus; Variola virus; Verocytotoxigenic *Escherichia coli* (including *E. coli* O157); *Vibrio cholera*; West Nile Virus; Yellow fever virus; *Yersinia pestis*.

Management

If a notifiable diseases is suspected the following must be submitted:

• Medical practitioner's name and contact details.
• Date of notification.
• Name, age, sex, ethnicity, and NHS number of the patient.
• The patient's address and contact details.
• The address of the premises where the patient is currently at.
• The patient's occupation and details of recent travel (if relevant).
• The patient's suspected disease or poisoning.
• The approximate date of onset and the date of diagnosis.
• The date of death if the patient has already died.

Further reading

The Health Protection (Notification) Regulations 2010. Available at: 🔗<http://www.hpa.org.uk>.

⑦ Infection control and isolation

Infection control procedures have a heightened significance within ICUs due to the relatively high proportion of both infected and immunocompromised patients. Detailed descriptions of infection control procedures are beyond the scope of this book, but some aspects common to ICU management are detailed here. Where there is any doubt as to how to manage a patient, hospital infection control teams should be involved.

Universal precautions

All staff should employ the following:
- Hand hygiene before and after any contact with patients or their immediate environment (hand washing or rubbing with alcohol gel).[1]
- Disposable gloves and protective equipment such as aprons for patient contact where fluid exposure is a risk (advisable for the majority of ICU patients).[2]
- Cohorting of staff and equipment to patients where possible.
- Appropriate disposal of 'sharps'.
- Staff with broken skin should cover breaks with waterproof dressings.
- Any contamination with body fluids (e.g. sharps injuries or blood splashes to eyes or mucous membranes) should be dealt with appropriately (see 📖 p.379).
- Items intended for single use should be used only once.

In addition, hospitals within the UK have adopted a 'bare below the elbows' policy where sleeves are rolled up, and wristwatches and jewellery are not worn.

Isolation

The ability to isolate patients within the ICU depends upon the available facilities. Where possible patients with the following should be isolated:
- Infections known to be easily transmissible within healthcare settings (e.g. *C. difficile*, norovirus, rotavirus).
- Easily transmissible airborne/droplet infections (e.g. influenza, SARS, TB, varicella zoster).
- Drug resistant organisms (e.g. MRSA, VISA/VRSA, ESBLs, multi-resistant *Pseudomonas* or *Acinetobacter*, VRE).
- Patients potentially infected with an epidemiologically important organism (e.g. patients transferred from another hospital; patients associated with a suspected outbreak).
- Patients requiring reverse-barrier nursing (e.g. immunocompromised patients).

Routine MRSA PCR screening of all ICU patients may allow early identification of those with incidental skin carriage, enabling isolation and decontamination (e.g. with topical treatments).

---

[1] Alcohol gel will not prevent the spread of *C. difficile* and its usage has been limited or stopped by some ICUs.
[2] For procedures where there is a high risk of blood contamination, full protective with gloves, gowns, facemasks, and eye-protection is advised.

Invasive procedures

Procedures that are performed within ICUs that are known to increase the risk of health-care associated infections include:
- Central venous catheterization.
- Peripheral cannula insertion and arterial line insertion.
- Mechanical ventilation after endotracheal intubation.
- Urinary catheterization.

'Care bundles' exist for many procedures in an attempt to decrease the risk of inadvertent inoculation of the patient with environmental or commensal organisms. It is often unclear which aspects of the bundle are efficacious, and so an all-or-nothing approach is advocated. Within the UK some care-bundles are termed 'high-impact interventions'.

Central venous catheter insertion bundles
- Full aseptic precautions should be used, which include hand washing, sterile gowns and gloves, and a sterile drape.
- Skin should be prepared using 2% chlorhexidine gluconate in 70% isopropyl alcohol.
- The subclavian site is the preferred point of access (femoral lines are the most susceptible to infection).
- Use of a sterile, semipermeable, transparent dressing to cover the insertion site—covering the insertion site with a chlorhexidine sponge may decrease the risk of infection (catheters with antimicrobial coatings may also decrease the incidence of catheter-related blood stream infection).
- Ongoing care should include aseptic technique when handling catheter lumens, and daily inspection of insertion site for evidence of infection.
- Removal of unused lines at the earliest opportunity.

Ventilator care bundles
- Elevation of the head of the bed to 30–40° (if possible).
- Oral hygiene with 1–2% chlorhexidine liquid or gel 6-hourly.[1]
- Tracheal cuff pressure maintained at 20–30 cmH$_2$O.
- Stress ulcer prophylaxis for high-risk patients only.
- Subglottic secretions are aspirated every 2 hours where an endotracheal or tracheostomy tube with an aspiration port has been used.[2]
- Patients are weaned from mechanical ventilation at the earliest safe opportunity—to facilitate this daily sedation holds should be undertaken where possible.

Endotracheal and tracheostomy tubes have been designed with various adaptations which are thought to decrease the incidence of VAP, these include cuffs which resist microaspiration, cuffs which maintain constant pressure, and silver-coated tubes.

[1] Selective decontamination of the digestive tract using oral and IV antimicrobials has been shown to reduce the incidence of VAP, but is not widely practised

[2] It has been suggested that patients who are expected to be intubated for >72 hours should have a tube with a subglottic port inserted.

Highly transmissible diseases

Diseases that are airborne or transmitted by small droplet particles can be easily transmitted to staff or other patients within the ICU environment, particularly during close contact (e.g. during endotracheal intubation), or if aerosol generating procedures are used (e.g. non-invasive ventilation. Diseases known to represent such a risk to a greater or lesser degree include:

• Influenza.
• SARS.
• Smallpox, monkey pox.
• TB.

Where the risk of transmission is associated with a high potential for morbidity (e.g. SARS, pandemic influenza) the following should be undertaken: isolation, avoidance of aerosol generating procedures, and strict adherence to PPE usage. The choice of facemask (surgical mask or FFP3 respirator) will depend upon the disease and the likelihood of aerosol contact; the infection control team should provide guidance.

Personal protective equipment guidelines

Donning PPE
• Put on a pair of non-sterile examination gloves.
• Put on a waterproof/water-repellent gown and apron ensuring that all ties are secure and clothing is completely covered.
• Put on disposable hair cover.
• Place mask on, ensuring that there is a good seal around the nose, sides and chin area (see later in list). Ask a 2nd person if present to check that there is a good fit.
• Put on eye protection, ensuring that they fit to the side of the head.
• Put on 2nd pair of non sterile gloves on and ensure they fit over the cuffs of the gown.

Correct fitting of a facemask
• Separate the 2 sides of the mask so the bottom is pulled out. Use the nose clip in the top panel to bend it into an approximate shape
• Place mask on the face by placing first under the chin. Lift the rest of the mask over the mouth and nose. Lift the headbands over the head with the upper band placed across the crown and the lower band below the ears.
• Adjust mask to produce a snug fit which is comfortable to wear.
• Shape the nose clip using both hands. Pinching the nosepiece with only one hand can result in less effective respirator performance.
• Cup both hands over the respirator. If the respirator is unvalved exhale sharply. If the respirator is valved inhale sharply. If air is felt around your nose re-adjust the nose piece.
• If air leaks at the sides, adjust the straps along the side of the head.

Removing PPE
• Rip the ties to the water-repellent gown and remove by rolling the gown forward, so as to turn inside out, removing the top set of gloves at the same time. Dispose of in the clinical waste bin.

- Remove eye protection and clean with alcohol (or dispose of if single use). If possible, use one hand to pull the eye protection forward from the centre and avoid touching the head.
- Remove facemask by breaking the ties. Remove hair cover. Dispose of both in clinical waste bin.
- Remove gloves:
  - Grasp outer edge near wrist
  - Peel away from hand, turning glove inside out
  - Hold in opposite gloved hand
  - Peel off 2nd glove, creating a bag for both gloves
  - Discard as clinical waste
- Clean hands using soap and water and/or an alcohol hand rub.

Dos and don'ts of PPE
- Work from Clean to Dirty.
- Limit opportunities for touch contamination, protect yourself, others and the environment:
  - Keep gloved hands away from face—do not touch your face or adjust PPE with contaminated gloves
  - Don't touch environmental surfaces except as necessary during patient care
  - Avoid touching or adjusting other PPE. Don't touch others unless necessary
  - Remove gloves if they become torn, perform hand hygiene before donning new gloves
- Discard PPE as clinical waste.

Reproduced from the Health Protection Agency Personal Protective Equipment guidelines, with permission.

Further reading

Department of Health. *Isolating patients with healthcare-associated infection. A summary of best practice.* London: Department of Health, 2007.

Marra AR, et al. Successful prevention of ventilator-associated pneumonia in an intensive care setting. *Am J Infection Control* 2009; **37**: 619–25.

Pronovost P, et al. An intervention to decrease catheter-related bloodstream infections in the ICU. *N Engl J Med* 2006; **355**: 2725–32.

Siegel JD, et al. *Guideline for isolation precautions: preventing transmission of infectious agents in health-care settings,* 2007. Available at: <http://www.cdc.gov/ncidod/dhqp/pdf/isolation2007.pdf>.

Surgical patients

① Postoperative sepsis

Patients commonly develop SIRS in the immediate postoperative period 2° to ↑cytokine levels caused by the surgical tissue trauma. This is normally a self-limiting response that subsides within 48 hours. Persistent SIRS, or the development of end-organ dysfunction, should prompt examination and investigations to elucidate the cause.

Causes

A number of factors predispose patients to developing postoperative sepsis, including:
- Preoperative:
  - Infection unrelated to the operation (e.g. LRTI, UTI)
  - Infection requiring surgery (e.g. bowel perforation, abscess)
  - Immunocompromised patients (e.g. RhA, malnutrition)
- Intraoperative:
  - Peritoneal contamination
  - Gut ischaemia (e.g. thromboembolism, volvulus)
  - Reperfusion injury (e.g. aortic cross-clamping)
  - GU surgery (especially if indwelling catheter/stent and/or mucosal damage by calculus or instrumentation)
  - Surgery of infected area (e.g. debridement of burns, incision and drainage of abscess)
- Postoperative:
  - Pneumonia (e.g. following thoracic/upper-GI surgery, prolonged immobility, or inadequate pain relief preventing deep breathing/coughing/mobilization)
  - Surgical wound infection

Presentation and assessment

(See also 🕮 p.322.)
- Pyrexia may be associated with other evidence of infection, including:
  - Tachypnoea, tachycardia, rigors, sweats
  - Complications of sepsis (see 🕮 p.322)
  - Raised WCC and inflammatory markers
- Features of sepsis and end-organ dysfunction may be present.
- After contaminated gut surgery, sepsis should be monitored for, particularly in the first 72 hours.

Investigations

- ABGs (metabolic acidosis, lactataemia suggest impaired perfusion).
- FBC (↑/↓WCC, ↑/↓ platelets).
- Coagulation screen (↑ APTT/PT and ↓ fibrinogen if DIC).
- CRP (raised in response to inflammation).
- Cultures:
  - Blood from indwelling lines and peripheral 'stab'
  - Samples from all drains and any effusions that can be tapped
  - Sputum: consider bronchoscopy/BAL
  - Urine: dipstick, MSU/CSU
  - Stool: C&S, *C. difficile* toxin if diarrhoea present
  - Wound swabs, if wound inflamed

- U&Es (raised urea/creatinine may suggest sepsis-induced AKI).
- LFTs (deranged if sepsis-induced hypoperfusion).
- Serum glucose, phosphate, magnesium, calcium.
- Serum amylase (raised in pancreatitis and other acute upper intra-abdominal conditions, e.g. cholecystitis).
- ECG (new onset AF).
- CXR (new shadowing/consolidation).
- Further imaging: consider US/CT of abdomen, pelvis, or chest (looking for evidence of perforation or collections) and plain films of joints if appropriate.

Differential diagnoses

- SIRS (no evidence of infection).
- MI (hypotension, tachycardia, hypoxia if LVF present, cool peripheries).
- PE (hypoxia, hypotension, tachycardia, cool peripheries).
- Haemorrhage (hypotension, tachycardia, cool peripheries).
- Ongoing ischaemia (e.g. bowel ischaemia).

Immediate management

(See also sepsis, 📖 p.325.)
- Give O₂ as required to maintain SpO₂ ≥95%, support airway, breathing, and circulation
- Invasive monitoring may be required to guide fluid management and deliver vasoactive support
- Keep the patient NBM initially in case surgery required
- Inform surgical team as urgent removal of infective source may be required
- Assess blood loss and crossmatch blood for transfusion if necessary

Further management

(See also sepsis, 📖 p.326.)
- Institute sepsis care management.
- Consider:
  - Open wound drainage
  - Continuous wound irrigation
  - Multiple laparotomies for repeated washouts
- In some conditions (e.g. necrotizing fasciitis) repeated surgical debridement may be required.
- Monitor for, and treat, complications of sepsis (e.g. AKI).

Pitfalls/difficult situations

- Multiple organ failure may occur if the source of infection is not aggressively treated.

Further reading

Monkhouse D. Postoperative sepsis. *Curr Anaesth Crit Care* 2006; **17**: 65–70.
Rivers E, et al. Early Goal-Directed Therapy Collaborative Group. Early goal-directed therapy in the treatment of severe sepsis and septic shock. *N Engl J Med* 2001; **345**: 1368–77.

① **Wound dehiscence**

This is partial or complete opening of the surgical wound. Presentation and management vary with the site.

Causes

Predisposing factors include:
- Wound infection.
- Poor surgical technique.
- Tension in the surgical incision site (ascites, ileus, obstruction).
- Bleeding/haematoma formation.
- Reduced tissue perfusion/oxygenation ('shock').
- Tissue oedema/poor tissue strength (obesity, hypoalbuminaemia, uraemia, heart failure, liver failure, chemotherapy, radiotherapy).
- Persistent coughing/vomiting.
- Diabetes.
- Smoking.
- Long-term or high-dose steroid use.
- Patient age >65 years.

Presentation and assessment

Early
- Open wound noticed at dressings change or removal of clips/sutures.
- Excessive soiling of dressings.
- Inappropriate pain.

Late
- Signs of shock: hypotension, tachycardia.
- Generalized sepsis.
- MOF/DIC.

Investigations

- ABGs (metabolic acidosis/↑ lactate suggest impaired tissue perfusion).
- FBC (↑/↓WCC, ↑/↓ platelets).
- Coagulation screen.
- U&Es (raised urea/creatinine may suggest sepsis or excessive fluid loss).
- LFTs (↓protein/albumin may occur with SIRS/malnutrition).
- Wound swabs.
- Blood cultures if there are signs of generalized sepsis.
- CXR or AXR may help identify alternate sources of infection.
- Further imaging: a CT scan or a US scan of wound area may detect any fluid collection, or other source of infection.

Immediate management

- Give O_2 as required to maintain $SpO_2 \geq 95\%$, support airway, breathing, and circulation.
- Invasive monitoring may be required to guide fluid management and deliver vasoactive support.
- Keep the patient NBM initially in case surgery required.

- Inform surgical team as urgent wound closure may be indicated.
- Assess blood loss and crossmatch blood for transfusion if necessary.
- Cover wound with sterile dressing.
- In mechanically ventilated patients consider deepening sedation or commencing neuromuscular blockade to decrease likelihood of expulsion of abdominal contents.

Further management

- Identify/avoid/treat any predisposing factors.
- Continued invasive monitoring and correction of:
  - Fluid status
  - Electrolytes
  - Coagulation status
- Antibiotic therapy may be required.
- Surgical management will be required:
  - Dressing changes as appropriate
  - Wounds may require debridement and/or closure (which may have to be delayed)
  - Drainage of any associated collection
- After re-closure of abdominal wound, pain relief will be extremely important; consider epidural infusion of local anaesthetics and opioids:
  - Involve the pain management team early
- Re-closure of abdominal wound may also cause splinting of diaphragm—respiratory support is likely to be required.

Pitfalls/difficult situations

- Sepsis and multiple organ failure may occur because the open wound is prone to infection. Strict sterile precautions are required.
- Insensible fluid losses may be difficult to assess.
- Patients are at high risk of developing resistant infections (e.g. MRSA, VRE, *C. difficile*).

Further reading

Menke NB, et al. Impaired wound healing. *Clin Dermatol* 2007; **25**: 19–25.
Penninckx FM, et al. Abdominal wound dehiscence in gastroenterological surgery. *Ann Surg* 1979; **189**(3): 345–52.

⚙ Major postoperative haemorrhage

The loss of blood from the site of surgery may be obvious (e.g. from drains) or concealed. Hypovolaemic shock rapidly leads to 2° organ impairment.

Causes

- Unnoticed haemostasis failure.
- Massive transfusion coagulopathy.
- Clip/suture migration.

Presentation and assessment

(See also Haemorrhage, 📖 p.112.)

- Blood loss in drains/blood-soaked dressings.
- Abdominal distension after intra-abdominal/pelvic surgery.
- Respiratory compromise following thoracic surgery.
- Signs and symptoms of compression near to the surgical site may appear (e.g. airway compression or compartment syndrome).
- Reduced GCS, raised ICP following neurosurgery.
- Clinical signs of hypovolaemic shock—hypotension, tachycardia,[1] vasoconstriction/reduced pulse pressure, oliguria, thirst, agitation.
- Development of organ failure is a late sign (e.g. reduced GCS).

Surgical drains

- Drainage >100 ml/hour over 3 hours should be reviewed, however:
  - Drains do not always drain
  - Large volumes of blood may be concealed in the abdomen/pelvis/ thorax
  - Abdominal signs may be unreliable in the post-op patient (i.e. if there is an epidural *in situ*)
- Decisions should be based on the clinical condition of the patient, not just the observed drainage.

Investigations

- Serial physical examinations.
- ABGs (metabolic acidosis, lactataemia suggest impaired perfusion).
- FBC (anaemia).
- Coagulation screen (↑APTT/PT, ↓ fibrinogen/platelets suggest DIC).
- Crossmatch blood/blood products as appropriate.
- U&Es (hyperkalaemia following massive transfusion).
- Ca^{2+} (may be ↓ following massive transfusion).
- ECG (cardiogenic shock from MI, right heart strain from PE).
- CXR (haemothorax).
- Consider imaging: US (unstable patient) or CT (stable patient).

Differential diagnoses

- Distributive shock (e.g. SIRS/sepsis, neuraxial blockade).
- Cardiogenic shock (e.g. MI, PE).

---

[1] Tachycardia may fail to develop in some patients.

Immediate management

(See also Haemorrhage, 🕮 p.112.)

- Give O_2 as required to maintain SpO_2 ≥95%, support airway, breathing, and circulation.
- Where peri-airway bleeding/swelling occurs, remove any clips and haematoma. Consider early endotracheal intubation (see 🕮 p.18).
- Intrathoracic bleeding may necessitate mechanical ventilation.
- Control any external bleeding with direct pressure.
- Call surgical team and haematologist/blood bank as required. Keep the patient NBM initially (in case surgery required).
- Restore intravascular volume using: crystalloids/colloids/blood (extra wide-bore peripheral access may be required).
- Aggressively correct any coagulopathy:
  - FFP (12 ml/kg) if PT or PTT > 1.5 × normal, or if >4 units of stored blood is transfused
  - Platelet concentrates (1–2 Adult Doses) if the count is <50 × 10⁹/L
  - Cryoprecipitate (1 pack/10 kg body weight) if fibrinogen <0.8 g/L
- Vasopressor/inotrope support may be required initially.
- Invasive monitoring will be required to guide fluid management—but should not delay urgent surgery.

Further management

- Continue with respiratory support until cardiovascular stability is established.
- Other haemostatic agents may be required:
  - Tranexamic acid (antifibrinolytic)
  - Vitamin K, prothrombin complex concentrate (warfarin reversal)
  - Protamine (heparin reversal)
  - Recombinant Factor VIIa
- Look for and manage other complications of massive transfusion:
  - Hypothermia (warm resuscitation fluids)
  - Hyperkalaemia, hypocalcaemia
  - Metabolic acidosis

Pitfalls/difficult situations

- Lack of improvement despite apparently adequate resuscitation should alert to:
  - Other sites of bleeding/continuing bleeding
  - Pneumothorax or cardiac tamponade
- Use of vasoactive support may mask ongoing hypovolaemia.
- Adhere strictly to the cross checking procedures for blood replacement to prevent inadvertent mismatched transfusion.
- Large volumes may be suddenly 'dumped' into drains on patient movement and do not necessarily indicate new/sudden haemorrhage.

Further reading

Dagi TF. The management of postoperative bleeding. *Surg Clin North Am* 2005; **85**(6): 1191–213.

:☺: Haemorrhage after cardiac surgery

Haemorrhage after cardiac surgery may be obvious (drains) or concealed (haemothorax). It may result in cardiac tamponade requiring chest re-opening on the ICU.

Causes
- Unnoticed failure of haemostasis.
- Rebound heparinization or post-bypass coagulopathy.
- Platelet dysfunction (2° to CPB and/or heparinization).

Presentation and assessment
- Haemodynamic instability, arrhythmias, shock.
- >400 ml blood loss in the first hour post-op, ongoing blood loss >100 ml/hour, >2 L blood loss in 24 hours post-op.
- Signs and symptoms of cardiac tamponade may rapidly appear (raised CVP/JVP, ↓ cardiac output, hypotension, acidosis).
- Clinical signs of hypovolaemic shock: hypotension, tachycardia,[1] vasoconstriction/reduced pulse pressure, oliguria, thirst, agitation.
- Development of organ failure is a late sign (e.g. reduced GCS).

Investigations
- ABGs (metabolic acidosis, lactataemia suggest impaired perfusion).
- FBC (anaemia).
- Coagulation screen (↑ APTT/PT, ↓ fibrinogen/platelets suggest DIC).
- TEG (if available offers rapid diagnosis of coagulation function).
- Crossmatch blood/blood products as appropriate.
- U&Es (hyperkalaemia following massive transfusion).
- Serum calcium (may be ↓ following massive transfusion).
- CXR (haemothorax, pneumothorax).
- Transthoracic/transoesophageal ECHO (tamponade, MI, LVF)
- Chest US (haemothorax, pneumothorax).

Differential diagnoses
- Cardiogenic shock (e.g. MI, PE, tension pneumothorax).
- Hypovolaemic shock (haemorrhage from elsewhere, e.g. GI bleed).
- Distributive shock (e.g. post-bypass SIRS).

Immediate management
- Give O_2 as required to maintain $SpO_2 \geq 95\%$, support airway and breathing (consider early endotracheal intubation).
- Restore intravascular volume using crystalloids/colloids/blood; extra wide-bore peripheral access may be required.
- Failure to respond/collapse/arrest are indications for chest reopening (see Fig. 11.1).
- Consider protamine IV (1 mg/kg) for rebound heparinization.

---

[1] Tachycardia may fail to develop in some patients.

Further management
- Continue with respiratory support until cardiovascular stability is established; vasopressor support may be required initially.
- Consider other haemostatic agents: tranexamic acid, aminocaproic acid (antifibrinolytics) or desmopressin (DDAVP).

Pitfalls/difficult situations
- Platelet dysfunction may not be revealed by standard coagulation screen; TEG may aid management of coagulopathy.
- Always involve haematology/blood bank for massive transfusions.
- Adhere strictly to cross-checking procedures.

Further reading
Dunning J, et al. Guideline for resuscitation in cardiac arrest after cardiac surgery. *Eur J Cardiothorcic Surg* 2009; **36**(1): 3–28.

Whitlock R, et al. Bleeding in cardiac surgery: Its prevention and treatment – an evidence-based review. *Crit Care Clinics* 2005; **21**(3): 589–610.

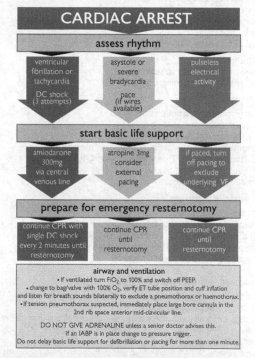

Fig. 11.1 Resuscitation after cardiac surgery algorithm. Reproduced with permission from the *European Journal of Cardiothoracic Surgery*.

:✪: TUR syndrome

TUR syndrome occurs when large volumes of hypotonic irrigating solution are absorbed rapidly into the circulation, resulting in rapid changes in serum osmolality and electrolyte concentrations. It most commonly occurs during transurethral resection of the prostate (TURP), but may be seen with bladder tumour resection (TURT), cystoscopy, lithotripsy, and transcervical endometrial resection (TCRE).

Causes
- Prolonged surgery.
- High irrigation pressures.
- Extensive surgical field.
- Inadequate haemostasis.

Presentation and assessment
Clinical features may include:
- Confusion, agitation, headache.
- Dyspnoea, tachypnoea, hypoxia.
- Hypertension.
- Nausea, vomiting.
- Visual disturbance, blurred vision.

Late signs include:
- ↓ level of consciousness, seizures.
- Hypotension, arrhythmias, cardiac arrest.

Investigations
- ABGs (hypoxia, metabolic acidosis).
- FBC (anaemia).
- U&Es (hyponatraemia).
- Ammonia (↑; major by-product of glycine metabolism).
- ECG (bradycardia, ST/T depression, wide QRS, SVT, VT).
- CXR (pulmonary oedema).
- Consider CT head if sodium normal.

Differential diagnoses
Other causes of respiratory failure/shock:
- Urosepsis (pyrexia, vasodilatory shock).
- MI (NSTEMI/STEMI, LVF, cardiogenic shock).
- PE (hypoxia, right heart strain, cardiogenic shock).
- Haemorrhage (hypovolaemic shock).

Immediate management
- Give O_2 as required to maintain SpO_2 ≥95%, support airway, breathing, and circulation.
- Hypoxia or frank pulmonary oedema may require treatment with external CPAP/NIV or endotracheal intubation and mechanical ventilation.
- Give furosemide IV 1 mg/kg (repeated doses may be required).
- Consider mannitol 50–100 ml IV if the patient is symptomatic but does not have pulmonary oedema.

- Correct hyponatraemia:
  - Raising the serum sodium concentration by 1 mmol/L/hour may be taken as a safe rate
  - Use saline 0.9% for gradual correction if Na^+ >120 mmol/L
  - Use hypertonic saline if Na^+ <120 mmol/L – ([body weight × 1.2] ml/hour of 3% saline should raise serum sodium by 1 mmol/L/hour)
- Correct hypokalaemia.
- Establish invasive monitoring in unstable patients.
- Consider bicarbonate if pH <7.2.
- Vasoactive support may be required if significant cardiac failure is present.
- Treat arrhythmias only if they are causing haemodynamic compromise (see 📖 pp.132 and 138).
- IV anticonvulsant therapy may be required if the patient has a seizure.

Further management
- Continue monitoring and correcting electrolyte imbalance.
- Consider renal replacement therapy if AKI 2° to prolonged hypotension occurs.
- Monitor for, and treat, hypothermia or DIC if they occur.

Pitfalls/difficult situations
- Neurological complications may lead to long-term sequelae (central pontine myelinolysis).
- Multiorgan failure may occur if the condition is not treated rapidly.

Further reading
Hahn RG. Fluid absorption in endoscopic surgery. *Br J Anaesth* 2006; **96**(1): 8–20.
Vijayan S. TURP syndrome. *Trends Anaesth Crit Care* 2011; **1**(1): 46–50.

:✪: **Bronchopleural fistula**

A bronchopleural fistula (BPF) is a communication between the pleural space and the bronchial tree. Although rare, BPFs represent a challenging management problem and are associated with important morbidity. After pulmonary resection, BPFs can be a life-threatening condition.

Causes

Predisposing factors to the development of postoperative bronchopleural fistulae include:

- Excessive/prolonged positive pressure ventilation after pulmonary resection.
- Infection of bronchial stump.
- Following empyema drainage.
- Patients who are immunocompromised or have poor tissue healing:
  - Following chemotherapy or radiotherapy
  - Steroids

Presentation and assessment

Clinical presentation is variable. Often subdivided into: acute, subacute, delayed, and chronic.

- Appearance of, or sudden increase in, air coming out from the chest drain on the side of operation.
- Subcutaneous (surgical) emphysema.
- Collapse of the remaining lung.
- Disappearance of post-pneumonectomy pleural effusion.
- Pneumothorax with or without tension (see 📖 p.80).
- Hypoxia.
- Dyspnoea and cough in awake patients.
- Persistent air leak in ventilated patients (this may result in an inability to deliver adequate tidal volumes using mechanical ventilation).
- Respiratory failure.
- Cardiovascular instability.

Investigations

- ABGs (hypoxia).
- FBC (raised WCC if infection present).
- CXR:
  - Subcutaneous (surgical) emphysema
  - Collapse of the remaining lung
  - Disappearance of post-pneumonectomy pleural effusion
  - Pneumothorax
- Consider CT scan in unclear cases.
- ECG (arrhythmias: AF, SVT if mediastinitis).

Differential diagnoses

Other causes of respiratory failure:

- MI (NSTEMI/STEMI, LVF, cardiogenic shock).
- PE (hypoxia, right heart strain, cardiogenic shock).

Immediate management

- Give O_2 as required to maintain SpO_2 ≥95%, support airway, breathing, and circulation.
- Exclude/treat any pneumothorax.
- Ensure patent intercostal drain.
- Positive pressure ventilation may be difficult to achieve:
  - Consider using larger than normal tidal volumes in the short term
  - Consider converting volume-controlled ventilation to pressure-controlled
- Involve the anaesthetist and the surgeon:
  - Bronchoscopy and insertion of a double-lumen tube may be required for independent lung ventilation (a range should be requested to be available: 37, 39, 41 Fr right or left sided)

Further management

- Repeated bronchoscopy may be required.
- Limiting ventilation pressures (PEEP, P_{INSP} and T_{INSP}) use of spontaneous breathing modes and weaning off positive pressure ventilation as soon as possible should be the initial goals.
- Treatment options of BPF include surgical procedures, as well as medical therapies such as glues, coils, or sealants.
- Surgical exploration and repair may be appropriate in cases of early BPF without obvious infection.

Pitfalls/difficult situations

- Maintenance of adequate tidal volumes may be difficult with standard ventilation strategies.
- High frequency oscillatory ventilation (HFOV) may allow ventilation to continue even in the presence of a large persistent air leak, and has been used with some success in difficult cases.

Further reading

Downs JB, et al. Treatment of bronchopleural fistula during continuous positive pressure ventilation. *Chest* (1976); **69**(3): 363–6.
Lois M, et al. Bronchopleural fistulas: an overview of the problem with special focus on endoscopic management. *Chest* 2005; **128**(6): 3955–65.

ⓘ **Postoperative pain**

Effective postoperative pain management not only minimizes patient suffering but also can reduce morbidity and facilitate rapid recovery and early discharge from hospital.

Postoperative pain can be divided into acute pain and chronic pain:
- Acute pain is experienced immediately after surgery (up to 7 days).
- Pain which lasts >3 months after the injury is considered to be chronic pain.

Causes

In general:
- Upper abdominal surgery and thoracic surgery cause severe pain.
- Major joint surgeries also cause significant pain, especially on mobilization.
- Unstabilized fractures are often severely painful.

A number of factors may predispose to ↑ postoperative pain:
- Pain tolerance of an individual patient.
- Opiate tolerance from preoperative exposure.
- Wound infection/wound tension.

Certain groups of patients are at ↑ risk of inadequate pain control, including paediatric patients, elderly patients, and patients with communication difficulties. Pain normally diminishes gradually over the first 72 hours following surgery.

Presentation and assessment

The awake, communicative patient will complain of pain, particularly during movement and coughing. Associated signs and symptoms are:
- Anxiety, agitation.
- Signs of sympathetic overactivity (sweating, tachycardia, hypertension, peripheral vasoconstriction).
- Tachypnoea, inadequate tidal volumes and respiratory insufficiency (particularly after abdominal/thoracic surgery).
- Inability to cough and/or mobilize.

Persistent inadequate analgesia can lead to:
- Depression, delirium.
- Respiratory failure.
- Poor mobility and/or delayed recovery.
- Impaired immunity and/or poor wound healing.

Differential diagnoses/investigations

Pain, especially when new, may be non-surgical in origin, consider investigating the following:
- Chest or abdominal pain: MI/angina, PE, pneumonia.
- Shoulder tip pain: diaphragmatic irritation (perforation/pneumothorax).
- Increasing abdominal pain: consider anastomotic leak, bowel ischaemia, obstruction, pancreatitis.
- Leg pain: compartment syndrome, ischaemia, DVT.

Immediate management
- Follow local guidelines, and involve the acute pain management team
- Analgesia should have been started intraoperatively and should be planned to continue into the postoperative period
- Evaluate and treat both the pain and the patient's response to treatment, and re-evaluate regularly (e.g. 4–8-hourly)
- Use a scoring system to assess pain (typically a 10 point verbal rating score where 0 is 'no pain' and 10 is 'severe pain'). Define the maximum pain score at which pain relief is offered (intervention threshold), for example, a verbal ratings score of 3 at rest and 4 on moving. As a minimum, patients must be able to cough and breathe deeply
- Prescribed regular adjunctive analgesics alongside opioids or regional techniques: paracetamol, gabapentin, and NSAIDs if appropriate

Parenteral opioids
- Patient-controlled analgesia (PCA) is the commonest mode of opioid delivery after major surgery
  - Check that the patient can use the handset, and understands the best way to use it
- Consider a bolus of opioid, discuss with the anaesthetist/pain team
- Give prophylactic antiemetics if required
- Monitor for sedation or respiratory depression
  - Remove the handset from any over-sedated patient.

Epidurals (or other regional anaesthesia infusions)
- Epidurals are normally a combined low-dose local anaesthetic (LA) (e.g. bupivacaine 0.125%) and opioid (e.g. fentanyl 4 µg/ml)
- Avoid concomitant IV opioids unless under specialist advice and in critical care environment
- If there is an inadequate block, check:
  - Height of block: if too low give bolus from the infusion and increase the rate
  - 'Depth' of block: if inadequate consider top-up of stronger LA
  - Unilateral block: consider withdrawing catheter and top-up with patient in lateral position ('unblocked' side down)
  - No block: consider resiting epidural
- Significant epidural-induced hypotension should be treated with fluids and/or vasopressor support, as appropriate

Further management
- Epidural sites should be checked daily: remove epidural if there are concerns about possible site infection. Site should be swabbed, catheter tip sent for culture, and, if possible, sample fluid should be aspirated from the catheter for culture.

Pitfalls/difficult situations
- Consider temporarily stopping epidural infusions if aggressive resuscitation for hypotension is required.
- LMWH doses should postponed if an epidural is due to be removed or resited.

- Stop epidural infusions if new arm or respiratory weakness occurs.
- A loss of leg motor and sensory function in patients with a thoracic or lumbar epidural may indicate an epidural haematoma or abscess; urgently inform the anaesthetic/acute pain teams.

Further reading

De Andres J et al: In consultation with European Society of Regional Anaesthesia and Pain Therapy (ESRA). *Postoperative pain management – good clinical practice general recommendations and principles for successful pain management.* ESRA, 2009.

Maund E, et al: Paracetamol and selective and non-selective non-steroidal anti-inflammatory drugs for the reduction in morphine-related side-effects after major surgery: a systematic review. *Br J Anaesth* 2011; **106**(3): 292–397.

Stone M et al. Patient-controlled analgesia. *BJA CEPD Rev* 2002; 79–82.

Chapter 12

Trauma, burns, and skin injury

☀ Trauma

Trauma is the biggest killer in the UK of those under the age of 45. Trauma deaths can be divided into 3 phases: those that occur at the time of injury, those that occur in the first few hours (and are largely preventable) and those occurring weeks later.

Critical care involvement may include:
• At the accident scene as part of a medical emergency response team (MERIT).
• In the ED as part of a trauma team.
• Receiving the trauma patient from theatre.
• Caring for the patient on the ICU.
• Admitting patients with complications from the ward.

Causes

Causes of trauma can be categorized into blunt and penetrating (most trauma in the UK is blunt). Knowledge of the mechanism of injury can help predict injury patterns.

Blunt mechanisms
• Road traffic collisions:
  • Pedestrian versus car; car versus car; motor bike accident (MBA)
  • Ejection from car; turned-over car
  • Fatality of others at the scene of the accident
  • Intrusion into the 'cockpit' of >30 cm
• Falls from height (>3 m, or 5 stairs); fall from a horse.
• Sporting injuries.
• Assaults.

Penetrating mechanisms
• Stabbings.
• Gunshot wounds (GSWs).
• Impalement.

Any patient with a significant mechanism should be transported to a major trauma centre where a trauma team is on standby to receive them.

Life-threatening injuries may have already been identified and managed in the 1° survey in the ED and operating theatre prior to the patient's admission to critical care. However, new pathologies can develop, or old ones recur. Always return to the ATLS style of management should a trauma patient become unstable.

Limb-threatening injuries (i.e. compartment syndrome) may not have been identified prior to ICU admission, or may have developed during resuscitative measures.

Life-threatening injuries

• Airway obstruction (e.g. laryngeal or tracheal injury):
  • Head injury with impaired consciousness
• Breathing injuries:
  • Pneumothorax (tension, open), or massive haemothorax
  • High spinal injury
  • Flail chest

- Cardiac injuries (tamponade or cardiac contusion).
- Severe haemorrhage:
  - Major arterial damage
  - Intra-abdominal bleeding
  - Pelvic fracture or bilateral femoral fractures
  - Acute coagulopathy of trauma
- Intracranial lesions.
- Hypothermia.

Limb-threatening injuries

- Traumatic amputation.
- Vascular injury/compromise.
- Open fracture.
- Compartment syndrome.
- Crush injury.

Approach

Assessment of trauma patients should follow a set routine, elucidating and treating life- and limb-threatening injuries as they are found, in the order in which they will harm the patient (an 'ATLS approach'). In all cases it is essential to ensure that those treating the patient are safe to carry out their work.

A 1° survey (following the ABC format) should be performed and life-threatening injuries treated simultaneously. For example, if there is catastrophic haemorrhage (e.g. major blast/ballistic injury, or traumatic amputation) the 1° survey is be modified to deal with this first.

Trauma primary survey: ABC approach

Primary survey

- Airway (and C-spine or other spinal immobilization)
- Breathing (and ventilatory control)
- Circulation (and haemorrhage control)
- Disability (and neurological care)
- Exposure (and temperature control)

Obtain a history and detailed information; the minimum should include an 'AMPLE' history (📖 p.2).

Obtain information from the patient, relatives, or paramedics concerning the mechanism of injury

Immediate investigations and decision-making

- Bloods, including crossmatch and β-HCG as needed
- CXR
- Pelvic X-ray
- Consider rapid US scan (focused assessment with sonography for trauma, 'FAST' scan)
- Decision-making: is there a need for urgent transfer (e.g. for a CT scan, urgent surgery, transfer to a major trauma centre)?

Immediate management

- Give 100% O_2, commence pulse oximetry, ECG, and BP monitoring.
- Commence C-spine/spinal control (Fig. 12.1).
- Perform 1° survey, initial resuscitation, and investigations.
- Obtain an AMPLE history (📖 p.2).

Primary survey

Airway

- Examine for: airway obstruction: ↓ conscious level, foreign body/matter, expanding neck haematoma, laryngeal fracture, stridor.
- If obstruction is present perform a jaw thrust and insert an oro/nasopharyngeal airway if required (chin lift and head-tilt should be avoided in patients with suspected C-spine injuries):
  - Avoid nasopharyngeal airways if BOS fracture is suspected
- Where obstruction is present, or likely to occur, consider endotracheal intubation or an emergency needle cricothyroidotomy/tracheostomy (see 📖 pp.522 and 528).

Breathing

- Look for evidence of respiratory compromise: hypoxia (reduced PaO_2 or SaO_2), dyspnoea, and/or tachypnoea, absent or abnormal chest movement, loss of chest wall integrity (flail segment), pulmonary aspiration, massive bleeding.
- Exclude/treat life-threatening conditions (e.g. tension pneumothorax, massive haemothorax[1]).
- Consider endotracheal intubation and mechanical ventilation in patients with actual or imminent respiratory distress.

Circulation

- Look for evidence of circulatory inadequacy: tachycardia, weak pulse, hypotension, cold peripheries, prolonged capillary refill (>2 seconds, but difficult to interpret in associated hypothermia).
- Look for obvious or concealed blood/fluid loss: palpate the abdomen, feel for blood pools (flanks, hollow of neck/back, groin), look for pelvic instability, look for long-bone fractures.
- Exclude life-threatening conditions such as cardiac tamponade (raised CVP/JVP, pulsus paradoxus, diminished heart sounds, low voltage ECG), tension pneumothorax,[2] haemorrhage or arrhythmia:
  - Assess degree of shock (📖 p.104)
  - Establish wide-bore IV access (2 × 16G cannulae), if not possible consider intraosseous or central access (📖 pp.536 and 542)
- Commence fluid/blood replacement and treatment of hypovolaemic shock; give 500 ml of colloid within 5–10 minutes and reassess:
  - Follow a major haemorrhage protocol (📖 p.115)
  - Permissive hypotension (📖 p.106) may be appropriate in some cases whilst awaiting definitive haemorrhage control

---

[1] The insertion of a chest drain to treat massive haemothorax may precipitate further catastrophic haemorrhage, obtain IV access first and have IV fluids prepared.

[2] Tension pneumothorax may present as a respiratory or circulatory emergency.

- Various initial resuscitation targets in trauma exist, one example is:
  - Head injury: systolic of 90 mmHg
  - Blunt trauma: systolic of 90 mmHg
  - Penetrating injury: systolic of 60–70 mmHg
  - Pre-existing hypertension: patient's usual MAP
- Haemorrhage control may require:
  - Direct pressure, or indirect pressure (e.g. femoral artery)
  - Elevation (where possible)
  - Wound packing
  - Windlass dressing, or tourniquets where required
  - Novel haemostatic agents (e.g. Celox®, Quickclot®)

Disability/neurology
- Rapidly assess the patient's neurological status using GCS or AVPU (**A**lert, responds to **V**oice, responds to **P**ain or is **U**nresponsive).
- Check for pupil signs and plantar responses.
- Check for Battle's sign and scalp, nose, or ear haemorrhage; perform otoscopy now or during 2° survey.

Exposure/general
- Measure the patient's core temperature:
  - Rewarming should be commenced if required[3]
- Establish full exposure of affected area.
- Provide analgesia as required.

[3] Where ROSC has occurred following cardiac arrest, active warming may be inappropriate.

Investigations
- ABGs may aid resuscitation.
- Finger-prick blood sugar test should be measured.
As soon as IV access is established take the following blood tests:
- Crossmatch.
- FBC (bedside Hb tests may be available).
- Coagulation test (especially during haemorrhage resuscitation; bedside coagulation screen may be available).
- U&Es, LFTs.
- Serum glucose.
- Consider paracetamol, salicylate, alcohol levels.
- βHCG (in women of childbearing age).
Also consider:
- Bench co-oximetry for carbon monoxide.
- ECG.
- Where severe abdominal bleeding is suspected consider performing diagnostic peritoneal lavage (DPL) to confirm the presence of blood (where scanning is not available).
Imaging of major trauma should include:
- Lateral C-spine, CXR, pelvis X-ray.
- Other long bones may be X-rayed as clinically indicated.
- AP and 'peg' views of the C-spine may also be considered, but CT of neck may be more appropriate (see pp.182 and 408).

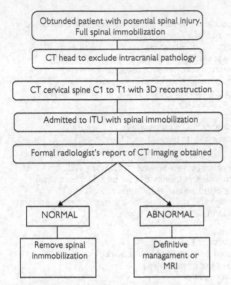

Fig. 12.1 Algorithm for ICU C-spine clearance. From Harrison P, et al. Clearing the cervical spine in the unconscious patient. *Continuing Education in Anaesthesia, Critical Care and Pain* 2008; 8: 117–20, by permission of Oxford University Press.

- CT of head, chest, neck, or abdomen/pelvis may be required.
- Rapid US scanning may be available to detect haemorrhage; FAST scan can be used to *rule in* pericardial, hepato-renal, spleno-renal and pelvic haemorrhage.

Other imaging that may be required:
- Long-bone X-rays.
- CT angiography.
- Retrograde urethrogram.

Chest X-ray findings associated with traumatic aortic disruption

- Widened mediastinum
- Distorted, poorly defined aortic knuckle
- Tracheal deviation (to the right)
- Loss of space between the pulmonary artery and the aorta
- Depression of the left main bronchus
- Oesophageal/nasogastric tube deviation (to the right)
- Paratracheal striping
- Left haemothorax

- Fractures of ribs 1 or 2; scapula fractures
- Pleural or apical caps
- Widened paraspinal interfaces

Specific injuries involving critical care

Spinal cord injuries

- In major trauma all patients should initially be assumed to have a spinal injury and spinal precautions used including hard collar, sand bags, head strapping, and log-rolling:
  - The patient must be moved from the long board, once stable, onto a mattress to prevent early pressure sores developing
- High spinal injuries (C1–C3) may present with dyspnoea, accessory muscle use, and ventilatory failure, necessitating early endotracheal intubation and ventilation:
  - Suxamethonium is safe to use within the first 48 hours of a spinal injury; once muscle atrophy occurs there is a risk of hyperkalaemia
- Spinal shock and autonomic disruption may occur; other causes of hypotension such as occult haemorrhage should be excluded:
  - Spinal shock may require vasopressors
  - Bradycardia may occur
- There is controversy about the use of high-dose steroids within the first 8 hours of spinal cord injuries: if used give methylprednisolone IV 30 mg/kg in 15 minutes, then 5.4 mg/kg/hour for 23 hours.
- Where it has not been possible to rule out spinal cord injury in an unconscious patient admitted to the ICU, carry out the investigations recommended on 📖 pp.182 and 408.
- Thermoregulation: patients are unable to regulate body temperature and require warming in the early phase of the injury.
- Urinary retention: all patients require catheterization.
- Autonomic dysreflexia: sudden peripheral stimuli may precipitate hypertensive crises.
- Considerations for the long-term care of paralysed patients may be found on 📖 p.197.

Airway damage

(See 📖 p.28.)

Pneumothorax/tension pneumothorax

(See 📖 p.80.)

- Open chest wounds have the potential to cause lung collapse and impaired gas exchange; sealing them completely risks development of a tension pneumothorax:
  - They should be sealed on 3 sides, with 1 side left free to allow air to escape; alternatively use Asherman or Bowlin chest seals.

Haemothorax

(See 📖 p.82.)

- This may occur early, at the time of the injury, or late if intercostal vessels are damaged by fractured ribs.

Rib fractures, flail chest, pulmonary contusion
- Severe pain may limit the ability of the patient to cough or deep breathe; a thoracic epidural may be required for pain relief:
  - Atelectasis and pneumonia may occur as a late complication of rib fractures, especially where respiration is limited by pain
- The presence of rib fractures increases the likelihood of pneumothoraces, especially in mechanically ventilated patients.
- The presence of multiple rib fractures, especially the upper 3–4 ribs, is associated with underlying lung, mediastinal, and C-spine injury.
- Flail chest occurs when a segment of chest wall loses continuity with the rest of the bony structure (usually as a result of 2 fractures) and effectively 'floats free':
  - In normal respiration the chest can expand and generate a negative pressure, where a flail segment is present *it* may be sucked in by the negative pressure, rather than air through the airways
- Paradoxical breathing may be obvious (flail segment moving in with respiration).
- Dyspnoea, tachypnoea may be present.
- Endotracheal intubation and mechanical ventilation are likely to be required.
- Pulmonary contusions may develop in the first 24 hours after blunt chest injury causing characteristic CXR changes:
  - Lung injuries with associated rib, T-spine, or clavicular fractures are more likely to be affected
  - Increasing O_2 requirement may indicate the need for endotracheal intubation and mechanical ventilation

Cardiac tamponade
(See 📖 p.146.)

Cardiac contusion
- Cardiac contusion may occur as a result of blunt chest injuries.
- Hypotension and ECG changes may occur: arrhythmias, VEs, sinus tachycardia, AF, RBBB, ST segment changes.
- ECG monitoring should be continued for 24 hours as severe arrhythmias may develop.
- Severe right-sided contusions may result in a raised CVP.
- Myocardial ischaemia may have *precipitated* the trauma.
- A troponin rise is common and does not usually represent ischaemic damage to the myocardium.
- Contusion usually settles without significant cardiac comorbidity.

Aortic disruption
- Rapid deceleration injuries affecting the chest may cause disruption of the great vessels, which may initially be contained by haematoma.
- Hypotension is normally caused by another bleeding site (as rapid aortic bleeding is mostly fatal).
- The presence of CXR changes (see 📖 p.408) should prompt CT angiography or TOE.
- If suspected, obtain vascular or cardiothoracic surgical advice.
- Avoid surges in BP; infusions of hypotensive agents such as labetalol or esmolol may be required.

Shooting
- 'Low'-velocity (handgun bullets) injuries cause damage along the bullet track; 'high'-velocity (rifle bullets) injuries may cause extensive cavitation areas within the wound.
- Entrance/exit wound size does not predict the degree of wound cavity.
- Bullet or bone fragments may cause further damage.
- The wound tract will be soiled by environmental contaminants:
  - Wound exploration, debridement and excision may be undertaken; delayed 1° suture (DPS) is likely to be necessary
- Antibiotic prophylaxis should be given.

Major haemorrhage
(See 📖 p.112.)
- Common sites of haemorrhage include: external wounds (blood on the floor), intrathoracic, abdominal/retroperitoneal (usually solid organ injury), pelvic fractures (especially 'open book'), femurs (can lose 1.5 L of blood each), scalp (especially in children).
- Diagnostic adjuncts for managing haemorrhage may include US or CT scanning (if the patient is stable enough to go to scan).
- Pelvic fractures should be splinted with a pelvic binder.
- Femoral fractures should be splinted with longitudinal traction.
- Open, or scalp, wounds may require temporary suture.
- Use a major haemorrhage protocol (📖 p.115).
- Following initial haemorrhage and hypoperfusion, an acute coagulopathy of trauma can occur; thromboelastography can help guide haemostatic resuscitation with blood coagulation products.
- Tranexamic acid may be given (1 g IV bolus followed by 1 g IV over 8 hours).
- Correction of hypothermia will improve haemostasis.

Intra-abdominal haemorrhage
- Intra-abdominal haemorrhage should be suspected in hypotensive victims of major trauma, especially where there is penetrating abdominal trauma, blunt trauma causing external abdominal bruising, signs of peritoneal irritation, haematuria, thoracolumbar fractures, pelvic fractures, or lower rib fractures.
- Investigations may include:
  - Laparotomy (or laparoscopy)
  - US of abdomen
  - Diagnostic peritoneal lavage (positive if ≥100,000 RBC/mm³, ≥500 WBC/mm³, bacteria present on Gram stain)
  - CT abdomen

Traumatic amputation
- Major traumatic amputations are particularly seen during ballistic injuries; there is extensive tissue disruption, major bony bleeding, and exposed blood vessels.
- Tourniquets applied on-scene at sites proximal to the amputation site can be life saving; they should only be removed by a surgeon as part of damage control surgery.

Traumatic brain injury
(See 🕮 p.178.)

Traumatic cardiac arrest
(See 🕮 p.98.)
- Cardiac arrest 2° to trauma has a poor prognosis.
- Management involves identifying/treating reversible causes:
  - Airway obstruction (requiring a definitive airway)
  - Tension pneumothorax (requiring decompression)
  - Cardiac tamponade (requiring pericardiocentesis and/or emergency thoracotomy)
  - Major haemorrhage (requiring haemostasis and resuscitation with blood and blood products)

Further management
- Once the patient has been stabilized a *2° survey* should be undertaken (a full history and head-to-toe examination looking for less severe injuries, some of which may still be limb threatening):
- Head:
  - Examine eyes, ears, nose, mouth, scalp, face, cranial nerves
- Neck and back (patient usually requires a log roll):
  - Examine for 'steps' or bony tenderness
  - Anal tone should be tested if spinal injury suspected
  - May be done early on to remove patient from spinal immobilization boards
- Chest, abdomen, and pelvis:
  - To identify simple pneumothorax, rib fractures, wounds
  - To monitor for signs of visceral perforation
  - Review the pelvis X-ray (avoid 'springing' the pelvis)
  - Examination of genitalia
- Full skeletal examination, looking for wounds, tenderness, and suspected fractures; X-rays as required.
- Check tetanus status.

Damage control surgery
- Damage control surgery is a combined anaesthetic and surgical concept which involves doing the minimum to the patient required to prevent bleeding and decontaminate wounds.
- Once physiology is stabilized, end-organ perfusion restored and acidaemia/temperature/clotting corrected, further staged surgical management may take place.

A *tertiary survey* should be undertaken once the patient has been resuscitated and is finally stabilized on the ward/ICU. On average, 10% of major trauma patients will have a missed injury. Commonly missed issues/injuries include:
- A history of comorbid illness.
- Eyes: corneal abrasions, contact lenses, vitreoretinal haemorrhage.
- Ears: tympanic perforation.
- Teeth: dental trauma.

- Wrist/hands: bony fractures (e.g. metacarpals, scaphoid):
  - Rings/jewellery should be removed to prevent distal ischaemia and pressure necrosis
- Foreign bodies, from the scene or from ED (e.g. caps or bungs which may cause pressure wounds)
- Compartment syndrome.

Pitfalls/difficult situations

- Missed injuries are common in the first 48 hours.
- Nerve damage is often difficult to detect in a sedated patient, a high level of suspicion should be maintained depending upon the mechanism of injury (penetrating/crushing trauma), or associated injuries (fractures/dislocations).
- Arterial injury usually presents with a cold, pale, pulseless limb; treatment may involve simply re-aligning a fractured limb, or vascular surgery.
- Compartment syndrome is often difficult to detect in sedated patients; a high level of suspicion must be maintained when there are high-risk injuries present (forearm/leg fractures, crush injuries).
- The tetanus immunization status of the patient should be established in case a further booster injection is required.
- Trauma may be associated with worse outcomes in the elderly, pregnant, malnourished; or those with severe comorbidities.
- Increasing inotropic requirements may indicate developing SIRS or occult haemorrhage or injury (e.g. tension pneumothorax).
- The signs of an acute abdomen may not be present, especially where a patient has been given neuromuscular blockade for endotracheal intubation and mechanical ventilation.
- Medical conditions may coexist with, or cause, trauma, including:
  - Alcohol intoxication
  - Syncope/seizures from any cause, especially SAH or cardiac arrhythmias
  - Diabetic hypoglycaemia

Further reading

American College of Surgeons Committee on Trauma. *ATLS Guidelines*, 8th edn. Chicago, IL: ACS, 2008.

Brooks A, et al. Missed injury in major trauma. *Injury* 2004; **35**(4): 407–10.

CRASH-2 trial collaborators. Effects of tranexamic acid on death, vascular occlusive events, and blood transfusion in trauma patients with significant haemorrhage (CRASH-2): a randomised, placebo-controlled trial. *Lancet* 2010; **376**(9734): 23–32.

CRASH-2 trial collaborators. The importance of early treatment with tranexamic acid in bleeding trauma patients: an exploratory analysis of the CRASH-2 randomised controlled trial. *Lancet* 2011; **377**(9771): 1096–101.

Deitch EA, et al. Intensive care unit management of the trauma patient. *Crit Care Med* 2006; **34**(9): 2294–301.

Houshian S, et al. Missed injuries in a level 1 trauma centre. *J Trauma* **52**(4): 715–19.

Morris CGT, et al. Clearing the cervical spine in unconscious polytrauma victims, balancing risks and effective screening. *Anaesthesia* 2004; **59**: 464–82.

Mowery NT, et al. Practice management guidelines for management of hemothorax and occult pneumothorax. *J Trauma* 2011; **70**(2): 510–18.

Smith J, et al. *Oxford desk reference of major trauma*. Oxford: Oxford University Press, 2010.

:⚙: Drowning

Drowning occurs after immersion in liquid resulting in cardiac arrest, or severe injury which may require critical care support. 'Near-drowning' is a term which has been used to describe cases who survived.

Causes

Drowning is associated with:
- Rural/coastal areas (especially where fishing or tourism are prevalent).
- Floods.
- Drug and alcohol use.
- Suicide or assault.
- Trauma, hypothermia, coexistent neurological, or cardiac injury.

There is little clinical difference between drowning in fresh or salt-water. 'Dry drowning' refers to cases where laryngospasm prevents aspiration.

Presentation and assessment

- Hypothermia may be present.
- Cardiovascular: cardiac arrest may occur, or:
  - Bradycardia may be present
  - Severe hypotension may occur due to myocardial dysfunction (2° to hypoxia, hypothermia, acidosis, electrolyte abnormalities), or hypovolaemia (associated trauma or fluid shifts)
- Respiratory: cough, tachypnoea, dyspnoea, wheeze:
  - ALI/ARDS may develop (development may be delayed)
  - Pneumonia may develop
- Neurological: anxiety, delirium, coma (2° to hypoxia or cerebral oedema).
- Metabolic acidosis and lactataemia are common.
- Electrolyte abnormalities are rare, but may occur after aspiration of >20 ml/kg water.
- Haemolysis, DIC, and AKI can also develop after massive aspiration.

Investigations

- Core temperature measurement.
- ABGs (hypoxia, hypercapnia, metabolic acidosis).
- FBC, coagulation screen, including fibrinogen (DIC).
- U&Es, LFTs, serum glucose, calcium, magnesium, phosphate, CK.
- Blood alcohol level (if intoxication suspected).
- ECG (to identify ischaemia or arrhythmias).
- CXR (if ALI or pneumonia is suspected).
- ECHO (if significant CVS instability is present).
- CT head (if cerebral oedema or infarction suspected).
- Trauma series X-rays (neck, chest and pelvis, if traumatic injury likely).
- Consider urine for toxicology (if intoxication suspected).

Differential diagnoses

The history of immersion is normally conclusive, but associated injuries may include: hypothermia, trauma, cardiac precipitant (e.g. arrhythmia, MI), neurological precipitant (e.g. epilepsy, stroke, SAH).

Immediate management

If the patient is in *cardiac arrest* follow the guidelines on 🔲 p.98 (this may be prolonged if hypothermia is present), otherwise:

- Give 100% O_2.
- If trauma suspected then assume C-spine injury and use collars and spinal stabilization.
- Endotracheal intubation may be required for respiratory support or airway protection.
- Respiratory support should be provided to maintain O_2 saturations of 94–98% (NIV or IPPV may be required).
- Fluid resuscitation with/without inotropes may be required to maintain a reasonable perfusion pressure (MAP ≥65 mmHg):
  - A CVC may be required to guide fluid resuscitation and allow vasoactive support if required
- Continuous ECG monitoring in view of risk of arrhythmias.
- Rewarm as appropriate to the degree of hypothermia (🔲 p.252).
- Consider inserting an NGT (or OGT if head or facial trauma are present) in order to drain ingested water or debris.

Further management

- In comatose patients institute measures to minimize cerebral oedema:
  - Nurse 15–30° head-up
  - Treat pyrexia and seizures
  - Maintain serum glucose of 6–10 mmol/L
  - If the patient is comatose after resuscitation from cardiac arrest rewarm to 34°C, and maintain at that temperature for 24 hours
- Bronchoscopy may be used to remove foreign bodies or debris.
- Insert a urinary catheter to monitor urine output.
- Consider inserting an arterial line for cardiovascular monitoring and repeated blood gas analyses.
- Treat any associated diseases or complications:
  - Traumatic injuries (🔲 p.404)
  - Seizures (🔲 p.160)
  - Cardiac disease and arrhythmias (🔲 pp.98, 132, and 138)
  - Hypothermia (🔲 p.250)
  - Hypoglycaemia (🔲 p.234)

Pitfalls/difficult situations

- Even where an apparently full recovery has rapidly occurred, patients should be monitored as delayed respiratory compromise may occur.
- In paediatric cases consider the possibility of non-accidental injury.

Further reading

Carter E, et al. Drowning. *Cont Educ Anaesth Crit Care Pain* 2011; **11**(6): 210–13.
Lord SR, et al. Drowning, near drowning and immersion syndrome. *J R Army Med Corps* 2005; **151**: 250–5.
Warner DS, et al. Drowning. Update 2009. *Anesthesiology* 2009; **110**: 1390–401.

☠ Severe burns

Causes
- Flame/dry heat contact (most commonly in adults).
- Wet heat contact (scalds, most commonly in children).
- Electricity (both current-induced injury and flash burns).
- Chemical damage (rare).

Presentation and assessment
Burn thickness may be:
- Epidermal (erythematous skin, not counted in % area).
- Superficial partial thickness (erythema, clear blisters, blanches).
- Deep partial thickness (erythema and white non-blanching areas; bloody blistering).
- Full thickness (leathery white or brown skin, painless centre).
- Full thickness burn+ (black/charred skin extending to deep structures).

Body surface area (BSA) coverage of burns should be assessed at presentation, ideally by a burns team. BSA can be difficult to assess in the initial stages and should be reassessed regularly. Methods include:
- Areas of burn equivalent in size to the patient's palm are ~1% of BSA.
- The 'Rule of 9's':
  - Chest   = 18%
  - Back   = 18%
  - Whole of head = 9%
  - Whole of arm   = 9% (each)
  - Front of leg   = 9% (each)
  - Back of leg   = 9% (each)
  - Genitalia   = 1%.
- Lund-Browder charts—these should be used where available.

The location of burns is also important:
- Airway involvement (see 🔲 p.30—singed nasal hair, hoarse voice, soot in airway).
- Special areas: head/neck, hands/feet, major joints, chest, perineum.
- Circumferential burns: limbs, neck, chest (risk of compartment syndrome, venous obstruction, airway obstruction, or chest restriction).

The mechanism of injury/associated trauma should assessed, especially:
- Cause of the burn, and duration of exposure to burning agent.
- Did the burn occur in an enclosed space (associated with smoke inhalation, airway damage, acute lung injury and CO poisoning)?
- Were toxins/accelerants present?

Investigations
- ABGs (hypoxia, metabolic acidosis), COHb by co-oximetry.
- FBC, coagulation studies, G&S.
- U&Es, LFTs, serum CK (renal indices and CK may be raised).
- Toxicology if appropriate.
- ECG (if feasible).
- Radiology: CXR, C-spine, pelvis, CT head if indicated.
- Urine for myoglobin/free Hb.

Immediate management

- Give 100% O_2, support airway, breathing, and circulation as required.
- Use spinal precautions if spinal trauma a possibility.
- Undertake a 1° survey and commence resuscitation.
- Obtain an AMPLE history (📖 p.2).
- Keep patients NBM.
- Alert the burns/plastics team.

Airway

(See also 📖 p.30 for inhalational injuries.)
- Early endotracheal intubation is likely to be necessary where:
  - GCS ≤8 or rapidly decreasing
  - Burns are widespread (>30% BSA)
  - There is facial or airway involvement
- Use an uncut oral tube to allow for facial swelling.
- Suxamethonium is safe to use in the immediate setting (unless there are other contraindications).

Breathing

- Ventilatory support may be required.
- Consider the possibility of associated chest trauma.
- Circumferential chest burns may require surgical escharotomy.
- Raised COHb levels will require 100% FiO_2 until COHb <6%.

Circulation

- Insert 2 × large (16-G) cannulae.
- If the patient is hypotensive consider a bolus of 20 ml/kg IV colloid.
- Estimate degree of burn and commence resuscitation using an appropriate formula (📖 p.418 and formulae in this section).
- Insert urinary catheter, arterial line, and CVP (avoid burned skin if possible).

Other

- Ensure adequate analgesia, titrate boluses of morphine IV.
- Monitor temperature; large area burns can result in rapid cooling:
  - Losses can be reduced by occlusive, watertight dressings and by nursing patients in a warm environment
  - Perform a 2° survey

Burns fluid resuscitation formulas

Parklands[1]

- Use IV Hartmann's.
- 1st 24 hours requirement = (body weight × BSA × 4 ml).
- Give ½ over 8 hours and ½ over next 16 hours.

Muir and Barclay[2]

- Use IV colloid (human albumin solution 4.5%).
- 1st 4 hours requirement = (body weight × BSA × ½ml).
- Give this fluid volume 6 times in the first 36 hours following the injury over the following lengths of time: 4, 4, 4, 6, 6, and 12 hours.

In addition to either of these formulas, patients require 1–1.5 ml/kg/hour of maintenance crystalloid (or NG feed).

[1] Reproduced from Charles R. Baxter & Tom Shires, 'Physiologic response to crystalloid resuscitation of severe burns', *Annals of the New York Academy of Sciences*, 150, pp.874–894, 1968, Wiley, with permission.

[2] Muir IFK, Barclay TL. Treatment of burn shock. In: Muir IFK, Barclay TL, editors. Burns and their treatment. London: Lloyd-Luke; 1962. pp. 13–47.

Further management

- Complete a tertiary survey in trauma cases once the patient is stable.
- Facial burns require ophthalmic assessment.
- Hypotension is common and may be due to hypovolaemia, low cardiac output, or, more commonly, low SVR:
  - Vasopressors use may be necessary, but may also compromise skin perfusion and increase tissue loss
  - Cardiac output monitoring is advised to ensure adequate filling and to assess the need for inotropic support (dobutamine)
  - Aim for a core-peripheral temperature gradient of <2°C
- Respiratory support:
  - ARDS is common, a lung protective ventilation protocol should be adopted
  - Airway involvement will produce severe oedema, the airway should be assessed prior to extubation (see 📖 p.21)
  - Fibreoptic bronchoscopy may be used to assess the degree of lower airway involvement
- Anticipate renal impairment, RRT is commonly required.
- Haemolysis can occur with full thickness burn, blood transfusions may be required to maintain an Hb 8–10 g/dl.
- Nutritional requirements in severely burned patients are ↑:
  - Gastric stasis is common, NG feeding should be established early, prokinetics may be required
  - NJ feeding is often necessary, PN is seldom required
  - Commence stress ulcer prophylaxis
- Monitor for developing sepsis (burns are initially sterile but rapidly become colonized). Regular surveillance cultures are helpful:
  - Typical organisms include *Staphylococcus aureus*, group-B *Streptococcus*, *Pseudomonas*, *Acinetobacter*
  - Sepsis can be difficult to identify in the presence of SIRS. It should be suspected in the presence of new organ failure, hyperpyrexia, or ↑WCC.
  - Empirical antibiotic therapy should include antipseudomonal and MRSA cover (e.g. piptazobactam IV 4.5 g 8-hourly and vancomycin IV 500 mg 6-hourly). Microbiological advice is essential
- Temperature control may become difficult, especially if full body dressings are required. If hyperpyrexia occurs consider:
  - Antipyretics (paracetamol and NSAIDs)
  - Neuromuscular blockade
  - Extracorporeal/intravascular cooling (e.g. CVVH or Coolguard®)
  - Taking down dressings

- Regular monitoring and correction of electrolytes is required.
- Surgery may be required for debridement, grafting, or synthetic skin cover:
  - Patients are often cardiovascularly unstable afterwards
  - Blood loss may be profound, exacerbated by coagulopathy
  - Antibiotic cover may be required
- Dressings changes are extremely painful, ketamine IV 1–2 mg/kg can provide suitable analgesia (alternatively consider a remifentanil infusion).

Indications for admission

To a burns unit

- >10% BSA burn or >5% full thickness burn.
- Burn to hands, feet, genitalia, perineum, joints.
- Burns to face.
- Electrical/chemical burns.
- Circumferential burns (limbs or chest).
- Extremes of age.

To a burns ICU

- Burns affecting >30% BSA.
- Burns affecting upper chest, neck, or face (affecting airway).
- Burns affecting the airway.
- Smoke inhalation.
- COHb >20%.
- 2° complications (e.g. sepsis, renal failure, major trauma).

Pitfalls/difficult situations

- Do not assume that patients have been adequately assessed or resuscitated prior to ICU admission, especially following inter-hospital transfers.
- Airway protection: if in doubt intubate—delay may make a difficult intubation impossible.
- Do not use suxamethonium >48 hours or <1 year after a major burn, severe hyperkalaemia and cardiac arrest may result.
- Some prolonged contact-burns are associated with overdose and/or compartment syndrome.
- Cyanide toxicity as a cause of unexplained metabolic acidosis is uncommon (see 📖 p.477)—the use of dicobalt EDTA is hazardous.
- Airway injuries are difficult to manage, where there is soot evident within the airways the following has been tried, although there is little evidence to support routine usage:
  - BAL with $NaHCO_3$ 1.4%
  - Nebulized unfractionated heparin
- Burns >60% have a high mortality, especially if associated with inhalation injury.
- Traditional prediction models overestimate mortality from burn injury.

Further reading

Hettiaratchy S, et al. Initial management of a major burn: I-overview *Br Med J* 2004; **328**: 1555–7.
Ipaktchi K, et al. Advances in burn critical care *Crit Care Med* 2006; **34**(9): S239–S244.
Treharne LJ, et al. The initial management of acute burns *J R Army Med Corps* 2004; **15B0**: 74–81.

:☢: Electrocution

Electrical injury can disrupt the normal electrical function of cells (e.g. causing arrhythmias or muscle tetany), or cause internal and external burns. Other injuries may result from muscle damage or contraction.

Causes

Contact with electrical sources can result in electrical injuries. The current involved is the major determinant of tissue damage.
- Lightning (immediate, ultra-high voltage and current, DC).
- High voltage (short-lived, >1000 V, high current, AC or DC).
- Low voltage (may be prolonged, <1000 V, <240 A, AC).
- Microshock (can occur when very low current, <1 mA, flows directly to the myocardium via indwelling catheter or pacing lines causing arrhythmia).

In general, DC shocks tend to 'throw' the victim clear, whilst AC is more likely to produce tetany. Some electrical burns cause flash burns (or arc-ing) without any electricity passing through the body.

Presentation and assessment

Signs and symptoms may include:
- General: burns are commonly seen (surface damage may be superficial compared with internal injuries):
  - Direct, arc and flame burns may be seen (from adjacent source)
  - Where the electrical path involves a limb the ↑ current density may cause greater tissue damage
  - Feathering/fern patterns (Lichtenburg figures) and 'spider' entry/exit wounds may be seen on the skin in lightning injuries
- Cardiac: asystole: VF/VT may occur with high currents (or microshock).
  - Myocardial injury or burns may occur causing ischaemia
  - Delayed presentation of arrhythmias (8–12 hours) can occur but is rare, especially if the shock is <1000 V and the initial ECG is normal
  - Small vessel coagulation ischaemia may occur
- Respiratory: respiratory muscle tetany may cause respiratory arrest.
  - Inhalational injury may occur with some flash burns
- Neurological: paraplegia, quadriplegia and/or autonomic instability may occur which often resolve over a period of hours.
- Musculoskeletal injuries (including long-bone fractures) may be caused by tetany or by associated falls:
  - There may be associated trauma (including C-spine) injuries
- AKI and/or rhabdomyolysis may occur as a complication.

Investigations

- ABGs (hypoxia, metabolic acidosis).
- U&Es (AKI, hyperkalaemia).
- LFTs, serum amylase.
- Serum CK (rhabdomyolysis).
- Cardiac enzymes (to detect myocardial injury).
- ECG (as a baseline, or to check for atrial arrhythmias or ischaemia).

- Urine myoglobin.
- CXR.
- Spinal or long-bone X-rays (if fractures suspected).
- CT head (if altered neurology is present).

Differential diagnoses

- Seizures.
- Spontaneous arrhythmia.

Immediate management

Ensure there is no risk of electrocution to staff or victim.
If the patient is in *cardiac arrest* follow the guidelines on 🕮 p.98 (prolonged resuscitation efforts may be appropriate), otherwise:

- Use spinal immobilization if trauma is suspected.
- Give 100% O_2, support airway, breathing, and circulation as required.
- Electrical burns may cause airway swelling, consider early
  endotracheal intubation even if patient has adequate ventilation.
- Use continuous ECG monitoring (continue for 12 hours in
  high-voltage injury, or any case with complications).
- Remove any burning/smouldering clothing.
- Commence burns resuscitation (see 🕮 p.416).
- Examine for evidence of tissue ischaemia or compartment syndrome.

Further management

- Fractures should be immobilized.
- Muscle tetany, or compartment syndromes 2° to muscle damage,
  fractures or burns may result in myoglobinuria and rhabdomyolysis:
  - Fasciotomy may be required
  - Monitoring/treating AKI may be required
- Ophthalmologic and otoscopic examination are required in cases of
  high-voltage injury.

Pitfalls/difficult situations

- Estimating BSA (and therefore fluid resuscitation requirements) can
  be difficult as there may be severe deep tissue injury with only limited
  superficial involvement.
- Occult trauma injuries (spinal cord injuries, or blunt abdominal/
  thoracic injury may be present).

Further reading

American Heart Association. Electric shock and lightning strike *Circulation* 2005; **112**: 154–5.
Bailey B, et al. Cardiac monitoring of high-risk patients after an electrical injury: a prospective
multicentre study. *Emerg Med J* 2007; **24**: 348–52.
Koumbourlis AC. Electrical injuries. *Crit Care Med* 2002; **30**(11, S1): S424– S430.
Luz DP, et al. Electrical burns: a retrospective analysis across a 5-year period. *Burns* 2009; **35**:
1015–19.

☼ Toxic epidermal necrolysis

Toxic epidermal necrolysis (TEN—also known as Lyell's syndrome) is a rare skin disorder characterized by extensive mucosal and epidermal sloughing. There is crossover between Stevens–Johnson syndrome (SJS) and TEN, with SJS involving <10% of BSA and TEN involving >30%. Severe systemic disturbance can occur before re-epithelization occurs, (which can take 14–21 days, often leaving only minimal scarring).

Causes

• Drugs (by far the most common cause) which have been introduced 2–6 weeks prior to onset of the prodrome, especially: anticonvulsants, antibiotics, antiretrovirals, and NSAIDS.
• Infections (HSV, *Mycoplasma*) and immunizations.

Presentation and assessment

• General: there is a prodromal phase of fever and malaise.
• Mucosal: often predates skin symptoms and can involve the mouth, eyes, and perineum (often mistaken for conjunctivitis or cystitis).
• Skin: acute coalescing macular exanthema, progressing rapidly to full thickness epidermal necrosis:
  • Prominent skin pain and tenderness
  • Bullae develop, followed by epidermal sloughing in large sheets
  • Lateral pressure on erythematous skin may induce epidermal separation (Nikolsky sign); this is not recommended in clinical practice
• Respiratory: bronchial tree desquamation can cause hypoxia, pneumonia and ARDS.

Investigations

• Skin biopsy showing full thickness epidermal necrosis, subepidermal separation, and sparse or absent dermal infiltrate is diagnostic:
  • Immunofluorescence is negative
  • A rapid diagnosis may be established by frozen section histology of the blister roof
• ABGs (lung involvement may cause hypoxia; metabolic acidosis may be present).
• FBC (WCC may be raised).
• U&Es, blood glucose, LFTs.
• Serum magnesium, phosphate, calcium, zinc may all be appropriate as large fluid shifts occur.
• CXR (to identify any lung involvement).
• Blood culture, sputum culture, and wound swabs (may need to be repeated as surveillance for infection is important).
• Mycoplasma serology.

Differential diagnoses

• Staphylococcal scalded skin syndrome.
• Erythema multiforme major.
• DRESS (drug rash with eosinophilia and systemic symptoms).
• Immunobullous diseases (e.g. paraneoplastic pemphigus).

Immediate management
- Give O_2 as required, support airway, breathing, and circulation.
- Withdraw all suspected and non-essential medications.
- Arrange dermatological review as soon as the condition is suspected.
- Consider early endotracheal intubation if there is hypoxia or respiratory involvement (NIV masks are likely to damage facial skin).
- Provide adequate analgesia, pain is likely to be severe.
- Patients with oropharyngeal involvement will be dehydrated, and IV rehydration will be required.
- Ideally patients with TEN should be nursed in an ICU with burns experience as the care is very similar.

Further management
- Careful protection of dermal surfaces and eroded mucosal surfaces is essential using emollients, burns dressings, and pressure area care.
- Core temperature readings are essential, and the patient should be nursed in a warm environment.
- The role of immunosuppressants in disease management is unclear:
  - IV immunoglobulin (0.4–1 mg/kg/day for 4 days) has been used
  - Ciclosporin has minimal evidence to support routine usage
  - Corticosteroids are suspected of worsening prognosis
  - Thalidomide is not currently recommended
- Sepsis, especially line-related sepsis, is a major cause of mortality; only essential venous access lines should be inserted.
- Careful fluid and electrolyte balance is required.
- Provide DVT/PE and stress ulcer prophylaxis.
- Provide nutritional support enterally. If absorption is limited due to protein-losing enteropathy, consider PN.
- Regular ophthalmological review will be required as eye involvement is common and may result in scarring:
  - Use of lubricants and topical antibiotics are usual
  - Amniotic membranes may be placed over corneas for protection
  - Complications may develop later so follow-up is essential

Pitfalls/difficult situations
- The diagnosis is often not considered until the patient is severely ill.
- Pyrexia is a feature of TEN and does not always represent infection.
- Dermatological review may help make the diagnosis in the early stages.
- SJS/TEN is more likely to triggered by antituberculous medication if HIV infection is also present.
- Despite the severity of the condition long-term scarring is unusual; ophthalmic scarring is the main cause of long-term morbidity.

Further reading
Chave TA, et al. Toxic epidermal necrolysis: current evidence, practical management and future directions. Br J Dermatol 2005; 153: 241–53.
Mukasa Y, et al. Management of toxic epidermal necrolysis and related syndromes. Postgrad Med J 2008; 84(988):60–5.

Chapter 13

425

Obstetric and fertility patients

① **Critical illness in pregnancy**

Any critical illness may complicate pregnancy, or the postpartum period; especially sepsis and thromboembolic disease. Pregnancy-related illnesses may also require critical care intervention, including: pre-eclampsia and eclampsia, the HELLP syndrome, major haemorrhage, and anaphylactoid syndrome of pregnancy (amniotic fluid embolism). As with any critical illness, life-threatening problems are identified and treated first.

Fetal well-being relies upon successful maternal resuscitation. Treating the maternal critical illness takes precedence, both in terms of investigations and therapies required. Occasionally it may be necessary to deliver the fetus so as to optimize maternal resuscitation (usually only after 20 weeks as caval compression becomes significant from this gestation).

In cardiac arrests, emergency Caesarean section should take place alongside CPR.

Assessment (physiological changes of pregnancy)

The physiological changes that occur in pregnancy must be considered when assessing and treating pregnant women, these are:

* Cardiovascular:
  * Plasma volume increases steadily up to 34 weeks' gestation, in late pregnancy a haematocrit of 30–35% is not uncommon
  * Significant blood loss may occur without apparent maternal compromise (fetal distress may still occur)
  * Maternal heart rate may be ↑ by 25% in late pregnancy with a resultant increase in cardiac output of up to 1.5 L/minute
  * Supine positioning reduces venous return and cardiac output in the second half of pregnancy due to significant aorto-caval compression
  * Blood pressure typically falls by 5–15 mmHg during the 2nd trimester, returning to normal levels in the 3rd trimester
* Respiratory:
  * Inspiratory capacity increases, FRC decreases; overall respiratory reserve reduces with pregnancy
  * Minute volume increases with ↑ tidal volume, leading to hypocapnia ($PaCO_2$ ~4 kPa) and compensated respiratory alkalosis
  * Oxygen consumption increases during pregnancy which, combined with the decrease in FRC, leads to rapid desaturation in the event of significant airway/breathing difficulties
* Renal:
  * Glomerular filtration rate and renal plasma flow increase during pregnancy; serum urea and creatinine levels decrease (by up to 50% of normal)
* GI tract:
  * Gastric emptying is delayed leading to ↑ risk of aspiration
* Drug handling:
  * Maternal drug handling may be altered by changes occurring in pregnancy (e.g. serum albumin levels fall to levels of 20–30 g/L)
  * Teratogenic/harmful effects of drugs to the fetus must be considered at different stages of the pregnancy

Immediate management

The use of an early warning scoring system, modified for obstetric patients, may facilitate the early detection of critical illness (Fig. 13.1; 🕮 p.428).

A multidisciplinary approach should be adopted with input from senior critical care/anaesthetic, obstetric, and midwifery disciplines.

• Give O_2 and support airway, breathing, and circulation as required.
• If endotracheal intubation is required a rapid sequence intubation will be needed to minimize the risk of aspiration:
  • If endotracheal intubation is becoming increasing likely consider giving prophylactic ranitidine 150 mg PO, or equivalent (sodium citrate 30 ml PO can be used but may increase maternal nausea)
  • The incidence of difficult intubation increases in late pregnancy, especially in patients with pre-eclampsia; immediate availability of intubation adjuncts and familiarization with difficult airway protocols is required (🕮 p.24)
  • Rapid desaturation at induction is likely (mentioned earlier)
• Mechanical ventilation may be difficult in heavily pregnant individuals; PEEP will be required to avoid further loss of FRC.
• Aggressive fluid resuscitation and/or inotropes may be required:
  • In a pregnant patient a right-sided wedge, or even lateral positioning, will decrease the effects of aorto-caval compression (even in the early stages of pregnancy)
  • Manual displacement of the uterus may useful in an emergency
• In cases of critical illness where pre-term delivery (23–34 weeks) is likely to occur, maternal steroids may improve fetal lung function post delivery (2 doses of betamethasone 12 mg 24 hours apart).

Further management

• The incidence of thrombotic events increases in pregnancy, thromboprophylaxis should be instituted where possible.
• It may be possible to facilitate the baby visiting the mother whilst she is in a critical care environment; this should be encouraged.
• Breastfeeding is more likely to succeed if established early, and where appropriate it should be encouraged within critical care.
• Drugs which are expressed in breast milk should be avoided if possible.
• Routine pre- or postpartum examinations by obstetricians or midwives should still be conducted in patients in critical care settings.
• Anti-D Rhesus immunization should be given to at-risk mothers.

Pitfalls/difficult situations

• Consider the possibility of epidural complications or local anaesthetic toxicity in the differential diagnosis.
• The management of patients with severe coexisting disease, particularly congenital cardiac abnormalities, will require specialist advice.

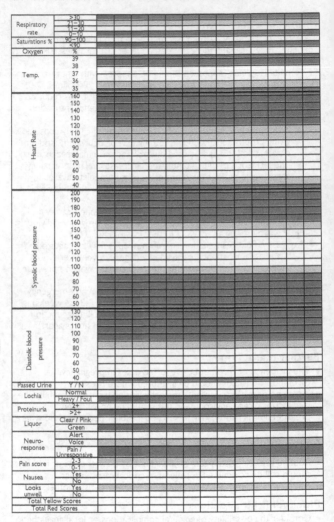

Fig. 13.1 Obstetric early warning scoring system. Contact doctor for early intervention if patient triggers 1 red or 2 pink scores at any one time.

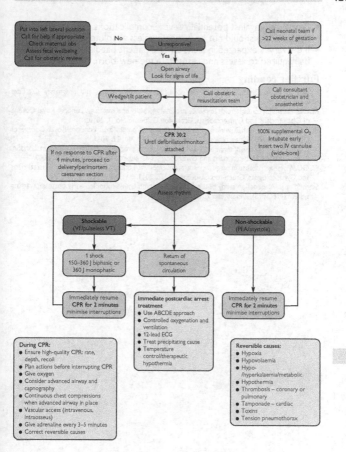

Put into left lateral position
Call for help if appropriate
Check maternal obs
Assess fetal wellbeing
Call for obstetric review

No ← Unresponsive?

Call neonatal team if >22 weeks of gestation

Yes

Open airway
Look for signs of life

Wedge/tilt patient ← Call obstetric resuscitation team → Call consultant obstetrician and anaesthetist

CPR 30:2
Until defibrillator/monitor attached

100% supplemental O₂
Intubate early
Insert two IV cannulae (wide-bore)

If no response to CPR after 4 minutes, proceed to delivery/perimortem caesarean section

Assess rhythm

Shockable (VF/pulseless VT)

Non-shockable (PEA/asystole)

1 shock 150–360 J biphasic or 360 J monophasic

Return of spontaneous circulation

Immediately resume CPR for 2 minutes minimise interruptions

Immediate postcardiac arrest treatment
● Use ABCDE approach
● Controlled oxygenation and ventilation
● 12-lead ECG
● Treat precipitating cause
● Temperature control/therapeutic hypothermia

Immediately resume CPR for 2 minutes minimise interruptions

During CPR:
● Ensure high-quality CPR: rate, depth, recoil
● Plan actions before interrupting CPR
● Give oxygen
● Consider advanced airway and capnography
● Continuous chest compressions when advanced airway in place
● Vascular access (intravenous, intraosseous)
● Give adrenaline every 3–5 minutes
● Correct reversible causes

Reversible causes:
● Hypoxia
● Hypovolaemia
● Hypo-/hyperkalaemia/metabolic
● Hypothermia
● Thrombosis – coronary or pulmonary
● Tamponade – cardiac
● Toxins
● Tension pneumothorax

KEY
ABCDE = airway, breathing, circulation, disability, exposure; CPR = cardiopulmonary resuscitation;
RCG = electrocardiogram; PEA = pulseless electrical activity; VF = ventricular fibrillation; VT = ventricular tachycardia

Fig. 13.2 Maternal collapse algorithm, Royal College of Obstetricians and Gynaecologists, *Maternal collapse in pregnancy and the puerperium*. Green-top Guideline No. 56, 2011. Reproduced with kind permission of the RCOG.

- Prophylaxis against potentially severe complications (e.g. anti-epileptic medications) should not be withheld unless absolutely necessary.
- If delivery is expected in a critical care patient paediatric support will be required to assess and resuscitate the new-born.

Further reading

Neligan PJ, et al. Clinical review: special populations – critical illness and pregnancy. *Crit Care* 2011; **15**: 227.

RCOG. *Antenatal corticosteroids to reduce neonatal morbidity and mortality.* London: Royal College of Obstetricians and Gynaecologists, Green-top Guideline No. 7, 2010.

RCOG. *The use of anti-D immunoglobulin for Rhesus D prophylaxis.* London: Royal College of Obstetricians and Gynaecologists, Green-top Guideline No. 22, 2011.

RCOG. *Reducing the risk of thrombosis and embolism during pregnancy and the puerperium.* London: Royal College of Obstetricians and Gynaecologists, Green-top Guideline No. 37a, 2009.

RCOG. *Maternal collapse in pregnancy and the puerperium.* London: Royal College of Obstetricians and Gynaecologists, Green-top Guideline No. 56, 2011.

Singh S, et al. A validation study of the CEMACH recommended modified early obstetric warning system (MEOWS). *Anaesthesia* 2012; **67**: 12–18.

Severe pre-eclampsia/eclampsia

Pre-eclampsia (...) to eclampsia (...) occurs after 20 weeks of pregnancy and (...) into the puerperium (...). It is (...) pregnancy-induced (...) with (...) and (...).

(...) a pre-eclamptic disease (...)

SBP (...) mmHg diastolic BP (...)

(...) occurs as (...) the VA (...)

(...)

Causes

- Risk factors for pre-eclampsia include:
  - first pregnancy
  - pre-eclampsia in a previous pregnancy
  - a family history of pre-eclampsia
  - Diabetes (?) pre-existing disease
  - (...)
  - Advancing maternal age
  - multiple pregnancy (...) polyhydramnios
  - (...) hypertension
  - new (...) partnership
  - (...) obesity
  - Renal disease
  - autoimmune disease such as SLE (...)

Presentation and assessment

(...) severe when fever (...)
(...) baseline blood pressure (...)

(...)

The (...) accompanied by one or more of:

- Headache (...)
- visual disturbances (retinal haemorrhages, papilloedema)
- hyper-reflexia/clonus (sustained)
- Seizures
- epigastric (...)
- oedema of (...)
- pulmonary oedema
- ARDS/ALI
- renal (...) oliguria (<400ml/24h)
- DIC
- Nausea and vomiting
- (...)
- Renal proteinuria (...)

:☼: Severe pre-eclampsia/eclampsia

Pre-eclampsia (or pre-eclamptic toxaemia, PET) occurs after the 20th week of pregnancy, and can occur into the postpartum period. It is defined as pregnancy-induced hypertension (PIH) with a systolic BP >140 mmHg and/ or diastolic BP >90 mmHg (on 2 separate occasions); with proteinuria of 0.3 g in a 24-hour period.

Severe pre-eclampsia is defined as pre-eclampsia with a systolic BP >160 mmHg or diastolic BP >110 mmHg and/or symptoms (e.g. altered neurology), and/or biochemical/haematological impairment. Death occurs as a result of CVA, hepatic failure, cardiac failure, or pulmonary complications.

Eclampsia is the occurrence of major seizure activity in the presence of pre-eclampsia (38% occur antepartum, 18% intrapartum, 44% postpartum). It may occur before the signs of hypertension or proteinuria.

Causes

Risk factors for pre-eclampsia include:
• First pregnancy.
• Pre-eclampsia in a previous pregnancy.
• A family history of PIH or PET.
• Diastolic BP >80 mmHg at booking.
• Obesity.
• Increasing maternal age.
• Multiple pregnancies or polyhydramnios.
• Underlying medical conditions:
  • Previous hypertension
  • Diabetes mellitus
  • Renal disease
  • Autoimmune disease such as SLE or antiphospholipid antibodies

Presentation and assessment

Pre-eclampsia, even when severe, may be asymptomatic and only discovered by routine blood pressure screening, or when complications such as eclampsia occur.

Signs and symptoms, when they occur, consist of:
• Neurological:
  • Headache and/or visual disturbance (cerebral oedema)
  • Hyper-reflexia/clonus (≥3 beats)
  • Seizures
  • Papilloedema
• Respiratory:
  • Dyspnoea on exertion
  • Pulmonary oedema
  • ALI, ARDS
• Cardiovascular: hypertension (>140/90 mmHg).
• GI:
  • Nausea and vomiting;
  • Epigastric discomfort (hepatic engorgement/ischaemia)
• Renal: proteinuria, marked oliguria (often <0.25 ml/kg/hour).

- General:
  - Peripheral oedema
  - Facial and laryngeal oedema (this may result in difficulty in endotracheal intubation)

Investigations

- FBC (thrombocytopaenia may be seen, platelets <100 × 10⁹/L).
- Blood film (if TTP suspected).
- Coagulation studies, including fibrinogen (DIC may occur with raised PT and APTT, thrombocytopaenia, hypofibrinogenaemia).
- U&Es (may be deranged as AKI can occur, a creatinine >80 µmol/L is likely to be abnormal, depending on maternal size).
- LFTs (may be deranged with ↑ALT and/or ↑AST; hypoproteinaemia may occur).
- Serum glucose (hypo/hyperglycaemia may be present).
- Serum urate is no longer recommended as a diagnostic test but may still be tested in some centres (previously thought to be associated with pre-eclampsia: >10 × the gestational age in weeks in µmol/L, or >360 µmol/L, or >6 mg/dL).
- Urinalysis, options include:
  - Urine dipstick (proteinuria: ≥++ seen; severe proteinuria: ≥+++ seen); ≥+ proteinuria seen requires further investigation
  - Spot protein: creatinine ratio (PCR) >30 mg/mmol
  - 24-hour collection (proteinuria: ≥0.3 g/24 hours; severe proteinuria: >1 g/24 hours)
- Blood, urine, and sputum cultures (if infection is suspected).
- US of the fetus, to examine for fetal well-being.

Differential diagnoses

- Seizures or altered neurology:
  - Epilepsy (prior history of seizures)
  - Encephalitis/meningitis (signs of sepsis)
  - CVA (CT findings, absence of proteinuria)
  - HUS/TTP (evidence of haemolysis)
- Hypertension:
  - Pre-existing hypertension (prior history)
  - Pain/agitation

Immediate management

A multidisciplinary approach should be adopted with input from senior critical care/anaesthetic, obstetric, and midwifery disciplines

- Give O_2 and support airway, breathing, and circulation as required.
- Overall aims include stabilization of BP, prevention of eclamptic seizures, and opportune delivery of the baby.

Hypertension treatment

- The aim should be to reduce diastolic BP to around 90–100 mmHg, precipitous drops in BP should be avoided.
- There is no consensus as to what constitutes first- or second-line therapy, a reasonable approach might be:

- First-line treatment: labetalol 200 mg PO, repeated after 30 minutes if required; if oral labetalol is ineffective consider labetalol 50 mg IV repeated every 5 minutes to a maximum of 200 mg, followed by infusion at 5–50 mg/hour
- Second-line: if labetalol is not tolerated or contraindicated (e.g. in asthmatics) give nifedipine 10 mg PO, which can be repeated after 30 minutes if required (*nifedipine should not be given sublingually*)
- Third-line: hydralazine 5–10 mg by slow IV bolus, repeated after 15 minutes, followed by an infusion at 5–15 mg/hour (consider a bolus of ≤500 ml crystalloid before, or at the same time as hydralazine given in the antenatal period)
- Atenolol, ACE inhibitors, ARBs, and diuretics should be avoided

Treatment and/or prevention of eclamptic seizures
- Magnesium sulphate IV 4 g (16 mmol $MgSO_4$) over 5–10 minutes, followed by an infusion of 1 g/hour (4 mmol/hour) for at least 24 hours:
  - A further dose of magnesium sulphate 2 g (8 mmol $MgSO_4$) over 15–20 minutes can be given if further seizures occur; or the infusion rate ↑ to 2 g/hour
- Close observation for evidence of magnesium toxicity is essential (see 📖 p.224).
- Second-line eclampsia treatments are only rarely required if BP control and magnesium have been used, but may include:
  - IV phenytoin or benzodiazepines (📖 p.161)
  - Induction of anaesthesia with endotracheal intubation and ventilation (the presence of upper airway oedema suggests difficult intubation will be more likely)
- The definitive treatment for severe pre-eclampsia/eclampsia is delivery of the baby:
  - The decision to deliver must weigh up the needs of the mother against the maturity of the baby
  - Seizures and other symptoms should be controlled prior to proceeding to delivery/Caesarean section if possible
  - Consider IV steroids for fetal lung development (📖 p.427)
  - Patients may be transferred to critical care for enhanced monitoring and vital organ support pre- or post-delivery

Further management
- The role of CVP monitoring is unclear, it can aid fluid management, but is not always required if urine output/fluid balance is strictly monitored; it is more difficult in the presence of agitation, dyspnoea, oedema, and coagulopathy.
- There is no evidence of benefit from fluid expansion and a fluid restriction regimen is associated with good maternal outcome:
  - Limit maintenance fluids to 80 ml/hour unless there are other ongoing fluid losses, such as haemorrhage
- There is no evidence that maintenance of a specific urine output is important to prevent renal failure (which is rare).

Pitfalls/difficult situations

- Endotracheal intubation may cause a profound hypertensive surge; short-acting IV opiates, or IV antihypertensives such as labetalol, should be used to blunt this effect.
- Up to 10% of women with severe pre-eclampsia, and 25–50% of women with eclampsia are affected by the HELLP syndrome.
- The key issue picked up in recent 'Confidential Enquiries' is the need to adequately treat BP; systolic BP >150 mmHg with pre-eclampsia should be treated to protect the maternal brain.

Further reading

Altman D, et al. Do women with pre-eclampsia, and their babies, benefit from magnesium sulphate? The Magpie Trial: a randomised placebo- controlled trial. *Lancet* 2002; **359**: 1877–890.

Duley L, et al. Management of pre-eclampsia. *Br Med J* 2006; 332; 463–468.

NICE. *Hypertension in pregnancy: the management of hypertensive disorders during pregnancy.* London: NICE, 2011.

:☼: HELLP syndrome

HELLP syndrome consists of **H**aemolysis, **E**levated **L**iver enzymes, and **L**ow **P**latelets. It may occur as an entity on its own, or in association with pre-eclampsia. The associated mortality is reported to be as high as 24% of patients.

Causes

HELLP is a multisystem disease consisting of generalized vasospasm and coagulation defects. No common precipitating factor has been identified.
- **H**aemolysis is due to a microangiopathic haemolytic anaemia (MAHA).
- **E**levated **L**iver enzymes are due to hepatic necrosis (in severe cases intra-hepatic haemorrhage, subcapsular haematoma or hepatic rupture may occur).
- **L**ow **P**latelets/thrombocytopaenia is due to ↑consumption.

Presentation and assessment

The signs and symptoms overlap with those of pre-eclampsia:
- Neurological: headache and/or visual disturbance (cerebral oedema), hyper-reflexia/clonus, seizures.
- Respiratory: dyspnoea on exertion, pulmonary oedema, ALI/ARDS.
- Cardiovascular: hypertension (>160/110 mmHg).
- GI: right upper quadrant tenderness, nausea and vomiting, epigastric discomfort (hepatic engorgement/ischaemia).
- Renal: proteinuria, marked oliguria (often <0.25 ml/kg/hour).
- General: malaise, bruising/petechiae, peripheral oedema, facial and laryngeal oedema.

Investigations

Investigations are used to confirm the diagnosis and monitor the progression of the disease; they should be taken early and repeated 6-hourly:
- FBC and blood film (**H**aemolysis will be evidenced by an abnormal film, spherocytes, schistocytes, burr cells; **L**ow **P**latelets will be confirmed by a thrombocytopaenia of $<100 \times 10^9$/L).
- Coagulation studies and fibrinogen (normal, unless DIC present).
- Serum haptoglobins (**H**aemolysis will reduce haptoglobins, <0.3g/L).
- U&Es (creatinine may be raised, AKI can occur).
- LFTs (**E**levated **L**iver enzymes will be seen, AST >70 iu/L; **H**aemolysis will also lead to a high bilirubin and an elevated LDH, >600 iu/L).
- Serum glucose (hypoglycaemia may be present).
- Urine, protein:creatinine ratio, 24-hour collection for proteinuria, or dipstick (as for pre-eclampsia).
- Abdominal and fetal US (to exclude differential diagnoses).

Differential diagnoses

Some of these alternative diagnoses are associated with a high maternal mortality and may cause long-term morbidity. Their differentiation from HELLP is difficult and careful diagnostic evaluation is required.
- Diseases related to pregnancy:
  - Acute fatty liver of pregnancy (AFLP)
  - Benign thrombocytopaenia of pregnancy

- Infectious and inflammatory diseases (e.g. viral hepatitis, cholangitis, cholecystitis, gastritis, peptic ulceration, pancreatitis).
- Thrombocytopaenia (e.g. idiopathic thrombocytopaenia, SLE, antiphospholipid syndrome).
- Rare diseases with MAHA (e.g. HUS/TTP).

Immediate management

The definitive treatment for severe HELLP syndrome is delivery of the baby; any decision to deliver must weigh up the needs of the mother against the maturity of the baby.

A multidisciplinary approach should be adopted with input from senior critical care/anaesthetic, obstetric, and midwifery disciplines:
- Give O_2 and support airway, breathing, and circulation as required.
- Correction of thrombocytopaenia may be required:
  - Patients with a platelet count >40 × 10⁹/L are unlikely to bleed
  - Transfusion is generally only required if the platelet count drops to less than 20 × 10⁹/L
  - Patients who undergo Caesarean section should be transfused to a platelet count >50 × 10⁹/L
- Patients with DIC should be given FFP and packed RBCs.
- See also section on pre-eclampsia management (□ p.432).
- Seizure prophylaxis: magnesium sulphate should be administered to prevent seizures, regardless of whether hypertension is present.
- Antihypertensives: should be administered according to the protocol for pre-eclampsia.
- Fluids: as for pre-eclampsia.
- If required betamethasone should be given to promote fetal lung maturation (□ p.427).

Further management
- Consider plasmapheresis after delivery.
- Epoprostenol and ketanserin have also been used as treatments.

Pitfalls/difficult situations
- Postpartum haemorrhage will require aggressive early treatment.
- High-dose steroids are no longer recommended as a treatment for HELLP.

Further reading
Haram K, et al. The HELLP syndrome: clinical issues and management. A review. *BMC Pregnancy Childbirth* 2009; 9: 8.

Hart E, et al. The diagnosis and management of pre-eclampsia. *BJA CEPD Rev* 2003; 3(2): 38–42.

:☹: Anaphylactoid syndrome of pregnancy

Anaphylactoid syndrome of pregnancy, also known as amniotic fluid embolism (AFE), is thought to be caused by amniotic fluid entering the maternal circulation, triggering an anaphylactoid reaction and/or DIC.

Causes

Risk factors include induction of labour and multiple pregnancy; older age and increasing parity may also be associated. It can occur at any time in late pregnancy, during or after labour/delivery (by vaginal delivery or Caesarean section), and also after termination.

Presentation and assessment

Anaphylactoid syndrome of pregnancy presents as collapse during labour or delivery (or within 30 minutes of delivery) with acute hypotension, respiratory distress and acute hypoxia. Presentation is typically biphasic.

Phase 1 signs/symptoms

- Dyspnoea, tachypnoea, pulmonary oedema, hypoxia, cyanosis:
  - Pulmonary hypertension and right heart failure (2° to pulmonary artery vasospasm/obstruction)
- Cardiovascular: hypotension, cardiovascular collapse, cardiac arrest.
- Neurological: tonic–clonic seizures.
- Other: fetal bradycardia.

Up to half of the survivors of phase 1 enter phase 2

- DIC with massive haemorrhage 2° to the coagulopathy (may occur as the presenting feature, without phase 1 features).

Investigations

- ABGs (acidaemia, hypoxia, hypercapnia).
- Crossmatch, FBC.
- Coagulation studies, including fibrinogen (DIC may occur with raised PT and APTT, thrombocytopaenia, hypofibrinogenaemia).
- U&Es, LFTs, serum glucose (exclude hypoglycaemia).
- Serum tryptase (if anaphylaxis suspected, see 📖 p.110).
- 12-lead ECG and/or cardiac echocardiography (differentials include cardiac ischaemic, arrhythmias; right-sided strain in PE).

Once the patient has been stabilized:
- CT pulmonary angiogram, or VQ scan (if PE suspected).
- CT head may be required.
- If a PAFC has been inserted a pulmonary artery blood sample may be examined for fetal cells or amniotic fluid (a finding associated with, but not diagnostic of, the syndrome); urine may also be examined.

Differential diagnoses

All differentials will be difficult to exclude/confirm in the acute situation:
- Occult haemorrhage (e.g. placental abruption, uterine rupture).
- Anaphylaxis (triad of hypotension, bronchospasm, and urticarial rash).
- PE (pleuritic chest pain and respiratory distress).
- Aortic dissection (tearing chest pain and hypotension).

- MI (crushing chest pain and hypotension).
- Septic shock (pyrexia and vasodilatory shock).
- Local anaesthetic toxicity, or regional anaesthesia complications.

Immediate management

A multidisciplinary approach should be adopted with input from senior critical care/anaesthetic, obstetric, and midwifery disciplines

- Give O_2 and support airway, breathing, and circulation as required
- Intubation and mechanical ventilation is often required:
  - NIV support may be considered in some cases
- Aggressive fluid resuscitation with vasopressor/inotropic support is likely to be required for haemodynamic instability.
- Anaphylaxis is often difficult to exclude, treatment with adrenaline, steroids, and antihistamine may be required (📖 p.110).
- Seizures occur as a result of cerebral anoxia and should be treated according to the protocol for status epilepticus (📖 p.160), with benzodiazepines as first line agent, *except*:
  - If eclampsia is a likely differential diagnosis consider using magnesium sulphate (see 📖 p.434) as the first line agent (eclampsia is associated with *hypertension*; anaphylactoid syndrome of pregnancy is associated with *hypotension*, which will be exacerbated by magnesium)
- The fetus should be delivered as soon as is practically possible to prevent further hypotensive episodes.
- If phase 1 is survived then transfer to critical care for close monitoring and vital organ support is likely to be required.
- Early invasive monitoring is advised.
- The coagulopathy/DIC which occurs in phase 2 should be corrected:
  - Packed red cells, platelets, FFP, and cryoprecipitate are all likely to be required
- ARDS commonly develops; a lung protective ventilation strategy should be adopted.

Further management

- Haemodialysis with plasmapheresis, and extracorporeal membrane oxygenation with IABP support have both been described in case reports with successful outcomes in treating anaphylactoid syndrome patients with cardiovascular collapse.

Pitfalls/difficult situations

- Until recently maternal mortality was thought to be 50–75%, more recent estimates of mortality are around 20%, although those who do survive are often left with significant neurological disability.

Further reading

Conde-Agudelo A, et al. Amniotic fluid embolism: an evidence-based review. *Am J Obs Gynaecol* 2009; **201**(5): 445.e1–13.

Knight M, et al. Incidence and risk factors for amniotic-fluid embolism. *Obstet Gynaecol* 2010; **115**(5): 91091–7.

O'Shea A, et al. Amniotic fluid embolism. *Int Anesthesiol Clin* 2007; **45**(1): 17–28.

:⚙: Massive obstetric haemorrhage

Major obstetric haemorrhage is defined as 1 or more of the following:
- Estimated blood loss ≥2000 ml.[1]
- Transfusion of 5 or more units of blood.
- 50% blood volume loss within 3 hours.
- Rate of blood loss ≥ 150 ml/minute.
- Blood loss precipitating treatment for coagulopathy (e.g. FFP, cryoprecipitate, platelets).

Haemorrhage may be antepartum (APH), occurring before delivery but after 24 weeks' gestation, or postpartum (PPH) occurring during or after delivery.

Causes
- Ectopic pregnancy.
- Placental abruption.
- Placenta praevia.
- Sepsis: septic abortion or puerperal sepsis.
- Uterine atony.
- Placenta accreta.
- Uterine/cervical/vaginal trauma.
- Uterine rupture.
- Retained products of conception.
- Coagulopathy, especially DIC.

Presentation and assessment
The definition of massive haemorrhage assumes that >20–30% of total blood volume has already been lost. The presentation is similar to haemorrhage from other causes (📖 p.112), and includes:
- Respiratory: dyspnoea, tachypnoea.
- Cardiovascular:
  - Tachycardia (may be obtunded by regional anaesthesia; bradycardia is generally a late/pre-terminal sign)
  - Delayed capillary refill, hypotension
- Renal: oliguria/anuria.
- Neurological: anxiety, thirst, drowsiness or unconsciousness.
- Other: pallor.

Bleeding PV or from the Caesarean section wound (or into the postoperative drains) may be seen. Occasionally bleeding is occult (e.g. uterine rupture, placental abruption, or postnatal vaginal or round ligament haematoma); abdominal pain may be present.
- Fetal CTG or blood gases may be abnormal.

Investigations
- ABGs (metabolic acidosis with/without respiratory compensation).
- FBC (↓haemoglobin; thrombocytopaenia in DIC).
- Coagulation studies, including fibrinogen (DIC may occur with raised PT and APTT, thrombocytopaenia, hypofibrinogenaemia).

---

[1] Blood loss may be difficult to estimate as it may be mixed with amniotic fluid during delivery.

- U&Es, LFTs.
- Serum calcium (↓with massive transfusion).
- Where bleeding is associated with suspected concealed pregnancy, β-HCG (urine or blood) or abdominal US may aid the diagnosis.

Differential diagnoses

- Anaphylactoid syndrome of pregnancy (dyspnoea, shock, possible seizures).
- Anaphylaxis (hypotension, bronchospasm and urticarial rash).
- Sepsis (pyrexia and vasodilatory shock).
- Vasovagal response (to uterine stimulation, causing profound bradycardia).
- Local anaesthetic toxicity, or regional anaesthesia complications.

Immediate management

A multidisciplinary approach should be adopted with input from senior critical care/anaesthetic, obstetric, midwifery, and haematology disciplines and the blood bank (Fig. 13.3):

- Give O_2 and support airway, breathing, and circulation as required.
- Intubation and mechanical ventilation are likely to be required, and will facilitate any surgery.
- Use the left lateral position or a wedge, to avoid aortocaval compression.
- Aggressive fluid resuscitation is required (warmed fluids if possible):
  - Accurate estimation of blood loss is essential
  - Large-bore IV cannulae will be required for rapid fluid infusion
  - Early packed red cell transfusion is likely to be needed, with O-negative blood if required
  - The use of bedside/portable Hb monitoring will guide transfusion
  - Consider cell salvage if trained staff and equipment available
  - Invasive monitoring, particularly CVP monitoring, may be required
- Ensure prompt recognition and aggressive treatment of coagulopathies:
  - Transfuse FFP, cryoprecipitate, and platelets as required
  - Consider vitamin K
  - Liaise with haematologists
  - Repeatedly check coagulation screen and fibrinogen
  - Consider recombinant factor VIIa for severe uncontrolled coagulopathy (see 📖 Pitfalls/difficult situations)
- Postpartum uterine atony may respond to:
  - Manual massage/bimanual compression
  - Oxytocin (5 units IV slow bolus, followed by an infusion at 10 units/hour)
  - Followed by ergometrine 500 mcg IM (unless there is a history of hypertension)
  - Additional agents include carboprost 250 mcg IM or intrauterine (non-licensed route of administration, avoid in asthmatics), every 15 minutes up to a maximum of 8 doses; or misoprostol 1000 mcg rectally

- Available surgical treatments depend upon the cause of the bleeding (see also 📖 Pitfalls/difficult situations, 📖 p.442) and include:
  - Traumatic tears may be repaired
  - Retained products of conception or retained placenta may be removed
  - Bleeding from placental site (e.g. placenta praevia) may respond to pressure from balloon tamponade
  - Uterine atony may respond to a brace suture (B Lynch), internal iliac artery ligation, hysterectomy or radiological intervention (e.g. angiographic embolization)
  - Temporary aortic compression may 'buy time'

Further management

- Postoperative monitoring should be in a critical care environment, ideally including arterial and CVP monitoring.
- Coagulopathy/DIC, clotting factor deficiency, or thrombocytopaenia may require treatment with platelets, FFP, or cryoprecipitate:
  - Where possible treatment should be guided by haematology
- Other complications of massive haemorrhage may include:
  - Hypothermia requiring active warming via a warm air blanket and warmed IV fluids (re-warming will also improve the efficacy of clotting factors)
  - Transfusion related acute lung injury (TRALI) may require support with non-invasive CPAP or ventilation; or with mechanical ventilation with a lung protective strategy
  - AKI: renal support may require volume resuscitation, maintenance of adequate perfusion pressure, or even renal replacement therapy
  - Hyperkalaemia (consider giving insulin/dextrose, or salbutamol)
  - Hypocalcaemia requiring calcium replacement if resistant hypotension is present

Pitfalls/difficult situations

- Recurrent haemorrhage can prove difficult to control, options include:
  - Returning to theatre for further surgical interventions
  - Further aggressive correction of coagulopathy
  - Recombinant factor VIIa (the use of recombinant factor VIIa in haemorrhage is an unlicensed indication with disputed efficacy)
  - Angiographic embolization
- Regional anaesthesia may 'hide' abdominal pain associated with concealed bleeding such as uterine rupture.
- The increase in circulating blood volume which occurs in pregnancy may delay the onset of symptoms associated with haemorrhage.

Further reading

Banks A, et al. Massive haemorrhage in pregnancy. Cont Educ Anaesth Crit Care Pain 2005; 5(6) 195–8.

RCOG. Blood transfusion in obstetrics. London: Royal College of Obstetricians and Gynaecologists. Green-top Guideline No. 47, 2007.

RCOG. Prevention and management of postpartum haemorrhage. London: Royal College of Obstetricians and Gynaecologists. Green-top Guideline No. 52, 2009.

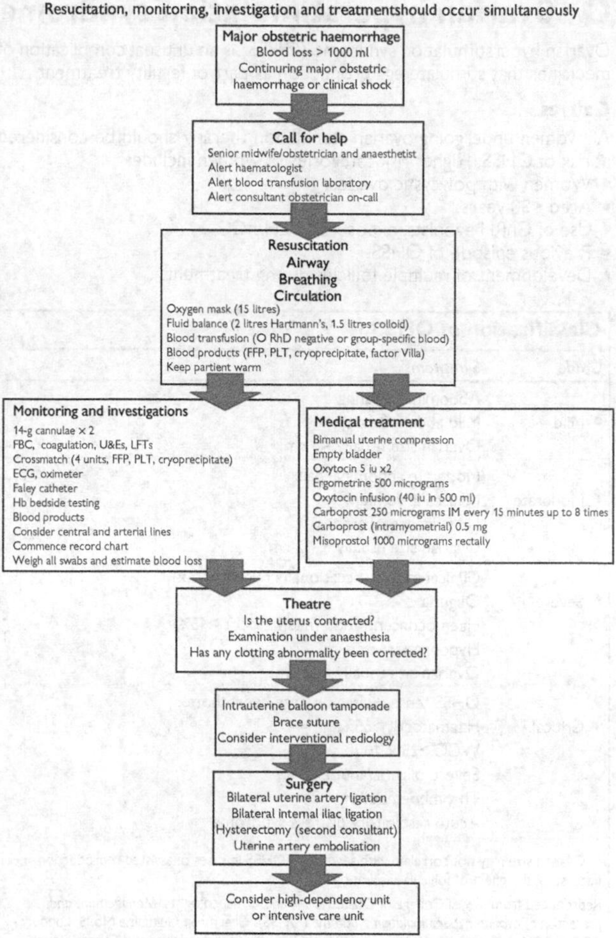

Resucitation, monitoring, investigation and treatmentshould occur simultaneously

Major obstetric haemorrhage
Blood loss > 1000 ml
Continuring major obstetric
haemorrhage or clinical shock

Call for help
Senior midwife/obstetrician and anaesthetist
Alert haematologist
Alert blood transfusion laboratory
Alert consultant obstetrician on-call

Resuscitation
Airway
Breathing
Circulation
Oxygen mask (15 litres)
Fluid balance (2 litres Hartmann's, 1.5 litres colloid)
Blood transfusion (O RhD negative or group-specific blood)
Blood products (FFP, PLT, cryoprecipitate, factor VIIa)
Keep partient warm

Monitoring and investigations
14-g cannulae × 2
FBC, coagulation, U&Es, LFTs
Crossmatch (4 units, FFP, PLT, cryoprecipitate)
ECG, oximeter
Faley catheter
Hb bedside testing
Blood products
Consider central and arterial lines
Commence record chart
Weigh all swabs and estimate blood loss

Medical treatment
Bimanual uterine compression
Empty bladder
Oxytocin 5 iu x2
Ergometrine 500 micrograms
Oxytocin infusion (40 iu in 500 ml)
Carboprost 250 micrograms IM every 15 minutes up to 8 times
Carboprost (intramyometrial) 0.5 mg
Misoprostol 1000 micrograms rectally

Theatre
Is the uterus contracted?
Examination under anaesthesia
Has any clotting abnormality been corrected?

Intrauterine balloon tamponade
Brace suture
Consider interventional rediology

Surgery
Bilateral uterine artery ligation
Bilateral internal iliac ligation
Hysterectomy (second consultant)
Uterine artery embolisation

Consider high-dependency unit
or intensive care unit

Fig. 13.3 Major postpartum haemorrhage algorithm. Royal College of Obstetricians and Gynaecologists. *Prevention and management of postpartum haemorrhage*. Green-top Guideline No. 52, 2009. Reproduced with kind permission from the RCOG.

:⚙: Ovarian hyperstimulation syndrome

Ovarian hyperstimulation syndrome (OHSS) is an unusual complication of medicines that stimulate egg production as part of fertility treatment.

Causes

All women undergoing ovarian stimulation therapy should be considered at risk of OHSS. Higher risk categories of women include:
- Women with polycystic ovaries.
- Aged <30 years.
- Use of GnRH agonists, exposure to LH/hCG.
- Previous episode of OHSS.
- Development of multiple follicles during treatment.

Classification of OHSS	
Grade	Symptoms
• Mild	Abdominal bloating
	Mild abdominal pain
	Ovarian size usually <8 cm[1]
• Moderate	Moderate abdominal pain
	Nausea ± vomiting
	US evidence of ascites
	Ovarian size usually 8–12 cm[1]
• Severe	Clinical ascites (occasionally hydrothorax)
	Oliguria
	Haemoconcentration (haematocrit >45%)
	Hypoproteinaemia
	Ovarian size usually >12 cm[1]
• Critical	OHSS tense ascites or large hydrothorax
	Haematocrit >55%
	WCC >25 × 10⁹/L
	Severe oliguria/anuria
	Thromboembolism
	Acute respiratory distress syndrome

[1] Ovarian size may not correlate with severity of OHSS in cases of assisted reproduction because of the effect of follicular aspiration.

Reproduced from: Royal College of Obstetricians and Gynaecologists. *Management and prevention of ovarian hyperstimulation syndrome (OHSS)*. Green-top Guideline No. 5. London: RCOG; 2006, with the permission of the Royal College of Obstetricians and Gynaecologists.

Presentation and assessment

OHSS typically occurs 1–2 days after follicular rupture/aspiration; only 5% of OHSS cases are moderate severity or worse. The features of OHSS are described in the classification of severity, but may also include:
- General: pyrexia (infection commonly occurs alongside OHSS).
- Cardiorespiratory: hypotension, tachycardia, pulmonary oedema.
- Renal: metabolic acidosis, hyperkalaemia hyponatraemia, AKI.

Investigations

- Measure weight and abdominal girth on admission, and daily thereafter.
- Abdominal/vaginal US (ascites, ovarian size).
- ABGs (metabolic acidosis).
- FBC (raised haematocrit; raised WCC), coagulation studies.
- U&Es (raised urea/creatinine; ↓Na may be seen in up to 50% of cases).
- LFTs (abnormal in up to 40%, but improve with disease resolution).
- Serum glucose, serum CRP.
- Blood, sputum, urine cultures (if infection suspected).
- CXR (basal atelectasis/pneumonia, pleural effusion, ALI/ARDS).
- ECG/ECHO (if pericardial effusion suspected).
- CTPA or VQ scan (if PE suspected).

Differential diagnoses

Several diseases may mimic OHSS, or coexist with it (e.g. acute abdomen, or intra-abdominal haemorrhage; PE or pneumonia).

Immediate management

A multidisciplinary approach should be adopted with input from senior critical care/anaesthetic, obstetric and midwifery disciplines:

- Give O_2 and support airway, breathing, and circulation as required.
- The rapid development of abdominal distension and ARDS may necessitate endotracheal intubation and mechanical ventilation:
  - In women requiring invasive respiratory support, a lung-protective strategy should be used (📖 p.53)
  - Hydrothorax may require drainage if present
- Women with severe haemoconcentration (Hb >14 g/dL, Hct >45%) will need intensive initial rehydration with 0.9% saline and/or colloid:
  - Potassium-containing solutions should be avoided due to the potential for hyperkalaemia
  - Invasive monitoring is indicated for severe OHSS with oliguria and haemoconcentration despite colloid volume expansion
- IAP should be monitored closely:
  - IAP >20 mmHg suggests the need for decompression
- Consider (US-guided) paracentesis where:
  - Abdominal distension is severe or impairs respiratory function
  - Oliguria persists despite adequate volume replacement
- IV fluid replacement should be considered in women who have large volumes of ascites drained (hypotension may occur).

Further management

- Thromboprophylaxis should be provided as there is a high risk of PE.
- Hyponatraemia should be corrected.
- Pelvic surgery should be restricted to cases with coincident problems requiring surgery or adnexal torsion (suspected if there is further ovarian enlargement, worsening unilateral pain, nausea, leucocytosis and anaemia; Doppler ultrasonography may help to diagnose torsion).

- Consider empirical antibiotic treatment, if infection is suspected, e.g. piptazobactam IV 4.5 g 8-hourly and gentamicin IV 5 mg/kg daily.
- Diuretics are generally avoided as they deplete intravascular volume; they may have a role with careful haemodynamic monitoring in cases where oliguria persists despite adequate intravascular volume expansion and a normal IAP.

Pitfalls/difficult situations

- Unusual neurology should raise the possibility of a thrombotic episode in an uncommon location.

Further reading

Budev MM, et al. Ovarian hyperstimulation syndrome. *Crit Care Med* 2005; **33**(10): S301–306.
RCOG. *The management of ovarian hyperstimulation syndrome*. London: Royal College of Obstetricians and Gynaecologists, Green top Guideline No. 5, 2006.

Chapter 14

Poisoning and overdose

☼ Emergency management

Poisoning or overdose (OD) may be intentional or unintentional. It can occur via ingestion, injection, or inhalation, and rarely by transdermal or other routes. It may be obvious from the history and presentation, but a high index of suspicion may also be required.

The emergency management of poisoning involves:
- Initial resuscitation.
- Identification, where possible, of likely agent.
- Specific treatments or antidotes.
- General supportive measures.

Causes

Common poisoning agents include:
- Pharmaceutical products including 'over-the-counter medications':
  - E.g. paracetamol (and paracetamol-containing products), aspirin (and other analgesics/NSAIDs), opiates/opioids, benzodiazepines and 'Z-drugs' (e.g. zopiclone), antidepressants (including SSRIs and tricyclics), and barbiturates
- Recreational drugs (including alcohol, the most common drug to be co-ingested either with recreational drugs or as part of self-poisoning):
  - E.g. opiates/opioids, cocaine, amphetamines, ecstasy, gammahydroxybutyric acid (GHB), hallucinogenics (e.g. LSD), glues or volatile chemicals
- Industrial chemicals, household chemicals, and environmental toxins including inhaled poisons (e.g. carbon monoxide and cyanide):
  - E.g. organophosphates, paraquat, methanol, ethylene glycol, household products (e.g. batteries, cleaning agents and detergents)
- Animal, fish, and insect bites/stings.

Presentation and assessment

- A history of attempted suicide, psychiatric illness, or substance abuse.
- Airway or respiratory signs and symptoms:
  - Respiratory depression
  - Aspiration, pneumonitis, or bronchospasm
  - Oropharyngeal burns
- Cardiovascular:
  - Hypotension, hypertension, cardiovascular collapse, cardiac arrest
  - ECG: tricyclics and antidepressants, amongst other drugs, cause conduction defects and arrhythmias, which may be resistant to treatment
- Neurological:
  - Agitation, confusion, or hallucinations
  - Unexplained unconsciousness, especially if associated with compartment syndrome or prolonged contact burns
  - Convulsions
  - Profound weakness, or conversely muscle rigidity or dystonia
  - Ataxia or nystagmus
- GI: vomiting or diarrhoea; liver failure.
- Renal: renal failure, rhabdomyolysis.

Other features that may be associated with poisoning include:
• Hypo- or hyperthermia.
• Self-harm injuries.
• Trauma, burns, drowning, and head injuries.
• Electrolyte imbalance, especially sodium, potassium, or glucose.
• Metabolic acidosis, especially with a raised osmolar or anion gap (see 📖 p.205).

Individual signs and symptoms are associated with certain poisons (Tables 14.1–14.4). Clusters of symptoms may occur together when poisoning with certain agents has occurred; these are commonly referred to as 'toxidromes' (Table 14.5).

Investigations

The investigations required will be dictated by the patient's severity of illness, and the most likely causative agent(s), but may include:
• ABGs (hypoxia, hypercapnia, metabolic acidosis, raised anion gap).
• FBC, coagulation studies (coagulation may be deranged).
• Blood methaemaglobin concentration (see 📖 p.453).
• RBC cholinesterase activity (in organophosphate poisoning).
• U&Es, LFTs.
• Serum calcium (in ethylene glycol poisoning) and phosphate.
• Serum CK (raised in rhabdomyolysis).
• Serum glucose.
• Blood alcohol levels (or expired air levels if possible).
• Paracetamol and salicylate levels (important to check timings).
• Specific drug serum levels may be indicated for other substances (e.g. ethylene glycol, digoxin, valproic acid, phenytoin, theophylline, iron, lithium, carbamazepine).
• Carboxyhaemoglobin (by co-oximetry).
• Urine for myoglobin.
• Consider taking blood, urine, and gastric aspirate samples for toxicology, or for storage in case later analysis is required.
• 12-lead ECG (may show ischaemia, evidence of hyperkalaemia or QT prolongation).
• CXR (if aspiration suspected or prior to hyperbaric oxygen therapy).
• AXR may be useful if ingestion of radiopaque substances is suspected (chloral hydrate, heavy metals, iron, enteric coated or sustained release preparations, 'body packing').
• Consider head CT or LP to exclude other causes of unconsciousness.

Differential diagnoses

• Conditions causing altered consciousness, altered behaviour, or respiratory depression (e.g. head injuries, meningitis/encephalitis, hypoglycaemia and post-ictal state).
• Conditions causing cardiovascular collapse (e.g. anaphylaxis).
• Conditions causing muscle weakness (e.g. Guillain–Barré and botulism)
• Conditions causing non-specific symptoms such as vomiting or hypothermia (e.g. infections/sepsis, neurological injury/SAH).

Table 14.1 Cardiorespiratory changes and associated poisons

Signs and symptoms	Potential poisons
Respiratory depression; hypoventilation	Alcohols, barbiturates, benzodiazepines, botulinum toxin, neuromuscular blocking agents, opioids, sedatives, strychnine, tranquillizers, tricyclic antidepressants
Tachypnoea	Ethylene glycol, isoniazid, methanol, pentachlorophenol, salicylates
Pulmonary oedema	Cocaine, chlorophenoxy herbicides, ethylene glycol, hydrocarbons, irritant gases, organic solvents, opioids, paraquat, phosgene, salicylates
Pneumothorax	Cocaine
Bradycardia	β-blockers, calcium-channel antagonists, carbamates, cholinergics, clonidine, digoxin, lithium, metoclopramide, opioids, organophosphates, phenylpropanolamine, physostigmine, propoxyphene, quinidine
Tachycardia	Amphetamines, anticholinergics, antihistamines, caffeine, carbon monoxide, cocaine, cyanide, hydralazine, hydrogen sulphide, phencyclidine, phenothiazines, sympathomimetics, theophylline, thyroxine, tricyclic antidepressants
Arrhythmias	β-blockers, chloroquine, cyanide, digoxin, phenothiazines, quinidine, theophylline, tricyclic antidepressants
Hypotension	β-blockers, calcium channel antagonists, ethanol, opioids, sedatives, tranquillizers
Hypertension	Anticholinergics, sympathomimetics

Table 14.2 Temperature, skin, and oral changes

Signs and symptoms	Potential poisons
Hyperthermia	Anticholinergics, amphetamines, antihistamines, cocaine, dinitrophenols, hydroxybenzonitriles, LSD, MAOIs, phencyclidine, phenothiazines, pentochlorophenols, procainamide, quinidine, salicylates, tricyclic antidepressants
Hypothermia	Barbiturates, carbon monoxide, colchicine, ethanol, lithium, opioids, phenothiazines, sedatives, tricyclic antidepressants
Excess salivation	Cholinesterase inhibitors, strychnine
Dry mouth	Anticholinergics, opioids, tricyclic antidepressants, phenothiazines
Sweating	Cholinergics, hypoglycaemics, sympathomimetics
Dry skin	Anticholinergics
Hair loss	Thallium
Acne	Bromide, organochlorine

Table 14.3 Neurological and eye changes

Signs and symptoms	Potential poisons
Coma, ↓consciousness	Alcohols, benzodiazepines, barbiturates, bethanechol, carbamates, clonidine, GHB, hypoglycaemic agents, lithium, nicotine, opioids, organophosphates, physostigmine, pilocarpine, salicylates, tranquillizers tricyclic antidepressants
Convulsions	Amphetamines, anticholinergics, antihistamines, antipsychotics, caffeine, camphor, carbamates, carbon monoxide, chlorinated hydrocarbons, cocaine, ethylene glycol, isoniazid, lead, lidocaine, lindane, lithium, methanol, nicotine, organophosphates, orphenadrine, phencyclidine, propranolol, salicylates, strychnine, theophylline, tricyclic antidepressants
Paraesthesia	Thallium
Ataxia/nystagmus	Antihistamines, bromides, barbiturates, carbamazepine, carbon monoxide, diphenylhydantoin, ethanol, phenytoin, piperazine, sedatives, thallium
Miosis	Barbiturates, carbamates, cholinergics, clonidine, ethanol, isopropyl alcohol, organophosphates, opioids, phencyclidine, phenothiazines, physostigmine, pilocarpine
Mydriasis	Amphetamines, anticholinergics, antihistamines, cocaine, dopamine, glutethimide, LSD, MAOIs, phencyclidine, tricyclic antidepressants
Blindness	Quinine, methanol

Table 14.4 Gastrointestinal and renal changes

Signs and symptoms	Potential poisons
Vomiting	Aspirin, iron, fluoride, theophylline
GI bleed	Anticoagulants, corrosive compounds, NSAIDs, salicylates
Liver failure	Carbon tetrachloride, paracetamol
Diarrhoea	Arsenic, cholinesterase inhibitors
Constipation	Lead, opioids, thallium
Urinary retention	Atropine, opioids, tricyclic antidepressants
Incontinence	Carbamates, organophosphates
Crystals in urine	Ethylene glycol, primidone
Renal failure	*Amanita* toxin, aminoglycosides, cadmium, carbon tetrachloride, ethylene glycol, oxalates, paracetamol, polymyxin, mercury, methanol.

Table 14.5 Toxidromes and combinations of symptoms and the likely associated poisons

Toxidromes	Constellation of signs and symptoms	Possible toxins
Anticholinergic activity	Agitation, delirium, diminished consciousness, mydriasis hyperthermia, dry skin and mucosal membranes, flushing, tachycardia, bowel stasis, urinary retention	Anticholinergic alkaloids (e.g. in plants such as belladonna), antihistamines, antiparkinsonian drugs, atropine, baclofen, cyclopentolate, phenothiazines, propantheline, scopolamine, tricyclic antidepressants
Cholinergic activity (muscarinic and/or nicotinic effects)	Miosis or mydriasis, blurred vision, sweating, excess salivation, lacrimation or bronchial secretions, wheezing or dyspnoea, tachycardia or bradycardia, hypertension, vomiting and diarrhoea, abdominal cramps, urinary and faecal incontinence, muscle weakness, fasciculations, paralysis	*Acetylcholinesterase inhibitors:* carbamates, neostigmine, organophosphates (pesticides or agents such as sarin), physostigmine, pyridostigmine
		Acetylcholine agonists: carbachol, choline, metacholine, pilocarpine
Sympathetic hyperactivity α and β-adrenergic activity	Agitation, mydriasis, sweating, flushing, pyrexia, tachycardia, hypertension	Amphetamines, cocaine, ecstasy, ephedrine, PCP, phencyclidine, pseudoephedrine
If predominantly β-adrenergic	Tremor, tachycardia, hypotension	Caffeine, salbutamol, terbutaline, theophylline
If predominantly α-adrenergic	Bradycardia, hypertension	Phenylephrine, phenylpropanolamine
Extrapyramidal	Cog-wheel rigidity, tremor, trismus, hyper-reflexia, dyskinesia, dystonia, posturing, opisthotonos, choreoathetosis	Haloperidol, olanzapine, phenothiazines, risperidone
Hallucinogenic	Agitation, psychosis, hallucinations, mydriasis, hyperthermia	Amphetamines, cannabinoids, cocaine, LSD
Narcotic	Decreased consciousness, miosis, bradypnoea, bradycardia, hypotension, hypothermia, bowel stasis	Clonidine, dextromethorphan, opiates, pentazocine, propoxyphene

Table 14.5 (Continued)

Toxidromes	Constellation of signs and symptoms	Possible toxins
Sedative	Confusion, slurred speech, ↓consciousness, normal or reduced respiratory rate, normotension, normocardia	Anticonvulsants, antipsychotics, barbiturates, benzodiazepines, ethanol, GHB, meprobamate
Volatile inhalation	Euphoria, confusion, slurred speech, headache, restlessness, ataxia, seizures, respiratory depression, arrhythmias	Acetone, chlorinated hydrocarbons, fluorocarbons, hydrocarbons (petrol, butane, propane), nitrites (isobutyl, amyl, butyl), toluene
Serotonin	Agitation, confusion, mydriasis, flushing, sweating, tremor, hyperreflexia, clonus, myoclonus, trismus, hyperthermia, tachypnoea, tachycardia, hypertension	Amphetamine, ecstasy, MAOIs, serotonin re-uptake inhibitors
Chemical pneumonitis	Cough, dyspnoea, wheeze, respiratory distress, cyanosis, fever *Can occur without aspiration or loss of consciousness*	Essential oils, petroleum distillates, turpentine, white spirit
Methaemaglobinaemia	Headache, diminished consciousness, dyspnoea, tachypnoea, severe hypoxia, tachycardia, chocolate coloured blood	Alanine dyes, benzocaine, chlorates, chloroquine, dapsone, nitrates and nitrites, nitrobenzene, nitrophenol, phenacetin, phenazopyridine, primaquine, sodium nitroprusside

Immediate management

Rapid simultaneous assessment of the patient, and of the likely agent(s) involved, may aid management.

Details of which agent(s), how much, and how long ago should be actively sought; the following may help:

- History from patient, family, other witnesses, or paramedics.
- History of repeat prescriptions from GP.
- Examination of patient for signs associated with certain drugs.
- Examination of pill bottles or tablets; a pill identification system such as the computer-aided tablet and capsule identification program (TICTAC) may be required.

Resuscitation
- Give O_2 and support airway, breathing, and circulation as required.

Airway support
- Endotracheal intubation may be required if the following is present:
  - Hypoxia
  - Diminished consciousnes (GCS ≤9, or rapidly deteriorating)
  - The patient is at risk of aspiration
  - The patient is agitated, or combative and not mentally competent
  - Any corrosive substances have been ingested

Breathing support
- Ensure ventilation is adequate, use mechanical ventilation if necessary:
  - Respiratory stimulants are unhelpful
  - In conditions where there is extreme acidosis it may be appropriate to hyperventilate the patient for a short period

Circulatory support
- Fluid loading may be required to treat hypotension:
  - Tachypnoea, sweating, and prolonged unconsciousness can lead to fluid depletion
  - Inotropes are occasionally required, but may interact with overdoses of cardiovascular drugs; where there is doubt discuss their use with an expert in poisonings
- Hypotension may be the result of arrhythmias requiring treatment; treat any cardiac arrhythmias and conduction defects which may compromise the circulation (see 🕮 p.132 and 138).
  - Correction of hypoxia, acidosis (both metabolic and respiratory), and electrolytes will be required
  - Where tricyclic antidepressants are involved a bolus of 50–100 ml sodium bicarbonate 8.4% IV may help
  - Where drugs have prolonged the QT interval resulting in torsade de pointes, it may be treated with magnesium sulphate 8 mmol (2 g) in 100 ml 5% glucose IV over 2–5 minutes followed by an infusion of 2–4 mmol/hour (0.5–1 g/hour) (10 mmol) and potassium supplementation (40 mmol in 100 ml 5% dextrose over 1–4 hours via a central line aiming for a plasma concentration of 4.5–5.0 mmol/L)

- Profound bradycardia may be caused by certain agents, and may be unresponsive to drug therapy, requiring:
  - Early transvenous or transcutaneous pacing
  - Chemical pacing with adrenaline or isoprenaline
  - β-blocker toxicity may require treatment with glucagon 2–10 mg IV/IM, and calcium channel antagonist toxicity may require calcium chloride 10 ml 10% IV; additional treatment for bradycardia and/or hypotension may also be necessary (see 🔲 pp.104 and 132)
  - In digoxin overdose treatment with Fab fragments may help
- Hypertension can occur with some drugs, particularly amphetamines and cocaine– hypotensive agents may be required.

Neurological support

- Convulsions are mostly brief and non-sustained; where status epilepticus occurs first-line treatment is with a short-acting benzodiazepine such as lorazepam 4 mg IV (see 🔲 p.160):
  - Be aware that many patients will have taken benzodiazepines as part of their overdose 'cocktail'
- Dystonic reactions can occur and may require treatment with procyclidine 5–10 mg IV.

Prevention of absorption

Activated charcoal

- 50–100 g PO of activated charcoal can be used if patients have ingested a potentially toxic dose of a poison within the past 1 hour:
  - Activated charcoal is contraindicated in patients at risk of aspiration, e.g. patients with ↓consciousness or after hydrocarbon ingestion; it is also relatively contraindicated in patients at risk of GI bleeding or perforation
  - In patients with diminished consciousness, charcoal can be safely delivered via a NGT if the airway is protected by cuffed ETT and the NGT position has been positively confirmed
  - It is ineffective against alcohols, solvents, metal salts (e.g. iron and lithium), petroleum distillates, DDT, and malathion
  - Do not give alongside an oral antidote
- Multiple-dose activated charcoal may be used for certain drugs, (phenobarbital, carbamazepine, dapsone, quinine, and theophylline) at a rate not less than 12.5 g/hour.

Gastric lavage

- Gastric lavage is not routinely recommended. It should only ever be considered in case of extreme risk from recent ingestion (<1 hour) of very toxic substances:
  - It is contraindicated in patients at risk of aspiration, and if corrosive substances or hydrocarbons (e.g. petrol) have been ingested due to the risk of gut perforation or pneumonitis

Forced emesis

- Forced emesis (e.g. with ipecacuanha) is no longer recommended.

Further management

Specific information on how to manage poisonings can be obtained from databases (e.g. Toxbase). Complex cases can be discussed with staff from a specialist poisons unit.

Agitation

- Look for and treat causes of agitation, e.g. hypoxia or full bladder.
- Sedation may be required in profoundly agitated patients, but may provoke a drop in consciousness requiring endotracheal intubation; sedation may also worsen any hypotension.
- Antipsychotics are sometimes used to treat agitation, but may lower the seizure threshold.

Coma

- If opioids or benzodiazepines are suspected of contributing to ↓level of consciousness naloxone (0.6–1.2 mg IV) or flumazenil (0.5 mg IV) may be administered as a diagnostic challenge:
  - Flumazenil may lower the seizure threshold, and can provoke arrhythmias (avoid in suspected tricyclic overdose)

Hypothermia

- Hypothermia is common following prolonged unconsciousness; or it can occur as a result of certain drugs (classically barbiturates).
- Hypothermia may be profound and require rewarming (📖 p.250); there may be an associated bradycardia (📖 p.132).

Hyperthermia

- Hyperthermia is associated with stimulants, neuroleptic and antimuscarinic drugs; cooling and specific antihyperthermic therapy may be required (📖 p.248).

Other

- Catheterization and urine output measurements may be required.
- Regular blood sugar measurements may be required in order to monitor/treat any hypoglycaemia.
- Invasive monitoring and continuous ECG monitoring are required for many poisonings and overdoses.

Antidotes and specific treatments

- Antidotes or treatments may be available for certain drugs and chemicals (see Table 14.6).

Active removal of drugs and poisons

- Haemodialysis or haemoperfusion may be useful in the removal of certain toxins (see 📖 p.457).
- Urinary alkalinization (often known as forced alkaline diuresis) using sodium bicarbonate can be used to encourage the renal excretion of specific acidic drugs (moderately severe aspirin/salicylate overdoses not requiring haemodialysis; 2,4-dichlorophenoxyacetic acid and chlorphenoxy herbicides; mecoprop):
  - Different regimens exist for achieving urinary alkalinization, an example is the infusion of 1000 ml 1.4% sodium bicarbonate in

water solution over 2.5 hours; urine should be tested to ensure a pH of 7.8–8.5
- Urinary alkalinization may also be of benefit in methotrexate, fluoride, or diflunisal poisoning, although the evidence for this is not clear
- It is not recommended for phenobarbital (multiple-dose activated charcoal is superior), or chlorpropamide (supportive care with glucose infusion mostly adequate)
- It is associated with hypokalaemia and alkalotic tetany (electrolytes should be monitored and replaced)
- It is relatively contraindicated in patients with incipient renal failure or significant pre-existing heart disease
- Urinary acidification has previously been considered for drugs such as amphetamines, quinine, and phencyclidine, but is generally not recommended because of associated complications.
- Whole bowel irrigation using balanced polyethylene glycol electrolyte solution (1500–2000 ml/hour NG) to promote bowel transit and liquefy stool has only limited evidence of effectiveness, but has been used in the following circumstances:
  - For sustained release drug preparations, and drugs not absorbed by charcoal (e.g. iron and lithium)
  - For 'body-packers' (drug couriers who have ingested packages/condoms filled with drugs)
  - Contraindications include: unprotected airway; bowel perforation, obstruction, or haemorrhage; haemodynamic instability

---

Extracorporeal removal of common poisons[1]

Haemodialysis[2]
- Alcohols (including ethylene glycol).
- Bromide.
- Lithium.
- Salicylates.
- Valproate.

Haemoperfusion[3]
- Barbiturates.
- Carbamazepine.
- Lipid soluble drugs.
- Paraquat.
- Theophylline.

[1] The elimination of many more drugs can be enhanced by extracorporeal techniques, but in many cases the clinical benefit is unknown, or there are more effective treatments (e.g. digoxin and fab fragments)

[2] CVVH is unlikely to be of benefit.

[3] Haemodialysis can also be used but is considered to be less effective.

Table 14.6 Specific antidotes and treatments

Drug or chemical	Antidote(s)
Anticholinergics	Physostigmine
β-blockers[1]	Glucagon
Benzodiazepines	Flumazenil
Calcium channel antagonists[1]	Calcium chloride/gluconate
Cyanide	Sodium-nitrate with sodium-thiosulphate
	Dicobalt edetate
	Hydroxycobalamin
Digoxin	Fab fragments
Ethylene glycol/methanol	Ethanol or fomepizole
Heavy metal poisoning	Sodium calcium edetate
	Penicillamine
	Dimercaprol
	DMSA/DMPS
Insulin/hypoglycaemics	Glucose, glucagon
Iron	Desferrioxamine
Isoniazid	Pyridoxine
Methaemoglobinaemia	Methylene blue
Opiates/opioids	Naloxone
Organophosphates/nerve agents	Atropine or pralidoxime
Paracetamol	Acetylcysteine or methionine
Rocuronium/vecuronium	Sugammadex
Snake bites	Antivenom (antivenin/antivenene)
Warfarin	Prothrombin complex
	Vitamin K

[1] β-blocker and calcium channel antagonist toxicity have also been successfully treated with high-dose insulin therapy. This therapy should only be used where there is an established protocol for its use.

NB Local anaesthetic agent toxicity has been successfully treated with IV lipid therapy (see 📖 p.493). This treatment is also being investigated for use with for other lipid-soluble drugs.

Pitfalls/difficult situations

- If a deliberate release of toxic agents, or a mass poisoning event, is suspected follow the guidelines on 📖 p.496.
- Accidental or deliberate self-poisoning is commonly associated with other injuries, including trauma.
- The use of multiple agents is common in self-poisoning, and signs and symptoms are often a mixture of those caused by various drugs.
- The combination of stimulant and sedatives (particularly GHB) taken together can result in profound fluctuations in consciousness.
- Where there is any doubt as to the aetiology of ↓consciousness or seizures a CT scan is indicated:
  - Alcohol is associated with head trauma and intracranial bleeding
- Paracetamol and salicylate are extremely common ingredients in overdose 'cocktails', check plasma levels for these agents in cases of self-poisoning, even if there is no evidence of ingestion.

- Prior to blood levels being available, or where no blood tests exist, treatment can be based upon the calculated maximum dose (e.g. if all the available pill bottles were full at the time of ingestion).
- Blood levels of toxins taken soon after ingestion may be falsely low.
- Identification of tablets, plants, or snakes brought in to hospital is often wrong, expert advice may be required either via direct contact or via programs such as TICTAC.
- Activated charcoal may sometimes be of use in cases where ingestion took place >1 hour prior to admission, or where the timing of ingestion is unknown; where there is doubt discuss the case with a poisons expert.
- 'Body-packers' (drug couriers who have ingested packages filled with drugs), require a surgical referral, treatment will depend upon the risks posed by the drug(s) involved and their position within the GI tract.
- Self-poisoning requires appropriate evaluation of any future suicide risk; ideally this should be arranged prior to ICU discharge.

Legal pitfalls

- Deaths from poisoning should be reported to the coroner.
- Most patients will cooperate with treatment though some, particularly those who have attempted suicide, may refuse it:
  - Patients who are mentally competent have the right to refuse any, and all, treatment, even if they risk death in doing so
  - Mental competency requires the ability to understand, retain, believe and evaluate information
- Life-saving treatments may be administered to patients against their will only if they are not mentally competent and have no legally binding advance directive.
- When in doubt ask for senior advice or psychiatric advice early.
- Carefully document any refusal of treatment, or any treatment against a patient's wishes.

Further reading

Brooks DE, et al. Toxicology in the ICU. Part 2: Specific toxins. *Chest* 2011; **140**(4): 1072–85.
Joint Formulary Committee. Emergency treatment of poisoning In *British national formulary*. London: BMJ Group and Pharmaceutical Press, latest edn September 2012.
Position paper on urine alkalinization. *Clin Toxicol* 2004; **42**(1): 1–26.
Position paper: gastric lavage. *Clin Toxicol* 2004; **42**(7): 933–43.
Position paper: whole bowel irrigation. *Clin Toxicol* 2004; **42**(6): 843–54.
Position paper: single-dose activated charcoal. *Clinical Toxicol* 2005; **43**: 61–87.
Position statement and practice guidelines on the use of multi-dose activated charcoal in the treatment of acute poisoning. *Clin Toxicol* 1999; **37**(6): 731–51.
Mental Capacity Act 2005. London: HMSO, 2005.
Levine M, et al. Toxicology in the ICU. Part 1: general overview and approach to treatment. *Chest* 2011; **140**(3): 795–80.
Levine M, et al. Toxicology in the ICU. Part 3: natural toxins. *Chest* 2011; **140**(5): 1357–70.
TICTAC tablet identification system: ℘ <http://tictac.vhn.net/home/>.
TOXBASE—web-based database of the National Poisons Information Service available to registered users (i.e. A&E departments): ℘ <http://www.spib.axl.co.uk/>.

Analgesics

! Paracetamol poisoning

Paracetamol (acetaminophen) is a common hepatotoxic agent in deliberate overdose. It is found in many over-the-counter medications.

Causes

- Paracetamol poisoning occurs when healthy individuals take moderate to large overdoses (10 g/20 tablets or 150 mg/kg within 24 hours).
- Certain patients have depleted stores of glutathione and are susceptible to hepatotoxicity at much lower doses, including:
  - Malnourished: anorexia, alcoholism, HIV
  - Taking enzyme inducing drugs: carbamazepine, phenobarbital, phenytoin, primidone, rifampicin, St John's wort
- In rare cases in high-risk individuals, poisoning may occur at normal doses administered over a prolonged time.

Presentation and assessment

- Initial presentation is mostly asymptomatic unless other agents are also involved, although nausea and vomiting may occur.
- In exceptionally high overdoses (>5000 µmol/L or 800 mg/L) acute deterioration in GCS may occur accompanied by lactic acidosis.
- Delayed presentation (12 hours–4 days) can be accompanied by RUQ pain with liver and/or renal failure.
- Liver damage is maximal at 4 days after the overdose, and may result in encephalopathy, cerebral oedema, haemorrhage, and hypoglycaemia.

Investigations

(See also 📖 p.449.)

- ABGs, if compromised (acidaemia).
- FBC and coagulation studies (deranged INR).
- U&Es, LFTs (raised transaminases).
- Serum glucose (hypoglycaemia may occur).
- Serum paracetamol levels (at 4 hours post ingestion if possible).

Immediate management

(See also 📖 p.454.)

- Give O_2 and support airway, breathing, and circulation as required.
- Treatment is guided by plasma levels taken >4 hours after ingestion, levels (earlier levels are misleading); high-risk patients require treatment at lower plasma levels (see Fig. 14.1).
- If history is suggestive of an overdose in the past 36 hours requiring treatment then commence IV N-acetylcysteine whilst awaiting levels.
- Methionine can be given if poisoning is <12 hours with no vomiting
- IV N-acetylcysteine (best started <8 hours after ingestion):
  - 150 mg/kg IV (diluted in 5% glucose) over 15 minutes, then
  - 50 mg/kg IV (diluted in 5% glucose) over 4 hours, then
  - 100 mg/kg IV (diluted in 5% glucose) over 16 hours

- Discontinue if overdose occurred <8 hours ago and serum paracetamol levels are under treatment levels, or
  - Overdose occurred >8 hours ago (or was staggered), serum paracetamol levels are under treatment levels, *and* AST normal.

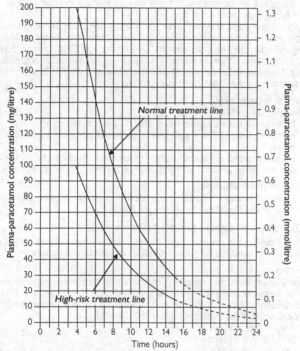

Patients whose plasma-paracetamol concentrations are above the **normal treatment line** should be treated with acetylcysteine by intravenous infusion (or, if acetylcysteine cannot be used, with methionine by mouth, provided the overdose has been taken **within 10–12 hours** and the patient is not vomiting).

Patients on enzyme-inducing drugs (e.g. carbamazepine, phenobarbital, phenytoin, primidone, rifampicin, alchohol, and St John's wort) or who are malnourished (e.g. in anonexia, in alcoholism, or those who are HIV-positive) should be treated if their plasma-paracetamol concentration is above the **high-risk treatment line**.

The prognostic accuracy after 15 hours is uncertain but a plasma-paracetamol concetration above the relevant treatment line should be regarded as carrying a serious risk of liver damage.

Graph reproduced courtesy of University of Wales College of Medicine Therapeutics and Toxicology Centre

Fig. 14.1 Paracetamol poisoning nomogram. Patients whose plasma-paracetamol concentrations are above the *normal treatment line* should be treated with acetylcysteine by IV infusion (or, if acetylcysteine cannot be used, with methionine by mouth, provided the overdose has been taken *within 10–12 hours* and the patient is not vomiting).

Patients at high-risk of liver damage, and who should be treated if their plasma concentration is above the high-risk treatment line, include:
* Those taking liver-enzyme-inducing drugs (e.g. carbamazepine, phenobarbital, phenytoin, primidone, rifampicin, efavirenz, nevirapine, alcohol, St John's wort).
* Those who are malnourished (e.g. anorexia or bulimia, cystic fibrosis, hepatitis C, in alcoholism, or those who are HIV positive); or who have not eaten for a few days.

The prognostic accuracy after 15 hours is uncertain but a plasma-paracetamol concentration above the relevant treatment line should be regarded as carrying a serious risk of liver damage. Graph reproduced with permission from Professor PA Routledge, All Wales Therapeutics and Toxicology Centre, Cardiff and Vale University Health Board. Text adapted from the *British National Formulary*.

Further management
(See also 📖 p.456.)
* Monitor for hepatotoxicity using serial PT/INR and bilirubin measurements; LFT changes often occur late; renal failure may also occur.
* Discuss impending hepatic failure with a specialist liver centre: INR >3, oliguria, raised creatinine, hypoglycaemia, acidosis and encephalopathy.

Pitfalls/difficult situations
* Medications may contain co-drugs needing treatment, in particular co-proxamol (available but no longer licensed).

☼ Aspirin/salicylate and NSAID poisoning
Most NSAIDs are benign in overdose, but salicylate overdoses can produce life-threatening, difficult-to-manage, complex clinical pictures.

Causes
NSAIDs are available as prescription and over-the-counter medicines and are commonly involved in multiple-drug overdoses. Salicylates overdoses have become less common than other NSAIDs but are far more toxic Salicylate (mild to moderate toxicity 150–200 mg/kg) is found in:
* Aspirin ingestion.
* Salicylic acid ingestion.
* Oil of wintergreen.

Presentation and assessment
NSAIDs
* GI pain, nausea, and vomiting are common.
* Seizures can occur, especially with mefanamic acid.
* GI bleeds, renal failure, coma, and arrhythmias can occur but are rare.

Aspirin/salicylates
* Respiratory: (hyperventilation; initially respiratory alkalosis, from respiratory stimulation, later metabolic acidosis which is an indicator of poor prognosis):
  * Pulmonary oedema (non-cardiogenic)
* Cardiovascular: tachycardia, dehydration, vasodilatation, cardiovascular collapse.

- Neurological: agitation, deafness/tinnitus, cerebral oedema, seizures, coma, tetany.
- Metabolic: hypokalaemia, hypoglycaemia (predominantly in children).
- Renal failure.
- Hyperpyrexia.
- Profound sweating.
- Nausea and vomiting.
- Petechiae or gastric erosions from platelet dysfunction (though major haemorrhage is rarely a problem).

Investigations
(See also 📖 p.449.)
- ABGs (respiratory alkalosis, raised anion gap acidaemia).
- FBC (leucocytosis).
- Coagulation studies (prolonged PT).
- U&Es (hypokalaemia), LFTs, CK (rhabdomyolysis).
- Serum glucose (hypoglycaemia).
- Serum salicylate levels (may rise for several hours post-ingestion).
- CXR (pulmonary oedema or ARDS in salicylate overdose; may also exclude other unrelated causes of respiratory compromise).

Differential diagnoses
- Subdural haematoma.
- Dehydration.
- Hyperthermia.
- Diabetic ketoacidosis, alcoholic ketoacidosis.

Immediate management
(See also 📖 p.454.)
- Give O_2 and support airway, breathing, and circulation as required.
- Give activated charcoal if safe to do so (📖 p.455), for:
  - Aspirin ingestion <1 hour ago of >125 mg/kg
  - Ibuprofen ingestion <1 hour ago of >400 mg/kg
- Multiple doses of activated charcoal may enhance aspirin elimination (there is mixed evidence).

NSAIDs
There is no specific treatment; indications for ICU/HDU admission include:
- Seizures, coma, encephalopathy.
- Arrhythmias, hypotension or shock.
- Respiratory failure, ARDS, pulmonary oedema.
- GI haemorrhage.

Aspirin/salicylates
- Aggressive IV fluid replacement will be required.
- Treatment is guided by plasma salicylate levels:
  - Delayed absorption may occur, repeat level after 4 hours
  - Levels >12 hours after ingestion may be misleading low
  - Acidaemia, or severe symptoms, also indicate high levels

- Levels >500 mg/L (3.6 mmol/L) are an indication for urinary alkalinization by giving 200–300 ml IV boluses of 8.4% sodium bicarbonate:
  - Bicarbonate may also be used to correct metabolic acidosis
- Levels >700 mg/L (5.1 mmol/L) are an indication for haemodialysis.
- Checked and replace potassium levels alongside urinary alkalinization.
- Serial blood glucose measurement (and correction) is required.
- Sedatives, or induction of anaesthesia, may decrease ventilation, and worsen acidaemia (encouraging further salicylate movement into the brain) prophylactic bicarbonate should be given in these situations.

Further management
(See also 📖 p.456.)
- FBC and U&E monitoring are advisable after large NSAID overdoses.
- Serial measurements of ABGs and U&Es will allow the monitoring of salicylate overdose progression.
- A salicylate level <25 mg/L should be aimed for.

Pitfalls/difficult situations
- Treat if salicylate blood levels are low, but symptoms are severe; also treat if asymptomatic but with high blood levels.
- Children and infants are much more sensitive to salicylate poisoning, use lower trigger level for treatment (see current edition of the *BNF*).
  - In pregnant patients consider elective Caesarean section

Further reading
Claridge LC, et al. Acute liver failure after administration of paracetamol at the maximum recommended the daily dose in adults. *Br Med J* 2010; **341**: 1269–70.
Daly FFS, et al. Guidelines for the management of paracetamol poisoning in Australia and New Zealand – explanation and elaboration. *Med J Aust* 2008; **188**(5): 296–302.
Joint Formulary Committee. *British national formulary*, 64. London: BMJ Group and Pharmaceutical Press, 2012.
Yip L, et al. Salicylate intoxication. *J Intensive Care Med* 1997; **12**(2): 66–78.

Antidepressants

Antidepressants

☼: Tricyclic antidepressants and SSRIs

Tricyclic antidepressants (TCAs) are commonly involved in self-poisoning. Alongside anticholinergic effects, they have neurological and cardiotoxic effects (caused by α-adrenergic receptor antagonism, sodium/potassium channel blockade, and other mechanisms).

Selective serotonin reuptake inhibitors (SSRIs) are safer in overdose. They have less anticholinergic effects; seizures and arrhythmias are uncommon. ECG monitoring for symptomatic cases is advisable.

Combinations of SSRIs or the inclusion of a MAOI can occasionally result in serotonin toxicity (🕮 p.468).

Causes

There are many tricyclics, modified tricyclics and related compounds. The more common ones include amitriptyline, clomipramine, dosulepin, imipramine, lofepramine, trimipramine, mianserin and trazadone. The most cardiotoxic is probably dosulepin.

SSRIs include: citalopram, escitalopram, fluoxetine, fluvoxamine maleate, paroxetine, sertraline, venlafaxine.

Presentation and assessment

Signs and symptoms of overdose are variable, but may include:
- Anticholinergic effects: dry skin, tachycardia, dilated pupils, blurred vision, urinary retention.
- Neurological: ↓consciousness, convulsions, hyper-reflexia, ataxia.
- Respiratory: bradypnoea, respiratory acidosis, pulmonary oedema.
- Cardiovascular: hypotension, tachycardia or bradycardia may develop.
- ECG changes, classic changes include:
  - PR and QT prolongation
  - Right axis deviation of terminal QRS in aVR
  - QRS >100 msec (associated with ↑ arrhythmia incidence)
- Other: hyperthermia, metabolic acidosis, hypokalaemia.

Investigations

(See also 🕮 p.449.)

Plasma levels do not aid management; qualitative drug screens may be affected by other drugs (e.g. carbamazepine and diphenhydramine)
- Core temperature
- ABGs (respiratory and/or metabolic acidosis)
- FBC, U&Es (hyperkalaemia, or hyponatraemia), LFTs
- Serum CK (rhabdomyolysis may occur)
- Serum glucose (exclude hypoglycaemia)
- 12-lead ECG (see above)
- Consider head CT scan to exclude other causes of unconsciousness.

Differential diagnoses

The combination of neurological and cardiac signs and symptoms are found in other illnesses including: intracranial haemorrhage/subarachnoid haemorrhage, meningitis/encephalitis, and sepsis.

Immediate management
(See also 📖 p.454.)
- Give O_2 and support airway, breathing, and circulation as required.
- ECG monitoring is essential.
- Markers of severe toxicity include: ↓consciousness or seizures, cardiac arrhythmias/conduction defects, hypotension, respiratory depression, QRS prolongation.
- If ingestion <1 hour ago, give activated charcoal, if safe to do so (see 📖 p.455):
  - Gastric lavage is not recommended as it may cause a bolus effect by pushing medication through the pylorus
- ↓consciousness may require intubation/ventilation
- Acidosis worsens cardiotoxicity:
  - If ↓consciousness, bradypnoea, and respiratory acidosis are present endotracheal intubation and ventilation are indicated
  - Temporarily increasing minute volume to create a respiratory alkalosis may 'buy time'
- Give 50 ml 8.4% sodium bicarbonate IV if there is evidence of:
  - A widened QRS, prolonged QTc, or RAD in lead aVR
  - Ventricular arrhythmias
  - Metabolic acidosis or hypotension
- Lidocaine or esmolol may be the best second-line antiarrhythmics (after bicarbonate); others may have marked cardiotoxic effects.
- Fluid replacement should be with 0.9% saline.
- Hypotension may occasionally require inotropes:
  - Resistant hypotension may respond to IV glucagon
- Seizures are best treated with benzodiazepines (phenytoin may worsen cardiotoxicity).

Further management
(See also 📖 p.456.)
- Patients with evidence of severe toxicity should be managed within an ICU/HDU environment.
- Serial ECG and ABG measurements will allow the monitoring of progression of illness.

Pitfalls/difficult situations
- Seizures often precede arrhythmias.
- Rhabdomyolysis may occur requiring treatment.
- Prolonged resuscitation for cardiac arrests associated with tricyclic overdose is associated with better-than-expected outcomes.
- Serotonin syndrome (📖 p.468) or hyponatraemia may occur with SSRI overdose.
- Fever may be an anticholinergic effect, serotonergic syndrome, or evidence of infection.
- Lipid therapy has been used, but there is no evidence to support routine usage at present.

- Ventricular arrhythmias may be resistant to treatment as many anti-arrhythmics (including amiodarone) are relatively contraindicated; torsade de pointes may be treated by lidocaine, magnesium sulphate, or overdrive pacing.
- Trazadone may cause priapism.

Monoamine oxidase inhibitors

The majority of MAOIs are non-selective (irreversibly binding to MAO A and MAO B). They are less commonly prescribed than other antidepressants, due to the risk of side effects and drug interactions, but they may be preferred in phobic or depressed patients with atypical features.

Causes

Non-selective MAOIs include phenelzine, isocarboxazid, and tranylcypromine. Moclobemide is a reversible MAO A inhibitor, but still carries the risk of interactions. Selegiline and rasagiline (used in Parkinson's disease) are both selective MAO B inhibitors which carry similar, but reduced, risks. Linezolid also has MAOI effects.

Overdose of MAOIs can result in noradrenergic and serotonergic effects, which can be severe.

MAOIs can also cause dangerous drug/food interactions:
- Combinations of SSRIs or the inclusion of a MAOI can occasionally result in serotonin toxicity.
- A hypertensive reaction can be triggered in patients on MAOIs by the ingestion of amine-rich foods such as certain cheeses and red wine (the 'cheese reaction').
- MAOIs interact with certain anaesthetic agents (see 📖 Pitfalls/difficult situations, p.469.)

Presentation and assessment

Signs and symptoms typically occur 12–24 hours after ingestion, and include:
- Neurological: agitation, dyskinesia, ↓consciousness, seizures.
- Autonomic instability: hypotension or hypertension, tachycardia or bradycardia:
  - Hypertension may be severe and symptomatic (with encephalopathy or intracerebral haemorrhage)
- Serotonergic toxicity: flushing, sweating, hyperthermia, tremor, hyperreflexia, clonus, myoclonus, trismus, tachypnoea.
- Rhabdomyolysis, DIC, acute renal failure, haemolysis, and metabolic acidosis are all recognized complications.

Investigations

(See also 📖 p.449.)
- Plasma levels do not aid management:
- Core temperature.
- ABGs (metabolic acidosis).
- FBC, coagulation studies (low platelets, prolonged PT in DIC).
- U&Es (renal failure), LFTs.
- Serum CK (rhabdomyolysis).
- Serum glucose (to exclude hypoglycaemia as a cause of symptoms).
- 12-lead ECG (bradycardia, tachycardia or arrhythmias).

Differential diagnoses
- Thyroid storm.
- Malignant hyperthermia/neurolept malignant syndrome.
- Withdrawal states.
- Tetanus.

Immediate management
(See also ▯ p.454.)
- Give O$_2$ and support airway, breathing, and circulation as required.
- ECG monitoring is essential.
- If ingestion <1 hour ago, give activated charcoal, if safe to do so (see ▯ p.455).
- Hypertension often responds to gentle sedation with benzodiazepines (see ▯ p.148 as a guide to management of hypertension):
  - If hypertension is resistant α blocking drugs may be started (phentolamine, phenoxybenzamine, doxazosin)
  - IV hydralazine or GTN if further antihypertensives are required
  - Do not use β blockers; they result in unopposed α stimulation
- Hypotension is a poor sign, avoid indirectly acting inotropes (e.g. dopamine, ephedrine).
- Hyperthermia can be treated with general cooling measures, including cooled IV fluids:
  - If hyperthermia is resistant to simple cooling consider giving IV dantrolene (1–10 mg/kg) and/or sedation, endotracheal intubation, and neuromuscular blockade
  - Drugs with indirect effects (e.g. ketamine and pancuronium) should probably be avoided

Further management
(See also ▯ p.456.)
- Admit all MAOI overdoses for ICU/HDU monitoring.
- Symptoms may persist for 1–2 days.
- Complications should be monitored and treated:
  - Serial ABG measurements will allow the monitoring of progression of illness
  - Serial U&Es and CK measurements may be required to monitor for rhabdomyolysis and renal failure
  - Serial FBC and coagulation studies will help monitor for DIC
- Bradycardia occurs late and may progress to asystole requiring pacing.

Pitfalls/difficult situations
- MAOIs are known to interact with:
  - Certain opioids, particularly pethidine to cause serotonergic symptoms—morphine would appear to be the drug of choice
  - Indirect acting sympathomimetics such as ephedrine and metaraminol may precipitate hypertensive crises
  - Drugs with indirect acting sympathomimetic effects (pancuronium, ketamine, cocaine) may also precipitate hypertensive crises

- Where inotropic support is required, direct acting drugs such as adrenaline, noradrenaline, and phenylephrine may be preferred.
- The effect of older MAOIs may persist for up to 3 weeks.

Further reading

Brent J, et al. *Critical care toxicology*. Philadelphia, PA: Moseby, 2005.

Eyer F, et al. Risk assessment of severe tricyclic antidepressant overdose. *Hum Exp Toxicol* 2009; **28**: 511–19.

Joint Formulary Committee. *British national formulary, 64*. London: BMJ Group and Pharmaceutical Press, September 2012.

Kerr GW, et al. Tricyclic antidepressant overdose: a review. *Emerg Med J* 2001; **18**: 236–41.

Sedatives

❁: Benzodiazepines and gamma-hydroxybutyric acid

Benzodiazepines are often taken along with other drugs in overdoses. Occasionally their presence may actually counteract the deleterious effects of other drugs (e.g. convulsions).

GHB is mostly a recreational drug and, like benzodiazepines, is sometimes used to 'spike' drinks as a 'date rape' drug.

Presentation and assessment

Benzodiazepines are relatively benign on their own. They cause sedative symptoms including respiratory depression, bradycardia and ↓consciousness; these rarely require active treatment.

GHB produces a 'high', but is sedative and is often taken with stimulants such as amphetamines. Individual responses are unpredictable but coma, seizures, bradycardia and hypotension may occur. Rapid swings in GCS can occur, as can rapid recovery from profound coma to self-extubation.

Investigations

(See also 🕮 p.449.)

Isolation of urinary metabolites is possible for some benzodiazepines. It may be worth considering if a criminal investigation may take place (see 🕮 Pitfalls/difficult situations). GHB may be detectable in urine in early samples (<12 hours):
* ABGs (hypercapnia; metabolic acidosis may occur with GHB).
* U&Es (hypernatraemia and hypokalaemia may occur with GHB).
* Serum glucose (hyperglycaemia may occur with GHB).
* CT head may be required to rule out other causes of ↓GCS.

Differential diagnoses
* Conditions causing altered consciousness/behaviour, or respiratory depression (e.g. head injuries, encephalitis, hypoglycaemia).

Immediate management

(See also 🕮 p.454.)
* Give O_2 and support airway, breathing, and circulation as required.
* Give activated charcoal if appropriate (🕮 p.455).
* For GHB ingestion temporary airway support is often all that is required as it is rapidly metabolized.
* For benzodiazepines consider flumazenil 500 mcg IV boluses, up to 3 mg:
    * Flumazenil may trigger agitation or convulsions, do not give to patients who are post-ictal or who have had head injuries
    * Flumazenil can also trigger arrhythmias and heart block, avoid if tricyclic overdose is suspected
    * Flumazenil is short acting so symptoms may return; an infusion (0.5–1 mg/hour) may be appropriate.

Further management
(See also 🕮 p.456.)

Pitfalls/difficult situations
• Benzodiazepines and GHB have been used as 'date rape' drugs, a low threshold of suspicion may be required.

☼: Barbiturates

Barbiturate overdose has become relatively uncommon, as drugs are no longer commonly prescribed as sedatives. Barbiturates such as phenobarbital or primidone are still prescribed as antiepileptics.

Presentation and assessment
Barbiturate poisoning presents with a similar clinical picture to that seen with benzodiazepines; certain symptoms may be more severe, including:
• Neurological: ↓consciousness, coma.
• Respiratory: bradypnoea, pulmonary oedema (occasional finding).
• Cardiovascular: hypotension, cardiovascular collapse.
• Other: hypothermia, skin blistering (barbiturate 'burns').

Investigations
(See also 🕮 p.449.)
• Urine assays are able to detect barbiturates to confirm the diagnosis:
• Core temperature.
• ABGs (metabolic acidosis), FBC, coagulation studies.
• U&Es (renal and electrolyte dysfunction), LFTs, serum CK (rhabdomyolysis), serum glucose.
• 12-lead ECG.
• CT head may be required to rule out other causes of ↓GCS.

Differential diagnoses
• Conditions causing ↓GCS (e.g. head injuries, hypoglycaemia).

Immediate management
(See also 🕮 p.454.)
• Give O_2 and support airway, breathing, and circulation as required.
• Give activated charcoal if appropriate; multiple doses are indicated (see 🕮 p.455).
• Treatment is supportive; intubation/ventilation may be required.
• Hypotension may be profound, requiring aggressive fluid resuscitation and/or inotropes.
• Hypothermia should be treated with aggressive re-warming measures (see 🕮 p.250).

Further management
(See also 🕮 p.456.)
• Serial barbiturate levels will help assess illness progression.
• If the patient's condition is severe (e.g. rising barbiturate levels, severe acidaemia, haemodynamic instability, metabolic derangement, or severe coexisting medical conditions), treatment options include urinary alkalinization or haemoperfusion/haemodialysis.
• Skin bullae may need dressing (and possibly tetanus immunization).

Pitfalls/difficult situations
- Brain death cannot be diagnosed whilst barbiturates are present.

Further reading

Brent J, et al. *Critical care toxicology*. Philadelphia, PA: Moseby, 2005.
Frenia ML, et al. Multiple-dose activated charcoal compared to urinary alkalinization for the enhancement of phenobarbital elimination. *J Clin Toxicol* 1996; **34**(2): 169–75
Kam PCA, et al. Gamma-hydroxybutyric acid: an emerging recreational drug. *Anaesthesia* 1998; **53**(12): 1195–8.

Inhaled poisons

☉: Carbon monoxide

Carbon monoxide (CO) is a colourless, tasteless and odourless gas. Poisoning may be intentional but is also often accidental.

Causes

It must always be considered in those trapped in an enclosed space with a fire (e.g. house-fire victims). It can also be an occult diagnosis (e.g. due to faulty boilers), and should be considered as a cause of unexplained unconsciousness, headache, confusion, or breathlessness.

Presentation and assessment

Carboxyhaemoglobin poisoning is strongly associated with severe burns and inhalational injuries (see ☐ pp.68 and 416). Other signs and symptoms are non-specific and a high index of suspicion is required:

- Cherry red skin is only sometimes present, cyanosis is more common.
- Minor neurological changes: headache, ataxia, nystagmus, hyper-reflexia, drowsiness.
- Major neurological: cerebral oedema, convulsions, coma.
- Cardiac: arrhythmias, myocardial infarct, cardiovascular collapse, ECG evidence of ischaemia.
- Other: pulmonary oedema, metabolic acidosis, rhabdomyolysis, or renal failure.

Routine clinical findings may become less reliable indicators of illness:
- PaO_2 is often normal; SaO_2 may be artificially high.

Investigations

(See also ☐ p.449.)
- COHb: the diagnosis can be confirmed using bench co-oximetry to measure levels of carboxyhaemoglobin, they are only a rough guide to the severity of poisoning.
- ABGs (metabolic acidosis; PaO_2 has minimal usage).
- FBC, U&Es (raised creatinine), LFTs.
- Serum CK, urine for myoglobin (rhabdomyolysis).
- Cardiac enzymes (cardiac ischaemia may occur).
- β-HCG (CO poisoning is very toxic to fetuses).
- 12-lead ECG (cardiac ischaemia may occur).
- CXR (inhalational injury, pulmonary oedema).
- Consider head CT scan to exclude other causes of unconsciousness.

Carboxyhaemoglobin levels[1]
- 3–5%: normal
- 6–10%: normal for smokers
- >25%: high risk of neurological derangement and cardiac ischaemia; late neurological complications likely
- >60%: highly likely to die

[1] Carboxyhaemoglobin levels do not always equate to severity of poisoning.

Differential diagnoses
- Simple viral infections.
- Any cause of metabolic acidosis, especially cyanide poisoning.
- Meningitis/encephalitis.

Immediate management
(See also 📖 p.454.)
- Support airway, breathing, and circulation as required.
- Assess and treat burns as appropriate (📖 p.416).
- *High concentration O_2 is required regardless of PaO_2:*
  - Treatment should be continued for at least 6 hours, longer if COHb remains above 5–10%
  - Alkalosis should be avoided if possible

Further management
(See also 📖 p.456.)
- Hyperbaric oxygen may be of benefit but is difficult to deliver:
  - Many patients are too unstable to transfer
  - In cases where COHb >25% the possibility of late-onset neurological complications may be lessened by hyperbaric oxygen
  - Other indications include COHb >40%, episode of unconsciousness, neurological disturbance, ECG changes, and pregnancy
- Cerebral oedema may require treatment with mannitol.

Pitfalls/difficult situations
- Inhaled gases from fires may cause other complications, including cyanide/cyanate poisoning or inhalational injury.

:⊙: Cyanide

Cyanide poisoning is associated with smoke inhalation injuries and with industrial accidents, as with CO a high index of suspicion is required. Signs and symptoms may include headache, convulsions, coma, tachypnoea cardiac ischaemia, arrhythmias, pulmonary oedema metabolic acidosis, and cardiac arrest.

Investigations
(See also 📖 p.449.)
- FBC, coagulation studies, U&Es, LFTs, ABGs, and ECG are all required.
- Blood should be taken for cyanide levels, but treatment should not be delayed if there is a clear history of exposure.

Immediate management

(See also 📖 p.454.)
- Patients should be decontaminated prior to examination/treatment
- Support airway, breathing, and circulation as required
- High concentration O_2 is required:
  - Inhaled amyl nitrite may provide a rapid temporary treatment
  - Consider IV sodium nitrite (10 ml of 3% over 3 minutes) followed by sodium thiosulphate (25ml of 50% over 10 minutes)
- Dicobalt edetate is toxic and reserved for confirmed severe cases.

Further reading

Ilano AL, et al. Management of carbon monoxide poisoning. *Chest* 1990; **97**: 165–9.

Industrial chemicals

⦂◉⦂ Organophosphates and carbamates

Industrial exposure and deliberate self-poisonings with organophosphates and carbamates are common, particularly in the developing world.

Causes

Organophosphates such as malathion, parathion, dichlorvos and phosmet are agricultural insecticides (malathion is also used for the treatment of body/head lice). Carbamates are also insecticides or insect repellents.

Organophosphates/carbamates inhibit acetylcholinesterase, allowing acetylcholine to accumulate/trigger autonomic and skeletal receptors. Carbamate poisoning is generally less severe and of shorter duration.

Chemical nerve agents (e.g. G-agents such as sarin, tabun and soman; V-agents such as VX gas) are similar to organophosphates, and require similar treatment (see also 📖 p.496).

Presentation and assessment

These agents can act via ingestion, inhalation or transdermally. A classic 'toxidrome' of cholinergic effects may be seen (📖 p.452) including:
- Excess salivation/secretions, sweating, miosis, and blurred vision.
- Vomiting, diarrhoea, abdominal cramps, faecal/urinary incontinence.
- Headaches, dizziness, tremors, ataxia, dystonia, seizures, coma.
- Muscle weakness, fasciculations, and paralysis (all occur late).
- Bradycardia, hypotension.
- Bronchorrhoea, bronchospasm, respiratory depression.

Investigations

(See also 📖 p.449.)
- RBC cholinesterase activity can be measured in suspected poisoning.
- ABG (hypoxia, hypercapnia).
- FBC, U&Es, LFTs.
- Serum glucose (hypoglycaemia or hyperglycaemia may occur).
- ECG (ST changes, peaked Ts, AV block, prolonged QT, arrhythmias).
- CXR (diffuse opacities, pulmonary oedema).

Immediate management

(See also 📖 p.454.)
- Patients should be decontaminated prior to examination/treatment.
- Give O_2 and support airway, breathing, and circulation as required.
- Intubation/ventilation may be required if there is respiratory distress.
- Atropine 2 mg IV should be given every 20 minutes until pupils dilate, skin is dry, and tachycardia occurs.
- In moderate to severe cases pralidoxime can be given (within 24 hours), 30 mg/kg IV with 1 to 2 further doses as required.
- Benzodiazepines may control agitation or seizures (📖 p.160).

Further management

(See also 📖 p.456.)
- Paralysis requiring ventilation may occur days after ingestion.
- Repeated pralidoxime doses may be required until atropine is no longer needed.

:Q: Phenoxyacetates

Phenoxyacetate pesticide poisoning signs and symptoms include:
- Neurological: diminished consciousness, seizures.
- Neuromuscular: myotonia, myositis, weakness, fasciculation.
- GI: burning mouth/throat, nausea, vomiting, diarrhoea.
- Other: sweating, hypertension, hyperthermia, rhabdomyolysis.

Investigations

(See also 🕮 p.449.)
- ABGs (metabolic acidosis is common).
- U&Es and serum calcium (hypocalcaemia is common).
- Serum glucose (hypoglycaemia is common).
- Serum CK, urine myoglobin will be required (rhabdomyolysis).

Immediate management

(See also 🕮 p.454.)
- Patients should be decontaminated prior to examination/treatment.
- Give O_2 and support airway, breathing, and circulation as required:
  - Neuromuscular weakness may require mechanical ventilation
- 2,4 dichlorophenoxyactic acid and meoprop may be treated with forced alkaline diuresis.
- Other phenoxyacetates may be treated by haemodialysis.

:Q: Paraquat

Paraquat poisoning initially presents as the ingestion of a corrosive agent. Cardiovascular collapse, pulmonary oedema, and metabolic acidosis may occur. Urine testing confirms the diagnosis, and plasma concentrations give prognostic information. Initial treatment is with oral/NG Fuller's earth. High O_2 concentrations may worsen pulmonary toxicity.

Later complications include liver or renal failure, but a progressive alveolitis over a few days is the most common cause of death.

:Q: Strychnine

Strychnine poisoning causes intense muscle spasms that may resemble tonic/clonic epilepsy (though the patient should be awake) or tetanus. Respiratory distress may occur, requiring endotracheal intubation and mechanical ventilation with neuromuscular blockade. U&Es and CK should be measured as rhabdomyolysis, renal failure, and hyperthermia may occur, requiring supportive treatment.

:Q: Chlorine

Chlorine exposure can cause haemoptysis, dyspnoea, bronchospasm, and pulmonary oedema. Toxicity can occur up to 24 hours after exposure, but is unlikely if the eyes have been exposed but are asymptomatic.

Laryngeal damage will necessitate early endotracheal intubation (see 🕮 p.30). Bronchodilators may help alleviate respiratory distress, but mechanical ventilation is likely to be required in severe cases.

Further reading

Eddlestome M, et al. Management of acute organophosphate poisoning. *Lancet* 2008; **371**: 597–607.

Alcohols and hydrocarbons

☼ Ethylene glycol and methanol

Ethylene glycol and methanol are both found in antifreeze solutions; methanol is found in household products and illegally produced spirits.

Presentation and assessment

- Intoxication, nystagmus/ataxia, seizures, ↓consciousness.
- Nausea, vomiting, flank (ethylene glycol) or abdominal pain (methanol).
- Tachycardia, hypotension, cardiogenic shock.
- Metabolic acidosis, tachypnoea, and respiratory distress.
- Methanol may produce marked visual disturbances.
- Ethylene glycol causes pulmonary oedema and renal failure.

Investigations

(See also 📖 p.449.)
- Serum methanol and ethylene glycol levels to confirm the diagnosis.
- ABGs and serum osmolality (methanol and ethylene glycol cause a very pronounced metabolic acidosis with a raised anion gap, >12 mmol/L, and raised osmolar gap, >10 mOsm).
- Serum U&Es (renal failure in ethylene glycol poisoning).
- Serum calcium, phosphate and magnesium (all ↓ with ethylene glycol).
- Serum glucose (hyperglycaemia occurs with methanol poisoning).
- Urine microscopy (oxalate crystals in ethylene glycol poisoning).
- CXR (infiltrates, pulmonary oedema).

Differential diagnoses

- Conditions causing altered consciousness/behaviour, or metabolic acidosis (e.g. alcohol intoxication, head injuries, sepsis).

Immediate management

(See also 📖 p.454.)
- Give O_2 and support airway, breathing, and circulation as required.
- Charcoal is ineffective, gastric lavage *may* be appropriate (📖 p.455).
- Ethanol should be given orally (loading dose 1 ml/kg 50%, ~50g or 1 cup of spirits), *or* IV (loading dose 7.5 ml/kg 10% over 30 minutes):
  - Serial serum ethanol levels will be needed (aiming for 0.8 g/L)
- Alternatively IV fomepizole may be used, if available (loading dose 15 mg/kg over 30 minutes, followed by 10 mg/kg 12-hourly).
- Folinic acid 30 mg IV 6-hourly should be given in methanol poisoning
- IV sodium bicarbonate may be required to treat acidosis.
- Haemodialysis should be commenced if ethylene glycol level is >500 mg/L, or acidaemia (pH <7.25), or renal failure occurs.
- The maintenance doses of ethanol or fomepizole should be ↑ if dialysis is used.

Further management
(See also 📖 p.456.)
- Serial osmolar gap measurements will guide treatment, as rebound increases in blood glycolic acid levels can occur after haemodialysis.
- Calcium replacement may cause oxalate crystal precipitation, it should be reserved for severe complications (e.g. seizures or cardiac failure).
- Serial U&Es should be performed.

☼ Ethanol/alcohol

As well as being found in alcoholic drinks ethanol can also be found in some household products (e.g. mouth-washes and aftershaves). It is often co-ingested with other poisons.

Presentation and assessment

Severe ethanol intoxication, particularly in relatively ethanol naïve individuals, may cause hypothermia, convulsions, coma, respiratory depression, and hypotension. Metabolic acidosis, hypoglycaemia, and hypokalaemia may also occur.

Investigations
(See also 📖 p.449.)
- Blood alcohol levels (<0.8 g/L = UK driving limit; > 5g/L = severe ethanol toxicity); but remember that other toxins are commonly present.
- Core temperature.
- ABGs (metabolic acidosis, hypoxia, hypercapnia).
- U&Es (hypokalaemia).
- Serum glucose (hypoglycaemia).
- Consider head CT scan to exclude other causes of unconsciousness.

Immediate management
(See also 📖 p.454.)
- Give O_2 and support airway, breathing, and circulation as required.
- Respiratory depression or loss of airway reflexes may necessitate endotracheal intubation and mechanical ventilation.
- Aggressive fluid resuscitation may be required to counteract ethanol induced vasodilatation.
- Correction of hypothermia may be required (📖 p.250).
- Correction of glucose and electrolytes may be required:
  - If there is doubt concerning the patient's nutritional status give thiamine as Pabrinex® vials 1 & 2 before administration of glucose to avoid precipitating Wernicke's syndrome
- Consider haemodialysis if blood alcohol is high or symptoms severe.

Further management
(See also 📖 p.456.)
- Consider performing a tertiary survey to look for evidence of occult trauma associated with acute alcohol intoxication.

☼ Petroleum, white spirit, other hydrocarbons

These can cause intoxication, agitation, depressed consciousness, and coma. Vomiting is common. Pneumonitis may occur up to 24 hours later, even in the absence of an obvious aspiration event. Arrhythmias may occur with volatile poisoning.

Consider ABGs and CXR if there are respiratory complications.

Activated charcoal is ineffective. Gastric lavage is not recommended. If laryngeal oedema is present, early intubation should be considered even if the patient is currently asymptomatic. ECG monitoring is advised. Bronchodilators may help in the treatment of hypoxia.

Further reading

Brent J. Current management of ethylene glycol poisoning. *Drugs* 2001; **61**(7): 979–88.

Recreational drugs

☼: Opiates/opioids

Opioid poisoning is associated with intentional overdose of prescription medications, or inadvertent overdose of illicit opioids (prescription or otherwise). In both cases they are commonly taken in combination with other drugs such as benzodiazepines.

Presentation and assessment

Opioid poisoning is classically associated with a narcotic 'toxidrome' (📖 p.452) including ↓consciousness, miosis, bradypnoea, bradycardia, hypotension, hypothermia, and bowel stasis.

Other signs and symptoms may include:
- Track marks and skin infections.
- Convulsions.
- Pulmonary oedema.

Investigations

(See also 📖 p.449.)
- Core temperature.
- ABGs (metabolic acidosis, hypoxia, hypercapnia).
- CXR (if pulmonary oedema suspected).
- Consider head CT scan to exclude other causes of unconsciousness.

Differential diagnoses

- Conditions causing ↓GCS (e.g. head injuries, hypoglycaemia).

Immediate management

(See also 📖 p.454.)
- Give O$_2$ and support airway, breathing, and circulation as required.
- Treatment is mainly supportive consisting of airway/respiratory support:
  - Pulmonary oedema may require the addition of PEEP or CPAP
- Hypotension may require aggressive fluid therapy and/or inotropes
- Opiate reversal with IV naloxone (0.4–2 mg) can be attempted
  - Naloxone is shorter acting than most opiates so repeat doses may be required
  - Consider a naloxone IV infusion (4 mcg/ml run at >1 mcg/kg/ hour, titrated to effect)

Further management

(See also 📖 p.456.)
- Trauma and compartment syndrome are associated with opioids.
- Unusual infections such as tetanus and botulism are associated with illicit IV or IM drug usage, as are HIV, HBV and HCV; appropriate precautions should be taken.

Pitfalls/difficult situations
• Paracetamol co-drugs contain opioids including codeine and dextropropoxyphene (co-proxamol, available but no longer licensed). Dextropropoxyphene has long-acting opioid effects and has a cardiotoxic metabolite, the treatment of which may require magnesium and/or bicarbonate.

☼ Cocaine

Severe poisoning with cocaine may cause:
• Severe hypertension, vasoconstriction, and hyperthermia.
• Hyper-reflexia, convulsions, coma, intracranial bleeds or infarcts.
• Myocardial ischaemia, arrhythmias, cardiogenic shock, cardiac arrest.
• Rhabdomyolysis and renal failure.

Investigations should include core temperature, U&Es, serum CK, cardiac troponins, 12-lead ECG, and possibly echocardiography or angiography.

> *Immediate management*
> (See also 📖 p.454.)
> • Give O_2 and support airway, breathing, and circulation as required.
> • ECG monitoring is essential.
> • Treat hypertension or cardiac ischaemia initially with benzodiazepines, α-blockers or IV nitrates:
>   • Ischaemic crises should be treated with aspirin
>   • Obtain cardiology advice in patients chest pain/ischaemia
>   • β-blockers may worsen hypertension
> • Hyperthermia should be treated by cooling and other treatments, including dantrolene if required (see 📖 p.248).

☼ Amphetamines and ecstasy

Amphetamines and MDMA (ecstasy) can cause agitation, convulsions, and coma. Arrhythmias are common, as is hypertension. Patients are often dehydrated, although in some patients excessive water consumption leads to a hypo-osmolar state. Investigations should include FBC, coagulation studies, U&Es, LFTs, serum CK, serum glucose, and ECG.

Hypertension caused by amphetamines or ecstasy should be treated in the same way as hypertension caused by cocaine.

An idiosyncratic hyperthermic reaction can occur and is associated with muscle rigidity, rhabdomyolysis, metabolic acidosis, renal failure, hepatic failure, convulsions, coma, and DIC. Cooling and other treatments for hyperthermia may be required (see 📖 p.248) along with dantrolene.

☼ Ketamine and LSD

Ketamine is sedative in nature. Airway support and, in severe poisoning, treatment for convulsions and raised ICP may be required. Emergence delirium/agitation may occur requiring treatment with benzodiazepines.

LSD is relatively benign. Hallucinations may lead to marked agitation or bizarre behaviour. Coma, convulsions, bleeding, and pyrexia sometimes occur. Sedation may be required with benzodiazepines.

:O: Cannabis

Cannabis is relatively safe except when injected. IV cannabis can cause hypotension, pulmonary oedema, DIC, and renal failure.

Further reading

Devlin RJ, et al. Clinical review: major consequences of illicit drug consumption. *Crit Care* 2008; 12: 202.

Miscellaneous poisons

☼ β-blockers and calcium channel antagonists

β-blockers and calcium channel antagonists are commonly prescribed in patients with cardiac conditions, which are likely to exacerbate the effects of inadvertent or deliberate overdose.

Presentation and assessment

Common signs and symptoms of β-blocker overdose include:
- Dizziness, syncope, bradycardia, complete heart block.
- Ventricular arrhythmias, torsade de pointes (particularly with sotalol).
- Hypotension, heart failure.
- Respiratory depression, bradypnoea, bronchoconstriction.
- Coma, seizures (particularly with propranolol).
- Hypoglycaemia, rhabdomyolysis, AKI, metabolic acidosis.

Signs and symptoms of calcium channel antagonist overdose include:
- Nausea, vomiting, hypotension, vasodilatation.
- Dizziness, agitation, confusion, coma.
- QT prolongation, bradycardia, complete heart block, asystole (verapamil, diltiazem).
- Respiratory distress, ARDS, metabolic acidosis, hyperglycaemia.

Investigations
(See also ⌑ p.449.)
- ABG (metabolic acidosis, hypoxia, hypercapnia).
- Serum glucose (hypoglycaemia or hyperglycaemia), serum CK.
- ECG (bradycardia, AV block, prolonged QT, arrhythmias).
- CXR (ARDS).
- Consider head CT scan to exclude other causes of unconsciousness.

Differential diagnoses
- Conditions causing hypotension and bradycardia (e.g. cardiac disease).

Immediate management
(See also ⌑ p.454.)
- Give O_2 and support airway, breathing, and circulation as required.
- ECG monitoring is essential.
- If ingestion <1 hour ago, give activated charcoal, if safe to do so (see ⌑ p.455).
- Respiratory compromise or bronchoconstriction may require intubation/ventilation.
- Bradycardia may respond to atropine (up to 3 mg IV):
  - If it does not resolve glucagon 2–10 mg IV, in 5% glucose, followed by an infusion (50 mcg/kg/hour) should be used
  - Third-line therapy involves isoprenaline and/or cardiac pacing
- Cardiogenic shock may be profoundly resistant to β agonists:
  - Inotropes, glucagon, or phosphodiesterase inhibitors may help

- Calcium channel antagonists may respond to calcium supplementation (10 ml 10% calcium chloride IV).
- Bradycardia and shock may respond to euglycaemic insulin infusions.
- Seizures and hypoglycaemia are managed with standard treatments.

☼ Lithium

Lithium poisoning may be an acute event, but is more often a complication of chronic therapy where levels are raised by the addition of diuretics, or by renal dysfunction. Lithium poisoning may cause agitation, ↓consciousness, convulsions, hyper-reflexia, myoclonus, ataxia, hypotension, arrhythmias and heart block, and renal failure.

Investigations

(See also 📖 p.449.)
- Serum lithium concentrations should be measured at 6 hours
  - 0.4–1.2 mmol/L is the therapeutic range
  - >2.5 mmol/L is associated with toxicity
- U&Es (to monitor for renal failure and hypernatraemia).
- Serum Ca^{2+} (to monitor for hypercalcaemia).
- 12-lead ECG (conduction abnormalities or ST/T wave changes).

Immediate management

(See also 📖 p.454.)
- Give O_2 and support airway, breathing, and circulation as required.
- Charcoal does not work, but gastric lavage may be of benefit (if appropriate).
- ECG monitoring is recommended.
- Volume replacement with isotonic saline fluids may be required
- Haemodialysis should be considered if:
  - Levels >7.5 mmol/L for acute overdoses in patients who are lithium naïve, or
  - Levels >2.5 mmol/L in patients on chronic treatment, or
  - In acute-on-chronic OD, or
  - Where symptoms are severe
- Haemofiltration may be used, but is less effective and will take longer to lower levels.

⑦ Lead

The acute presentation of lead poisoning is an encephalopathy with ataxia, convulsions, and coma; associated with abdominal pain and vomiting. A peripheral motor neuropathy (foot and wrist drop) may occur.

Investigations

(See also 📖 p.449.)
- Blood lead levels can be estimated.
- FBC (anaemia with basophilic stippling, and RBC fluorescence).
- U&Es (reveal renal dysfunction).

Immediate management
(See also 🕮 p.454.)
- Give O_2 and support airway, breathing, and circulation as required.
- Charcoal does not work.
- Chelation therapy with IV EDTA or oral DMSA (preferred) should be considered.

Further management
(See also 🕮 p.456.)
- An ingested source should be looked for, as should any environmental contaminants.

☼ Iron
Iron poisoning usually occurs as a result of deliberate or accidental ingestion of large quantities of iron tablets.

Presentation and assessment
Iron initially acts as a GI irritant and may cause nausea and vomiting, abdominal pain, and GI bleeding. ↓consciousness and convulsions may occur if overdose is severe, accompanied by hypotension, pulmonary oedema, and metabolic acidosis.

Further complications may occur up to 48 hours after ingestion and can include: liver failure and/or renal failure, with accompanying metabolic acidosis, hypoglycaemia, and cardiovascular collapse.

Investigations
(See also 🕮 p.449.)
- Serum iron levels should be taken at 4 hours post ingestion (or just prior to desferrioxamine if given at <4 hours)—later iron levels may be artificially low.
- ABGs (to monitor for acidosis).
- FBC, coagulation screen.
- U&Es, LFTs.
- Serum glucose.
- AXR (may be useful to identify tablets).

Immediate management
(See also 🕮 p.454.)
- Give O_2 and support airway, breathing, and circulation as required.
- Charcoal does not work but gastric lavage is likely to be of benefit (if within 1 hour of ingestion or if AXR reveals intra-gastric tablets).
- Cardiovascular support with fluids/inotropes may be required.
- Desferrioxamine (15 mg/kg/hour IV, up to 80 mg/kg/day) may be indicated:
  - For patients with severe symptoms (do not delay whilst waiting for iron levels)
  - If serum iron >90 μmol/L (5 mg/L)
  - Desferrioxamine causes hypotension
- Whole bowel irrigation may be indicated for large overdoses.

Further management
(See also 📖 p.456.)
• Bowel ischaemia may occur requiring surgical treatment.
• Pyloric stenosis causing gastric outlet obstruction is a late
  complication.

☼: Corrosives, acids, alkalis, bleaches
The main acute risk with these agents is airway or pharyngeal damage. If
laryngeal oedema is present, early intubation should be considered even
if the patient is currently asymptomatic. Early ENT or thoracic surgical
involvement should be considered.

Activated charcoal does not work and gastric lavage should not be
attempted. Later complications include GI burns, which may require surgical intervention.

☺: Local anaesthetic toxicity
Local anaesthetic toxicity within critical care can occur if IV injection/infu-
sion occurs (e.g. a local anaesthetic epidural infusion bag is mistaken for
IV fluids), or if the soft-tissue dose given exceeds the maximum recommended dose.

Maximum recommended local anaesthetic doses
• Bupivacaine/levobupivacaine: 2 mg/kg
• Ropivacaine: 3 mg/kg
• Lidocaine: 3 mg/kg
• Lidocaine with adrenaline: 6 mg/kg
• Prilocaine: 6 mg/kg.

Presentation and assessment
Signs and symptoms include:
• Orofacial tingling/numbness, tinnitus, blurred vision, fasciculations.
• ↓consciousness, seizures, respiratory arrest.
• Circulatory collapse with resistant arrhythmias.

Immediate management
(See also 📖 p.454.)
• Stop giving the drug.
• Give O_2 and support airway, breathing, and circulation as required.
• Endotracheal intubation and mechanical ventilation may be required.
• Treat seizures as appropriate (📖 p.160).
• Consider treating cardiovascular collapse/arrest with:
  • Intralipid® 20% IV 1 ml/kg over 1 minute, repeated every 3–5
    minutes to a maximum of 3 ml/kg

☼ Bites and stings

Many snakebites are 'dry' (no injected venom), requiring no treatment, and many other bites or stings are of low toxicity. Expert advice is required to identify animals/insects and to direct treatment.

Toxicity is generally either local (tissue necrosis) or systemic (cardiotoxic, neurotoxic, or coagulopathic, either via direct inhibition or consumption of clotting factors).

Initially a compression lymph bandage may be applied (not a tourniquet) to slow the spread of any toxins. Antivenom may be advised for the treatment of certain snakebites, otherwise treatment is supportive.

Bites, stings, and antivenom may cause anaphylaxis or anaphylactoid reactions (see 📖 p.110).

Further reading

Joint Formulary Committee. *British national formulary, 64*. London: BMJ Group and Pharmaceutical Press, September 2012.

Odedra D, et al. Local anaesthetic toxicity. *Curr Anaesth Crit Care* 2010; **21**: 52–4.

Shepherd G. Treatment of poisoning caused by β-adrenergic and calcium-channel blockers. *Am J Health Syst Pharm* 2006; **63**: 1828–35.

Incidents and adverse events

:O: Suspected outbreaks

Suspected outbreaks may be associated with infections, biological agents, or poisonings (chemical, nutritional, or radioactive). Suspicious circumstances include: intelligence of a threat, multiple cases, simultaneous outbreaks elsewhere, and illness affecting a particular community.

Presentation and assessment

- Illnesses which do not fit any recognizable clinical condition.
- A known illness that is not expected in the setting where observed, or follows an unexpected course.

Illnesses that should arouse suspicion include:

- Clusters (>2) of patients with similar symptoms.
- Signs and symptoms inappropriate to patient's history/location.
- Signs/symptoms of syndromes/toxidromes (see 📖 p.452), such as:
  - Cholinergic activity: see 📖 p.480 (G and V nerve agents)
  - Respiratory symptoms: chest tightness, pulmonary oedema, associated eye irritation (phosgene, chlorine, mustard gases)
  - Unexplained severe metabolic acidosis (cyanides)
  - Skin blistering, unexplained 'thermal' type burns
  - Fever with paralysis, mediastinal lymphadenopathy, or haemorrhagic thrombocytopaenia, see 📖 pp.358 and 370 (anthrax, VHFs, tularaemia, pneumonic plague)
  - Aplastic anaemia, hair loss, severe GI loss

Investigations

For biological agent exposure, the following samples may be requested:

- Serum and whole blood EDTA (paired sample if recovery occurs).
- Blood cultures (at least 1 sample prior to antibiotics if possible).
- Sputum or bronchoalveolar lavage (if safe to do so).
- Biopsy or aspiration samples of necrotic lesions or vesicles (vesicle swabs should be placed in viral transport medium).
- Pus and/or swabs (take multiple samples).
- Urine and other body fluids.
- Stool or vomitus sample (if food contamination suspected).

Take HPA advice on sample precautions. The specimen should be labelled with surname/forename/DOB, and transported to a clinical microbiology laboratory as soon as possible.

Further actions

- Decontaminate before ICU admission; if unsure contact the HPA.
- Make list of all staff who may have been exposed; treat waste, property and samples as hazardous until advised otherwise.
- Use personal protective equipment as advised by HPA; if uncertain, use gloves, gown, cap, mask and eye protection (see 📖 p.384 for instructions on how to don protective equipment in high-risk cases).
- Give appropriate treatments where they are available:
  - Chemical poisoning: atropine and oximes, see 📖 p.480
  - Cyanide, see 📖 p.458
  - Anthrax/plague, see 📖 p.358
  - Tularaemia: doxycycline

- VHFs, see 📖 p.370)
- Radiation: potassium iodide may be appropriate; in cases of internal exposure: chelation, ion exchange, or lavage may be possible

Further reading

Health Protection Agency. *CBRN incidents: clinical management and health protection.* London: HPA, 2005.

Health Protection Agency. *Initial investigation and management of outbreaks and incidents of unusual illnesses: A guide for health professionals*, 2010. Available at: 🔗 <http://www.hpa.org.uk/webc/HPAwebFile/HPAweb_C/1201265888951>.

White SM. Chemical and biological weapons. Implications for anaesthesia and intensive care. *Br J Anaesth* 2002; **89**(2): 306–24.

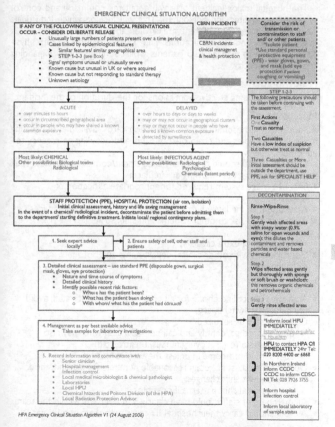

Fig. 15.1 Algorithm for the management of outbreaks. Reproduced with permission from the Health Protection Agency.

⚠ Major incidents

A major incident may be external (a disaster in the community) or internal (e.g. a fire). It is loosely defined as any incident that generates sufficient numbers/types of casualties as to require special arrangements.

Every hospital (and ICU) should have a major incident plan of which staff should be aware. A major incident should trigger involvement of senior management within the hospital to co-ordinate an effective response from different clinical departments. ICU staff may have to work closely with operating theatres, A&E, and other high dependency areas within the same hospital and/or other hospitals.

The hospital major incident plan will detail the command and control structure (both sites and personnel). This will include which individuals have responsibility for different areas/roles, including 'on scene', A&E, triage, theatres, and communications. The 1° role of intensive care physicians is usually to manage ICU patients whilst simultaneously expanding critical care capacity.

Major incidents and ICU

Consider suspending elective admissions for the duration of the incident.

Management

All areas of the hospital should have 'action cards' available, designating major incident roles and chain-of-command; and detailing emergency telephone numbers.

Senior ICU staff should take over management/coordinating roles. They should ensure that the following are in place:

• Effective triage system required for appropriate allocation of resources.
• Assessment of the likely burden and its impact on existing services.
• Assessment of risk to other patients and staff; strategies for risk containment.
• Identification of extra capacity.
• Coordination with other clinical departments and hospital management.

Staff

• Activate a direct-line phone for all communications with staff; avoid using hospital switchboard.
• Call extra staff as required:
  • Be prepared to identify and call non-ICU staff who may also provide help (e.g. recovery nurses, theatre staff)
  • Staff should not come in unless they are contacted
• Do not call in *all* staff; retain reasonable numbers for second, third, and subsequent shift changes:
  • Keep original shift patterns if possible
• All members of staff should have clearly defined roles within the team.
• All staff should carry their hospital ID cards with them at all times.

Identifying extra capacity

ICUs should have 'surge' plans that can be activated in the event of a sudden increase in demand for ICU beds. Actions include:
- Identify patients who may be safely discharged from critical care.
- Identify patients who may be safely transferred to other units.
- Identify capacity in nearby hospitals and keep them on alert.
- Identify other areas where extra patients can be managed (e.g. theatres, recovery).
- Identify and check equipment which can be used (e.g. syringe drivers, theatre ventilators).

Allocating roles

- Where possible, task-specific roles may be allocated (i.e. 1 member of staff preparing all IV infusions).
- Use flexible dependency systems (i.e. 1 critical care trained nurse to 2 level three patients).
- Where possible cohort patients with similar pathology to be cared for by 1 team.
- Allocate staff to transfer teams if required.

Communication

- The hospital internal telephone system may become overrun; a runner should be allocated to ICU.
- Keep families informed as much as possible, but only where face-to-face communication is possible; do not give out details over the phone.
- Do not communicate directly with the press, direct them to appropriate designated personnel (communication officer).
- Keep all channels of communication open.
- Arrange regular updates with other clinical departments (A&E, theatres) and senior hospital management.

Intensive care triage

In times of extreme pressure on resources it may become necessary to actively triage patients in order to maximize the delivery of healthcare to those patients most likely to benefit. Various systems of triage exist, but most attempt to categorize patients into 3 broad groups: those with critical illness who are unlikely to survive; those who are not critically ill, and for whom definitive treatment can be safely delayed; those who are critically ill, but are deemed salvageable (the group to whom resources are preferentially allocated).

Further reading

Mahoney EJ, et al. Mass-casualty incidents: how does an ICU prepare? *J Intensive Care Med* 2008; **23**: 219–35.

:Ö: Adverse events, managing the aftermath

Adverse events may lead to severe patient harm or death. Such a catastrophe has a major impact on patients, relatives, and staff. Providing appropriate care to the patient, and practical help and support to the relatives and the staff, are part of good clinical governance and risk management.

Immediate actions

- Consult departmental/hospital guidelines on the actions required in the event of an adverse incident.
- Accurate and contemporaneous records are vital:
  - A full retrospective account must be recorded as soon as possible
  - Records should be legible, timed, dated, and signed
  - Where possible, electronic copies of monitoring be printed and filed
  - Original charts and notes must not be altered in any way; amendments, if any, must be recorded separately
  - If possible, make personal notes for reference at a later date

Dealing with the patient

- In cases where death has resulted, leave all lines, tubes, and equipment in place, and inform the coroner.
- In case where the patient survives, consider asking a colleague to help and take over their care.

Dealing with relatives

- Do not break bad news over the telephone if at all possible; invite the relatives to come to the hospital; inform them that some complication had occurred, but provide no further details.
- Be polite with them all the time; if possible get a senior colleague or member of the team to help deal with relatives.
- Any interview with relatives should be a team approach; other members of the team could be surgeons, physicians, nurses, and colleagues.
- Offer a full explanation of any events, as far as they are known:
  - Avoid 'underplaying' the severity or seriousness of events
  - If the facts are not clear, avoid speculation (e.g. as to the cause of any event, or regarding any events which may have occurred before your involvement)
- Inform relatives that a full investigation will take place, and that this may take some time.
- Further interviews may be necessary.
- In cases where death has occurred, involve the hospital bereavement services.

Dealing with staff

- A senior colleague should attend the hospital and help in dealing with the aftermath.

- A decision will need to be made as to whether the members of staff involved are in a reasonable condition to continue with their duties.
- The clinical director should be involved at an early stage.
- The staff involved should contact their medical protection organizations at the earliest possible opportunity.
- Staff should cooperate with investigation, and not isolate themselves.

'Later' actions

Communications

- The clinical director, or a consultant not involved with the incident, should talk to senior hospital management, if necessary.
- The incident should be reported to local and national incident reporting channels.
- The communications officer, and complaints manager, within the hospital will require briefing of the adverse event.

Equipment and drugs

- The clinical director, or a consultant not involved with the incident, should check the patient, drugs, equipment, and records.
- Any faulty equipment should be de-commissioned.
- All pieces of equipment, records, imaging, and drug ampoules should be stored in a secure place for further investigation, if required.
- An accurate record of any equipment/drug checks should be maintained.

The ICU team

- A debriefing should be organized with the team to provide information and gain feedback.
- Any anxieties and misconceptions should be allowed to be aired, and then dealt with appropriately.
- The services of a trained counsellor may be required to assist staff.

The media

- Media enquiries, if they arise, should be directed to the communications officer within the hospital.

The role of the department

- Colleagues should allow the member of staff involved in the incident, to 'talk about it', without being judgemental.
- A group of colleagues may be required to lead a root cause analysis of the event.
- A senior colleague may be informally assigned to provide mentorship and support to the staff involved in the incident.
- Individuals involved are likely to need further support, e.g. from occupational health:
  - Where staff are severely affected by the event, they may suffer daydreams, flashbacks, restlessness, apathy, anger, fear, guilt, relationship problems, alcohol dependence and physical manifestations of stress

Possible outcomes (depending on the severity of the event and the circumstances involved)
- Local route cause analysis, including presentation of 'lessons learnt' in a meeting.
- Suspension of the staff involved in the incident, pending investigation.
- Involvement of deaneries and royal colleges in the case of trainees.
- Disciplinary actions by the General Medical Council or other regulatory body, which may involve retraining, and/or further assessment.
- Criminal prosecution or civil litigation.

Reporting an incident

In the majority of critical incidents, individual error is only a small fraction of the problem. The main problems are the latent factors inherent in unsafe systems (i.e. faulty design, poor resources, poor communication) which create conditions in which a simple mistake leads to the incident.

A system of reporting critical incidents, and learning from them, is central to patient safety and clinical governance within a hospital. All hospital staff should report any critical incident, at least at local level, in which they may have been involved.

Incident reporting in ICU

Each ICU should have robust incident reporting systems and a clinical governance lead. Ideally this system should also feed in to the hospital systems and/or national systems. All staff should be aware of the system, how to access it, what to report and then what to expect.

Periodic meetings, case discussions, root cause analysis, and initiatives to improve systems will be required to keep all staff engaged. Systems should also be in place to support the patient, relatives, and staff involved in the incident.

Core principles of an incident reporting system

- The main aim is to learn from incidents, so that systems can be improved to prevent incidents from recurring.
- In order to encourage staff to report, the system should be based on a non-punitive approach; i.e. rather than looking at 'who' was involved in the incident, we should be looking at 'how' the incident was caused and 'what' system improvements can be made to prevent it from recurring in future.
- It should allow free text so that staff can narrate what actually happened, with very few, if any, closed questions.
- If the reporter so desires, it should allow anonymity.
- The reporter should be able to submit it anytime, although early submission should be encouraged.
- It should be easy for the staff to report without worries of any punitive action.
- It should not take more than few minutes to report a typical incident.

- All incidents should be analysed, exploring institutional, organizational, environmental, team, individual, and patient factors:
  - Analysis should define the problem and suggest solutions
  - Analysis of incidents should be fed back using multiple channels (e.g. newsletters, e-mails, networking, safety meetings)

Training for emergencies (human factors)

Individuals are more likely to make mistakes when the demand on their cognition exceeds their capacity to handle (i.e. during emergency situations in a busy ICU). Systems should be in place whereby the chances of mistakes made by an individual member of the team are minimized (e.g. checklists, team working, protocols, alerts). Training for emergencies for ICU staff should have 2 components:
- Technical skills
- Non-technical skills

Training in non-technical skills should have the following components:

Situational awareness
- Information gathering: structured handovers; good communication; visible monitoring and alarms.
- Recognizing and understanding of the situation and its burden, resources, capacity, and priorities.
- Anticipating likely changes.

Decision-making
- Identifying options.
- Balancing risks and selecting options.
- Seeking opinions of the team members.
- Re-evaluating.

Team working and leadership
- Exchanging information.
- Assessing capabilities and supporting other members of the team
- Coordinating activities of the team members:
  - Confirm roles and responsibilities of individual team members
  - Discuss case with colleagues, and other specialists (e.g. radiologist, surgeon, microbiologist)
  - Consider requirements of others before acting
  - Focus on goals, and cooperate with others to achieve them

Task management
- Planning and preparing.
- Prioritizing.
- Maintaining standards.
- Resource management.

Training for emergencies:
- Should have an educational lead in the unit.
- Should ideally be undertaken in teams, involving all members of staff (e.g. physicians, nurses, managers).

- Utilize simulation centre facilities whenever possible.
- Practice case scenarios and major incidents on regular basis.
- Should incorporate de-briefing, reflection, and constructive feedback.
- Must incorporate training in non-technical skills.
- Evaluate non-technical skills of individual members of staff using standardized framework.
- Should emphasize a systems-approach to errors.
- Should incorporate strategies to improve systems to deal with emergencies (e.g. design, layout, resources, equipment, staff capacity and skill mix, channels of communication).
- Should incorporate strategies to improve performance during an emergency (e.g. team approach, roles and responsibilities, non-technical skills, leadership and priority, structured handovers/communication, protocols, and checklists).

Further reading

Association of Anaesthetists of Great Britain and Ireland. *Catastrophes in anaesthetic practice – dealing with the aftermath.* London: AAGBI, 2005.
Buckley TA, et al. Critical incident reporting in the intensive care unit. *Anaesthesia* 1997; **52:** 403–9.

Communication and organ donation

⊕ Breaking bad news

Communication with patients and their relatives should be part of ongoing care, and should, where possible, be provided at regular intervals or whenever the clinical situation changes.

Given the severity of illness and high probability of death of patients requiring critical care, communicating bad news with patients and/or their families is a common occurrence. Breaking bad news can be difficult and distressing for all concerned. Where possible, the breaking of bad news should be led by a consultant who has received training in how to do this, but the speed with which patients deteriorate may mean that this is not possible, and what follows is a simplified template for ensuring that this is done as professionally as possible. It may need to be adapted for certain situations and according to the individuals involved.

Breaking bad news

Preparation

- Confirm you have the right patient and check the latest details regarding their condition and ongoing management.
- Maintain relatives'/patient's privacy if possible by using a quiet room or pulling curtains around bed.
- Ensure you are not interrupted (if possible hand pagers and phones to someone else).
- Where possible have the nurse caring for the patient present at the interview to ensure good continuity of information.
- Introduce yourself to the patient or their relatives and confirm who you are talking with.
- Sit at the same level as the person you are talking to and maintain appropriate eye-to-eye contact.

What do the relatives or the patient know?

- Enquire as to what information has already been passed on to the patient or their relatives.
- Confirm their understanding of what they have already been told.

What information is wanted?

- Enquire as to what information they want to know next.

Give a 'warning shot'

- Give patients and relatives time to prepare for any bad news by giving a 'warning shot' such as: 'I'm afraid I have some bad news' or 'I'm afraid the situation is very serious'.

Allow relatives/patient to refuse further information

- Some patients or relatives may not want to hear bad news at this point, and they should be allowed to refuse to hear any more at this time; if they refuse then inform them that they can always ask for more information in the future.
- Relatives are not allowed to refuse on behalf of a relative who has *capacity*; it should be made clear that if the patient asks for information it will be given to them.

Give explanation (if requested)

- Give an honest explanation of the patient's clinical condition and likely prognosis.
- Use language which is clear and avoids, or simplifies, medical terms wherever possible.
- Avoid euphemisms, where it is appropriate to use words such as 'death' or 'dying' then do so.
- Do not provide false reassurance.
- If you do not know the diagnosis or likelihood of injury/death then it is appropriate to say so, it is also appropriate to explain in terms of what you *suspect* the most likely diagnosis/outcome will be.
- Re-iterate important points and confirm that they are understood: 'Does that make sense?'

Listen to concerns

- Enquire as to whether the patient/relatives have questions they want to ask. Time must be provided for them to absorb information and to ask questions—their agenda may be very different from what you are expecting and it is important to listen to any concerns.

Encourage expression of feelings

- A phrase such as 'How does that news leave you feeling?' may allow the relatives or patient to express their feelings and emotions which may be therapeutic in its own right.

Summarize explanation and explain plan, then offer availability and support

- Ensure that the patient or their relatives are aware that you, or a member of your team, will be available to provide further information as and when it is requested.

Communicate with team

- A summary of the conversation should be recorded in the patient's medical records; this should include any key points along with any specific concerns raised.

Adapted from Guidelines for communicating bad news with patients and their families, East Midlands Cancer Network (2010) by P Costello and G Finn, with permission ℗ http://www.eastmidlandscancernetwork.nhs.uk/Library/BreakingBadNewsGuidelines.pdf

Pitfalls/difficult situations

- Communication is a process. The severity of a situation may require several conversations with different clinicians before it is fully accepted.
- Patients/relatives may be angry about the situation or about previous management. This anger should be acknowledged, and where appropriate an apology offered. Do not enter into criticism of previous management.

Further reading

Buckman R. *How to break bad news*. Baltimore, MD: John Hopkins University Press, 1992.
Fallowfield L, et al. Communicating sad, bad, and difficult news in medicine. *Lancet* 2004; **363**: 312–19.
Kaye P. *Breaking bad news: A ten step approach*. Northampton: EPL Publications, 1996.

☠ Referral to the coroner

It is not uncommon to be required to discuss the deaths of critically ill patients with a member of the coroner's office, or to the procurator fiscal in Scotland

The role of the coroner is to investigate deaths that are unexpected, unexplained, violent or unnatural, occur whilst in custody, or occur as the result of a medical mishap. The coroner is tasked with establishing who the deceased was, as well as where, when, and how they died.

Deaths requiring referral to the coroner

- Where the cause is unknown or unclear.
- Any sudden or unexpected death, including:
  - Sudden infant death
  - Stillbirths where there was a possibility of the child being born alive
- Any death which is 'unnatural', including:
  - Deaths associated with poisoning (deliberate or accidental)
  - Death associated with therapeutic or recreational drug usage, including alcohol overdose
  - Death which may be related to an accident
- Any death which may be related to industrial disease.
- Any death associated with violence, including:
  - Death connected with a crime, or suspected crime
  - Suspected suicide
- Any death associated with neglect, including:
  - Self-neglect, including chronic alcoholism
  - Neglect by others
- If the deceased was not seen professionally by a doctor during their last illness, within 14 days of death (28 days in Northern Ireland), or after death.
- Death occurring during an operation, or before recovery from an anaesthetic.
- Any death in custody or detention, or occurring shortly after release.

Referral inclusion criteria are deliberately broad, and in practice the list should be interpreted as including any unexpected hospital death, death from a complication of routine treatment, or trauma-related death.

After discussion, the coroner may ask whether or not, as the reporting medical practitioner, you are able to issue a death certificate (e.g. where potentially life-saving surgery has been attempted in an otherwise dying individual). Alternatively (or in cases where you are not able to issue a death certificate), the coroner will take over the case.

The coroner may require a postmortem examination in order to ascertain the cause of death (this cannot be refused), and may hold an inquest (or fatal accident inquiry in Scotland), for which you may be required to write a factual report and/or attend and give evidence.

Verdicts (or Findings, Northern Ireland, or Determinations, Scotland) may be narrative in form, analysing the context and causes of the death. Alternatively 'short form' verdicts may be used, of which the commonest are:
- Natural causes.
- Accidental death, or death by misadventure.
- Suicide.
- Unlawful or lawful killing.
- Industrial disease.
- Open verdicts (there is insufficient evidence for any other verdict).

Coroners are independent of government, and are not part of the civil or criminal courts. The coroner does not attribute culpability or liability. The coroner can, however, draw the case to the attention of an appropriate authority (for instance, if a further death could be prevented).

Pitfalls/difficult situations
- Organ donation may still be possible in brain-dead individuals or potential 'non-heart beating donors' who require referral to the coroner; contact the coroner, who may allow donation to go ahead.
- There are no time limits as to when a death may be attributable to a violent or medical cause.
- The rules regarding what should be reported to the procurator fiscal in Scotland are essentially the same as those in England and Wales, but a previous publication includes a list which is much more specific in certain areas:
  - Possible or suspected suicide
  - Accidents: any death arising from the use of a vehicle including an aircraft, a ship, or a train; any death by drowning; any death by burning or scalding or as a result of a fire or explosion
  - Certain deaths of children: any death of a newborn child whose body is found, any death from apparent sudden infant death syndrome (cot death), any death of a child from suffocation including overlaying, any death of a foster child
  - Occupational: any death at work, whether or not as a result of an accident; any death related to occupation, e.g. industrial disease or poisoning
  - Any death following an abortion or attempted abortion
  - Any death as a result of a medical mishap, and any death where a complaint is received which suggests that medical treatment or the absence of treatment may have contributed to the death
  - Any death due to notifiable infectious disease, or food poisoning
  - Any death of a person of residence unknown, who died other than in a house

Further reading
Crown Office. *Death and the procurator fiscal*. London: Crown Office Publication, November 1998.
Crown Office and Procurator Fiscal Service. *The role of the procurator fiscal in the investigation of deaths*. London: Crown Office and Procurator Fiscal Service, 2009.
General Medical Council. *Treatment and care towards the end of life*. London: GMC, 2010.
Ministry of Justice. *A guide to coroners and inquests*. London: Ministry of Justice 2010.

:O: The potential organ donor

Patients may be considered for organ donation after brainstem death or after cardiac death ('non-heart-beating donors').

Brainstem death

Two doctors (one a consultant) are required to perform brainstem death tests. Both must be competent to perform the tests and be registered with the GMC for 5 years. Neither may be connected with transplant team. Two sets of tests are required with a gap in between (there is no set time period). Both doctors should be present at both tests.

Death is confirmed after the 2nd set of tests, *but* time of death is after the 1st test.

Criteria for brainstem death

Exclusions

- Is the core temperature <35°C?
- Could any narcotics, hypnotics, tranquillizers, or muscle relaxant drugs still be affecting the patient (e.g. been given within the past 12 hours or 24 hours if renal/hepatic failure present)?
- Is there a metabolic, circulatory or endocrine cause for the coma?

If the answer to any of these questions is **yes** then brainstem death cannot be said to exist (*do not perform tests*)

Brainstem death tests

- Do the pupils react to light, either directly or consensually?
- Are corneal reflexes present when a cotton bud is gently pressed to the cornea?
- Is there any eye movement following slow injection of 50 ml iced water over a period of 1 minute into both ears with the head flexed at 30°?[1]
- Is there any limb, facial, or neck movement in response to bilateral supraorbital nerve pressure? Is there any limb, facial, or neck response to a painful stimulus to any other somatic area?
- Is a gag reflex present (contraction of the soft palate when the uvula is stimulated)?
- Is a cough reflex present on tracheal suctioning (with the suction catheter passed via the ETT as far as the carina)?
- Is there any eye movement during the 'Doll's eye' manoeuvre?[2]
- Is there any respiratory effort during an apnoea test (patient given 100% O_2 for 10 minutes, $PaCO_2$ allowed to rise to ≥5 kPa, then the patient is disconnected from the ventilator and $PaCO_2$ allowed to rise to >6.65 kPa with a pH <7.4)?

If the answer to any of these questions is **yes** then brainstem death is *not present*.

Ancillary tests (4-vessel cerebral angiography, cerebral radioisotope scanning, or transcranial Doppler) may help in confirming brainstem death, but are not required.

[1] Tympanic membranes should be examined by otoscopy first.

[2] Not required but still used by some practitioners.

Brainstem death potential donors

Where a patient is expected to be brain dead, and testing is planned, the local transplant coordinator (or specialist nurse for organ donation) should be informed. The timing of any discussion with donor's relatives depends upon the individual circumstances. One approach is to perform the 1st set of brainstem death tests and approach the relatives to obtain assent if organ donation is likely to be possible.

If assent is granted, life-sustaining ICU treatment may continue until organ donation, providing it doesn't risk harm or distress to the patient.

Cardiac death donors

Where a patient is expected to die (either as result of disease progression, or more likely as a result of treatment withdrawal where ongoing treatment is considered futile) they may be considered for organ donation after death. This is often only possible where cause of death is unlikely to be systemic and organ damaging (i.e. after head injuries, but not after fulminant systemic sepsis). The local transplant coordinator should again be contacted and familial assent obtained.

If assent is granted, life-sustaining ICU treatment may continue until organ donation, providing it does not risk harm or distress to the patient. Once organ donation is ready to proceed (i.e. the team is present), treatment is discontinued and the patient is allowed to die. Once death is confirmed (following an external examination and 5–10 minutes of monitored asystole) organ donation may proceed *provided* no measures capable of resuscitating the brain are taken.

Potential organ donors

Many contraindications to organ donation are relative; a full discussion with the transplant coordinator is essential. Aside from lack of consent other potential contraindications include fulminant sepsis, extra CNS malignancy, hepatitis B or C, HIV, CJD, and direct myocardial toxicity. In potential thoracic donors, donor age, smoking status, inotrope requirements, organ damage, and a PaO_2 <19 kPa on FiO_2 of 30% (or PaO_2 <33 kPa on a FiO_2 of 50%) may affect the decision. Renal and liver retrieval decisions may be affected by the presence of IDDM, renal/reno-vascular disease, liver disease, fatty liver, or a history of alcohol abuse.

The management of potential organ donors

Be guided by the transplant coordinator and the organ retrieval team
- Continue ICU management, including: lung protective ventilation, physiotherapy, aseptic precautions, antibiotic treatment, nutrition.
- Prevent/correct hypothermia, biochemical and endocrine derangement.
- Maintain cardiovascular status; teat hypovolaemia, but avoid excessive volume replacement; correct anaemia and coagulopathy.
- Take blood samples as advised.

Further reading

Academy of Medical Royal Colleges. *A code of practice for the diagnosis and confirmation of death.* London: Academy of Medical Royal Colleges, 2008.
Department of Health. *Legal issues relevant to non-heartbeating organ donation.* London: DoH, 2009.
General Medical Council. *Treatment and care towards the end of life.* London: GMC, 2010.

Common emergency procedures

⑦ Transfers and retrievals

Types of transfer/retrieval
- Intrahospital transfer (e.g. to ICU or to CT scan).
- Interhospital transfer (e.g. because the patient requires a specialist investigation or intervention; there is a lack of critical care beds in the referring hospital; to repatriate the patient).
- 1° retrieval (e.g. from the roadside).[1]
- 2° retrieval (an interhospital transfer using a specialist team from another healthcare facility to retrieve the patient).

Decision to transfer
- Is the transfer necessary?
- Is further stabilization required; will further stabilization delay urgent treatment (e.g. surgical decompression of intracranial haematomas)?[1]
- Is everything that might be needed to treat any reasonably predictable complication available to accompany the patient?
- Are the correct staff, equipment, and transfer apparatus available?

Organization of transfer
- Transfers should be organized using the *ACCEPT* format.
- **A**ssessment:
  - Review the history and assess the need for transfer
  - Clinically reassess the patient (following **A, B, C, D, E,** format)
- **C**ontrol:
  - Identify team members and allocate roles and tasks
- **C**ommunication:
  - Ensure relatives and clinicians are aware of the transfer
  - For interhospital transfers, telephone the receiving unit before leaving
- **E**valuation:
  - Ensure transfer is appropriate, and decide the urgency of transfer
  - Decide what transfer vehicle and escort requirements are needed
  - Air transfer may be appropriate for long distances, or where speed is required, but may worsen hypoxia
- **P**reparation:
  - Ensure the patient is appropriately 'packaged'
  - Check equipment and reserves of O_2, drugs, and battery life
  - Ensure all necessary notes and imaging are packaged
- **T**ransportation:
  - Confirm the route and the final destination
  - Continue monitoring during transit
  - Recheck the patient just before leaving, and just before arriving
  - Ensure handover of crucial information

---

[1] With the exception of 1° retrievals, and transfers for urgently required treatments, there will be sufficient time to fully stabilize the patient. A 'scoop and run' policy should only be adopted where there are insufficient resources available to resuscitate A, B, and C.

Stabilization and preparation prior to transfer
- Most procedures are difficult to undertake en route; if there is a probability of deterioration then anticipate and prepare for it.
- Reassess the patient's history, treatment, and examination findings.
- Use a checklist wherever possible.

Airway
- Consider endotracheal intubation if the airway may obstruct (especially in facial burns or trauma, or where GCS may drop to <8).
- Confirm the ETT position and ensure it is secured firmly in place.
- Decide whether C-spine precautions are required for transfer.
- Some centres replace ETT cuff air with saline prior to air transport.

Breathing
- If oxygenation/ventilation is poor consider elective intubation and mechanical ventilation prior to transfer:
  - NIV is rarely possible to deliver during transport
- In ventilated patients with refractory hypoxia it may be possible to use portable ECMO for the transfer, this is provided by specialist centres.
- Establish the patient on the transport ventilator *prior to transfer* and check ABGs:
  - Transport ventilators often only produce basic levels of respiratory support
- Check for any chest problem, review CXR for evidence of pneumothoraces (difficult to treat in transit; may expand during air transfer)
  - Consider prophylactic chest drains in cases of chest trauma
  - Fluid-locked chest drains may be replaced with Heimlich valves

Circulation
- Avoid transferring hypotensive patients where possible.
- Ensure a minimum of 2 secure, working large-bore (16-G cannulae).
- Control haemorrhage and fluid resuscitate.
- If required, establish on inotropes/vasopressors prior to transfer:
  - Avoid using high concentration inotrope solutions where possible (>16 mg adrenaline/noradrenaline in 50 ml) as low volume siphoning from syringe drivers may occur
- An invasive arterial line is preferable for BP monitoring:
  - NIBP monitoring is possible during road and air transport, but is less reliable and uses more battery power
- If a PAFC is *in situ* and the waveform cannot be monitored in transit, consider withdrawing it to the RA to avoid inadvertent 'wedging'.
- Where arrhythmias are a problem place adhesive defibrillator pads on the patient prior to 'wrapping'.
- Check last measured Hb and K^+ results.
- Stabilize long-bone/pelvic fractures.

Neurological
- Re-check GCS and neurological status.
- Commence any required/recommended treatment for raised ICP.
- Establish mechanically ventilated patients on sedative infusions.

Other
- Check available equipment for transfer:
  - Assemble and check critical pieces (e.g. self-inflating bags)
- 'Mummy-wrap' the patient with blankets (strap in all lines/tubes).
- Ensure pressure point care and eye protection.
- Remove/stop any unnecessary equipment or infusions.
- If using air travel consider inserting an NGT and splitting plaster casts.
- Consider the mode of transfer (ground versus air):
  - Air transfers may be high risk for patients with high O_2 requirements, recent altitude sickness, recent diving injury, pneumothorax, bullae, pneumoperitoneum, or pneumocranium
  - Do they really need to fly; can the aircraft be pressurized to ground level equivalent?
- Discuss morbidly obese patients with ambulance control as specialist bariatric equipment may be required.
- Avoid using transfer oxygen/batteries until the last minute.

Communication and documentation
- All notes, X-rays, CT scans, and blood results should be taken.
- A patient summary sheet should be prepared where possible.
- Ensure that all parties involved are aware of the transfer: the receiving hospital/unit, the patient/relatives, ambulance control:
  - Confirm the destination and obtain directions if appropriate
  - Consider a police escort for 'life or death' transfers

Transfer practices
- 'Intensive care' monitoring and management should be continued throughout the transfer process.
- A minimum of 2 staff should accompany the patient, 1 of whom should be trained in advanced airway techniques for any patient who is, or may require to be, intubated; both staff should be familiar with transfer equipment.
- Phone the receiving unit immediately prior to transfer.
- Before leaving review the patient's condition for a final time and check all the drugs and equipment needed are going with the patient.
- Take money and an emergency phone with you (and the telephone numbers of the transferring and receiving units).

Monitoring
- *Minimum* standard monitoring should include:
  - Continuous presence of appropriately trained staff
  - ECG, non-invasive BP, oxygen saturation (SpO_2)
  - $ETCO_2$ in ventilated patients
  - Ventilator pressure, disconnect/FiO_2 failure alarms
  - Temperature (preferably core *and* peripheral)

Management
- Allocate any task-specific roles early (e.g. who is responsible for monitoring specialist equipment such as ICP monitoring).

Airway
- Disconnect the ventilator tubing from the ETT whenever the patient is moved from one bed to another to avoid accidental extubation.
- The person in charge of the head and airway controls when any patient movements occur.
- ETCO$_2$ monitoring provides an essential disconnect alarm.

Breathing
- Mechanically ventilated patients often need to be sedated and given neuromuscular blocking drugs to facilitate safe transfer.
- Transport ventilators are often less efficient, necessitating ↑ventilation pressures or higher FiO$_2$ especially during air transport.
- Special attention needs to be paid to chest injuries:
  - Do not clamp chest drains
  - Where pneumothoraces occur in mechanically ventilated patients during air/road transfers consider doing a mid-axillary line blunt-dissection thoracocentesis without inserting a chest drain (air should be released, the lung should be palpable confirming re-expansion, a sterile chest drain may be inserted upon arrival)
- Calculate the volume of O$_2$ required for the transfer:
  - Switch to ambulance/aircraft O$_2$ supply as soon as appropriate

Circulation and neurological
- Where possible keep infuser pumps at the same level as the patient (some pumps siphon).
- Vibration in aircraft (particularly rotary wing) may interfere with gravity IV infusions, pressure infusers should be available.
- Invasive BP monitoring is often more reliable than non-invasive techniques during transfer.
- Infusion pumps, monitors and any associated transfer equipment must be attached to either the transfer trolley or the vehicle during transfers (to avoid them becoming projectiles in crash situations).
- Maintain access to pupils (for assessment).

Environment
- Keep the ambulance/aircraft warm.
- Keep all monitoring within view.
- Ensure IV access is always within reach.

Movement
- Perform a visual sweep prior to the patient moving from any location to ensure lines, NGTs, urinary catheters are not going to catch.
- Always ensure that the team are prepared and know exactly *how* (i.e. log roll, slowly) and *which way* the patient is going to be moved:
  - A recognized 'count' is: 'ready, steady, slide/roll'
- Secure the patient to any transfer trolley (cot-sides up, safety belts attached) prior to moving trolley; ensure trolley is secured to ambulance/aircraft prior movement.

Transport vehicles
- Once inside a vehicle secure all equipment.
- Staff should be securely seated during travel.
- If possible the head and one side of the patient should be accessible.
- Consider providing antiemetics to the patient (and staff).
- Special considerations for aircraft:
  - *Never* approach/enter an aircraft without permission from the pilot or load-master; follow their instructions at all times
  - *Never* approach the rear of a rotary wing aircraft with a tail rotor
  - Consider providing ear-defenders, or other protection, to the patient during air transfers
  - 'Hot' unloads are rarely necessary, full engine shutdown should normally be allowed to happen before departure from rotary wing aircraft; if a 'hot' unload is required make sure everyone knows their roles and responsibilities prior to landing (and that ground crew are aware)
  - Defibrillation in aircraft: most modern aircraft are defibrillation-safe, check first
  - Take-off, landing, and banking will increase physiological stresses (hypotension or raised ICP may be temporarily worsen); infusion pumps above or below the patient may have slightly altered rates
- Air expansion at altitude:
  - Air-filled splints should be opened, plaster casts may need splitting, NG decompression may be required
  - Some guidelines recommend inflating endotracheal and catheter cuffs with saline rather than air (alternatively monitor pressures)
  - Air bubbles in invasive monitoring sets will expand and dampen pressure monitoring traces

Documentation
- Take all relevant patient documents with you.
- Document the patient's condition during the transfer.
- Perform a detailed handover of the patient to the receiving team.

Transfer equipment
- Ensure you are familiar with available equipment
- When retrieving patients assume that no equipment will be available: take your own
- Use dedicated trolleys for interhospital transfers where available
- Where transfer may be weight-limited (e.g. in rotary wing aircraft)—discuss any requirements with the crew.

Airway and ventilation
- Guedel and nasopharyngeal airways (assorted sizes).
- ETTs (assorted sizes); laryngoscopes (spare bulbs and battery); intubating stylet; lubricating gel; Magill's forceps; tape for securing tracheal tube; sterile scissors; stethoscope; laryngeal mask airways (assorted sizes).

- Portable suction; Yankauer sucker; suction catheters (assorted sizes); NG tubes (assorted sizes) and drainage bag.
- Self-inflating bag and mask with O_2 reservoir; high-flow breathing circuit; chest drains (assorted sizes); Heimlich flutter valves.
- Ventilators: check prior to use; spare valves for portable ventilator.

Oxygen

- Calculate O_2 requirements for trip, ensure that 2–3 hours of 'back-up' O_2 is available (discuss with ambulance crew the O_2 they have available) (Table 17.1).
- Many ventilators display their O_2 consumption.

Table 17.1 British Oxygen Company cylinder sizes and volume

Standard valve	Integral valve	Handwheel
C (170 L)	CD (460 L)	ZA (300 L)
D (340 L)	ZD (600 L)	ZB (300 L)
E (680 L)	HX (2300 L)	ZC (300 L)
F or AF (1360 L)	ZX (3040 L)	AD (460 L)
G (3400 L)	ZH (2400 L)	DD (460 L)
J (6800 L)	DF (1360 L)	

Circulation and drugs

- Syringes (assorted sizes); needles (assorted sizes); alcohol wipes; IV cannulae (assorted sizes); arterial cannulae (assorted sizes); central venous cannulae; IV fluids; infusion sets/extensions; 3-way taps; dressings/tape; pressure infusers.
- Emergency drugs for cardiac arrest and intubation/reintubation should be available; spare infusions should be prepared for any inotropes, sedatives, or muscle relaxants; predictable emergency drugs should also be available (e.g. anti-seizure medication); spare IV fluid should be available.
- Infusion pumps should be checked (and spares taken where transfer will be long, or an infusion is critical); a defibrillator may be required (ambulance crews may be able to provide this).

Other equipment

- Consider the need for: blood, minor instrument/cut-down set, tracheostomy set.
- Specialist protective clothing should be available for interhospital transfers or retrievals; individuals roles should be clearly identifiable.

Pitfalls/difficult situations

- Most problems during transfer result from inadequate stabilization prior to departure, or failure to continue optimal treatment and monitoring during transfer.

Further reading

Ahmed I, et al. Risk management during inter-hospital transfer of critically ill patients: making the journey safe. *Emerg Med J* 2008; **25**: 502–5.

Association of Anaesthetists of Great Britain and Ireland. *Interhospital transfer, AAGBI safety guideline.* London: AAGBI, 2009.

Intensive Care Society. *Guidelines for the transport of the critically ill adult.* London: Intensive Care Society, 2011.

Macartney I, et al. Transfer of the critically ill adult patient. *Br J Anaesth CEPD Rev* 2001; **1**(1): 12–15.

Rapid sequence intubation

ⓘ **Rapid sequence intubation**

Rapid sequence endotracheal intubation (RSI) is a complex skill, which should not be attempted without training. Even if you are not competent to perform the procedure you may be called upon to assist or prepare the equipment.

Indications for endotracheal intubation

To protect the airway
- From risk of aspiration (e.g. blood/vomit).
- From risk of airway obstruction.
- Where sedation/anaesthesia is required to allow assessment or treatment (particularly in agitated or combative patients).

To permit mechanical ventilation
- Apnoea or bradypnoea.
- Hypoxia or inadequate respiratory effort.
- Hypercapnia or requirement for hyperventilation.
- Cardiovascular instability, to optimize oxygen supply/demand.

Indications for rapid sequence intubation

RSI is the preferred technique for endotracheal intubation where there is a risk of aspiration:
- Aspiration of gastric contents is strongly associated with unstarved patients, pregnancy, oesophageal disease, obesity, ileus/bowel obstruction.

Contraindications

- When attempted as an absolute emergency (i.e. impending or actual cardiac arrest) there are no contraindications to attempting endotracheal intubation.
- In all other situations (i.e. urgent or semi-elective endotracheal intubation) the operator must be experienced in the technique and the likelihood of the patient being difficult to intubate must be assessed (📖 p.24) and appropriate preparations made.
- Suxamethonium should not be used in patients with a known allergy to suxamethonium, a history of MH, hyperkalaemia, recent burns (>2 days, <18 months), or paralysis.

Equipment
- One assistant (preferably more) is required to monitor the patient, administer drugs, pass equipment to the operator, and apply cricoid pressure (allocate roles beforehand, in case of difficult intubation).
- Full monitoring (PaO_2, ECG, BP).
- A range of facemasks and a means of ventilating (i.e. self-inflating bag).
- Airway adjuncts (OPAs NPAs).
- Cuffed ETT; as a rough guide size 8 for adult females, size 9 for males:
  - Range of cuffed ETTs (sizes 6.5–10)

- Spare ETTs should be prepared in the sizes above and below the chosen size
- ETTs may be pre-cut to a length of 26–28 cm; *do not cut ETTs if oro-facial swelling is likely (e.g. burns)*
- Lubricant gel (to facilitate passage of ETT through vocal cords).
- 10-ml syringe (for inflating ETT cuff).
- Laryngoscope (plus spare) with Mackintosh blades size 3 and 4.
- Gum elastic bougie, stylet.
- Tape or tie (to secure ETT post-intubation).
- Stethoscope.
- Yankauer sucker, suction catheters and suction apparatus, and a bed/trolley that can tilt head down if possible.
- Magill forceps.
- ETCO$_2$ monitoring.
- Intubation drugs (e.g. ketamine, thiopental, or propofol; suxamethonium or rocuronium).
- Emergency drugs, immediately available:
  - Resuscitation drugs (e.g. metaraminol, atropine, adrenaline)
- Failed intubation equipment, readily accessible:
  - Microlaryngel tubes (size 5–6)
  - Special laryngoscopes (e.g. McCoy, short-handled, polio blade)
  - LMAs/supraglottic airway devices (sizes 3, 4, 5) (intubating LMA if available)
  - Airway exchange catheters
  - Intubating fibreoptic scope
  - Berman airways
  - Emergency cricothyroidotomy kit
  - Jet ventilator
- Consider having an NGT available.

Anatomical landmarks

- The cricoid cartilage may be identified immediately inferior to the thyroid cartilage; it feels like a wedding ring below the skin (Fig. 17.1).

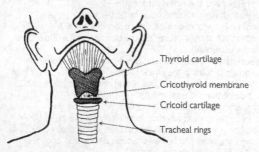

Thyroid cartilage

Cricothyroid membrane

Cricoid cartilage

Tracheal rings

Fig. 17.1 Anatomy of the cricoid cartilage.

Technique

* Briefly assess the patient's airway (see 📖 p.24); and check any pertinent history (e.g. allergies, previous anaesthetic reactions).
* Check equipment (suction, laryngoscope bulb, ETT cuff).
* Mentally prepare a plan A, B, and C in case of failed intubation (see 📖 p.25), ensure staff are informed of key aspects.
* Establish IV access.
* Aspirate NGT if one is in place.
* Ensure the patient is positioned with their head on a pillow (often removed during CPR) so that the head is raised just above the shoulders.
* Attach all monitoring; check that the bed/trolley head tilt mechanism is working.

Head positioning is not possible where trauma is suspected; in such cases an assistant is required to apply manual in-line stabilization to the head. The anterior aspect of the hard collar can then be undone or removed prior to attempting tracheal intubation. Where possible a bougie should be used for trauma intubations in order to minimize the degree of neck movement required.

* Pre-oxygenate with 100% O_2 for 3–5 minutes if possible, using a facemask and ventilating circuit (gently assisting ventilation is best avoided if possible, but may be necessary in critically ill patients).
* Remove false teeth.
* Have suction turned on and within reach.
* Administer induction agents over 20–30 seconds, any of:
  * Thiopental IV 2–5 mg/kg
  * Propofol IV 1–5 mg/kg
  * Ketamine IV 1–3 mg/kg
  * Thiopental and propofol commonly cause hypotension requiring fluid and/or inotropic support; in cardiovascularly unstable patients consider using ketamine (may cause hypertension, tachycardia or raised ICP)
* Apply cricoid pressure (do not release until ETT is in position, $ETCO_2$ is present and the cuff is inflated[1]).
* Immediately administer suxamethonium IV 1–2 mg/kg (where suxamethonium is contraindicated use rocuronium IV 0.6–1 mg/kg):
  * Suxamethonium should cause fasciculation within 15–30 seconds (not always observed).
* After 30 seconds (or when fasciculations cease, or 60 seconds if using rocuronium), holding the laryngoscope in your left hand (close to the angle between the handle and blade), insert the blade into the right-hand side of the patients' mouth:
  * Bring the laryngoscope back to the midline, pushing the tongue aside beneath it; advance forwards until the tip of the laryngoscope is in the vallecula space, then lift vertically until the vocal cords are seen (do not lever scope backwards onto teeth)
* Pass a size 8–9 ETT through the cords.
* Inflate the ETT cuff and attempt ventilation.

- Confirm correct position of the ETT within the trachea by:
  - Presence of $ETCO_2$[2]
  - Obvious chest movement
  - Presence of misting/clearing of the ETT/catheter mount
  - Bilateral chest sounds on auscultation (listen to the chest in the mid-axillary line on both sides)
  - Absence of 'bubbling' sounds over the stomach on auscultation
- Secure the ETT in position using tape or tie; make a note of the ETT length at the teeth/gums.
- If intubation is successful and the patient stable consider inserting an NGT or OGT.
- Commence a sedative infusion.
- Consider a bolus dose of non-depolarizing muscle relaxant (unless rocuronium already used).
- Confirm the distal position of the ETT on CXR (above the carina).
- Check ABGs.

In the event of a failed/difficult intubation
- If unable to intubate adjust the head and neck position and have one more attempt; if still unable to intubate follow the failed intubation protocol (🕮 p.27).
- 'Declare' the situation, so that members of the team know that it is an emergency and can adopt the previously assigned role.
- Proceed to plans A, B, and C as previously decided (see 🕮 p.25).
- Never forget that *the priority is oxygenation not intubation; be prepared to maintain oxygenation by any technique available.*

[1] Cricoid pressure may have to be released in the event of a failed intubation, see 🕮 p.27.
[2] CO_2 will not be present if there is no cardiac output, i.e. cardiac arrest.

Special considerations/complications
- Oesophageal intubation may be difficult to spot, signs include:
  - Absent $ETCO_2$ trace
  - Poor chest expansion, or abdominal distension
  - 'Distant' breath sounds
  - Progressive cyanosis
- *If in doubt remove ETT and re-intubate.*
- Endobronchial intubation: commonly right-sided causing unilateral chest expansion and breath sounds; withdraw the ETT to 21–23 cm listening for bilateral chest sounds; check position with a CXR.
- Etomidate is no longer routinely recommended as an induction agent for critically ill patients (although it is a cardiovascularly stable drug, it may cause adrenal suppression); if etomidate has been used consider giving hydrocortisone 50 mg 8-hourly for 24 hours.

① Laryngeal mask airway insertion

Indications

Laryngeal mask airways (LMAs) are the most commonly used supra-glottic airway device. Less training is required to insert LMAs than for endotracheal intubation, and the skill is retained over a long period.

Within critical care the indications for insertion of an LMA are:
- To obtain an airway in an emergency, as a bridge to endotracheal intubation.
- As an alternative to endotracheal intubation during CPR.
- To obtain an airway as a last resort (e.g. failed intubation).

Contraindications

- In an emergency situation there are no contraindications.
- LMAs do not provide a definitive airway, and do not protect from aspiration; the intention should always be to proceed to endotracheal intubation or tracheostomy as soon as appropriate.

Equipment

- LMAs (sizes 3, 4, and 5):
  - Size 3 for a small female, size 5 for a large male
- Lubricant.
- Tape or ties.
- 20- or 50-ml syringe.
- Yankauer sucker and suction apparatus.
- Stethoscope.

Technique

- Check equipment (no blockage within the tubing; LMA cuff is intact when inflated).
- Deflate cuff; apply lubricant to the smooth surface of the cuff/mask.
- Position the patient's head on a pillow if possible.
- If possible, ask an assistant to pull the lower jaw downwards.
- Insert the cuff/mask end of the LMA into the mouth so that its smooth surface is against the patient's palate.
- Using your first 2 fingers, against the point where the 'mask' and tube connect, the LMA should be advanced until it has moved behind the tongue and in front of the vocal cords (Fig. 17.2).
- Gently inflate the mask with air (size 3: 20 ml; size 4: 30 ml; size 5: 40 ml), the protruding tube end of the LMA usually rises 1–2 cm.
- Attach means of ventilation (e.g. a self-inflating bag) to the 15-mm connection and attempt gentle ventilation:
  - Check that air entry is present by the presence of $ETCO_2$; obvious chest movement; presence of misting/clearing of the ETT/catheter mount; chest sounds present on auscultation
  - A small air leak is acceptable
- Consider inserting an oropharyngeal airway as a 'bite block'.

Special considerations/complications
- Obstruction or leak:
  - The LMA may curl back on itself during placement, causing it to be malpositioned (attempt to ensure the smooth surface of the LMA does not curl back as it moves from the soft palate to the posterior pharyngeal wall)
- LMAs provide only minimal protection against aspiration.
- The seal produced by an LMA may not be good enough to provide adequate levels of PEEP.
- Laryngospasm may be provoked.
- Sore throat is common.

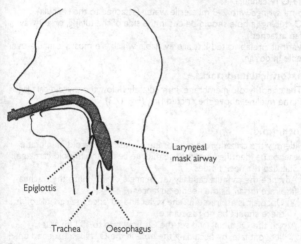

Fig. 17.2 Positioning of a laryngeal mask airway.

:☠: Needle cricothyroidotomy

Indications
- To obtain an airway and oxygenate the patient in the event of an obstructed upper airway
- The last resort following a failed intubation where oxygenation is impossible by other means

Contraindications
- When done as an emergency procedure there are no contraindications

Equipment
- 14-G IV cannula.
- 5-ml syringe with 2–3 ml sterile water (attached to the cannula).
- O_2 tubing (a hole should be cut in the side of the tubing, or a 3-way tap attached).
  Various prefabricated kits are available which are mostly cannula-over-needle in design.

Anatomical landmarks
- The cricothyroid membrane: immediately below the thyroid cartilage in the midline, above the cricoid ring (Fig. 17.3).

Technique
- Identify the cricothyroid membrane (if the cricothyroid membrane cannot be identified aim for the midline below the thyroid cartilage).
- Stabilize the neck tissues.
- Advance the cannula caudally (at an angle of ~45°) into the trachea (aspirate for air as the needle advances):
  - Once air is aspirated fix the stylet and advance the cannula off it; there should be no resistance
- Attach the O_2 tubing and set the O_2 flow rate to 15 L/minute:
  - 'Jet ventilate' by occluding the hole in the O_2 tube (1 second on, 4 seconds off)
- Proceed to a definitive airway as soon as possible (arrange for anaesthetic assistance with/without ENT cover).

Complications
Needle cricothyroidotomies are a temporary means of maintaining oxygenation. The intention should be to proceed to endotracheal intubation or tracheostomy as soon as possible:
- An escape route for insufflated air is required if the upper airway is completely obstructed, otherwise barotrauma will occur, if necessary:
  - Turn down the O_2 flow rate
  - Inserted further needle cricothyroidotomies to allow gas to escape
  - Even without airway obstruction the high pressures involved may cause barotrauma

- The cannula is easily kinked or misplaced; paratracheal gas insufflation may result.
- CO_2 will accumulate.

Surgical cricothyroidotomy

Should a needle cricothyroidotomy prove inadequate, and there is no other means of securing an alternative airway, then a larger surgical cricothyroidotomy may be attempted using the same landmarks as before:

- Make a 2-cm transverse incision through skin and cricothyroid membrane.
- Dilate the tract with artery forceps (or the handle of the scalpel).
- Insert an endotracheal or tracheostomy tube (the smallest size immediately available, typically size 6.5).
- Inflate the cuff and ventilate as normal (confirming position within the trachea as per normal endotracheal intubation).

This technique is technically more demanding, but does provide a definitive airway through which full ventilatory support can be provided.

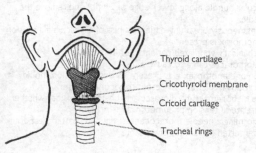

Thyroid cartilage

Cricothyroid membrane

Cricoid cartilage

Tracheal rings

Fig. 17.3 Anatomy of the cricothyroid membrane.

☠ Needle thoracocentesis

Indications
- Suspected tension pneumothorax.

Contraindications
- Where the anterior chest wall cannot be accessed consider performing a needle thoracocentesis in the mid-anterior axillary line (at the 5th intercostal space).

Equipment
- 14 or 16-G cannula.

Anatomical landmarks
- Anterior chest wall, mid-clavicular line, 2nd intercostal space (commonly at, or just below, the level of the angle of Louis) (Fig. 17.4).

Technique
- Insert the cannula just above top edge of 3rd rib (in order avoid the neurovascular bundle along lower edge of 2nd rib) and remove the stylet/needle:
  - In spontaneously breathing patients a hiss of air occurs if a tension pneumothorax is present
  - In mechanically ventilated patients non-tensioning pneumothoraces can also cause a hiss
- If a tension pneumothorax was present its decompression should improve cardiovascular and/or respiratory compromise:
  - If the patient remains cardiovascularly unstable consider whether a contralateral tension pneumothorax is present
- After performing a needle thoracocentesis, an intercostal chest drain should be inserted as soon as practicable.

Complications
- A needle thoracocentesis performed where no pneumothorax was present will cause a pneumothorax to occur; proceed to intercostal chest drain insertion in all cases.
- The cannula may kink, allowing the tension pneumothorax to re-accumulate (further decompression may be required).
- Tension pneumothoraces requiring needle decompression can still occur with chest drains in place (e.g. if the drains get kinked).
- Bleeding/haemothorax.
- Lung laceration/bronchopleural fistula.

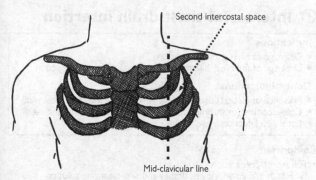

Fig. 17.4 Anatomy of the 2nd intercostal space in the mid-clavicular line.

① **Intercostal chest drain insertion**

Indications
- Drainage of air (e.g. pneumothorax)
- Drainage of fluid (e.g. haemothorax, pleural effusion, empyema)

Contraindications
- Presence of pleural adhesion (lung which is stuck to the chest wall)
- Coagulopathy (or thrombocytopaenia) is a relative contraindication
- Local skin infection

Equipment
- Full sterile preparation:
  - Hat, mask, gown, gloves, drapes and skin-cleansing solution
- Syringe, 25-G needle and lidocaine 2% or 1%.
- Underwater drain chamber and sterile water, or Heimlich valve assembly; and connection tubing.
- Sutures and sterile adhesive dressings.
- Biochemistry/microbiology sample tubes (if draining fluid).

Surgical chest drain
- Scalpel and chest drain (sizes 20–32 Fr); remove the trocar.
- Spencer-Wells forceps (or needle holders):
  - 'Load' the chest drain onto the forceps using the distal side-hole.

Seldinger chest drain
- Seldinger chest drain set (typically 12–14 Fr drains) with syringe, needle, guidewire, dilator, and 3-way tap.
- US (if thoracic fluids are present this allows safer needle insertion by identifying diaphragm and thoracic structures; it will not identify thoracic structures if pneumothorax present).

Anatomical landmarks
- 5th intercostal space, mid-anterior axillary line (Fig. 17.5).
- Occasionally an anterior drain (2nd intercostal space mid-clavicular line) is required.
- US-guided Seldinger drains can be placed where fluid depth is greatest, and the risk of hitting the diaphragm is minimized (in patients who are able to sit this may require a more posterior approach).

Technique
- Prepare the skin with sterilizing solution.
- Infiltrate 4–5 ml lidocaine subcutaneously and down into muscle.

Surgical chest drain
- Perform a 2–3-cm transverse skin incision.
- Perform blunt dissection down to pleura over top edge of 6th rib (to avoid the neurovascular bundle along lower edge of 5th rib).
- Pierce the pleura with a fingertip and perform a finger sweep.

- Guide the chest drain into the pleural space using the attached Spencer Wells forceps.
- Detach and withdraw the forceps and then advance the drain by 10–15 cm (depending upon patients' body-habitus).

Seldinger chest drain
- If fluid is thought to be present confirm the position with US, and ensure that myocardium and diaphragm are not in the needle's path.
- Insert the needle through skin (perpendicular to the chest cavity), with negative pressure on the syringe until fluid is aspirated.
- Gently insert the guidewire through the needle, then remove the needle and insert the dilator, followed by the chest drain.

Once the drain is inserted
- Take any samples required (samples may include: pH, protein, LDH, glucose, amylase, cytology, microscopy and culture).
- Hold in place and attach the underwater drain, or Heimlich valve assembly (in mechanically ventilated patients the chest drain may be anchored with sutures first).
- Insert anchoring sutures at either end of the skin incision, and tie them off leaving long 'tails'; wrap the tails around the chest drain throwing ties every 2–3 turns to indent the drain.
- Place sterile dressings either side of the drain and fix in place with adhesive dressings.
- Obtain a post-insertion CXR.

Complications
- Bleeding/haemothorax, lung laceration.
- Surgical emphysema.
- Failure of the lung to re-expand.
- Damage to the diaphragm or intra-abdominal organs.

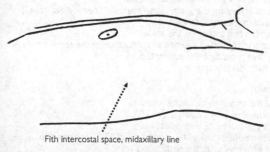

Fith intercostal space, midaxillary line

Fig. 17.5 The fifth intercostal space, mid-anterior axillary line.

⊕ **Arterial line insertion**

Indications
- Where beat-to-beat monitoring of BP is desirable (e.g. during the titration of inotropes in cardiovascularly unstable patients)
- Where regular blood sampling is required (particularly ABG sampling)
- To allow pulse wave contour analysis to calculate cardiac output and systemic vascular resistance

Contraindications
- Where blood supply to the associated limb is already compromised
- Coagulopathy (or thrombocytopaenia) is a relative contraindication
- Where there is localized infection at the site of insertion

Equipment
- Full sterile preparation:
  - Hat, mask, gown, gloves, drapes, and skin-cleansing solution (2% chlorhexidine in 70% isopropyl alcohol)
- Syringe, 25-G needle and lidocaine 2% or 1%.
- Arterial cannula of choice (commonly 20 G):
  - Both Seldinger-style insertion and cannula-over-needle arterial lines are available
- Transducer set (run through and zeroed).
- Suture.
- Sterile dressing.

Anatomical landmarks
- The radial artery is palpable at the wrist, and is preferred because of the presence of a collateral circulation.
- Other palpable arteries include:
  - Dorsalis pedis (on the dorsum of the foot)
  - Brachial artery (in the antecubital fossa)
  - Femoral artery (in the groin); longer arterial lines are available if required for femoral cannulation
  - Posterior tibial artery (at the ankle)
- The ulnar artery is often avoided as cannulation of the radial artery is likely to have recently been attempted.
- US may help identify arteries.

Technique
- Prepare the skin with cleansing solution.
- Identify the artery by palpation (or US).
- Infiltrate puncture site with lidocaine.
- Insert the needle/arterial line at an angle of 45–60° to the skin, pointing proximally, until a flashback is seen:
  - If a Seldinger kit is being used then the guidewire is advanced; there should be no resistance

- • If the line is a cannula kit then advance the cannula off the needle; again no resistance should be felt
- For difficult arteries the 'transfixion technique' may be more reliable. Following initial flashback the needle/cannula is advanced through the artery, then slowly withdrawn until blood flows—and then the guidewire/cannula is advanced.
- Attach the transducer set, suture the line in place, and cover with a sterile dressing.

Allen's test (not routinely used)

- Compressing the radial artery at the wrist will result in blanching of the hand in the absence of a patent ulnar artery; this is considered a contraindication to using the radial artery.
- The test is not very reliable: absence of blanching does not preclude ischaemia; arterial lines have been safely placed in radial arteries in the absence of collateral circulation.

Complications

- Inability to palpate the artery may occur, particularly in shutdown patients. Consider using the femoral or brachial arteries, or giving a small bolus of ephedrine (3–6 mg IV) or metaraminol (0.5–1.0 mg IV) to cause a transient rise in BP.
- Should ischaemia occur distal to the arterial line, remove it.
- Carefully label the arterial line to avoid inadvertent injections.
- Bleeding/haematoma.
- Infection (skin or CRBSI).

ⓘ Central venous access

Indications
- To insert a CVC, or:
  - Dialysis catheter
  - Pulmonary artery flotation catheter
  - Transvenous cardiac pacing wire
- The indications for inserting a CVC include:
  - Emergency venous access in 'shut-down' patients
  - To measure CVP and guide fluid resuscitation
  - To administer fluids or drugs (especially irritant fluids/drugs such as inotropes/vasopressors, concentrated potassium, amiodarone, PN, chemotherapy)
- Where multiple or long-term IV access is required.
- For frequent blood sampling.

Contraindications
- Uncorrected coagulopathy or thrombocytopaenia.
- Damaged or infected skin at the point of insertion.
- Being unable to lie supine (or head down) is a relative contraindication to superior vena cava territory access.

Equipment
- Full sterile preparation: hat, mask, gown, gloves, drapes and skin-cleansing solution (2% chlorhexidine in 70% isopropyl alcohol).
- Syringe, needle, and lidocaine 2% or 1%.
- CVC set (or dialysis catheter, PAFC sheath), which commonly contains:
  - A needle, a 5-ml syringe, and a Seldinger wire
  - A scalpel
  - Adjustable clamp which is attached to the catheter at the point of skin insertion
- 20–30 ml sterile saline 0.9%.
- 20-ml syringe (and blood culture bottles if required).
- Transducer (run through and zeroed).
- Suture.
- Sterile transparent dressings.
- US machine (with sterile sheath and gel).
- Many CVCs have antimicrobial-resistant coatings, which may reduce the incidence of CRBSI.

Anatomical landmarks
Common sites for insertion of central venous access include:
- The subclavian vein (potentially the lowest infection rate).
- The internal jugular vein.
- The external jugular vein (occasionally used in emergency situations).
- Femoral vein (safer in coagulopathic patients, or patients who cannot lie flat/head-down; but more prone to infection).

Anatomical identification
- Subclavian: may be approached at any point along the middle 1/3 of the clavicle (Fig. 17.6):
  - Not recommended in emergency situations, unless the operator is skilled in its use
  - US guidance can be used, but is of little use for the standard approach
- Internal jugular: lateral to the carotid artery at the level of the thyroid cartilage (high approach) or at the point where the lateral and medial heads of sternocleidomastoid meet (low approach) (Fig. 17.6):
  - US guidance is recommended, typically for the low approach (vein is compressible, less pulsatile, and typically triangular or oval in shape)
- External jugular: identified by pressing across the base of the lateral side of the neck; occluding the flow of blood allows the vein to fill.
- Femoral vein: medial to the femoral artery, distal to the inguinal ligament (Fig. 17.7); it is the safest major vein to cannulate in an emergency (especially if coagulation status is not known) as inadvertent arterial puncture may be easily controlled.
  - US guidance is recommended (vein is compressible, and less pulsatile).

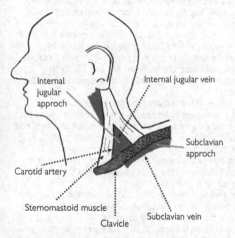

Fig. 17.6 Anatomy of the internal jugular and subclavian veins.

Technique
- Check coagulation studies.
- Place the patient in a head-down position for internal jugular or subclavian approaches; slightly head-up for femoral.
- Prepare the skin with cleansing solution and drape the patient.
- Infiltrate the puncture site with lidocaine.

- Prepare the CVC by flushing all the lumens through with saline.
- Half fill the 5-ml syringe with saline and attach the needle.

Internal jugular or femoral vein access
- Identify the vein using US where possible (veins are compressible, less pulsatile, and dilate during Valsalva manoeuvres):
  - US-guided techniques may be in-plane (where the needle is viewed throughout its entire passage), or out-of-plane (where the needle is not directly visualized, but the tissue distortion created by the needle passage is seen); out-of-plane is more commonly used
- When out-of-plane US guidance is used the needle should be 10° from the perpendicular (angled proximally); short, jabbing movements will help identify the position of the needle tip on the US image through tissue distortion.
- The needle should be gently advanced with a continuous, gentle, negative pressure maintained on the syringe until flashback is obtained (this may occur as the needle is withdrawn due to the vein being compressed on insertion).
- Once a flashback occurs the syringe should be disconnected with the needle stabilized:
  - If there is doubt as to whether the needle is in a vein or artery a blood gas sample may be obtained and compared with SpO_2 (venous saturations will be lower than arterial)
- Advance the Seldinger guidewire (20–25 cm at the needle hub is all that is required in most patients); no resistance should be felt.
- Withdraw the needle and incise the skin entry point with a scalpel.
- The dilator is then be inserted to between 1/2 and 2/3 its length, before being removed (this is often easiest using a gentle 'screwing' or twisting motion).
- The central line is then threaded over the guidewire to the appropriate depth; when initially threading the central line onto the guidewire there must be guidewire protruding through the 'hub' side of the catheter before the catheter is inserted into the patient, in order to prevent accidental loss of the wire into the vein.
- Check that blood can be aspirated from all lumens, and flush them with saline (in septic patients take this opportunity to take sterile blood cultures prior to flushing the line).
- The guidewire is then removed and the CVC sutured in place; both the hub *and* adjustable clamp (if used) should be sutured; cover the insertion site with a transparent sterile dressing.
- Obtain a CXR for IJ, EJ, or SC lines to confirm correct position (the tip should be in the SVC just above/at the level of the carina), and to exclude pneumo/haemothorax.

When US is not used (not recommended) the relevant anatomy should be established. It is suggested for the internal jugular and femoral routes that once the artery has been identified the palpating fingers are only gently rested on the skin during venous puncture so as not to compress the vein.

Subclavian access
- Typically approached at the junction of the middle 1/3 of the clavicle with the needle under the clavicle (inferiorly):
  - Once in this position the needle is placed as flat to the skin as is possible and gently inserted towards the suprasternal notch or the contralateral shoulder (gently aspirating on the syringe)
  - Once venous access is confirmed by flashback, Seldinger guidewire and catheter insertion is as described earlier

Catheter insertion lengths
- Right IJ, EJ, or subclavian lines: 12–14 cm.
- Left IJ, EJ, or subclavian lines: 16–20 cm.
- Femoral lines: fully inserted.

Complications
- Arterial puncture.
- Arrhythmias.
- Pneumothorax or haemothorax (more common with subclavian lines).
- Cardiac tamponade.
- Infection (skin or CRBSI).
- Venous thrombosis.

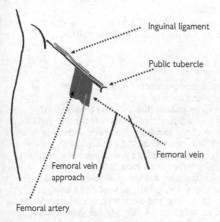

Fig. 17.7 Anatomy of the femoral vein.

:☢: Intravenous cutdown

Indications
- Where emergency IV access is required for fluid resuscitation and no other IV access is obtainable:
  - Also consider alternatives such as central venous or IO access

Contraindications
- Injuries proximal to, or overlying, the ankle (or other cutdown site)
- If the saphenous vein at the ankle is not accessible consider using the median basilic vein at the antecubital fossa, 2.5 cm lateral to the medial epicondyle

Equipment
- Syringe, 25-G needle, and lidocaine 2% or 1%.
- Scalpel.
- Artery clips (or similar).
- Surgical ties.
- IV cannula (15–18-G stylet removed).
- IV fluid and giving set.
- Suture.

Anatomical landmarks
- The long saphenous vein at the ankle (Fig. 17.8):
  - 2 cm anterior and 2 cm superior to the medial malleolus

Technique
- Clean the area with antiseptic solution.
- Infiltrate incision site with lidocaine.
- Make a 2–3-cm transverse incision (full thickness through skin).
- Use blunt dissection (using artery clips) to identify the vein and lift away a 2–3-cm portion of the vein from the tissues underlying it.
- Pass 2 ties behind the vein, one caudal and one cephalad:
  - This is most easily done by gripping the mid-point of a length of suture using artery forceps, this loop can then be passed underneath the vein and then divided to leave 2 ties
  - Tie off the caudal end and keep the cephalad tie as a sling
- Make a small incision in the vein and dilate it using the artery forceps.
- Introduce the plastic cannula into the vein and use the sling/tie to secure it in place.
- Attach the giving set to the cannula and infuse fluid.
- Close the incision with interrupted sutures or dress the wound with a sterile dressing.
- Remove the cannula as soon as the patient is stable and alternative IV access is available.

Complications

- The vein may be difficult to identify; the artery or nerve may be damaged.
- Bleeding/haematoma.
- Wound infection or thrombophlebitis.

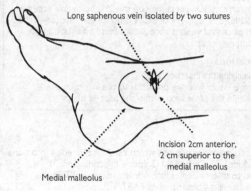

Long saphenous vein isolated by two sutures

Incision 2cm anterior, 2 cm superior to the medial malleolus

Medial malleolus

Fig. 17.8 Anatomy of the long saphenous vein.

⊕ Intraosseous access

Indications
- Where emergency vascular access is required for fluid resuscitation or drug administration and no IV access is obtainable:
  - Also consider alternatives such as central venous access or venous cutdown
  - In cardiac arrests, IO access may be the 2nd choice if IV access is not available (ETT delivery of drugs is no longer advocated; the insertion of central venous access may cause interruptions in chest compressions)

Contraindications
- Infection overlying the insertion site.
- Fracture in the insertion bone proximal to the insertion site.
- IO access within the same limb within the past 48 hours.

Equipment
- Proprietary sets are manufactured which can 'drive' needles into bone. Examples include: EZ-IO® and B.I.G. (Bone Injection Gun™).
- Sets designed to insert needles into non-standard sites (e.g. the sternum) are also available, including FAST-1™.
- For small adults trocar-sets (normally used in paediatrics) may be used.
- Other equipment:
  - IV fluid and giving set
  - Syringe, needle, and lidocaine 2% or 1%

Anatomical landmarks
- The preferred site is the proximal tibia, 2 cm distal to the tibial tuberosity, on the anteromedial aspect (Fig. 17.9).
- Alternative sites include:
  - The distal tibia, 2 cm proximal to the medial malleolus
  - The proximal humerus, into the greater tuberosity
  - The sternum (using specialized equipment)
  - The iliac crest and the femur (anterior midline, 1–3 cm above the tibial plateau) have also been used

Technique
- Clean the area with antiseptic solution.
- Palpate the anatomical landmarks.
- Infiltrate incision site with lidocaine if appropriate.
- 'Fire' the needle into the bony site, following the manufacturer's guidelines, using an appropriate pre-set needle depth:
  - The direction of insertion is typically 90° to the surface of the skin
- Connect a flushed giving set directly to the needle.
- Remove after 24 hours of use, after obtaining alternative access.

Where trocar sets are used these should be pushed into the bone using a drilling motion:
- The trochar should be removed once the set has pushed through into the cortex.

Complications
- Extravasation into surrounding tissues.
- Compartment syndrome.
- Embolism (including fat embolism).
- Bone fracture during insertion.
- Infection/osteomyelitis.
- Needle dislodgement.
- Infusion pain.

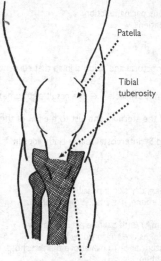

Patella

Tibial tuberosity

Insertion point: anteromedial 2 cm below the tibial tuberosity

Fig. 17.9 Anatomy of proximal tibia for insertion of intraosseous needles.

:☹: External pacing

Indications
- Complete heart block with associated hypotension (or cardiac arrest).
- Ventricular standstill.
- Profound bradycardia.
  External pacing is indicated in peri-arrest situations. The management of peri-arrest arrhythmias is detailed on 🕮 p.132.

Contraindications
- The skin must be dry, and it must be safe to approach the patient.
- Remove GTN patches.
- Avoid placement near an implanted pacemaker.

Equipment
- A defibrillator with transcutaneous pacing function.
- Adhesive pads to attach to the patient.
- Resuscitation equipment.

Anatomical landmarks
- Pads should be placed over the pectoral and apical skin so that current traverses the heart (Fig. 17.20).

If the pectoral/apical positions are not available (i.e. as a result of trauma) then alternatives include:
- Anterior posterior: to the left of the sternum and just to the left of the midline on the back.
- Side to side: overlying the 4th and 5th intercostal spaces both sides in the mid-axillary line.

Technique
- Ensure pads are attached to clean, dry skin if possible.
- Choose *fixed* mode (consider *demand*, if available, once stable).
- Set the rate for 60–90/minute.
- Increase the *output* (start at 70 mA) until *capture* occurs: pacing spikes are seen and QRS complexes are triggered by them.
- Once capture occurs set the output at 5–10 mA above the threshold.
- If no capture occurs at 120 mA then:
  - Consider resiting the electrodes
  - Exclude biochemical abnormality (e.g. hyperkalaemia)
- Ensure there is a pulse present with QRS complexes, otherwise treat for PEA.
- Muscle twitching is normal; provide sedation or analgesia if there is associated pain.

Complications

- Transcutaneous pacing is a temporary measure only, if the arrhythmia does not resolve proceed to transvenous pacing.
- Minor burning may occur, review the skin areas afterwards and treat as appropriate.

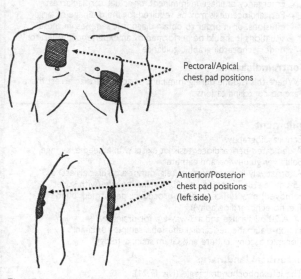

Pectoral/Apical chest pad positions

Anterior/Posterior chest pad positions (left side)

Fig. 17.20 Positioning of transcutaneous pacing pads.

☠ **Pericardiocentesis**

Indications
- Cardiac tamponade:
  - Emergency drainage in imminent, or actual, cardiac arrest
  - Pericardiocentesis may be required for the drainage of large effusions, or in order to obtain diagnostic samples; in these situations it should be performed by an experienced operator under echocardiographic guidance

Contraindications
- Where this is done during imminent or actual cardiac arrest there are no contraindications

Equipment
- Echocardiography.
- A dedicated pericardiocentesis kit exists with a needle, syringe, Seldinger guidewire, and catheter.
- Alternatively in an emergency (e.g. during a cardiac arrest) a 15-cm 16–18-G cannula or a 20-G spinal needle (with stylet removed) may suffice; and the procedure performed 'blind' (i.e. no echocardiography):
  - A 20-ml syringe and a 3-way-tap for drainage
- In non-traumatic pericardial effusions, sample containers (for microscopy, culture and Gram stain; cytology).

Anatomical landmarks
- The left xiphochondral angle (Fig. 17.21).

Technique
- Monitor patients' ECG continuously.
- Prepare the sub-xiphoid area with antiseptic solution if time allows.
- Insert the cannula at an angle of 30–45° to the skin, near the left xiphochondral angle, aiming towards the tip of the left scapula.
- Advance slowly, aspirating gently at all times.
- When fluid/blood is aspirated stop advancing the cannula, advance the catheter over the needle, and remove the needle.
- Attach the 3-way-tap and aspirate as much blood/fluid as possible.
- Aspirating as little as 100 ml of blood is likely to make a dramatic difference to cardiac output, even in chronic, massive effusions.
- Secure the cannula in place as blood may re-accumulate.
- Arrange formal drainage or surgery as soon as possible.

Complications

- ECG changes may be seen (QRS widening, ST–T-wave changes or ventricular ectopics) if the cannula is advanced too far; withdraw the needle and redirect more posteriorly.
- Ventricular fibrillation (or other form of cardiac arrest) may occur during drainage.
- A new haemopericardium or haematoma may be generated (by myocardial or coronary artery puncture); or blood may be aspirated directly from the right or left ventricles, further compromising cardiac output.
- Pneumothorax.
- Always perform under echocardiographic guidance unless there is imminent/actual cardiac arrest.

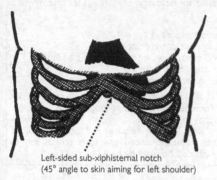

Left-sided sub-xiphisternal notch
(45° angle to skin aiming for left shoulder)

Fig. 17.21 Anatomy of the xiphochondral angle.

① Fibreoptic bronchoscopy

Indications
- Confirmation of ETT or tracheostomy position
- To facilitate a difficult intubation (fibreoptic intubation, FOI)
- To facilitate percutaneous tracheostomy placement (by confirming intratracheal guidewire placement)
- To obtain microbiological samples (either a bronchoscopy-protected deep respiratory sample, or BAL)
- To localize and control haemoptysis
- To remove secretions, mucous plugs, blood clots, or foreign bodies
- To examine for strictures, tumours, or tracheobronchial trauma (including burns or smoke inhalation damage):
  - Biopsies may be taken for histology, or washings for cytology

Contraindications
- Relative contraindications include:
  - Moderate/severe hypoxia or hypercapnia
  - Coagulopathy, SVC obstruction, or other risk of bleeding
  - Near-complete tracheal obstruction
  - Myocardial ischaemia, arrhythmias or hypotension

FOI or bronchoscopy in awake, unintubated patients is a complex skill that requires practical fibreoptic and anaesthetic experience.

Fibreoptic bronchoscopy in patients who already have an endotracheal or tracheostomy tube in place requires the acquired skill of bronchoscope manipulation. Inexperienced operators are unlikely to perform bronchoscopy unaided, but may be asked to assist.

Equipment
- An assistant to monitor the patient and provide sedation if required.
- Gown, gloves, and mask.
- A fibreoptic bronchoscope (already sterilized); various different bronchoscopes are available, including:
  - Small-bore, 'intubating' bronchoscopes, ideal for intubation, and placing/positioning ETTs (including double-lumen tubes)
  - Large-bore bronchoscopes, with a large suction/biopsy channels which are better for removing secretions or performing biopsies (these typically fit through a size 8 ETT or larger)
- Light source.
- Suction source and suction tubing (attach this to the bronchoscope).
- Angle-piece/catheter mount adapter through which the bronchoscope can pass; and lubricant.
- Sputum traps, syringes (luer slip variety), 0.9% saline for lavages.
- Bronchial brushes or biopsy forceps (if required).

Anatomical landmarks
- A knowledge of the tracheobronchial tree is required (Fig. 17.22).

Technique

For patients who already have an ETT or tracheostomy tube in place:

- Pre-oxygenate patient by increasing FiO_2 to 100%.
- Ensure the ETT is a size 8 or greater (for a standard bronchoscope).
- Consider deepening sedation and/or adding neuromuscular blockade.
- Check the bronchoscope, light source, and suction.
- Scrub and use gown/gloves; technique should be as sterile as possible.
- Attach the angle-piece adapter to the ETT and pass the lubricated bronchoscope through it.
- Identify the carina and systematically explore the tracheobronchial tree, starting on the 'good' side where possible.
- If secretions are present, attach the suction trap to collect specimens.
- If a BAL is required, identify the appropriate site (in most cases the furthest point the bronchoscope will safely pass, in the affected lobe); inject 20–40 ml sterile water through the suction channel, then suction back up into a sputum trap:
  - The total volume which should be injected is unclear, but large volumes may result in hypoxia
  - BAL samples may be sent for different tests, including: microscopy and Gram stain, culture (and fungal culture), immunofluorescence, PCP or viral PCR
- Clean and sterilize the bronchoscope after use.

Complications

- Hypoxia during or after the procedure, and/or pneumothorax.
- Tracheobronchial trauma/bleeding.

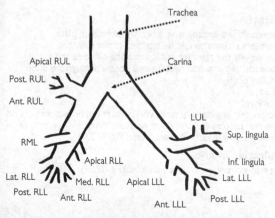

Fig. 17.22 Anatomy of the bronchial tree. RUL, right upper lobe; RML, right middle lobe; RLL, right lower lobe; LUL, left upper lobe; LLL, left lower lobe; post., posterior; ant., anterior; med., medial; lat., lateral; sup., superior; inf., inferior.

① Intra-abdominal pressure measurement

Indications

- The detection of IAH and ACS in patients with:
  - Blunt abdominal trauma (ACS can develop in up to 15% of patients)
  - Abdominal surgery with 1° closure
  - Severe burns with eschar formation
  - Prone positioning
  - Bowel obstruction
  - Haemoperitoneum, pneumoperitoneum
  - Ascites or visceral oedema, infection, liver failure, pancreatitis, massive fluid resuscitation
  - Peritonitis, intra-abdominal abscesses
  - Tumour, haematoma, surgical packs
  - Pelvic fracture
- Intra-abdominal pressure monitoring is indicated in any of these conditions where abdominal pressure is causing, or likely to cause, renal impairment or respiratory embarrassment

Contraindications

- The catheter must be patent; clot retention/bladder irrigation is a relative contraindication (discuss with a urologist as irrigation may be temporarily suspended)
- Intra-vesical pressures are not an absolute measure of IAP, and should be interpreted in conjunction with clinical findings

Equipment

- The patient should already have a urinary catheter in place.
- A manometry column should be attached to the catheter:
  - Alternatively the catheter outflow may be clamped and a transducer set attached to it (using a needle through the urine sampling port)
- Sterile water.
- 20 ml syringe.
- Proprietary sets are manufactured which utilize either manometers or pressure transducers (e.g. AbViser® pressure monitoring system, or UnoMeter Abdo-Pressure™ manometer; Fig. 17.23).

Anatomical landmarks

- The mid-axillary line is the zero-point (Fig. 17.24).

Technique
- The patient should be supine.
- 20–25 ml of sterile water is instilled into the bladder via the catheter.
- After 30–60 seconds the pressure should be measured (at end-expiration).
- Pressure is expressed in mmHg (1 mmHg = 1.36 cmH$_2$O).

Complications
- Artificially high readings may be measured; recheck IAP before considering treatment to ensure that any increase is sustained.

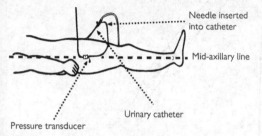

Needle inserted into catheter

Mid-axillary line

Urinary catheter

Pressure transducer

Fig. 17.23 Abdominal pressure measurement using a transducer.

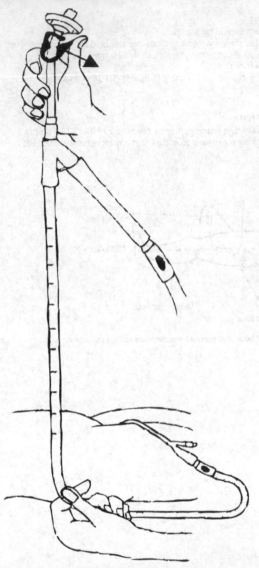

Fig. 17.24 UnoMeter Abdo-Pressure™ manometer.

① **Lumbar puncture**

Indications
- To sample CSF:
  - Infection (e.g. suspected meningitis/encephalitis)
  - SAH
  - Inflammatory neuropathy (e.g. GBS)
  - Malignant infiltration.

Contraindications
- Raised ICP/focal neurology (perform head CT beforehand)
- Uncorrected coagulopathy or thrombocytopaenia
- Damaged or infected skin at the point of insertion

Equipment
- Full sterile preparation:
  - Hat, mask, gown, gloves, drapes, and skin-cleansing solution
- Syringe, 25-G needle and lidocaine 2% or 1%.
- Introducer needle.
- 20–24-G spinal needle (e.g. Whittacre or Quincke).
- A CSF manometry set with a 3-way tap:
  - Manometry sets take a long time to fill with small-gauge needles
- 3 sterile universal containers and a glucose measurement bottle.

Anatomical landmarks
- L3/4 interspace: the gap between the spinous processes of L3 and L4, approximately level with the iliac crests (Fig. 17.25).

Technique
- Position the patient on their side, with their chin on their chest and their knees drawn up (the 'fetal' position).
- Identify the L3/4 interspace (if the patient is able to speak, and spinous processes are hard to palpate, ask them to confirm when you are touching the midline).
- Scrub, gown (mask, hat,) drape the area, and prepare the skin.
- Infiltrate lidocaine around the previously indented area.
- Insert the introducer needle into the indented area staying perpendicular to the skin.
- Advance the spinal needle through the introducer until a 'give' is felt as it passes through the dura; stop (withdraw and redirect if the patient complains of 'shooting' pains at any point).
- Remove the stylet and observe for CSF.
- If the subarachnoid space is not found withdraw the spinal needle into the introducer needle, redirect the introducer needle, and advance again.

- If using a manometer, attach it (with the 3-way tap in the appropriate position) and let fluid collect to measure the opening pressure; then use the fluid within the manometer and collect further fluid for samples (see later in list).
- Samples: collect 1–1.5 ml in each of the 3 universal containers (and also in the glucose bottle) and send for:
  - Microscopy and culture, protein, glucose, PCR (and consider cytology, AFBs, cryptococcal antigen, India ink stain, fungal culture, and oligoclonal bands)
- Remove the needle and dress the wound.
- Send a serum glucose sample as well (for comparison).

Complications

- The commonest complication is failure to identify the subarachnoid space—repositioning the patient to increase the lumbar kyphosis often helps.
- Postdural puncture headache is common with larger needles and multiple attempts. If it occurs, discuss treatment options with an anaesthetist.
- Nerve damage (rare); stop and withdraw if shooting pain occurs
- Infection (as meningitis or as an epidural abscess) or bleeding may occur, but are uncommon.
- Coning may occur if raised ICP is present (i.e. not identified beforehand); *if in doubt perform a CT head beforehand.*

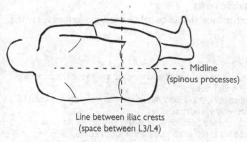

Midline
(spinous processes)

Line between iliac crests
(space between L3/L4)

Fig. 17.25 Lumbar puncture anatomical landmarks.

ⓘ Sengstaken–Blakemore tube insertion

> Indications
> * Severe upper GI haemorrhage due to varices when other methods (e.g. endoscopic sclerotherapy) cannot be used
>
> Contraindications
> * Oesophageal perforation
> * Previous oesophageal surgery

Equipment
* A SBT, or equivalent:
    * SBT tubes have 3 ports (oesophageal and intragastric balloons and gastric aspirate ports)
    * Minnesota tubes have 4 ports (as for SBT tubes, with extra oesophageal aspirate port)
    * Linton–Nachlas tube (has a larger intragastric balloon)
    * Check all balloons prior to use
* 50-ml syringe.
* Lubrication.
* Mouth guard.
* Lidocaine spray 4%.
* Marker pen.
* Non-toothed clamps (e.g. Kelly clamps).

Anatomical landmarks
* The intragastric balloon should be below the diaphragm on X-ray (Fig. 17.26).

Technique
* Most patients will be intubated and mechanically ventilated to allow insertion of the SBT tube:
    * In awake patients, if available and time allows, spray the back of the mouth with 4% lidocaine
    * The patient should be supine or in the left lateral position
* Insert the tube via the mouth using the mouth guard:
    * In anaesthetized patients use laryngoscopy to aid oesophageal insertion
* Pass the tube until the gastric balloon is in the stomach then gently inject 50–100 ml of air in to the intragastric balloon port listening with a stethoscope over the stomach to check for sounds of insufflation (also use pressure monitoring to confirm that pressure does not exceed 15 mmHg).
* Inject further air to a total of 200–300 ml of air (stop if there is patient discomfort) and clamp the port.
* Gently apply traction on the tube to bring the gastric balloon up to the fundus.

- Check the tube position with a thoracoabdominal X-ray.
- Inflate the oesophageal balloon to a pressure of 20–30 mmHg and clamp.
- Return the patient to a 30–40° head-up position.
- Mark the position of the tube at the teeth using a marker pen.
- Apply 250g of traction to the tube.
- SBT tubes can stay in place for 1–3 days.
- Deflate the oesophageal balloon for 10 minutes every 2–4 hours to decrease the likelihood of oesophageal ischaemia.

Complications
- Re-bleeding.
- Oesophageal ischaemia.

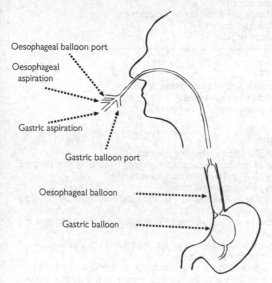

Oesophageal balloon port

Oesophageal aspiration

Gastric aspiration

Gastric balloon port

Oesophageal balloon

Gastric balloon

Fig. 17.26 Minnesota tube (similar to a Sengstaken–Blakemore tube, but with an extra channel for oesophageal suction).

⊙ **Prone positioning**

Indications
- To improve oxygenation in ALI or ARDS
- To improve the mobilization of secretions and decrease basal atelectasis

Contraindications
- Facial injuries or burns where loss of airway may occur
- Unstable spinal or pelvic fractures
- Raised IAP; recent abdominal trauma or surgery
- Pregnancy
- Seizures; head injuries with raised ICP
- Raised IOP
- Relative contraindications include
  - Morbid obesity
  - Cardiovascular instability or hypotension
  - Recent tracheostomy
  - Agitation or pain

Equipment
- Liquid paraffin and gel pads for eye protection.
- 5 staff (ideally 1 airway trained).
- 4 extra pillows.

Technique
- Check ABGs prior to changing position.
- Remove all non-essential monitoring (keep pulse oximetry attached).
- Aspirate NGT and perform tracheal suctioning.
- Apply eye protection (gel pads).
- Ensure analgesia is adequate; ↑sedation and neuromuscular blockade may be required.
- Check the airway (ensure the ETT is secure and check position at teeth/gums).
- Position 2 staff at either side of the patient and 1 at the head ('head' controls the timing of all movement).
- Disconnect ventilator tubing from the patient prior to all moves.
- Place the patient's arms by their side (palms in) and place a pillow between the patient's legs.
- 'Mummy-wrap' the patient in the sheets they are lying on and slide them to the edge of the bed.
- Place pillows beside the patient at the level of the upper chest, the pelvis, and the ankles.
- Roll the patient over onto the pillows and ensure that the abdomen 'hangs' free; bring 1 arm forward and turn the head towards 1 side, adopting the 'swimmer's' position.

- Reconnect the ventilator tubing, all monitoring, and lines.
- Position the whole bed 30–45° head up.
- Check all pressure or stress areas (toes, knees, genitalia, elbows, wrists, breasts, neck, chin, lips, nose, eyes, ears); make sure pressure points are hanging free or are very well padded, make sure joints are in physiological acceptable positions.

Complications
- Loss of airway: re-intubation in the prone position is difficult, should it occur rapidly return the patient to the supine position; if this is impossible an LMA may be inserted as a temporary measure.
- Hypotension may occur immediately after turning.
- Skin joint or nerve damage may occur.
- Dependent facial oedema may occur.

Emergency drug doses

See Table A.1.

Table A.1 Emergency drug doses

Adenosine	
Narrow complex tachycardia	6 mg IV (rapid bolus), repeat if required after 3 minutes with 12mg (up to 3 times). *Caution with WPW syndrome, asthma, or patients with transplanted hearts*
Adrenaline/epinephrine	
Cardiac arrest	1 mg (10 ml 1 in 10,000, or 1 ml 1 in 1000) IV or IO after 3rd shock (VF/VT) or immediately (PEA/asystole) then every 3–5 minutes
Anaphylaxis/angio-oedema	500 mcg (0.5 ml 1 in 1000) IM
Stridor or severe bronchospasm	1–3 mg nebulized
Infusion for hypotension, bradycardia or bronchospasm	0.05–1mcg/kg/minute (made up as 4 mg in 50 ml starting rate for; 70 kg: 2.6 ml/hour)
Alteplase (r-tPA)	
Cardiac arrest caused by pulmonary embolism	10 mg IV over 2minutes followed by 90 mg IV over 90 minutes; *alternatively tenecteplase 500–600 mcg/kg IV over 10 seconds*
Aminophylline	
Bronchospasm	250 mg IV slow (if not already on theophyllines), then 0.5 mg/kg/hour
Amiodarone	
Cardiac arrest VF/VT	300 mg (in 20 ml dextrose 5%) IV or IO after 3rd shock
Broad complex tachycardia, narrow complex tachycardia, fast AF	300 mg (in 50 ml dextrose 5%) over 10–60 minutes depending on severity of symptoms, followed by 900 mg (in 50 ml dextrose 5%) over 24 hours
Aspirin	
Acute coronary syndromes	300 mg PO/NG/PR
Atracurium	
Difficulty ventilating/raised intracranial pressure (ONLY if intubated)	50 mg IV (give anaesthetic agents as well to prevent awareness)
Atropine	
Severe or symptomatic bradycardia	500 mcg IV, repeated up to 3 mg maximum

(continued)

Table A.1 (Continued)

Organophosphate/nerve agent poisoning	2 mg IV every 20 minutes until pupils dilate, skin is dry, and tachycardia occurs
Benzylpenicillin	
Meningitis/meningococcal septicaemia	1.2 g IV
Calcium	
Hyperkalaemic cardiac arrest	Calcium chloride 10 ml 10% (6.8 mmol) IV
Severe hyperkalaemia, or hyperkalaemia with ECG changes	Calcium chloride 3–5 ml 10% (≤3.4 mmol) IV or calcium gluconate 10 ml 10% (2.2 mmol) IV. *Caution in patients taking digoxin, may need to be given slowly over 20 minutes*
Ceftriaxone	
Meningitis/meningococcal septicaemia	2 g IV
Chlorphenamine	
Anaphylaxis/angio-oedema	20 mg IV (slow) *after* adrenaline
Dantrolene	
Malignant hyperpyrexia	2.5 mg/kg IV and repeat with 1 mg/kg as needed up to 10 mg/kg. *For a 70-kg adult initial bolus – 9 vials of dantrolene (20 mg) each mixed with 60 ml sterile water*
Diamorphine	
Pulmonary oedema	2.5–5 mg IV
Severe pain	2.5–5 mg IV/IM/SC
Digoxin	
Fast AF	500 mcg IV (over 30 minutes)
Dobutamine	
Hypotension/heart failure	2.5–10 mcg/kg/minute (made up as 250mg in 50 ml starting rate for; 70 kg: 2.1 ml/hour)
Ephedrine	
Hypotension	3–6 mg IV repeat every 2–3 minutes as required
Esmolol	
Narrow complex tachycardia	Loading dose 500 mcg/kg over 1 minute
	Followed by infusion of 50–200 mcg/kg/minute
Etomidate	
Induction of anaesthesia	0.1–0.4 mg/kg

(continued)

Table A.1 (Continued)

Flumazenil	
Benzodiazepine overdose	200 mcg IV (repeat every minute as required up to 1 mg)
Furosemide	
Pulmonary oedema	20–40 mg IV
Glycopyrronium bromide	
Severe/symptomatic bradycardia	300–600 mcg IV
Glucagon	
Hypoglycaemia	1 mg IV/IM/SC
Glucose	
Hypoglycaemia	25–50 ml of 25–50% IV (via a large cannula/vein if possible)
Glyceryl trinitrate (GTN)	
Angina	300–600 mcg sublingual tablet or spray
Unstable angina, left ventricular failure, or severe hypertension	10–200 mcg/minute IV
Haloperidol	
Severe agitation	2.5–5 mg IM/PO (always consider other causes, repeat up to 15 mg, continually review sedation/airway)
Hydrocortisone	
Anaphylaxis	200 mg IV (slow) *after* adrenaline
Severe bronchospasm	200 mg IV (slow)
Addisons/hypoadrenalism	200 mg IV (slow)
Insulin and glucose	
Severe hyperkalaemia	15–20 units soluble insulin in 50 ml 50% glucose IV over 30–60 minutes
Ipratropium bromide	
Bronchospasm	500 mcg nebulized
Ketamine	
Induction of anaesthesia	1–4 mg/kg IV or 4–10 mg/kg IM
Maintenance of anaesthesia	10–45 mcg/kg/minute or 1–3 mg/kg/hour IV (may provide additional bronchodilatory effects in patients with severe bronchospasm)
Lidocaine	
Broad complex tachycardia	50 mg IV (over 2 minutes) repeat as required up to 200 mg

(continued)

Table A.1 (Continued)

Lorazepam	
Status epilepticus	4 mg IV (slow)
Magnesium sulphate	
Cardiac arrest (VF/VT) with possible hypomagnesaemia	8 mmol (2 g or 4 ml MgSO$_4$ 50%) IV
Bronchospasm	8 mmol (2 g or 4 ml MgSO$_4$ 50%) IV over 20 minutes
Eclampsia	Loading dose: 20 mmol (4 g) IV over 3–5 minutes, followed by infusion of 5–10 mmol/hour
Mannitol	
Raised ICP/intracranial mass effect	0.5–1 g/kg (~200–400 ml 20% solution)
Metaraminol	
Hypotension/vasodilatation	0.5 mg IV
Midazolam	
Sedative infusion	0–3 mcg/kg/minute (made up as 50 mg in 50 ml, ~dose 0–20 ml/hour)
Morphine	
Pulmonary oedema	2.5–10 mg IV
Severe pain	2.5–10 mg IV/IM/SC
Sedative infusion (combined with propofol or equivalent)	0–3 mcg/kg/minute (made up as 50 mg in 50 ml, ~0–20 ml/hour)
Naloxone	
Opioid overdose	400 mcg IV (repeat every minute as required up to 2 mg; SC or IM routes can be used in extremis)
Noradrenaline/norepinephrine	
Hypotension requiring vasoconstriction	0.05–1 mcg/kg/minute (made up as 4 mg in 50 ml, starting rate for 70 kg: 2.6 ml/hour)
Phenylephrine	
Hypotension/vasodilatation	50 mcg IV, or 30–60 mcg/minute
Phenytoin	
Status epilepticus	Loading dose 15 mg/kg (in 0.9% saline) IV infusion at a rate not exceeding 50 mg/minute (ECG monitoring required)
Procyclidine	
Oculogyric crisis/acute dystonia	5–10 mg IV/IM

(continued)

Table A.1 (Continued)

Propofol	
Induction of anaesthesia	2–5 mg/kg IV
Sedative infusion	0–4 mg/kg/hour
Salbutamol	
Bronchospasm	5 mg nebulized
Bronchospasm IV infusion	250 mcg IV over 10 minutes, then 5–30 mcg/minute
Sodium bicarbonate	
Cardiac arrest & tricyclic overdose or hyperkalaemia	50 ml 8.4% IV
Suxamethonium	
Rapid sequence intubation	1–2 mg/kg IV
Terlipressin	
Severe refractory septic shock	1 mg IV 8-hourly
Thiopental	
Induction of anaesthesia	3–5 mg/kg
Vasopressin	
Severe refractory septic shock	0.01–0.04 units/minute IV infusion (made up as 20 units in 50 ml starting rate 1.5 ml/hour)

Reference values

See Tables A.2–A.10.

Table A.2 Cardiovascular and haemodynamic variables

Heart rate and cardiovascular pressures		
Heart rate	60–100/min	
Mean arterial pressure (MAP)	75–105 mmHg	
Central venous pressure (CVP)	0–8 mmHg	0–10 cmH$_2$O
Right atrial pressure (RAP)	0–8 mmHg	
Right ventricle pressure, systolic	14–30 mmHg	
Right ventricle end-diastolic pressure (RVEDP)	0–8 mmHg	
Pulmonary artery pressure (PAP), systolic	15–30 mmHg	
Pulmonary artery pressure, diastolic	5–15 mmHg	
Pulmonary artery pressure, mean (MPAP)	10–20 mmHg	
Pulmonary artery occlusion pressure, mean (PAOP, or PAWP)	5–15 mmHg	
Left atrial pressure (LAP)	4–12 mmHg	
Left ventricular pressure, systolic	90–140 mmHg	
Left ventricular end-diastolic pressure (LVEDP)	4–12 mmHg	
Haemodynamic variables		
Estimated circulating blood volume (adult)	65–70 ml/kg	
Cardiac output (CO)	4.5–8 L/min	
Cardiac index (CI)	2.7–4 L/min/m^2	
Stroke volume	60–130 ml/beat	
Stroke volume index (SVI)	38–60 ml/beat/m^2	
Systemic vascular resistance (SVR)	770–1500 dyn s/cm^5	
Systemic vascular resistance index (SVRI)	1860–2500 dyn s/cm^5/m^2	
Pulmonary vascular resistance (PVR)	100–250 dyn s/cm^5	
Pulmonary vascular resistance index (PVRI)	225–315 dyn s/cm^5/m^2	
Left ventricular stroke work index (LVSWI)	50–62 g/m^2/beat	
Rate-pressure product (RPP)	9600	

(continued)

Table A.2 (Continued)

Ejection fraction (EF)	>60%	
Oxygen delivery (DO_2)	950–1300 ml/min	
Systemic oxygen consumption (VO_2)	180–320 ml/min	

Formulae for cardiovascular variables

$CO = SV \times HR$

$CI = SV/BSA$

$SVR = 79.9 \times ((MAP - CVP)/CO)$

$DO_2 = 0.134 \times CO \times Hb \times SaO_2$

$VO_2 = 0.134 \times CO \times Hb (SaO_2 - SvO_2)$

Haemodynamic variables associated with transoesophageal Doppler (TOD)

Flow time, corrected (FTc)	330–360 ms	
Peak velocity	at 20 years old	90–120 cm/s
	at 50 years old	70–100 cm/s
	at 70 years old	50–80 cm/s
	at 90 years old	30–60 cm/s

Haemodynamic variables associated with pulse contour analysis

Intrathoracic blood volume index (ITBVI)	850–1000 ml/m²
Extravascular lung water index (EVLWI)	3–7 ml/kg
Stroke volume variation (SVV)	<10%
Global end diastolic volume index (GEDVI)	681–800 ml/m²
Left ventricular contractility	1200–2000 mmHg/s
Cardiac function index (CFI)	4.5–6.5 L/min

Electrocardiogram (ECG) values

Recording speed	25 mm/s	1 mm = 0.04 s
Amplitude	1 cm = 1 mV	
Normal axis	−30° to +120°	
PR interval	0.12–0.2 s	
QRS width	<0.12 s	
ST interval	0.27–0.33 s	
Corrected QT (QTc)	380–440 ms	

Table A.3 Blood gases

Arterial blood gases (ABGs)		
pH	7.35–7.45	
H^+	35–45 nmol/L	
PaO_2	12–14.67 kPa	90–110 mmHg
$PaCO_2$	4.53–6.13 kPa	34–46 mmHg
O_2 saturation (SaO_2)	95–98%	
Bicarbonate	24–30 mmol/L	
Base excess	±2 mmol/L	
Anion gap	8–16 mmol/L	
Carboxyhaemoglobin (COHb)	Non-smokers 1–2%	Smokers 2–6%
Venous blood gases		
pH	7.32–7.42	
PaO_2	4.93–5.6 kPa	37–42 mmHg
$PaCO_2$	5.33–6.93 kPa	40–52 mmHg
O_2 saturation (SvO_2)	70–75%	
PaO_2/FiO_2 ratio		
Normal	≥67 kPa	≥500 mmHg
Acute lung injury	≤40 kPa	≤300 mmHg
Acute respiratory distress syndrome	≤26.7 kPa	≤200 mmHg

Table A.4 Respiratory variables

Respiratory rate (RR)	12–18/min
Peak expiratory flow rate (PEFR)	See Fig. 17.27
Tidal volume (V_T)	7–10 ml/kg
Minute ventilation (V_E)	85–100 ml/kg/min
Vital capacity (VC)	50–55 ml/kg
Forced expiratory volume in 1 second (FEV_1)	70–83% of VC
Functional residual capacity (FRC)	2300–2800 ml
Total lung capacity (TLC)	5000–6500 ml
Lung compliance, total (C_T)	
Awake, erect	~100 ml/cmH$_2$O
Anaesthetized, supine (static)	~70–80 ml/cmH$_2$O
Anaesthetized, supine (dynamic) (Tidal volume/inflation pressure)	~50–60 ml/cmH$_2$O
Diffusing capacity transfer coefficient (K_{CO})	1.25–1.75 mmol/min/kPa/L
Airway occlusion pressure at 0.1 s ($P_{0.1}$)	3.5–4.5 cmH$_2$O

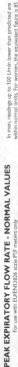

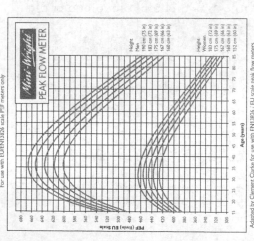

Fig. A.1 Peak flow chart—normal values. Adapted from Clement Clarke International Ltd. for use with EN13826/EU Scale peak flow meters. Adapted from British Medical Journal, 'New regression equations for predicting peak expiratory flow in adults'; Nunn AJ, et al., 298, pp. 1068–1070. Copyright 1989, with permission from BMJ Publishing Group Ltd.

In men, readings up to 100 L/min lower than predicted are within normal limits. For women, the equivalent figure is 85 L/min. Values are derived from Caucasian populations.

Mini-Wright
(Standard Range)
EU scale
(EN 13826)

Blue text
on a yellow
background

Single Patient Use
Part Ref: 3103388

Multiple Patient Use
Part Ref: 3103387

HS Logistics
Code : FDD 609

Mini-Wright
(Low Range)
EU scale

Blue text
on a yellow
background

Single Patient Use
Part Ref: 3104708

Multiple Patient Use
Part Ref: 3104710

Clement Clarke has developed mathematical equations that will allow conversion of P.E.F. readings from Wright-McKerrowscale to EN 13826 scale, and vice-versa. Contact us directly, or visit the website www.peakflow.com

CLEMENT CLARKE INTERNATIONAL
Clement Clarke International Ltd. Edinburgh Way, Harlow, Essex.
England CM20 2TT U.K.
Tel. +44 (0) 1279 414969 Fax. +44 (0) 1279 456304
www.clement-clarke.com email: resp@clement-clarke.com

(Issue 1. Date of preparation: 23rd July 2004)

PEAK EXPIRATORY FLOW RATE - NORMAL VALUES
For use with EU/EN13826 scale PEF meters only

Adapted by Clement Clarke for use with EN13826 : EU scale peak flow meters
from Nunn AJ Gregg I. Br Med J 1989;298:1068-70

Table A.5 Pulmonary function tests

Age		Height (cm)								
		150	155	160	165	170	175	180	185	190
38–41	FVC	♀2.69	♀2.91	♂3.81 ♀3.13	♂4.10 ♀3.35	♂4.39 ♀3.58	♂4.67 ♀3.80	♂4.96 ♀4.02	♂5.25	♂5.54
	FEV$_1$	♀2.30	♀2.50	♂3.20 ♀2.70	♂3.42 ♀2.89	♂3.63 ♀3.09	♂3.85 ♀3.29	♂4.06 ♀3.49	♂4.28	♂4.49
42–45	FVC	♀2.59	♀2.81	♂3.71 ♀3.03	♂3.99 ♀3.25	♂4.28 ♀3.47	♂4.57 ♀3.69	♂4.86 ♀3.91	♂5.15	♂5.43
	FEV$_1$	♀2.20	♀2.40	♂3.09 ♀2.60	♂3.30 ♀2.79	♂3.52 ♀2.99	♂3.73 ♀3.19	♂3.95 ♀3.39	♂4.16	♂4.38
46–49	FVC	♀2.48	♀2.70	♂3.60 ♀2.92	♂3.89 ♀3.15	♂4.18 ♀3.37	♂4.47 ♀3.59	♂4.75 ♀3.81	♂5.04	♂5.33
	FEV$_1$	♀2.10	♀2.30	♂2.97 ♀2.50	♂3.18 ♀2.69	♂3.40 ♀2.89	♂3.61 ♀3.09	♂3.83 ♀3.29	♂4.04	♂4.26
50–53	FVC	♀2.38	♀2.60	♂3.50 ♀2.82	♂3.79 ♀3.04	♂4.07 ♀3.26	♂4.36 ♀3.48	♂4.65 ♀3.71	♂4.94	♂5.23
	FEV$_1$	♀2.00	♀2.20	♂2.85 ♀2.40	♂3.07 ♀2.59	♂3.28 ♀2.79	♂3.50 ♀2.99	♂3.71 ♀3.19	♂3.93	♂4.14

Age

Age	Test		♀	♀	♂/♀	♂	♂	♂	♂	♂	♂
54–57	FVC	♀	2.27	2.49	2.72	2.94	3.16	3.38	3.60		
		♂			3.39	3.68	3.97	4.26	4.55	4.83	5.12
	FEV₁	♀	1.90	2.10	2.29	2.49	2.69	2.89	3.09		
		♂			2.72	2.94	3.16	3.38	3.60	3.81	4.03
58–61	FVC	♀	2.17	2.39	2.61	2.83	3.06	3.28	3.50		
		♂			3.29	3.58	3.87	4.15	4.44	4.73	5.02
	FEV₁	♀	1.80	2.00	2.20	2.39	2.59	2.79	2.99		
		♂			2.62	2.84	3.05	3.27	3.48	3.70	3.91
62–65	FVC	♀	2.07	2.29	2.51	2.73	2.95	3.17	3.39		
		♂			3.19	3.47	3.76	4.05	4.34	4.63	4.91
	FEV₁	♀	1.70	1.90	2.10	2.29	2.49	2.69	2.89		
		♂			2.51	2.72	2.94	3.15	3.37	3.58	3.80
66–69	FVC	♀	1.96	2.18	2.40	2.63	2.85	3.07	3.29		
		♂			3.08	3.37	3.66	3.95	4.23	4.52	4.81
	FEV₁	♀	1.60	1.80	2.00	2.19	2.39	2.59	2.79		
		♂			2.39	2.60	2.82	3.03	3.25	3.46	3.68

≥70

FVC
$$\text{♂} = (0.0576 \times \text{height}) - (0.026 \times \text{age}) - 4.34$$
$$\text{♀} = (0.0443 \times \text{height}) - (0.026 \times \text{age}) - 2.89$$

FEV₁
$$\text{♂} = (0.043 \times \text{height}) - (0.029 \times \text{age}) - 2.49$$
$$\text{♀} = (0.0395 \times \text{height}) - (0.025 \times \text{age}) - 2.60$$

Table A.6 Cerebrospinal fluid and neurological variables

Normal CSF values		
Pressure	7–18 cm H_2O	
Specific gravity	1.0062–1.0082	
Protein	0.15–0.45 g/L	
Chloride	120–130 mmol/L	
Glucose	2.8–4.2 mmol/L	75% of blood glucose
Cell count		
Lymphocytes	≤ 5/mm^3	
Neutrophils	Nil	
Xanthachromia index	<0.015	

CSF findings associated with disease				
	Pressure	Cell count /mm3	Protein	Glucose
Bacterial meningitis	↑	1000–60,000 Neutrophils	↑	↓ (<60%)
TB meningitis	↑	<1500 Neutrophils initially lymphocytes later	↑	↓ (<60%)
Viral meningitis	Normal or ↑	Normal or ↑ (<500) Mononuclear cells may be seen	Mildly ↑ (< 2 g/L)	Normal (>60%)
HSV meningitis	↑	↑ Lymphocyte count	↑	Normal (>60%)
Fungal meningitis	↑	<500 mostly lymphocytes	↑	↓ (<60%)
Abscess	↑	Variable	↑	Normal (>60%)
Tumour	↑	Mononuclear or blast cells may be seen	Sometimes >5 g/L	Normal or ↓

Neurological variables		
Jugular venous bulb saturations (SjO_2)	55–75%	
Intracranial pressure (ICP)	0–10 mmHg	0–14 cm H_2O
Transcranial Doppler (TCD) temporal windows		
MCA, mean flow velocity	55 ± 12 cm/s	
ACA, mean flow velocity	50 ± 11 cm/s	
PCA, mean flow velocity	40 ± 10 cm/s	
TICA, mean flow velocity	39 ± 09 cm/s	

(continued)

Table A.6 *(Continued)*

Electroencephalogram (EEG)		
Cerebrofunction monitor (CFM)	Abrupt spikes in epilepsy	Up to 50μV
Bispectral index (BIS)	Indicates anaesthesia	<50

Table A.7 Haematological results

Full blood count (FBC)		
Haemoglobin (Hb)	♂ 13–18 g/dl	♀ 12–16 g/dl
Haematocrit (Hct)	♂ 0.4–0.54	♀ 0.35–0.47
Mean cell volume (MCV)	76–96 fl	
Mean cell haemoglobin (MCH)	27–32 pg	
White cell count (WCC)	4–10 × 10⁹/L	
Differential white cell count		
Neutrophils	2–7.5 × 10⁹/L	
Lymphocytes	1.3–3.5 × 10⁹/L	
Eosinophils	0.04–0.44 × 10⁹/L	
Basophils	0–0.1 × 10⁹/L	
Monocytes	0.2–0.8 × 10⁹/L	
Platelet count	150–400 × 10⁹/L	
Coagulation studies		
Prothrombin time (PT)	10–14 s	
INR	0.9–1.2	
Activated partial thromboplastin time (APTT)	35–45 s	
APTT ratio	0.9–1.2	
Thrombin time (TT)	14–16 s	
Fibrinogen	1.5–4 g/L	
Fibrin-degradation products (FDPs)	0–10 mg/L	
D-dimers	<500 mcg/L	<500 ng/ml
Haptoglobins	0.7–3.8 g/L	
Thromboelastography (TEG®)	(Whole blood)	
R-time	15–30 mm	
K-time	6–12 mm	
α-angle	40–50°	
maximum amplitude	50–60 mm	
LY30	<7.5%	

Table A.8 Blood chemistry

Urea and electrolytes (U&Es)—plasma	
Sodium (Na$^+$)	135–145 mmol/L
Potassium (K$^+$)	3.5–5 mmol/L
Urea	2.5–6.7 mmol/L
Blood urea nitrogen (BUN)	6–20 mg/dL
Creatinine	70–150 µmol/L
Chloride	90–105 mmol/L
Bicarbonate	24–30 mmol/L
Osmolality	278–305 mOsmol/kg
Glomerular filtration rate	>90 ml/min/1.72m^2

Urea (mmol/L) = 0.375 × BUN (mg/dl)

Estimated GFR (eGFR) = 186 × (age in years) $^{-0.203}$ × (serum creatinine µmol/L × 0.01131)$^{-1.154}$ × 0.742 if female and × 1.2 if African American

Liver function tests (LFTs)		
Alkaline phosphatase (ALP)	30–300 iu/L	
Alanine aminotransferase (ALT)	5–35 iu/L	
Aspartate aminotransferase (AST)	5–35 iu/L	
Gamma-glutamyl transpeptidase (GGT)	♂ 11–51 iu/L	♀ 7–33 iu/L
Bilirubin	3–17 µmol/L	
Albumin	35/50 g/L	
Total protein	60–80 g/L	

Cardiac enzymes and markers of tissue damage		
Troponin I	<0.04 mcg/L	
Creatine kinase (CK)	♂ 25–195 iu/L	♀ 25–170 iu/L
CKMB	<25 iu/L	CKMB/CK ratio <5%
Lactate dehydrogenase (LDH)	70–250 iu/L	

Thyroid function tests (TFTs)	
Thyroid-stimulating hormone (TSH)	0.5–5.7 mu/L
Tri-iodothyronine (T$_3$)	1.2–3 nmol/L
Thyroxine (T$_4$)	70–140 nmol/L
Thyroxine (free)	9–22 pmol/L

Markers of inflammation/infection	
Erythrocyte sedimentation rate (ESR)	<20 mm/hour

(continued)

Table A.8 *(Continued)*

C-reactive protein (CRP)	<10 mg/L	
Procalcitonin (PCT)	<0.5 ng/ml	Systemic infection unlikely
	0.5–2 ng/ml	Systemic infection possible
	>2 ng/ml	Systemic infection likely
Other biochemistry—plasma		
Ammonia	<50 μmol/L	
Amylase	<180 Su/dL	(Su: Somogyi units)
B$_{12}$	0.13–68 nmol/L	
Calcium (ionized)	1–1.25 mmol/L	
Calcium (total)	2.12–2.65 mmol/L	
Cortisol (random level)	450–700 nmol/L	(0800h)
	80–280 nmol/L	(2400h)
Ferritin	12–200 mcg/L	
Folate	2.1 mcg/L	
Glucose	3.5–5.5 mmol/L	(fasting)
Glycosylated haemoglobin (HbA$_{1C}$)	2.3–6.5%	
Iron (Fe)	♂ 14–31 μmol/L	♀ 11–30 μmol/L
Iron binding capacity (IBC)	54–75 μmol/L	
Lactate (arterial)	0.5–1.6 mmol/L	(venous 0.5–2.2)
Lipase	0.2–1.5 iu/L	
Magnesium	0.75–1.05 mmol/L	
Parathyroid hormone	12–72 ng/L	
Phosphate	0.8–1.45 mmol/L	
Tryptase	<1 ng/mL	
Urate	♂0.21–0.48 mmol/L	♀0.15–0.39 mmol/L
Zinc	11–24 μmol/L	

Table A.9 Urine biochemistry

pH (minimum)	4.5
Osmolality	350–1000 mOsmol/kg
Potassium	14–120 mmol/24 hours
Sodium	100–250 mmol/24 hours
Protein	<150 mg/24 hours
Urinary tests for phaeochromocytoma/carcinoid	
Catecholamines	<0.36 µmol/24 hours
Hydroxy-indole acetic acid (5HIAA)	16–73 µmol/24 hours
Hydroymethylmandelic acid (HMMA, VMA)	16–48 µmol/24 hours

Table A.10 Drug levels

Therapeutic drug levels		
Amikacin (pre-dose trough level)	5–10 mg/L	
Carbamazepine	4–10 mg/L	17–51 µmol/L
Digoxin	0.8–2 mcg/L	1–2.6 nmol/L
Gentamicin (pre-dose trough level)	<2 mg/L	
Lithium	0.6–1 mmol/L	
Phenytoin	10–20 mg/L	40–80 µmol/L
Theophylline	10–20 mg/L	55–110µmol/L
Vancomycin (pre-dose trough level)	5–10 mg/L	
Drug levels associated with poisoning		
Blood alcohol levels		
UK driving limit	<0.8 g/L	
Severe ethanol toxicity	>5 g/L	
Carboxyhaemoglobin (COHb)	See 📖 p.476	
Methaemaglobin	<1.5%	
Salicylate	>350 mg/L	>2.5 mmol/L

'Malnutrition Universal Screening Tool' ('MUST') MAG

BAPEN
Advancing Clinical Nutrition   *BAPEN is registered charity number 1023927   www.bapen.org.uk*

Alternative measurements: instructions and tables

If height cannot be obtained, use length of forearm (ulna) to calculate height using tables below
(See The 'MUST' Explanatory Booklet for details of other alternative measurements (knee height and demispan) that can also be used to estimate height).

Estimating height from ulna length

Measure between the point of the elbow
(olecranon process) and the midpoint of the prominent
bone of the wrist (styloid process) (left side if possible).

HEIGHT (m)													
Men (<65 years)	1.94	1.93	1.91	1.89	1.87	1.85	1.84	1.82	1.80	1.78	1.76	1.75	1.73	1.71
Men (>65 years)	1.87	1.86	1.84	1.82	1.81	1.79	1.78	1.76	1.75	1.73	1.71	1.70	1.68	1.67
Ulna length (cm)	32.0	31.5	31.0	30.5	30.0	29.5	9.0	28.5	28.0	27.5	27.0	26.5	26.0	25.5
Women (<65 years)	1.84	1.83	1.81	1.80	1.79	1.77	1.76	1.75	1.73	1.72	1.70	1.69	1.68	1.66
Women (>65 years)	1.84	1.83	1.81	1.79	1.78	1.76	1.75	1.73	1.71	1.70	1.68	1.66	1.65	1.63

HEIGHT (m)													
Men (<65 years)	1.69	1.67	1.66	1.64	1.62	1.60	1.58	1.57	1.55	1.53	1.51	1.49	1.48	1.46
Men (>65 years)	1.65	1.63	1.62	1.60	1.59	1.57	1.56	1.54	1.52	1.51	1.49	1.48	1.46	1.45
Ulna length (cm)	25.0	24.5	24.0	23.5	3.0	22.5	22.0	21.5	21.0	20.5	20.0	19.5	19.0	18.5
Women (<65 years)	1.65	1.63	1.62	1.61	1.59	1.58	1.56	1.55	1.54	1.52	1.51	1.50	1.48	1.47
Women (>65 years)	1.61	1.60	1.58	1.56	1.55	1.53	1.52	1.50	1.48	1.47	1.45	1.44	1.42	1.40

Estimating BMI category from mid upper arm circumference (MUAC)

The subject's left arm should be bent at the elbow at a 90 degree angle,
with the upper arm held parallel to the side of the body. Measure the
distance between the bony protrusion on the shoulder (acromion) and
the point of the elbow (olecranon process). Mark the mid-point.

Ask the subject to let arm hang loose and measure around
the upper arm at the mid-point, making sure that the tape
measure is snug but not tight.

If MUAC is < 23.5 cm, BMI is likely to be <20 kg/m².
If MUAC is > 32.0 cm, BMI is likely to be >30 kg/m².

Fig. A.2 BAPEN alternative height measurement tool. Reproduced with
the kind permission of BAPEN (British Association for Parenteral and Enteral
Nutrition). For further information on the 'Malnutrition Universal Screening Tool'
('MUST') see 🖰 www.bapen.org.uk

Index